AF443095

MEDICINE MEETS VIRTUAL REALITY 14

Studies in Health Technology and Informatics

This book series was started in 1990 to promote research conducted under the auspices of the EC programmes' Advanced Informatics in Medicine (AIM) and Biomedical and Health Research (BHR) bioengineering branch. A driving aspect of international health informatics is that telecommunication technology, rehabilitative technology, intelligent home technology and many other components are moving together and form one integrated world of information and communication media. The complete series has been accepted in Medline. Volumes from 2005 onwards are available online.

Series Editors:
Dr. J.P. Christensen, Prof. G. de Moor, Prof. A. Famili, Prof. A. Hasman, Prof. L. Hunter,
Dr. I. Iakovidis, Dr. Z. Kolitsi, Mr. O. Le Dour, Dr. A. Lymberis, Prof. P.F. Niederer,
Prof. A. Pedotti, Prof. O. Rienhoff, Prof. F.H. Roger France, Dr. N. Rossing,
Prof. N. Saranummi, Dr. E.R. Siegel, Dr. P. Wilson, Prof. E.J.S. Hovenga,
Prof. M.A. Musen and Prof. J. Mantas

Volume 119

Recently published in this series

ISSN 0926-9630

Medicine Meets Virtual Reality 14

Accelerating Change in Healthcare: Next Medical Toolkit

Edited by

James D. Westwood

Randy S. Haluck MD FACS

Helene M. Hoffman PhD

Greg T. Mogel MD

Roger Phillips PhD CEng FBCS CIPT

Richard A. Robb PhD

and

Kirby G. Vosburgh PhD

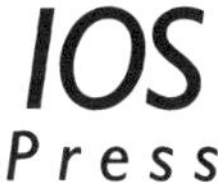

IOS Press

Amsterdam • Berlin • Oxford • Tokyo • Washington, DC

ISBN 1-58603-583-5
Library of Congress Control Number: 2005937901

Publisher
IOS Press
Nieuwe Hemweg 6B
1013 BG Amsterdam
Netherlands
fax: +31 20 687 0019
e-mail: order@iospress.nl

Distributor in the UK and Ireland
Gazelle Books
Falcon House
Queen Square
Lancaster LA1 1RN
United Kingdom
fax: +44 1524 63232

Distributor in the USA and Canada
IOS Press, Inc.
4502 Rachael Manor Drive
Fairfax, VA 22032
USA
fax: +1 703 323 3668
e-mail: iosbooks@iospress.com

LEGAL NOTICE

The publisher is not responsible for the use which might be made of the following information.

PRINTED IN THE NETHERLANDS

Medicine Meets Virtual Reality 14
J.D. Westwood et al. (Eds.)
IOS Press, 2006

v

Preface
Accelerating Change in Healthcare: Next Medical Toolkit

James D. WESTWOOD and Karen S. MORGAN
Aligned Management Associates, Inc.

Machine intelligence will eclipse human intelligence within the next few decades – extrapolating from Moore's Law – and our world will enjoy limitless computational power and ubiquitous data networks. Today's iPod® devices portend an era when biology and information technology will fuse to create a human experience radically different from our own.

Between that future and the present, we will live with accelerating technological change. Whether predictable or disruptive, guided or uncontrollable, scientific innovation is carrying us forward at unprecedented speed. What does accelerating change entail for medicine?

Already, our healthcare system now appears on the verge of crisis; accelerating change is part of the problem. Each technological upgrade demands an investment of education and money, and a costly infrastructure more quickly becomes obsolete. Practitioners can be overloaded with complexity: therapeutic options, outcomes data, procedural coding, drug names…

Furthermore, an aging global population with a growing sense of entitlement demands that each medical breakthrough be immediately available for its benefit: what appears in the morning paper is expected simultaneously in the doctor's office. Meanwhile, a third-party payer system generates conflicting priorities for patient care and stockholder returns. The result is a healthcare system stressed by scientific promise, public expectation, economic and regulatory constraints, and human limitations.

Change is also proving beneficial, of course. Practitioners are empowered by better imaging methods, more precise robotic tools, greater realism in training simulators, and more powerful intelligence networks. The remarkable accomplishments of the IT industry and the Internet are trickling steadily into healthcare. MMVR participants can readily see the progress of the past fourteen years: more effective healthcare at a lower overall cost, driven by cheaper and better computers.

We are pleased that this year's conference has an increased emphasis on medical education. In many ways, education is the next medical toolkit: a means to cope with, and take advantage of, accelerating change. Through interaction with novice students, medical educators are uniquely equipped to critique existing methods, encourage fresh thinking, and support emerging tools. Each new class of aspiring physicians stimulates flexibility in problem solving and adaptation within technological evolution. As an earlier generation of physicians trains its successors, experience can guide innovation so that change accelerates for the better.

As always, we wish to thank all the participants who make MMVR possible each year. It is our privilege to work with you.

MMVR14 Proceedings Editors

James D. Westwood
MMVR Program Coordinator
Aligned Management Associates, Inc.

Randy S. Haluck MD FACS
Director of Minimally Invasive Surgery
Director of Surgical Simulation
Associate Professor of Surgery
Penn State, Hershey Medical Center

Helene M. Hoffman PhD
Assistant Dean, Educational Computing
Adjunct Professor of Medicine
Division of Medical Education
School of Medicine
University of California, San Diego

Greg T. Mogel MD
Assistant Professor of Radiology and Biomedical Engineering
University of Southern California;
Deputy Director, TATRC
U.S. Army Medical Research & Materiel Command

Roger Phillips PhD CEng FBCS CIPT
Research Professor, Simulation & Visualization Group
Director, Hull Immersive Visualization Environment (HIVE)
Department of Computer Science
University of Hull (UK)

Richard A. Robb PhD
Scheller Professor in Medical Research
Professor of Biophysics & Computer Science
Director, Mayo Biomedical Imaging Resource
Mayo Clinic College of Medicine

Kirby G. Vosburgh PhD
Associate Director, Center for Integration of Medicine and
Innovative Technology (CIMIT)
Massachusetts General Hospital
Harvard Medical School

MMVR14 Organizing Committee

Michael J. Ackerman PhD
Office of High Performance Computing & Communications,
National Library of Medicine

Ian Alger MD
New York Presbyterian Hospital;
Weill Medical College of Cornell University

David C. Balch MA
DCB Consulting LLC

Steve Charles MD
MicroDexterity Systems;
University of Tennessee

Patrick C. Cregan FRACS
Nepean Hospital,
Wentworth Area Health Service

Henry Fuchs PhD
Dept of Computer Science,
University of North Carolina

Walter J. Greenleaf PhD
Greenleaf Medical Systems

Randy S. Haluck MD FACS
Dept of Surgery,
Penn State College of Medicine

David M. Hananel
Surgical Programs,
Medical Education Technologies Inc.

Wm. LeRoy Heinrichs MD PhD
Medical Media & Information Technologies /
Gynecology & Obstetrics,
Stanford University School of Medicine

Helene M. Hoffman PhD
School of Medicine,
University of California, San Diego

Heinz U. Lemke PhD
Institute for Technical Informatics,
Technical University Berlin

Alan Liu PhD
National Capital Area Medical Simulation Center,
Uniformed Services University

Greg T. Mogel MD
Dept of Radiology, University of Southern California;
TATRC/USAMRMC

Kevin N. Montgomery PhD
National Biocomputation Center,
Stanford University

Makoto Nonaka MD PhD
Foundation for International Scientific Advancement

Roger Phillips PhD CEng FBCS CIPT
Dept of Computer Science,
University of Hull (UK)

Carla M. Pugh MD PhD
Center for Advanced Surgical Education,
Northwestern University

Richard A. Robb PhD
Mayo Biomedical Imaging Resource,
Mayo Clinic College of Medicine

Jannick P. Rolland PhD
ODA Lab at School of Optics / CREOL,
University of Central Florida

Ajit K. Sachdeva MD FRCSC FACS
Division of Education,
American College of Surgeons

Richard M. Satava MD FACS
Dept of Surgery, University of Washington;
DARPA; TATRC/USAMRMC

Steven Senger PhD
Dept of Computer Science,
University of Wisconsin – La Crosse

Ramin Shahidi PhD
Image Guidance Laboratories,
Stanford University School of Medicine

Don Stredney
Interface Laboratory,
OSC

Julie A. Swain MD
Cardiovascular and Respiratory Devices,
U.S. Food and Drug Administration

Robert M. Sweet MD
Dept of Urology,
University of Minnesota

Kirby G. Vosburgh PhD
CIMIT/Brigham & Women's Hospital /
Harvard Medical School

Dave Warner MD PhD
MindTel LLC;
Institute for Interventional Informatics

Suzanne J. Weghorst MA MS
Human Interface Technology Lab,
University of Washington

Mark D. Wiederhold MD PhD FACP
The Virtual Reality Medical Center

Contents

Medicine Meets Virtual Reality 14
J.D. Westwood et al. (Eds.)
IOS Press, 2006

Centerline-Based Parametric Model of Colon for Colonoscopy Simulator

Woojin Ahn[a], Jae Kyoung Joo[a], Hyun Soo Woo[a], Doo Yong Lee[a], and Sun Young Yi[b]
[a]*Department of Mechanical Engineering, Korea Advanced Institute of Science and Technology, Daejeon, Republic of Korea*
[b]*Department of Internal Medicine, Ewha Womans University, Seoul, Republic of Korea*

Abstract. This paper presents a centerline-based parametric model of colon for collision detection and visualization of the colon lumen for colonoscopy simulator. The prevailing marching cubes algorithm for 3D surface construction can provide a high resolution mesh of triangular elements of the colon lumen from CT data. But a well organized mesh structure reflecting the geometric information of the colon is essential to fast and accurate computation of contact between the colonoscope and colon, and the corresponding reflective force in the colonoscopy simulator. The colon is modeled as parametric arrangement of triangular elements with its surface along the centerline of the colon. All the vertices are parameterized according to the radial angle along the centerline, so that the triangles around the viewpoint can be found fast. The centerline-based parametric colon model has 75,744 triangular elements compared to 373,364 of the model constructed by the marching cubes algorithm.

Keywords. Colonoscopy simulator, collision detection, haptic rendering

Introduction

Collision detection and force rendering is required to maintain the viewpoint of the colonoscopy simulators inside the virtual colon. The viewpoint moves mostly along the centerline of the colon as the inserted depth of the virtual colonoscope increases. A well-organized mesh structure exploiting this particular geometric feature can allow fast computation of collision check between the viewpoint and the surface of the colon. The prevailing marching cubes algorithm for 3D surface construction [1], which does not consider the geometric features of colonoscopy, can provide a high resolution triangular mesh structure from CT data of patients. However, there are two limitations in applying the algorithm to the colonoscopy simulator. First, it becomes inefficient to build the hierarchical data representation of primitives such as vertex, edge and triangle [2], and store the massive data for online collision detection and response, especially for the large models as in the colonoscopy simulator. The second limitation results from contact behavior of the colonoscopy simulator. Free-motion-to-collision contact, rather than successive resting contacts, occurs frequently during the colonoscopy simulation. Thus, the primitive-based hierarchical data structure, that is efficient for the successive resting contacts, has no advantage in the colonoscopy simulator.

This paper proposes a centerline-based parametric model of colon that efficiently computes the collision detection and response as well as visualization of internal colon. The colon is modeled as parametric arrangement of triangular elements with its surface along the centerline of the colon, and cross-sectional rings defined at every sampled point in the centerline. This allows more efficient graphic rendering in comparison with the marching cubes algorithm, and successful collision detection and response in the developed colonoscopy simulator.

1. Centerline-based parametric model of colon

The colon model is constructed in two stages. First, the boundary of the colon is segmented from abdomen CT data of patients. Second, the centerline of the colon is extracted. The extracted centerline is further processed to obtain smooth and continuous B-spline curve. The cross-sections orthogonal to the centerline are computed for all the sampled points in the centerline during the second stage. We will denote the sampled point as *centerline node*. The pre-determined number of rays is traced in the cross-section plane. The intersection points between the rays and the boundary of the colon define the cross-sectional rings as shown in Figure 1. Hence the surface of the colon is parameterized along both the centerline and the rays.

Figure 2 depicts the interference among the cross-sectional rings occurring in the high-curvature areas. A new method, simpler than the nonlinear ray-tracing [3], is developed to compute successively the orientation of the cross-sectional rings until there is no more interference. Figure 3 illustrates how to modify the intersected cross-sectional ring to keep away from the interference. If at least two intersection points between rays in the cross-sectional ring R2 and the orthogonal plane including the R1 are located inside the circle of the radius defined as the maximum length among rays in R1, the interference occurs. *ray1* and *ray2* are the boundary rays of the intersected rays. The vector *L=ray1-ray2* specifies the direction of rotation axis, and *i*, which coincides with a centerline node, is the center of rotation. Rotation angle is gradually increased until the two cross-sectional rings are separated.

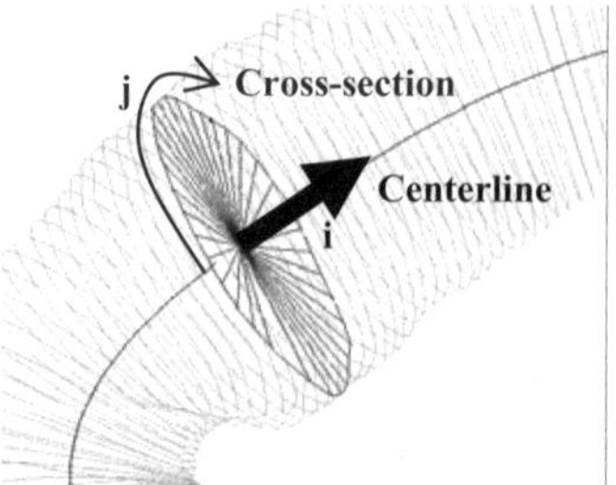

Figure 1. Cross-sectional rings along the centerline.

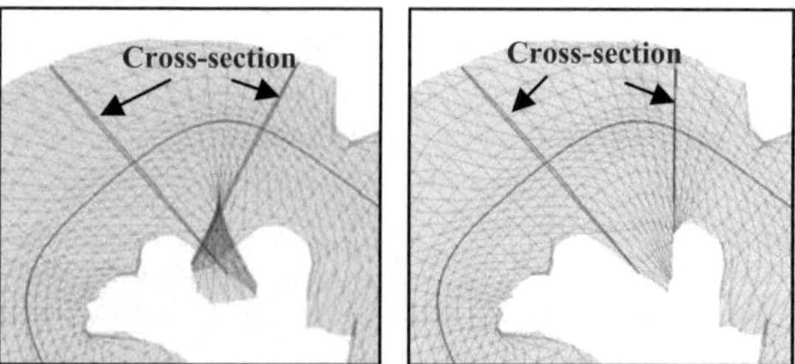

Figure 2. Resolution of the interference.

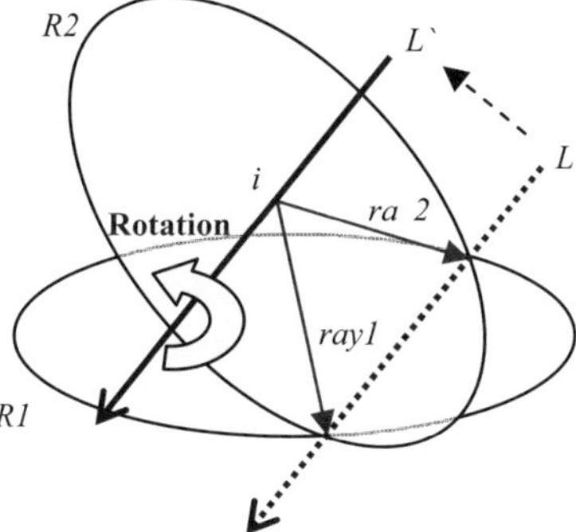

Figure 3. Rotation of intersected cross-sectional ring.

The colon model is parameterized by using the centerline and the radial angle. The set of all vertices V on the surface of the colon is composed of the parameterized vertices $v(i,j)$ according to their cross-sectional ring i and the radial angle j.

$$V = \left\{ v(i,j) \mid i = 1,\cdots,n_c, \ \ j = 1,\cdots,n_\theta, \ \ v(i,j) \in \Re^3 \right\}, \tag{1}$$

where n_c is the sampled number of the centerline nodes, and n_θ is the sampled number of the rays traced in each cross-sectional ring.

Hierarchical data representations of primitives such as vertex, edge, and triangle are generally used for fast collision detection between a moving point and 3D objects. To alleviate computational burden and the memory space associated with vertices and edges, our collision detection technique exploits only parameterized triangle primitives. This approach does not require the relationship between a triangle and its neighbors such as vertices and edges, as hierarchical representations do. A set of the triangle elements is defined as using the two parameters.

$$T = T^L \bigcup T^U$$

$$T^L = \left\{ \begin{array}{l} t^L(i,j) \mid t^L(i,j) = \Delta v(i,j)v(i+1,j)v(i,j+1), \\ i = 1,\cdots,n_c, \ \ j = 1,\cdots,n_\theta \end{array} \right\}, \tag{2}$$

$$T^U = \left\{ \begin{array}{l} t^U(i,j) \mid t^U(i,j) = \Delta v(i+1,j)v(i+1,j+1)v(i,j+1), \\ i = 1,\cdots,n_c, \ \ j = 1,\cdots,n_\theta \end{array} \right\}$$

where superscript L and T mean upper and lower triangle in Figure 4, respectively. Figure 4 illustrates unfolded colon surface to describe relationship between the parameters and the triangular mesh structure. The parameter of radial angle $n_\theta + 1$ is equivalent to 1 so that $v(i, 1)$ and $v(i, n_\theta + 1)$ are collocated, since the unfolded colon is sewed to form a hollow cylindrical structure. This parametric representation of the surface of the colon does not need any pre-computation for building hierarchical data structure, but makes possible to easily find triangles around the viewpoint by simple operations such as addition and subtraction of the parameters. As a result, it can be efficiently utilized for fast collision detection and response.

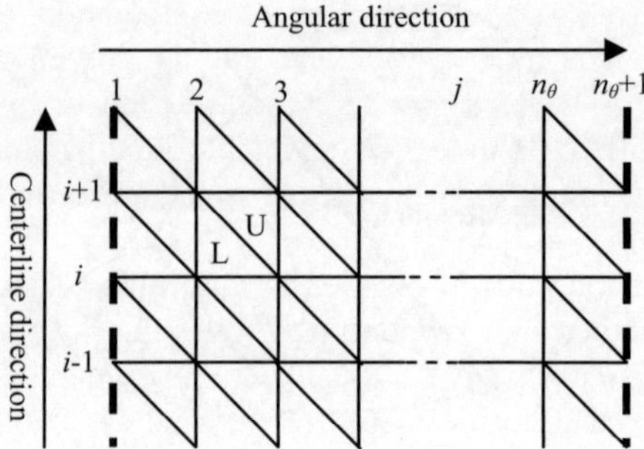

Figure 4. Unfolded triangular mesh.

2. Collision detection and response

Figure 5 illustrates four steps for collision detection between the viewpoint and the centerline-based parametric colon model. The collision detection algorithm keeps tracking the position of the viewpoint, and updates the group of triangles assigned by the parameters i and j around the viewpoint.

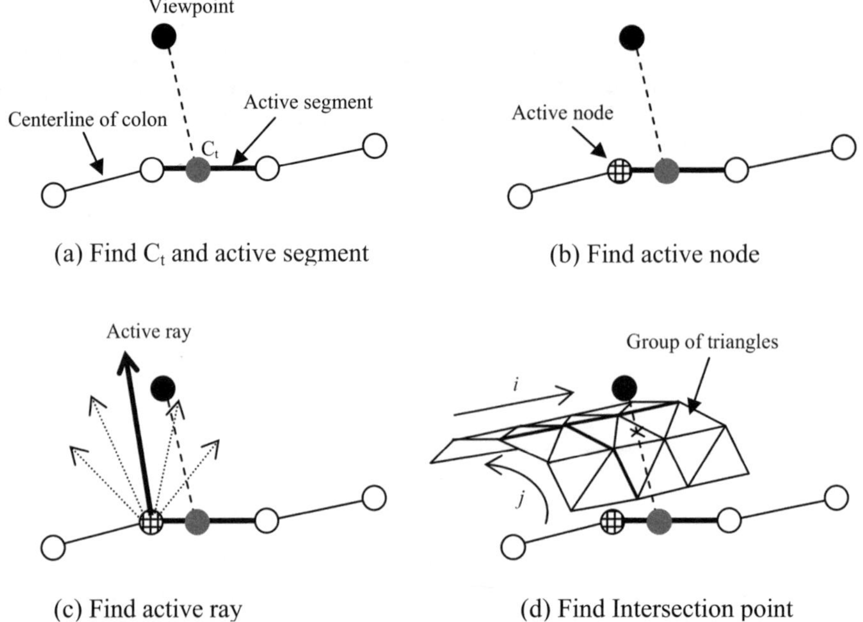

(a) Find C_t and active segment   (b) Find active node

(c) Find active ray   (d) Find Intersection point

Figure 5. Collision detection

The first step finds the closet point C_t to the viewpoint (figure 5(a)). The centerline is a piecewise linear curve connecting the centerline nodes that are uniformly sampled from the B-spline curve. Hence the C_t is obtained by checking the smallest distance between the viewpoint and centerline segments. We will denote the centerline segment containing the C_t as *active segment*. For efficient computation, the centerline segments that will be tested at the next time step include only the previous active segment and its neighbors. *Active node* is defined as nearer node to the C_t among two nodes in the active segment (figure 5(b)). Its index is equivalent to the parameter *i*. *Active ray* is the closet to the viewpoint among rays in the cross-sectional ring corresponding to the active node (figure 5(c)).

In the final step of the collision detection algorithm, detailed intersection test is carried out to check whether the viewpoint penetrates the surface of the colon using the active node and the active ray (figure 5(d)). Common collision detection algorithms for a moving point and fixed 3D objects utilize the line segment joining two points at previous and current time step. Instead, our algorithm uses different line segment that is formed by the current viewpoint VP and the C_t as shown in figure 6. This approach reduces extra computation and, as subsequent explanation will clarify, this line segment gives further benefits for computation of contact force and adjustment of the penetrated viewpoint. A small set of triangles for intersection test is defined as

$$T_t = \left\{ t^L(i,j), t^U(i,j) \mid i_a - \alpha \le i \le i_a + \alpha, \;\; j_a - \beta \le j \le j_a + \beta \right\}, \tag{3}$$

where i_a and j_a denote the active node and the active ray, respectively. α and β define ranges of two parameters to specify the group of the triangle. The first triangle satisfying intersection condition is set to the contact triangle during procedure of intersection test in order to avoid the unnecessary test associated with edges and vertices. VP` denotes the intersection point between the line segment and the contact triangle.

Ho *et al.*[2] and Zilles *et al.*[4] propose constraint-based haptic rendering algorithms to compute contact force. They determine the constrained point remaining on the surface of the object by iteratively computing the shortest distance from the haptic interface point, corresponding to the viewpoint, to the surface. We employ a simple non-iterative collision response algorithm that adjusts the viewpoint to keep it inside colon and computes contact force during contact with the surface of the colon. If collision is detected, the viewpoint VP is modified to coincide with the contact point VP` determined in the preceding collision detection procedure as in figure 6. As a result, the viewpoint can be continuously remained inside the colon without additional computation during contact. The contact force proportional to the collision depth is transmitted to the user by the haptic device [5].

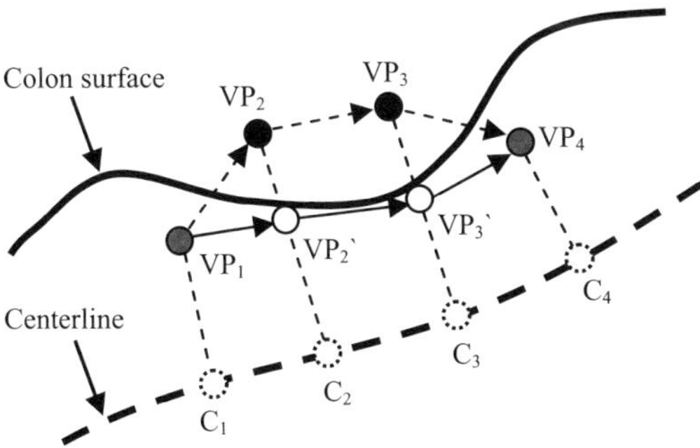

Figure 6. Collision response

3. Conclusion and future work

Figure 7 shows the colonoscope view inside the colon using the centerline-based parametric model and the collision detection algorithm in the developed colonoscopy simulator. The centerline-based parametric model of colon has 75,744 triangular elements compared to 373,364 of the model constructed by the marching cubes algorithm. The specialized collision detection and response technique for the colonoscopy simulator provides successful control of the viewpoint and stable contact force during simulation. The proposed resolution method for the interference among the cross-sectional rings should be further improved to reduce the distortion of the surface of the colon.

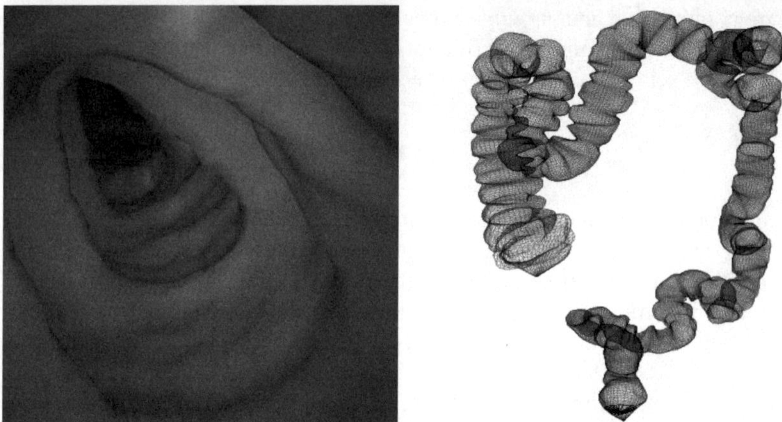

Figure 7. Centerline-based parametric model of colon

References

[1]   W. E. Lorensen, and H. E. Cline, "Marching Cubes: A High Resolution 3D Surface Construction Algorithm," *Computer Graphics*, vol. 21, no. 3, pp. 163-169, 1987.
[2]   C. Ho, C. Basdogan, and M. A, Srinivasan, "Efficient Point-Based Rendering Techniques for Haptic Display of Virtual Objects," *Presence*, vol. 8, no. 5, pp. 477-491, 1999.
[3]   A. V. Bartrolí, R. Wegenkittl, A. König, and E. Gröller, "Virtual Colon Unfolding," *in Proceedings of the conference on Visualization 2001*, pp. 411-420, 2001.
[4]   C. B. Zilles and J. K. Salisbury, "A Constraint-based God-object Method for Haptic Display," *in Proceedings of International Conference on Intelligent Robots and Systems*, vol.3, pp.146-151,1995.
[5]   J. Y. Kwon, H. S. Woo, and D. Y. Lee, "Haptic Device for Colonoscopy Training Simulator," *Medicine Meets Virtual Reality 13*, pp. 277-279, 2005.

Medicine Meets Virtual Reality 14
J.D. Westwood et al. (Eds.)
IOS Press, 2006

New Tools for Sculpting Cranial Implants in a Shared Haptic Augmented Reality Environment

Zhuming Ai [a,1], Ray Evenhouse [a], Jason Leigh [b], Fady Charbel [c], and
Mary Rasmussen [a]

[a] *VRMedLab*
Department of Biomedical and Health Information Sciences
University of Illinois at Chicago
1919 W. Taylor St, AHP, MC 530
Chicago, IL 60612
[b] *Electronic Visualization Laboratory*
University of Illinois at Chicago
851 S. Morgan St., MC 152, 1120 SEO
Chicago, IL 60607
[c] *Department of Neurosurgery*
University of Illinois at Chicago
912 South Wood Street (MC 799)
Chicago, IL 60612

Abstract. New volumetric tools were developed for the design and fabrication of
high quality cranial implants from patient CT data. These virtual tools replace time
consuming physical sculpting, mold making and casting steps. The implant is designed by medical professionals in tele-immersive collaboration. Virtual clay is
added in the virtual defect area on the CT data using the adding tool. With force
feedback the modeler can feel the edge of the defect and fill only the space where no
bone is present. A carving tool and a smoothing tool are then used to sculpt and refine the implant. To make a physical evaluation, the skull with simulated defect and
the implant are fabricated via stereolithography to allow neurosurgeons to evaluate
the quality of the implant. Initial tests demonstrate a very high quality fit. These
new haptic volumetric sculpting tools are a critical component of a comprehensive
tele-immersive system.

Keywords. Implant Design, Virtual Reality, Augmented Reality, Haptic Rendering

1. Introduction

The incidence of large cranial defects is on the rise. Dujovny and Evenhouse et al. have
developed a technique for cranial implant design using patient CT data, which builds
patient-specific implants with near perfect fit.[1] However this method is expensive and

---

[1] Correspondence to: Zhuming Ai, E-mail: zai@uic.edu.

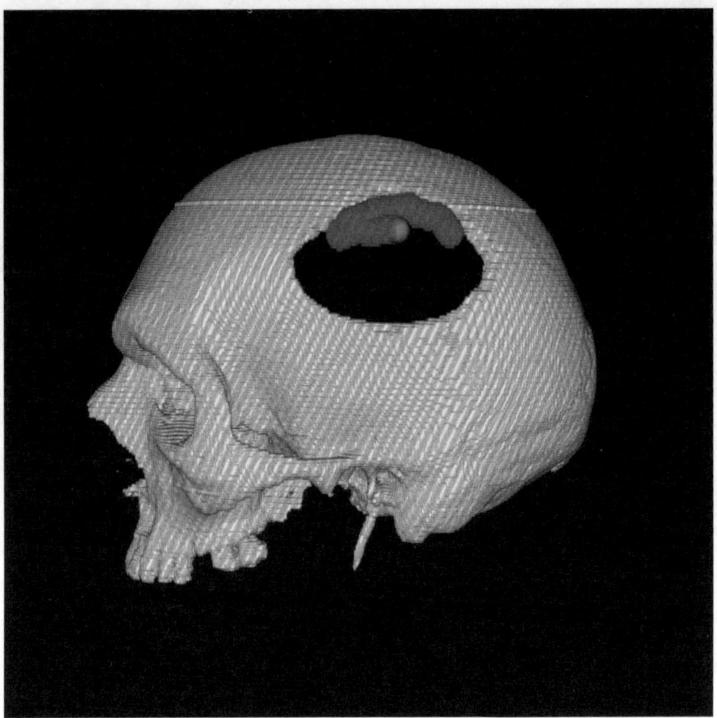

Figure 1. Implant design on a simulated defect.

time consuming because many traditional sculpting steps such as physical sculpting, mold making and defect stereolithography are involved.

Good visual feedback and the sense of touch are as crucial in virtual sculpting as in traditional physical sculpting. The goal of this research is to develop a networked augmented reality sculpting system with tactile feedback to replace as many physical steps as possible in the process.

2. Methods

The process of implant design begins with CT data of the patient and the Personal Augmented Reality Immersive System (PARIS^{TM})[2]. The implant is designed by medical professionals in tele-immersive collaboration.[3] In this design process the medical modeler creates a virtual implant that precisely fits a defect generated from patient CT data. A PHANTOM desktop haptic device supplies the sense of touch.

2.1. Sculpting Tools with Haptics

A proxy-based haptic rendering algorithm that can be used directly on volumetric data has been developed.[4] The proxy used is a sphere so the forces can be calculated according to the size of the tool and its relation to the data.

Virtual clay is added in the virtual defect area using the toothpaste-like adding tool. With force feedback the modeler can feel the edge of the defect and fill only the space

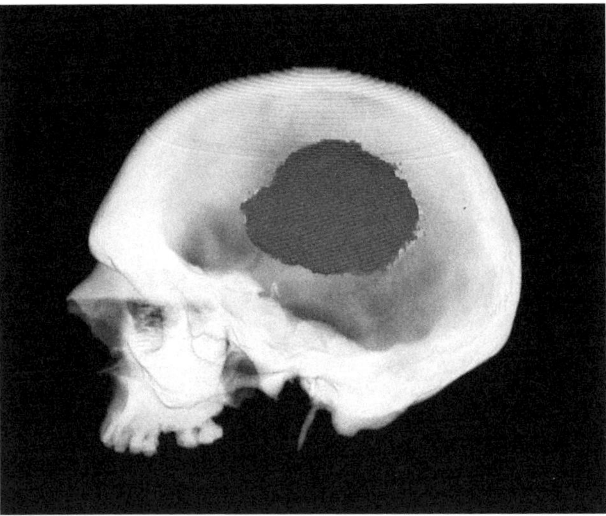

Figure 2. The virtual skull with virtual implant.

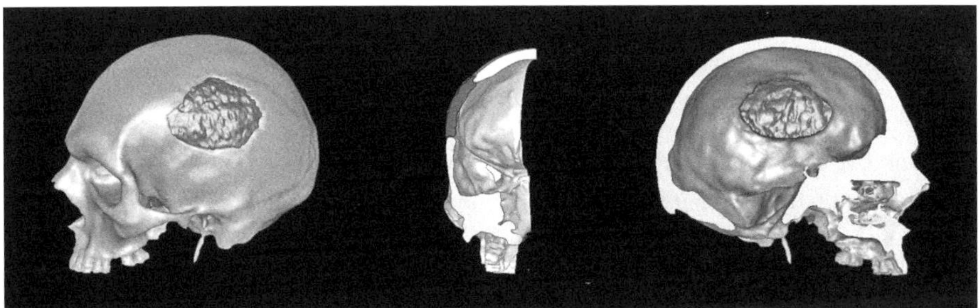

Figure 3. Implant fits in the defect.

where no bone is present. When the defect is filled with clay, a carving tool is then used to sculpt the implant and a smoothing tool is used to refine the surface. Fig. 1 shows that an implant is being designed on the simulated defect.

A surface refinement tool has been developed for volume sculpting. When the smoothing tool moves along the surface of the implant, the value of each voxel inside the spherical tool is recalculated. The new value is determined by averaging the voxels in a small neighboring volume. The designer can move the tool on rough surface areas of the implant, and the smoothing algorithm will be applied. Smoothness is limited only by the resolution of the volumetric data. The resulting implant together with the skull is shown in Fig. 2.

The volume is then segmented and the marching cubes algorithm is used to convert the implant volumetric model to a stereolithography (STL) model ready for fabrication. The STL model of the skull and implant are viewed with a cutting plane to analyze the fit (Fig. 3) and if no modifications are needed sent for stereolithography fabrication.

A hardware assisted fast direct volume rendering algorithm using three-dimensional texture mapping has been implemented. Incorporated with level of detail, this algorithm minimizes the latency between visual and force feedback.

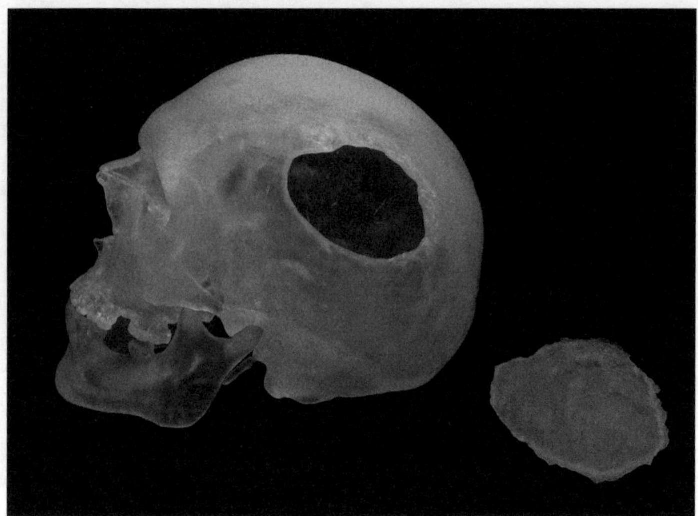

Figure 4. Stereolithography fabricated skull with a simulated defect and the implant.

2.2. *Sculpting in a Networked Shared Environment*

Collaborative consultation and implant design is an important part of this project. Audio communication over the network has been implemented in the system. A tele-immersive server has been setup in the VRMedLab, UIC. Data are shared among collaborators.

The network protocol for tele-immersive collaboration has been defined. Currently it contains the following parts: audio communication, state data sharing, and volumetric data sharing. All the participants in the collaborative session will share their viewing angle, transformation matrix, and sculpting tools information over the network. Any change made by any one participant will be transferred to all other participants. Any changes to the volumetric data will also be shared among collaborators

The network component is implemented using The Quality of Service Adaptive Networking Toolkit (QUANTA)[5]. QUANTA is developed at the EVL, UIC. It is a toolkit for supporting Optiputer applications over optical networks. Quanta is a cross-platform adaptive networking toolkit for supporting the diverse networking requirements of latency-sensitive and bandwidth-intensive applications. It seeks to develop an easy-to-use system that will allow programmers to specify the data transfer characteristics of their application at a high level, and let Quanta transparently translate these requirements into appropriate networking decisions.

During collaborative implant design, the changes to the volume are shared in real-time among all participants. Only a sub-volume that contains the modified data is transferred to other collaborators in order to save bandwidth. A tool will be added in the future that allows one to push the whole volumetric data to all the others. If someone joins the session in the middle, this tool will allow him/her to obtain the up-to-date data.

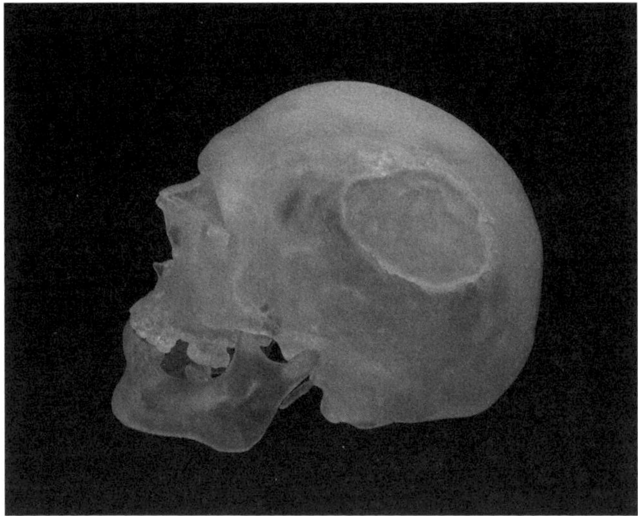

Figure 5. Stereolithography fabricated skull with implant in place.

3. Results

For initial testing purposes, the Visible Human Project®[6] CT data was used. The CT data was segmented to remove soft tissue, and a simulated defect was created. An implant was designed using the system based on this CT data. The designed model was converted to triangles and saved as a stereolithography (STL) model ready for fabrication. The STL model of the skull and implant were loaded into a computer program, and it shows that they fit well (Fig. 3). To make a physical evaluation for quality of fit and shape, this skull with simulated defect was fabricated via stereolithography. The implant was fabricated via stereolithography as well to allow neurosurgeons to evaluate the quality of the implant (Fig. 4). Fig. 5 shows the stereolithography skull model with implant in place. Initial tests demonstrate a very high quality fit.

4. Discussion and Conclusion

New volumetric tools were developed for the design and fabrication of high quality cranial implants from patient CT data. These virtual tools replace time consuming physical sculpting, mold making and casting steps. These new haptic volumetric sculpting tools are a critical component of a comprehensive tele-immersive system. An augmented reality system (PARIS) is used by a medical modeler to sculpt cranial implants. A conference-room-sized system (C-Wall) is used for tele-immersive small group consultation and an inexpensive, easily deployable networked desktop virtual reality system (the Physician's Personal VR Display)[7] supports surgical consultation, evaluation and collaboration.

5. Acknowledgments

This publication was made possible by Grant Number N01-LM-3-3507 from the National Library of Medicine/National Institutes of Health.

References

[1] M. Dujovny, R. Evenhouse, C. Agner, F.T. Charbel, Sadler L., and D. McConathy. Preformed prosthesis from computed tomography data: Repair of large calvarial defects. In Benzel E.C. Rengachary SR, editor, *Calvarial and Dural Reconstructuion*, pages 77–88. American Association of Neurological Surgeons, Park Ridge, Ill, 1999.

[2] A. Johnson, D. Sandin, G. Dawe, Z. Qiu, S. Thongrong, and D. Plepys. Developing the paris: Using the cave to prototype a new vr display. In *CDROM Proceedings of IPT 2000: Immersive Projection Technology Workshop*, Ames, IA, Jun 2000.

[3] C. Scharver, R. Evenhouse, A. Johnson, and J. Leigh. Designing cranial implants in a haptic augment reality environment. *Communications of the ACM*, 27(8):32–38, August 2004.

[4] Zhuming Ai, Ray Evenhouse, and Mary Rasmussen. Haptic rendering of volumetric data for cranial implant modeling. In *The 27th Annual International Conference of the IEEE Engineering in Medicine and Biology Society*, Shanghai, China, Sept 2005.

[5] J. Leigh, O. Yu, D. Schonfeld, R. Ansari, et al. Adaptive networking for tele-immersion. In *Proc. Immersive Projection Technology/Eurographics Virtual Environments Workshop (IPT/EGVE)*, Stuttgart, Germany, May 2001.

[6] MJ Ackerman. Accessing the visible human project. *D Lib Mag*, Oct 1995.

[7] Zhuming Ai and Mary Rasmussen. Desktop and conference room vr for physicians. *Stud Health Technol Inform*, 111:12–4, 2005.

Medicine Meets Virtual Reality 14
J.D. Westwood et al. (Eds.)
IOS Press, 2006

13

Reification of Abstract Concepts to Improve Comprehension Using Interactive Virtual Environments and a Knowledge-Based Design: A Renal Physiology Model

Dale C. ALVERSON[a], Stanley M. SAIKI Jr.[e,f], Thomas P. CAUDELL[b], Timothy GOLDSMITH[c], Susan STEVENS[c], Linda SALAND[a], Kathleen COLLERAN[a], John BRANDT[a], Lee DANIELSON[a], Lisa CERILLI[a], Alexis HARRIS[a], Martin C. GREGORY[g], Randall STEWART[a], Jeffery NORENBERG[a], George SHUSTER[a], PANAOITIS[d], James HOLTEN, III[b], Victor M. VERGERA[b], Andrei SHERSTYUK[5], Kathleen KIHMM[5], Jack LUI[5], Kin Lik WANG[5]

[a]Health Sciences Center, [b]School of Engineering, and [c]Department of Psychology, [d]School of Music, University of New Mexico, Albuquerque, NM 87131 U.S.A., [e]John A. Burns School of Medicine University of Hawaii, Honolulu, HI 96822, [f]Pacific Telehealth and Technology Hui, Tripler Army Medical Center, Honolulu, HI 96859, School of Medicine, [g]University of Utah, Salt lake City, UT 84132 U.S.A.

Abstract. Several abstract concepts in medical education are difficult to teach and comprehend. In order to address this challenge, we have been applying the approach of reification of abstract concepts using interactive virtual environments and a knowledge-based design. Reification is the process of making abstract concepts and events, beyond the realm of direct human experience, concrete and accessible to teachers and learners. Entering virtual worlds and simulations not otherwise easily accessible provides an opportunity to create, study, and evaluate the emergence of knowledge and comprehension from the direct interaction of learners with otherwise complex abstract ideas and principles by bringing them to life. Using a knowledge-based design process and appropriate subject matter experts, knowledge structure methods are applied in order to prioritize, characterize important relationships, and create a concept map that can be integrated into the reified models that are subsequently developed. Applying these principles, our interdisciplinary team has been developing a reified model of the nephron into which important physiologic functions can be integrated and rendered into a three dimensional virtual environment called Flatland, a virtual environments development software tool, within which a learners can interact using off-the-shelf hardware. The nephron model can be driven dynamically by a rules-based artificial intelligence engine, applying the rules and concepts developed in conjunction with the subject matter experts. In the future, the nephron model can be used to interactively demonstrate a number of physiologic principles or a variety of pathological processes that may be difficult to teach and understand. In addition, this approach to reification can be applied to a host of other physiologic and pathological concepts in other systems. These methods will require further evaluation to determine their impact and role in learning.

Keywords. Virtual reality, simulation, education, physiology, reification

Introduction

There are many abstract concepts in medical education that are difficult to teach and comprehend [1]. In order to address this challenge; we have been applying the approach of reification of abstract concepts using interactive virtual environments and a knowledge-based design.

Reification is the process of making abstract concepts and events, beyond the realm of direct human experience, concrete and accessible to teachers and learners [2]. Entering virtual worlds and simulations not otherwise easily accessible provides an opportunity to create, study, and evaluate the emergence of knowledge and comprehension from the direct interaction of learners with otherwise complex abstract ideas and principles by bringing them to life.

One example of applying this approach is in the area of renal physiology and pathophysiology, where aspects of acid-base, water, electrolyte balance, and the concentrating mechanisms in the nephron are important concepts to understand. These types of concepts, such as the counter-current concentrating mechanism in the loop of Henle, have been ranked as some of the most difficult for students to learn and apply as well as important for further research [1]. Applying these principles, our interdisciplinary team have begun developing a reified model of the nephron into which important physiologic functions could be integrated and rendered into a three dimensional virtual environment called Flatland, a virtual environments development software tool, within which a learners can interact using off-the-shelf hardware [3]. The nephron model can be driven dynamically by a rules-based artificial intelligence engine, applying the rules and concepts developed in conjunction with the subject matter experts. In the future, the nephron model can be used to interactively demonstrate a number of physiologic principles or a variety of pathological processes that may be difficult to teach and understand. In addition, this approach to reification can be applied to a host of other physiologic and pathological concepts in other systems. These methods will require further evaluation to determine their impact and role in learning.

1. Methods/Tools

1.1. Knowledge –based Design

Using a knowledge-based design process and appropriate subject matter experts, knowledge structure methods are applied in order to prioritize, characterize important relationships, and create a concept map that can be integrated into the reified models that are subsequently developed [4,5]. Generally 4-5 subject matter experts first prepare a list of the most important concepts related to the learning goals and objectives of the topic of interest that will be incorporated into the virtual reality simulation model and the artificial intelligence that supports it. Those concepts are averaged, prioritized and culled to the 20-40 most important concepts and presented to the subject matter experts for final review and agreement. That list is then used in the Pathfinder software [5] to allow the experts to determine the relatedness of those concepts, from which the expert knowledge structure and concept map is created. The expert knowledge structure is used as the gold standard against which the novice knowledge structure can be compared and statistically correlated before and after any simulation experience. If the simulation experience has had a positive impact on the learner's knowledge structure, a significant improvement in the correlation with the experts' knowledge structure should be demonstrated [6, 7].

We begun by focusing upon the water and electrolyte concentration functions of the nephron and asked six experts to list the most important related concepts. Initially a list of nearly 200 potentially related concepts was presented to the experts based on several references. That list was then decreased to 90 concepts and then finally culled to 34 to incorporate into the relatedness ratings needed to create the knowledge structure and concept map. Each structure network can be compared to the previously defined expert network resulting in a similarity index*(s)* that ranged from zero to one and used to determine any changes in knowledge structure after the learning experience.

Those concepts are built into the model design and used to program the rules-based artificial intelligence that drives the simulation and the responses to the user as they interact with the simulation in the virtual environment. The subject matter experts work with the computer programmers to develop the rules coded into the simulation, as well as the graphic artists that create the three dimensional model and its components. Subject matter experts confirm the face and content validity of the reified model, the artificial intelligence controlling the model and the responses to the user programmed into the simulation.

1.2. Flatland Platform

Flatland serves as the virtual reality platform [3]. It is a visualization application development environment, created at the University of New Mexico. Flatland allows software authors to construct, and users to interact with, arbitrarily complex graphical and aural representations of data and systems. It is written in C/C++ and uses the standard OpenGL graphics language to produce all graphic models. In addition, Flatland uses the standard libraries for window, mouse, joystick, and keyboard management. It is object oriented, multi-threaded and uses dynamically loaded libraries to build user applications in the virtual environment. The end result is a virtual reality immersive environment with sight and sound, in which the operator using joy wands and virtual controls can interact with computer-generated learning scenarios that respond logically to user interaction.

In the context of Flatland, an application is a relatively self-contained collection of objects, functions and data that can be dynamically loaded and unloaded into the graph of an environment during execution. Thus an application is responsible for creating and attaching its objects to the graph, and for supplying all object functionality. It is added to Flatland through the use of a configuration file. This structured file is read and parsed when Flatland starts, and contains the name and location of the libraries that have been created for the application, as well as a formal list of parameters and an arbitrary set of arguments for the application. All sound is emitted in Flatland from point sources in the 3D space. The author specifies the location of the sounds in the same model coordinate system used for the graphics.

Using the reification approach, graphic models are created that can represent the objects, concepts, or data of interest in a visually understandable manner and with which the user can interact. In the case of the nephron, a mechanical motif was created, similar to a plumbing circuit and duct-like system, with sliding openings representing passive diffusion that can be manipulated manually or integrated active pumps powered by through energy dependent systems. The molecular elements are represented as different shapes and colors. The user can choose to also visualize the relative concentration of these elements graphically, superimposed upon the nephron model. To assist the user in orientation to the more typical anatomic depiction of the nephron, the user can also chose to switch to an organic model within the virtual environment.

1.3. Tracking in the Flatland Environment

Flatland is designed to integrate any position-tracking technology. A tracker is a multiple degree of freedom measurement device that can, in real time, monitor the position and orientation of multiple receiver devices in space, relative to a transmitter device. In the standard immersive Flatland configuration, trackers are used to locate hand held wands and to track the position of the user's head. Head position and orientation are needed in cases that involve the use of head mounted displays or stereo shutter glasses.

User interaction is a central component of Flatland, and as such, each object is controllable in arbitrary ways defined by the designer. Currently there are four possible methods for the control of objects: 1) Pop up menus in the main viewer window, 2) the keyboard, 3) 2D control panels either in the environment or separate windows, and 4) external systems or simulations.

The immersed user or avatar interacts with the virtual models using a joy wand equipped with a six degree of freedom tracking system, buttons, and a trigger. The wand's representation in the environment is a virtual human hand. The user may pick up and place objects by moving the virtual hand and pulling the wand's trigger.

In the context the non-immersed metaphor, the user can locomote, navigate and manipulate objects in the virtual environment using a gaming interface device or using the computer mouse and keyboard. This approach eliminates the need for the head mounted display, which often constitutes the most expensive component of the fully immersive system.

1.4. Artificial Intelligence (AI)

The artificial intelligence (AI) is a forward linking "IF-THEN" rulebase system and contains knowledge of how objects interact. The rules, which are determined by subject matter experts, are coded in a C computer language format as logical antecedents and consequences, and currently have limited human readability. The AI loops over the rulebase, applying each rule's antecedents to the current state of the system, including time, and testing for logical matches. Matching rules are activated, modifying the next state of the system. Time is a special state of the system that is not usually directly modified by the AI, but whose rate is controlled by an adjustable clock. Since the rate of inference within the AI is controlled by this clock, the operator is able to speed up, slow down, or stop the action controlled by the AI. This allows the operator to make mistakes and repeat a simulation scenario as a way to learn from those mistakes.

Results

The nephron model has created a platform that can be driven dynamically by a rules-based artificial intelligence engine, applying the rules and concepts developed in conjunction with the subject matter experts.

The nephron model can be displayed in either a reified mechanical or organic motif (Figure 1). The simulation artificial intelligence engine dynamically governs changes in physiology and responses to interactions or interventions of the user. Elements such as water, sodium, potassium and urea are depicted as various shaped and colored objects

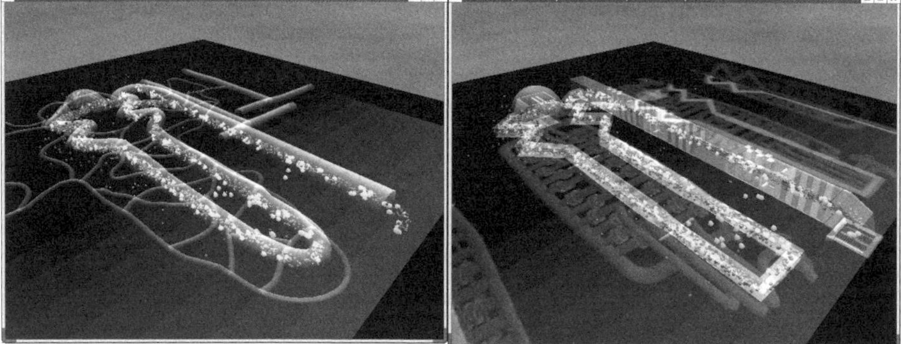

Figure 1. Reified nephron in an organic or mechanical motif

Participants can interact with this model in either a fully immersive virtual reality environment using a head-mounted display or non-immersive interface using a computer monitor with a mouse or video-game interface (Figure 2).

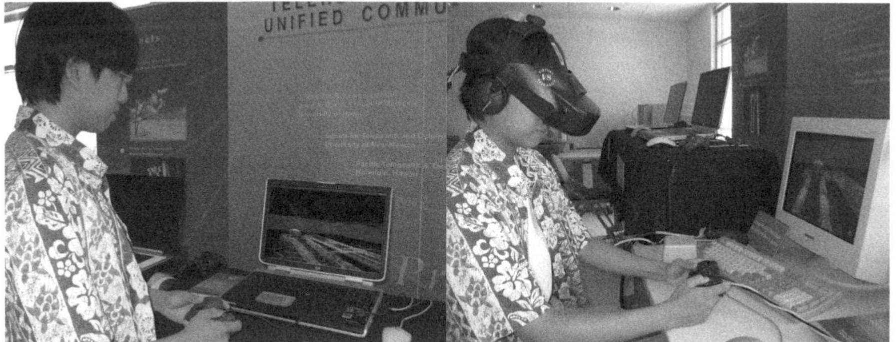

Figure 2. Student using non-immersion or full immersion system

The expert knowledge structure and associated concept map is being completed and will be used to develop the integrated artificial intelligence needed to demonstrate the critical concepts and responses to the user. That expert knowledge structure will be used as the gold standard against which the novice learner can be compared and the impact on knowledge acquisition and learning can be evaluated after the simulation experiences.

Conclusion/Novelty/Discussion

Using a knowledge-based design, appropriate subject matter experts and a virtual reality environment, we have developed a process for creating reified versions the nephron in which abstract concepts are embedded and can be driven by an artificial intelligence engine. It is within these virtual reality environments that participants interact can interact, providing a means to improve understanding of these concepts through experiential learning. In the future, the nephron model can be used to interactively demonstrate a number of physiologic principles or a variety of pathological processes that may be difficult to teach and understand. In addition, this approach to reification can be applied to a host of other physiologic and pathological concepts in other systems. These methods will require further evaluation to determine their impact and role in learning.

References

[1]   Dawson-Saunders, B., Feltovich, PJ, Coulson, R.L., and Steward, D.E. A survey of medical school teachers to identify basic biomedical concepts medical students should understand. *Academic Medicine*. 1990; Volume 65, Number 7:448-454

[2]   Winn, WD. A conceptual basis for educational applications of virtual reality. *Human Interface Technology Laboratory Technical Report TR-93-9*. Seattle, WA: Human Interface Technology Laboratory, University of Washington; August 1993

[3]   Caudell TP, Summers KL, Holten J IV, Takeshi H, Mowafi M, Jacobs J, Lozanoff BK, Lozanoff S, Wilks D, Keep MF, Saiki S, Alverson D: A Virtual Patient Simulator for Distributed Collaborative Medical Education. Anat Rec (Part B:New Anat) 270B:16-22, 2003

[4]   Johnson PJ, Goldsmith TE and Teague KW. Structural knowledge assessment: Locus of the predictive advantage in Pathfinder-based structures. *Journal of Educational Psychology*. 1994; 86:617-626

[5]   Schvaneveldt RW (Ed.). *Pathfinder Associative Networks: Studies in Knowledge Organization*. Norwood, NJ. Ablex; 1990

[6]   Stevens SM, Goldsmith TE, Summers KL, Sherstyuk A, Kihmm K, James R. Holten JR III, Davis C, Speitel D, Maris C, Stewart R, Wilks D, Saland L, Wax D, Panaiotis, Saiki S Jr, Alverson D and Caudell TP. Virtual Reality Training Improves Students' Knowledge Structures of Medical Concepts. in Medicine Meets Virtual Reality 13; The Magic Next Becomes the Medical Now, Volume 111 Studies in Health Technology and Informatics Edited by: James D. Westwood, Randy S. Haluck, Helene M. Hoffman, Greg T. Mogel, Roger Phillips, and Richard A. Rob. IOS Press, Amsterdam, The Netherlands; 519-525, 2005

[7]   Alverson DC, Saiki SM Jr, Caudell TP, Summers K, Panaiotis, Sherstyuk A, Nickles D, Holten J, Goldsmith T, Stevens S, Kihmm K, Mennin S, Kalishman S, Mines J, Serna L, Mitchell S, Lindberg M, Jacobs J, Nakatsu C, Lozanoff S, Wax DS, Saland L, Norenberg J, Shuster G, Keep M, Baker R, Buchanan HS, Stewart R, Bowyer M, Liu A, Muniz G, Coulter R, Maris C, Wilks D. Distributed immersive virtual reality simulation development for medical education. Journal of International Association of Medical Science Educators; 15:19-30, 2005

Medicine Meets Virtual Reality 14
J.D. Westwood et al. (Eds.)
IOS Press, 2006

A Surgical and Fine-Motor Skills Trainer for Everyone? Touch and Force-Feedback in a Virtual Reality Environment for Surgical Training

Christoph ASCHWANDEN[1,2], Andrei SHERSTYUK[2],
Lawrence BURGESS[2], Kevin MONTGOMERY[3]
[1]*caschwan@hawaii.edu*
[2]*Telehealth Research Institute (TRI)*
[3]*Stanford-NASA National Biocomputation Center*

Abstract. Access to the laboratory component of a class is limited by resources, while lab training is not currently possible for distance learning. To overcome the problem a solution is proposed to enable hands-on, interactive, objectively scored and appropriately mentored learning in a widely accessible environment. The proposed solution is the Virtual-Reality Motor-Skills trainer to teach basic fine-motor skills using Haptics for touch and feel interaction as well as a 3D virtual reality environment for visualization.

Keywords. Surgery, Trainer, Simulator, Virtual Reality, Haptics, Force-Feedback, Touch, Fine-Motor Skills, Simulation, Laparoscope, Suction, Extraction, Implantation, Bimanual, 3D, VR, Human-Computer Interaction, SPRING

1. Introduction

Didactic learning is taught to large audiences in a conventional classroom setting with the lecture hall further expanded for distance learning, using either live teleconference or archived video to provide wider educational access for students. However, this luxury is not afforded to the teaching of motor skills or manual tasks, as an expert instructor traditionally interacts with students in a laboratory environment. Access to the laboratory component of a class is limited by resources, while lab training is not currently possible for distance learning.

To overcome the problem a solution is proposed to enable hands-on, interactive, objectively scored and appropriately mentored learning in a widely accessible environment. The ultimate goal of such a solution is to preserve faculty resources, which would in turn provide either wider access to live laboratory exercises, or the ability to expand the curriculum for the same number of students. Likewise, with distance learning possible, geographically isolated rural populations or persons with confining disabilities will have greater access to training.

The addition of Haptics (Touch & Feel) to computer-assisted learning has broader societal implications, as auditory and visually impaired persons with disabilities would have a new tool to enhance learning for all disciplines and all age groups. The proposed solution is the Virtual-Reality Motor-Skills trainer (VRMS) to teach basic laparoscopic skills using Haptics for interaction and a 3D virtual reality environment for visualization.

2. Related Work

Computer assisted VR simulation has successfully been applied to various fields in medicine. Simulation systems exist for microsurgery [1], sinus surgery [3] and operative hysteroscopy [10] among others. Surgical simulation has found to support learning in numerous studies conducted [4][6][11]. The SPRING software framework used for this research has successfully been applied to various projects [8][9]. SPRING is specialized in soft-tissue modeling and Haptics.

Previously, costs for a dual-handed Haptics station were in the area of $20,000. Laparoscopic simulators are in the neighborhood of $100,000. However, efforts are underway to produce a low-cost Haptics interface device targeted at the consumer market for under $100 a piece[1]. This makes the system very affordable. Distributed capabilities of the software framework further allow for easier access as well as centralized data collection.

3. Motor-Skills Trainer

The goal of this interdisciplinary research is to move toward an understanding of human performance in skills development through computer assistance as well as to increase laboratory access and distributed learning.

The Virtual-Reality Motor-Skills trainer created is specifically designed to teach baseline fine-motor skills used in surgery, in a non-threatening abstract environment. Bead-like objects of various sizes are manipulated in 3D virtual space. Complexity is increased or decreased by changing the following factors: requirement for non-dominant or bimanual hand use with and without wrist rotation; environmental changes (depth of field, decreased exposure, smaller objects, and obstacles). Haptics is utilized for touch and force-feedback to provide more human-computer interaction and realism then previously possible for personal-computer applications. Figure 1 depicts the surgical simulator incorporating hinge operation and blood suction.

The performance measures being scored include motor skills (speed, accuracy, efficiency of motion) and cognitive skills (appropriate procedure selection). Dominant, non-dominant hands working in tandem will be trained and evaluated. The learning outcome will be progressive learning improvement and successful task acquisition based on expert and peer standards.

---

[1] Novint Technologies, http://www.novint.com/ (Novint Falcon)

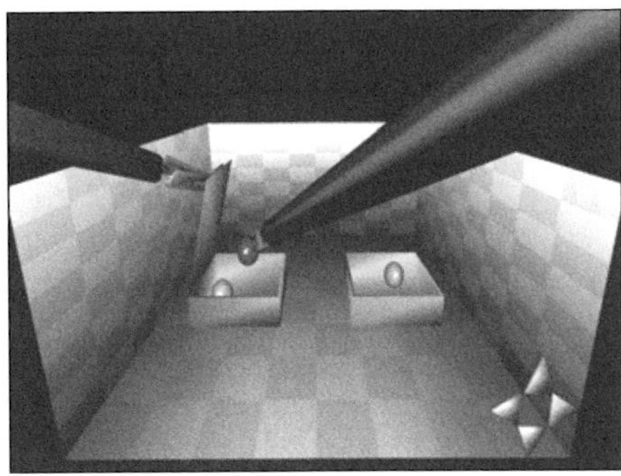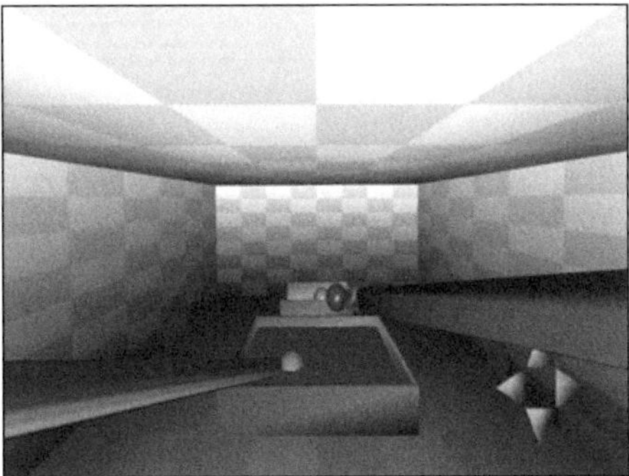

Figure 1 - Virtual Reality Motor-Skills Trainer

4. Contributions and Future Directions

The surgical trainer created is designed to teach surgical extraction and implantation skills focusing on motor, surgical and cognitive proficiency. Currently, no empirical studies were conducted, which are planned next to evaluate learning and usability of the system.

References

[1]　Brown, J., Montgomery, K., Latombe, J. C., Stephanides, M. (2001). A Microsurgery Simulation System, Medical Image Computing and Computer-Assisted Interventions (MICCAI 2001), Utrecht, The Netherlands, October 14-17, 2001.

[2]　Dev P, Montgomery K, Senger S, et al. Simulated medical learning environments over the Internet. J Am Med Inform Assoc.

[3]　Edmond CV (2002). Impact of the Endoscopic Sinus Surgical Simulator on Operating Room Performance, Laryngoscope, 112, 1148-58.

[4]　Grantcharov TP, Bardram L, Funch-Jensen P, Rosenberg J (2003). Learning curves and impact of previous operative experience on performance on a virtual reality simulator to test laparoscopic surgical skills. Am. J. Surg.,185(2), 146-149.

[5]　Heinrichs, W. L., Srivastava, S., Montgomery, K., and Dev, P. (2004). The Fundamental Manipulations of Surgery: A Structured Vocabulary for Designing Surgical Curricula and Simulators, J Am Assoc Gynecol Laparasoc, 11(4), 450-456.

[6]　McNatt, S. S. and. Smith, C. D. (2001). A computer-based laparoscopic skills assessment device differentiates experienced from novice laparoscopic surgeons, Surg. Endoscopy, 15, 1085-1089.

[7]　Montgomery, K., Bruyns, C. (2003). Virtual Instruments: A Generalized Implementation. 11th Medicine Meets Virtual Reality Conference, January 22-25, 2003.

[8]　Montgomery, K., Bruyns, C., Brown, J., Sorkin, S., Mazzella, F., Thonier, G., Tellier, A., Lerman, B., Menon, A. (2002). Spring: A General Framework for Collaborative, Real-time Surgical Simulation, In: Westwood, J., et. al. (eds.): Medicine Meets Virtual Reality, IOS Press, Amsterdam, 2002.

[9]　Montgomery, K., Bruyns, C., Wildermuth, S. (2001). A Virtual Environment for Simulated Rat Dissection: A Case Study of Visualization for Astronaut Training, 12th IEEE Visualization 2001 Conference, October 24-26, 2001, San Diego, CA.

[10]　Montgomery, K., Bruyns, C., Wildermuth, S., Heinrichs, L., Hasser, C., Ozenne, S, Bailey, D. (2001). Surgical Simulator for Operative Hysteroscopy, IEEE Visualization 2001, San Diego, California, October 14-17, 2001.

[11]　Seymour, N. E., Gallagher, A. G., Roman, S. A., O'Brien, M. K., Bansal, V. K., Andersen, D. K. and Satava, R. M.(2002). Virtual reality training improves operating room performance: results of a randomized, double-blinded study, Ann. Surgery, 236(4), 458-464.

Medicine Meets Virtual Reality 14
J.D. Westwood et al. (Eds.)
IOS Press, 2006

A Topologically Faithful, Tissue-Guided, Spatially Varying Meshing Strategy for the Computation of Patient-Specific Head Models for Endoscopic Pituitary Surgery Simulation

M.A. Audette[1], H. Delingette[2], A. Fuchs[3] and K. Chinzei[1].
[1]: *AIST, Surgical Assist Group, Tsukuba, 305-8564, Japan.*
Email: m.audette@aist.go.jp. [2]: *INRIA, Sophia-Antipolis, France.*
[3]: *KF^2Strategy GmbH, Stuttgart, Germany.1.*

Abstract. This paper presents a method for tessellating tissue boundaries and their interiors, given as input a tissue map consisting of relevant classes of the head, in order to produce anatomical models for finite element-based simulation of endoscopic pituitary surgery. Our surface meshing method is based on the simplex model, which is initialized by duality from the topologically accurate results of the Marching Cubes algorithm, and which features explicit control over mesh scale, while using tissue information to adhere to relevant boundaries. Our mesh scale strategy is spatially varying, based on the distance to a central point or linearized surgical path. The tetrahedralization stage also features a spatially varying mesh scale, consistent with that of the surface mesh.

1. Introduction

Virtual reality (VR) based surgical simulation involves the interaction of a user with an anatomical model representative of clinically relevant tissues and endowed with realistic constitutive properties, through virtual surgical tools. This model must be sufficiently descriptive for the interaction to be clinically meaningful: it must afford advantages over traditional surgical training in terms of improving surgical skill and patient outcome. Our simulation application, *endoscopic transnasal pituitary surgery*, is a procedure that typically involves removing mucosa, enlarging an opening in the sphenoid sinus bone with a rongeur, making an incision in the dura mater, and scooping out the pathology with a curette, while avoiding surrounding critical tissues. This entails anatomical meshing capable of an accurate depiction of the pituitary gland and of the arteries and cranial nerves surrounding it, as well as the brain, relevant sinus bones, dura mater, and any imbedded pathology, as shown in figure 1. This paper presents a method for tessellating tissue boundaries and their interiors, featuring surface and volume meshing stages, as part of a *minimally supervised* procedure for computing patient-specific models for neurosurgery simulation.

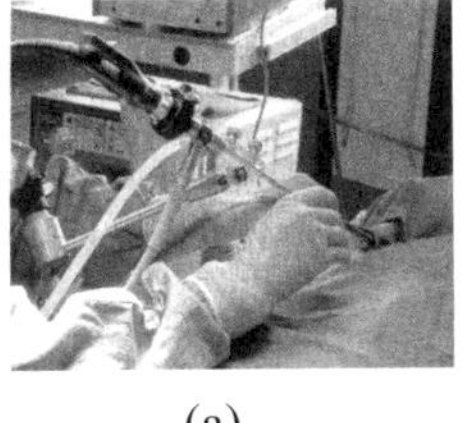
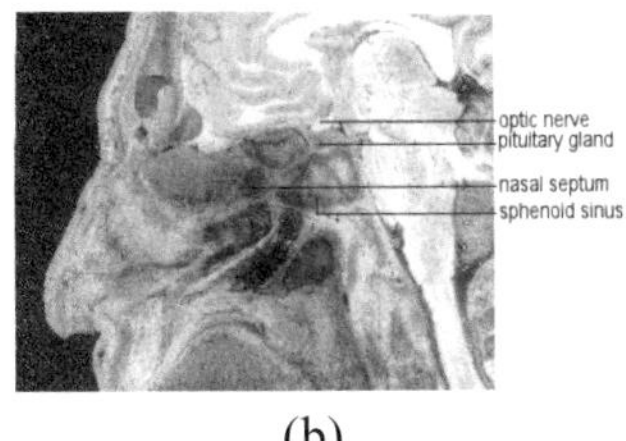

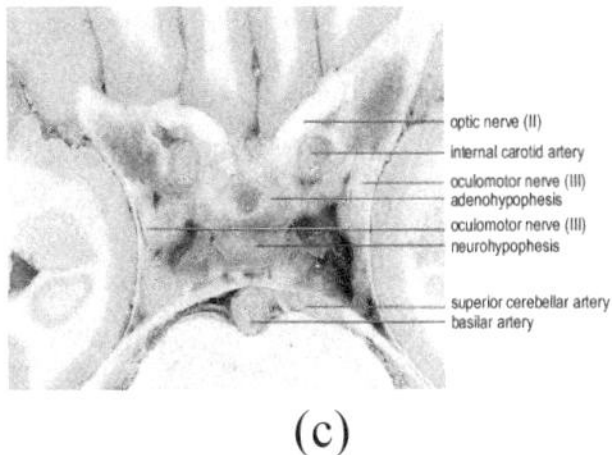

(a)   (b)   (c)

Figure 1. Illustration of endoscopic trans-nasal pituitary surgery: (a) OR setup; (b) sagittal image of the head featuring the pituitary gland, parasellar bones, brain and cranium; (c) oblique image featuring pituitary gland and surrounding critical tissues (reproduced with permission [3]).

Our clinical application, in light of the presence of surrounding critical tissues and the correlation between lack of experience and surgical complications [4], is a good candidate for simulation. Our meshing objectives are the following:

- The method must produce *as few elements as possible*, to limit the complexity of the real-time problem, while meeting our requirements for haptic, visual and constitutive realism. Therefore, *mesh scale must be spatially flexible*, to allow small elements near the surgical target, particularly if an endoscopic view is required, while producing significantly larger elements far away, thereby limiting the number of elements overall, and still maintaining the conformality of the mesh. The hierarchical multirate FE model of [1] suggests a way of treating this mesh that alleviates adverse effect on the condition number of the system.

- The *meshing must reflect the topology* of the underlying tissue: if a tissue features one or more inner boundaries, as well as an outer boundary, these boundaries must be accounted for, if the constitutive realism of the simulation requires it.

- Next, the method should *afford both 2D and 3D elements*, as some tissues are better modeled as collections of surface elements, such as the dura mater, thin cranial bones and vasculature[1], while others are inherently volumetric. Existing methods that are purely volumetric [11] suffer from their inability to model tissues that are inherently curviplanar.

- Last, the meshing method must *produce high-quality triangles and tetrahedra*: within each 2D or 3D element the edges should be of near-equal length, as opposed to 1 or 2 edges significantly shorter than the others, for the sake of rapid convergence of the FE method [9]. It should also produce smooth boundaries where anatomically appropriate.

The goal of the surface meshing procedure is to establish the topologically faithful tissue surfaces bounding each class or contiguous subset of classes, where each surface mesh exhibits the required edge scale pattern. Given our objectives, we have opted for a surface model-based approach to tessellating anatomical boundaries, featuring the well-known *simplex* model [5]. Its topological operators provide explicit control over individual faces and edges. This surface meshing stage is followed by a tetrahedralization stage that also meets our mesh scale objectives and that uses as input the triangular boundaries produced by the surface meshing stage.

---

[1] The latter might be simplified as a curvilinear element, were it not for the requirement that cutting through it should appear realistic and be appropriately penalized in our simulation.

2. Materials and Methods

2.1 Topologically Accurate Tissue-guided Simplex Mesh with Spatially Varying Scale

The m-simplex mesh is a discrete active surface model [5], characterized by each vertex being linked to each of m+1 neighbours by an edge. A surface model in 3D is realized as a 2-simplex, where each vertex has 3 neighbours, and this representation is the dual of a triangulated surface, with each simplex vertex coinciding with a center, and each simplex edge being bisected by an edge, of a triangle. Furthermore, this surface model also features *image-based balloon forces* as well as *internal forces* [7] that nudge each face towards having *edges of locally consistent length* and towards C_0, C_1 or C_2 *continuity*.

This model has been limited by its topological equivalence with a sphere, in the absence of topological adaptivity. While topological adaptivity is achievable, based on operators published in [5], the convergence of the surface to the intended boundary, involving hundreds of iterations of a model integrating internal and image forces, is fraught with local extrema, a situation exacerbated by the capability of splitting or fusing. To alleviate this issue, we instead *initialize the simplex model with a dense surface mesh of high accuracy and topological fidelity, resulting from Marching Cubes (MC)* [7], based on the duality between a triangular surface and a 2-simplex mesh.

We then decimate the simplex mesh in a highly controlled, spatially varying manner, while exploiting a previously computed tissue map to guide the model on a tissue-specific basis. The final simplex boundaries can be converted to triangulated surfaces by duality. This way of proceding allows us more control over the decimation than existing algorithms not based on surface models, as our spatially varying control over mesh scale allows us to resolve the relevant anatomical surfaces densely enough for endoscopic simulation, while still limiting the number of triangles and tetrahedra enough to make real-time interaction feasible.

Control over mesh size is typically implemented through the *Eulerian T_1 and T_2 operators* [5], as triggered by geometric measurements of each simplex face or edge. For example, if the smallest edge of a face is smaller than the edge scale objective at that position, in order to produce a sparser mesh we delete that edge by a T_1 operation. Also, if a simplex face has more than k vertices ($k = 7$ usually), coinciding with a triangular mesh vertex with more than k incident, typically elongated, triangles, we also use T_1 and T_2 to reduce the number of simplex vertices and improve mesh quality.

It should also be emphasized that our procedure identifies anatomical surfaces prior to volumetric meshing, rather than proceed directly from the classification to tissue-guided volumetric meshing, because some tissues are inherently curviplanar rather than volumetric and are more efficiently modeled by shell elements than tetrahedra or hexahedra. Also, a purely volumetric approach will in general not produce a mesh that is as smooth and that closely agrees with the anatomical boundary: from a haptic and visual rendering standpoint, an anatomical model with jagged or badly localized boundaries would detract from the realism and clinical relevance of a surgical simulator as well as confuse the user.

We start from a densely triangulated surface produced by Marching Cubes, post-processed by an existing, topology-preserving, decimation method [8], which is somewhat more computationally efficient than ours and in order to reduce the number of triangles to a manageable number, as well as with identification and area-thresholding of contiguous structures, all VTK-based [10]. This stage produces a set of triangulated surfaces that we convert to simplex meshes by duality. From geometric tests to ascertain the shortest edge of each face, we iteratively perform T_1 operations on those faces whose shortest edge are furthest from their respective objective. We note that when the curvature of the boundary may be sufficiently pronounced, with respect to the edge scale objective, T_1 operations lead to faces whose center lies too far from the boundary. At that point, the optimal representation may be a trade-off between the desired edge scale and the desired proximity of the face center to the boundary. This trade-off entails the use of T_2 operators to partition each ill-fitting face into two.

2.2 Spatially Varying Edge Scale Strategies: Radial and Surgical Path-Based Distance

Control over simplex mesh edge scale can be exercised with a *Radially Varying Surface Mesh Scale* function $L_{sm}(d_R (x, p_c))$. This function is defined at any x in the volume spanned by the mesh, based on the Euclidian distance $d_R (x, p_c) = \| x - p_c \|$ from a user-provided central point p_c (e.g.: on the pituitary gland). This function produces small edges near the pituitary gland and longer edges away from it.

Alternately, we can specify at any x a *Surgical Path Based Mesh Scale* function $L(d_{SP} (x, S))$, substituting d_{SP} for d_R in expression (1), where $S = \{ E_i (p_i, p_{i+1}) \}$ is a set of linear edges E_i. Each edge E_i connects 2 user-provided points p_i and p_{i+1}, and together they approximate a planned surgical path: $d_{SP} (x, S) \equiv min_{\{E_i \in S\}} d_{edge} (x, E_i)$, where $d_{edge} (x, E_i) \equiv min_{i, \{ u + v = 1 \}} \| u\, p_i + v\, p_{i+1} - x \|$. We seek the minimum distance from x to the set of edges S that approximates the surgical path.

This notion of using proximity to a point or to an intended surgical path to optimize mesh size can be extended to choices about constitutive and clinical realism. For example, within a distance threshold ε_d from a point or a path we may elect to model soft tissues as *nonlinearly elastic*, beyond which we are content with *linearly elastic* behaviour. Or, for any x where $d_{SP} (x, S) > \varepsilon_d$ we may model skin, muscle, fat and bone as having a *prescribed null displacement*, thereby effectively eliminating them from the real-time FE problem, whereas closer to the surgical path, we can account for the material properties of mucosa, muscle and even bones.

2.3 Almost-regular Volumetric Meshing with Spatially Varying Resolution Control

The last stage in our procedure partitions each volume bounded by a triangulated mesh, coinciding with a tissue class or contiguous subset of tissue classes, into tetrahedral elements consistent with the FE method. The volumetric meshing stage is a published technique [6] that automatically produces an optimal tetrahedralization from a given polygonal boundary, such as a triangulated surface. This method features the optimal positioning of inner vertices, expressed as a minimization of a penalty functional, followed by a Delaunay tetrahedralization. Moreover, based on the relationship between the number of simplex and triangle vertices $V_t \approx V_{sm}/2$ [5], a target simplex mesh size of L_{sm} works out to a triangle or a tetrahedral mesh size of $L_t (x) \approx \sqrt{2}\, L_{sm} (x)$. We modify this technique by integrating into the penalty functional the spatially varying scale, specified as a target edge length $L_t (x)$ for each tetrahedron.

3. Results and Discussion

Figures 4 and 5 contrast an existing, curvature-sensitive (but otherwise spatially consistent) decimation algorithm [8] with our spatially varying, simplex-based surface mesh decimation. Figure 4 displays a synthetic cube with 4 tubular openings through it, along axes x and y, to which we've added a synthetic hemispherical "gland" in its inner ceiling: (a) surface as originally identified by MC, (b) as decimated by the existing method. We choose a proximity threshold that is tight at the gland and looser far away. Figure 5 shows results for a brain surface, going from the prior method in (a) to the results of our method in (b) and (c), while (d) illustrates the flexibility and clinical applicability of the surface meshing method, in its ability to characterize relevant critical tissues.

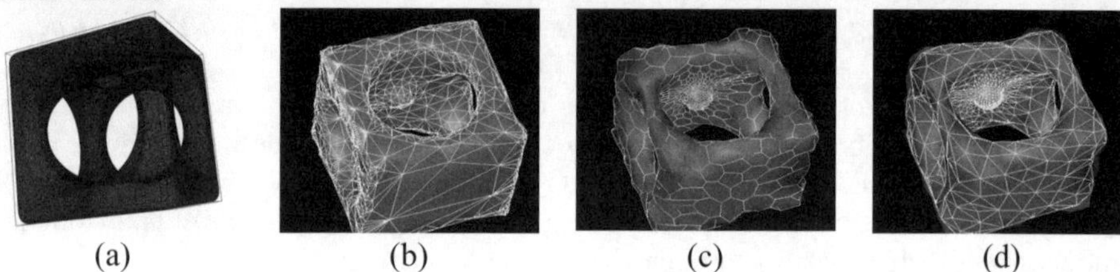

(a)   (b)   (c)   (d)

Figure 4. Contrasting decimation methods on synthetic invaginated cube surface, featuring a hemispheric inner gland: (a) wireframe of MC results; (b): existing decimation method; (c) and (d): radially varying simplex mesh, featuring final simplex and dual triangular results.

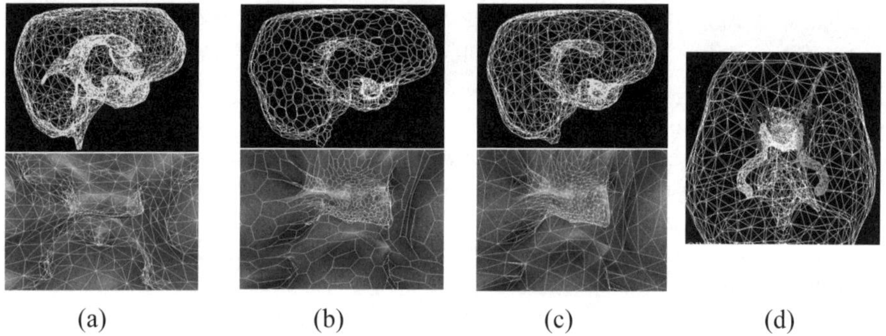

(a)   (b)   (c)   (d)

Figure 5. Anatomical results. (a)-(c) Contrasting decimation methods on brain surface: (a) existing method, featuring wireframe of overall brain surface mesh and closeup of wireframe overlaid on rendering of brain surface, centered on pituitary gland; (b) radially varying simplex mesh, featuring wireframe and overlay closeup views as in (a); (c) radially varying triangular surface, dual to simplex mesh in (b). (d) Superposition of relevant critical tissue meshes with brain surface: basilar arteries, optic and oculomotor nerves.

Figure 6 depicts how a combination of path-based ($\varepsilon_{d,SP}$ = 10mm) and radial ($\varepsilon_{d,R}$ = 25mm) distance allows us to convert "distant" extra-cranial tissue to "null displacement" tissue to exclude it from the real-time biomechanical problem. These two distances are then used to determine the mesh scale. Finally, figure 7 illustrates our topologically accurate, radially varying tetrahedralization results, on the cube and brain volumes. The former meshing is visualized as a wireframe composed of all tetrahedral edges. The brain tetrahedral meshing is shown a semi-transparent volume whose intersection with a clipping plane is shown as a set of triangles, as well as a wiremesh of all edges in a manner comparable to the cube.

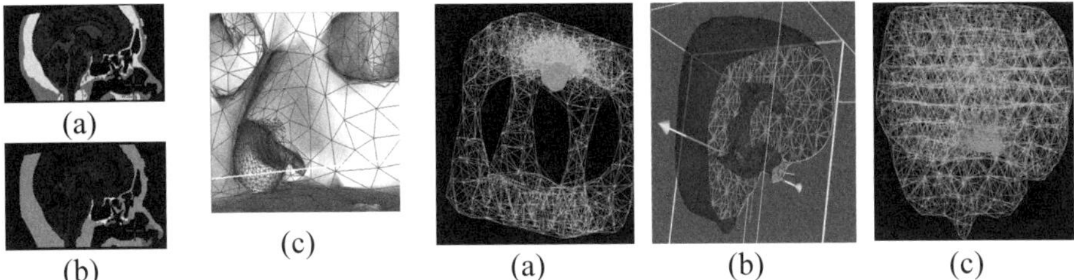

Figure 6. Illustration of use of radial and path-based distance to convert "distant" extra-cranial soft tissue to tissue of null displacement and determine edge scale: (a) original tissue map [2]; (b) null-displacement tissue in orange; (c) final triangulated surface.

Figure 7. Illustration of tetrahedralization: (a) invaginated cube visualized as 3D wireframe of all tetrahedral edges; (b) semi-transparent boundary of clipped volume, where triangular intersections of tetrahedra with clipping plane shown as white wireframe, and (c) 3D wireframe rendering.

4. Conclusions

This paper presented a new meshing strategy for computing patient-specific anatomical models comprised of triangles and tetrahedra coinciding with, or for computational efficiency idealized as, homogeneous tissue, in a manner that addresses the requirements of endoscopic pituitary surgery simulation. Our strategy offers promise for dealing with the conflicting requirements of narrowly focused, and especially endoscopic, visualization and haptic rendering as well as the computation of body forces and displacements over large volumes, particularly if combined with hierarchical multirate finite elements. This method is conceived to be extensible to surgery simulation in general, and it appears able to deal with any tissue shape as well as most practical requirements for tissue mesh size.

5. References

[1] O. Astley & V. Hayward, Multirate Haptic Simulation Achieved by Coupling Finite Element Meshes Through Norton Equivalents, *IEEE Int. Conf. Rob. Auto.*, 1998.

[2] M.A. Audette and K. Chinzei, The Application of Embedded and Tubular Structure to Tissue Identification for the Computation of Patient-Specific Neurosurgical Simulation Models, *Int. Symp. Med. Sim, LNCS 3078*, PP. 203-210, 2004.

[3] P. Cappabianca et al., *Atlas of Endoscopic Anatomy for Endonasal Intracranial Surgery*, Springer, 2001.

[4] I. Ciric et al., Complications of Transsphenoidal Surgery: Results of a National Survey, Review of the Literature, and Personal Experience, *Neurosurg.*, Vol. 40, No. 2., pp. 225-236, Feb. 1997.

[5] H. Delingette, General Object Reconstruction Based on Simplex Meshes, *Int. J. Comp. Vis.*, Vol. 32, No. 2, pp. 111-146, 1999.

[6] A. Fuchs, Almost Regular Triangulations of Trimmed NURBS-Solids, *Eng. w. Comput.*, Vol. 17, pp. 55-65, 2001.

[7] W. Lorensen & H. Cline, Marching Cubes: a High Resolution 3D Surface Construction Algorithm, *Comput. Graph.s*, Vol. 21, No. 4, pp. 163-170, 1987.

[8] W. Schroeder et al., Decimation of Triangle Meshes, *Comput. Graph. SIGGRAPH '92*, 26(2):65-70,1992.

[9] J.R. Shewchuk, What is a Good Linear Element? Interpolation, Conditioning and Quality Measures, *11th Int. Meshing Roundtbl.* pp. 115-126, 2002.

[10] VTK: Visualization Toolkit, *http://public.kitware.com/VTK*.

[11] Y. Zhang, C. Bajaj & B.S. Sohn, 3D Finite Element Meshing from Imaging Data, *Comput. Meth. in Appl. Mech. & Engng..*, to appear, 2005.

Medicine Meets Virtual Reality 14
J.D. Westwood et al. (Eds.)
IOS Press, 2006

Determination of Face Validity for the Simbionix LAP Mentor Virtual Reality Training Module

ID AYODEJI [a,1], MP SCHIJVEN [b], JJ JAKIMOWICZ [c]

a Department of General Surgery, Maxima MC, Eindhoven
b Department of General Surgery, IJsselland Hospital, Capelle aan den IJssel
c Department of General Surgery, Catharina Hospital, Eindhoven

[1] Corresponding Author: Petrus Dondersstraat 119, 5613LT Eindhoven, The Netherlands; E-mail segun@ayodeji.com

Abstract. This study determines the expert and referent face validity of LAP Mentor, the first procedural virtual-reality (VR) trainer. After a hands-on introduction to the simulator a questionnaire was administered to 49 participants (21 expert laparoscopists and 28 novices). There was a consensus on LAP Mentor being a valid training model for basic skills training and the procedural training of laparoscopic cholecystectomies. As 88% of respondents saw training on this simulator as effective and 96% experienced this training as fun it will likely be accepted in the surgical curriculum by both experts and trainees. Further validation of the system is required to determine whether its performance concurs with these favourable expectations.

Keywords. Laparoscopic skills, virtual reality, face validation, laparoscopic trainer, assessment, skills training

Introduction

Aspiring laparoscopists need very specific basic skills training in order to acquire unique psychomotor skills as well as procedural training [1-7]. While laparoscopic surgery has been embedded in general surgery's repertoire the surgical curriculum has evolved little to accommodate this.

The historically applied apprenticeship model essentially sees future surgeons trained in the operating room on actual patients. A hoax of detrimental effects results from this practice: a higher risk to the patient, loss of valuable OR time, a stressful leaning environment, an unpredictable incidence of learning opportunities, and variance in the teaching capacities of the supervising surgeon. Until recently, lacking validated alternatives for surgical training, these negative aspects of training full surgical procedures exclusively on patients had to be tolerated. For endoscopic surgery in particular this has changed due to the evolution of training simulations.

Simbionix USA Corp (www.simbionix.com) launched LAP Mentor in 2003, simulating a complete laparoscopic cholecystectomy on the Xitact LS500 haptic platform (www.xitact.com) that has been systematically validated [8-11].

The first step in LAP Mentor's systematic validation is determining face validity: for successful integration into a curriculum both potential teachers and potential trainees must accept a model as valid and be inclined to work with it.

1. Materials and methods

LAP Mentor consists of a basic skills trainer and a procedural trainer. The first simulates abstract tasks for training dexterity; the second offers a realistic model with anatomic variations on which an entire procedure can be performed.

Participants having performed fifty laparoscopies or more were classified as 'experts' (n=21), others –representing trainees- as were 'referent' (n=28). Each was given a twenty-minute hands-on introduction to LAP Mentor and then asked to fill out a structured questionnaire using Likert scaled questions focussed on the application of training simulators in general and LAP Mentors' validity specifically, touching on aspects as design, realism and effectivity was used to collect data which was subsequently analyzed. The responses of the two distinct groups were compared using the Mann Witney U test to determine significance.

2. Results

When requested to judge the realism of the Lap Mentors simulation, only one single expert and one single referent respondent rated it less that 6 out of 10, with half of all respondents rating it 8 or more. The results of our enquiry into the various aspects of face validity are listed in Table 1.

There is no significant difference of opinion between the expert and referent groups, reflected by a high P-value indicating consensus. Both groups feel basic skills should be acquired before attempting live laparoscopic surgery and find procedural training an important aspect of the curriculum.

	Referent Mean	Expert Mean	Total Mean	SD	P
LM as a valid training mode l for laparoscopic surgery	8.57	8.29	8.45	1.542	0.391
Realism of the cholecystectomy procedure	8.19	8.00	8.11	1.451	0.571
Realism of basic skills module	7.62	7.90	7.74	1.594	0.652
Realism of peritoneal cavity anatomy	7.48	7.25	7.38	1.664	0.759
Realism of force feedback (haptics)	6.64	6.00	6.37	2.028	0.243
Software design	7.52	8.44	7.91	1.571	0.070
Choice of exercises	7.76	7.68	7.73	1.531	0.910

Table 1. Face validity ratings (1: very bad, to 10: very good)

The LAP Mentor is:	Referent Mean	Expert Mean	Total Mean	SD	P
Effective for practicing basic skills	8.57	8.48	8.53	1.138	0.724
Effective for training laparoscopic cholecystectomy	8.69	8.63	8.67	1.206	0.815
Suitable for evaluation during training	7.29	7.80	7.50	1.957	0.512
A user friendly learning environment	8.86	8.60	8.75	1.345	0.579
Simply fun to practice on	8.71	8.48	8.61	1.643	0.432
Effective in shortening learning curves in the OR	8.29	8.57	8.41	1.731	0.810
Effective in reducing the incidence of complications	7.50	7.50	7.50	2.000	0.799
The LAP Mentor shall reduce expenses of training after purchase	6.00	6.22	6.09	2.091	0.623

Table 2. Applicability in the curriculum (1: very bad, to 10: very good)

3. Conclusion

Both experts and trainees see training on LAP Mentor as effective and fun so they will likely accept it in the surgical curriculum. Further validation of the system is required to determine whether its performance concurs with these expectations.

References

1. Club, T.S.S., *The learning curve for laparoscopic cholecystectomy*, in *Am J Surg*. 1995. p. 55-59.
2. Dent, T.L., *Training, credentialling and granting of clinical privileges for laparoscopic general surgery*. Am J Surg, 1991. **161**: p. 399-403.
3. Deziel, D., et al., *Complications of laparoscopic cholecystectomy: a national survey of 4,292 hospitals and an analysis of 77,604 cases*. Am. J. Surg., 1993. **165**: p. 9-14.
4. Figert, P.L., et al., *Transfer of training in acquiring laparoscopic skills*. J Am Coll Surg, 2001. **193**(5): p. 533-537.
5. Torkington, J., et al., *The role of the Basic Surgical Skills course in the aquisition and retention of laparoscopic skill*. Surg Endosc, 2001. **15**: p. 1071-1075.
6. Rosser, J.C., L.E. Rosser, and R.S. Savalgi, *Skill acquisition and assessment for laparoscopic surgery*. Arch Surg, 1997. **132**(2): p. 200-4.
7. Chung, J.Y. and J.M. Sackier, *A method of objectively evaluating improvement in laparoscopic skills*. Surg Endosc, 1998. **12**: p. 1111-1116.
8. Schijven, M. and J. Jakimowicz, *Face-, expert, and referent validity of the Xitact LS500 laparoscopy simulator*. Surg Endosc, 2002. **16**(12): p. 1764-70.
9. Schijven, M. and J. Jakimowicz, *Construct validity: experts and residents performing on the Xitact LS500 laparoscopy simulator*. Surg Endosc, 2003. **17**: p. 803-810.
10. Schijven, M.P. and J. Jakimowicz, *The learning curve on the Xitact LS 500 laparoscopy simulator: profiles of performance*. Surg Endosc, 2003.
11. Schijven, M.P. and J.J. Jakimowicz, *Introducing the Xitact LS500 Laparoscopy Simulator: Toward a Revolution in Surgical Education*. Surg Technol Int, 2003. XI: p. 32-36.

Medicine Meets Virtual Reality 14
J.D. Westwood et al. (Eds.)
IOS Press, 2006

Enhancing the Visual Realism of Hysteroscopy Simulation

Daniel Bachofen [a,1], János Zátonyi [b], Matthias Harders [b], Gábor Székely [b],
Peter Früh [a], Markus Thaler [a]

[a] *Inst. for Applied Information Technology, ZHW Winterthur, Switzerland*
[b] *Virtual Reality in Medicine Group, Computer Vision Lab, ETH Zurich,
Switzerland*

Abstract. Visualization is a very important part of a high fidelity surgical simulator. Due to modern computer graphics hardware, which offers more and more features and processing power, it is possible to extend the standard OpenGL rendering methods with advanced visualization techniques to achieve highly realistic rendering in real-time. For an easy and efficient use of these new capabilities, a stand-alone graphics engine has been implemented, which exploits these advanced rendering techniques and provides an interface in order to ensure the interoperability with a software framework for surgical simulators.

Keywords. surgical simulation, visualization, graphics engine

1. Introduction

The target of our current research is the development of a high fidelity simulator for hysteroscopic interventions. Hysteroscopy is the standard procedure for the endoscopic inspection of the inner surface of the uterus. It belongs to the most often performed procedures in gynecology, even though serious complications might arise. Repetitive training is the only way for a surgeon to acquire sufficient experience. Surgical simulation using virtual reality is a promising alternative to apprenticeship providing appropriate training environment and so patient involvement can be avoided. As opposed to existing systems [1,2,3,4] we aim at achieving the highest possible realism. More specifically, our goal is to go beyond exercising of basic manipulative skills and enable procedural training. Therefore the highest possible realism needs to be provided by all of the components (surgical tool, haptics and visualization) of the entire system.

A typical view into the uterine cavity during an intervention is shown in Figure 11. In order to reproduce this complex scene virtually, a comprehensive set of visual cues has to be captured. These comprise the photo-realistic rendering of the different materials and surfaces present in the scene (such as organ, pathologies and cut surfaces, consisting of tissues with different appearance showing of-

---

[1]Correspondence to: bachofen@vision.ee.ethz.ch

ten specular reflections), the endoscopic camera model with lens distortion and proper illumination of the scene with emphasis on the spotlight effect. Moreover, the representation of floating endometrial material, tissue fibres, debris, air bubbles and the realistic simulation of the intra uterine bleeding are also among the essential needs for a fully realistic hysteroscopy simulator.

We have developed a graphics framework, which is able to handle all these needs for a high-fidelity visual appearance. Furthermore, all these effects are generated with interactive speed and are therefore adaptable in real-time according to user input.

2. Tools and Methods

The actual surgical scene is created based on a statistical framework allowing to obtain variable geometries of the healthy anatomy, which can be extended by adding different pathologies, e.g. polyps or myomas [5]. Two different models of the geometries are maintained in the simulation - a high resolution triangular model representing the surface and a lower resolution tetrahedral model used for the computation of the deformation and for the collision detection.

To achieve a highly realistic rendering of the virtual scene, we have a set of different computer graphics tools at hand. Multi-texturing, multipass rendering and programmable shaders can be used for an extended OpenGL illumination. Bump mapping and environment mapping can help us to visualize the different material properties. The use of billboarding technique allows to simplify the visualization of complex objects so that thousands of them can be rendered in real-time. Finally, pixel buffer and render-to-texture techniques can be used for postprocessing the resulting image. This can be done by the central processing unit or even by the graphics processing unit, if programmable shaders are used.

The appropriate combination of these available resources enable to build up a realistic graphics engine for a hysteroscopy simulator. To keep the system compatible to any older graphics hardware, we currently do not use any programmable shader techniques. Thus, we make use of multi-texturing and multipass rendering for implementing the illumination model as well as different texture mapping techniques for the materials. For organ surfaces including cuts we use enhanced texturing with images from our extensive database, which was established from intra-operative recordings of hysteroscopic interventions. Billboards are used for floating tissues, fibres and bubbles, while bleeding is modeled by a particle system that makes use of animated billboards. The lens distortion and depth of field effect of the camera is realized by using a render-to-texture strategy. The visualization pipeline of the graphics engine is depicted in Fig. 1.

The graphics engine, as a standalone unit within a surgical simulator, is not only responsible for the visualization, but also for the handling of the surface data. In our solution, the data handling is driven by a scene graph, which provides an organized hierarchy of the triangle surfaces and visual properties of the models. It allows using different triangle surfaces and materials for a single organ. Furthermore the scene tree is fully dynamic, meaning that data structures can be modified at runtime, which is an important issue, e.g. when pieces of deformable objects are cut off during surgery.

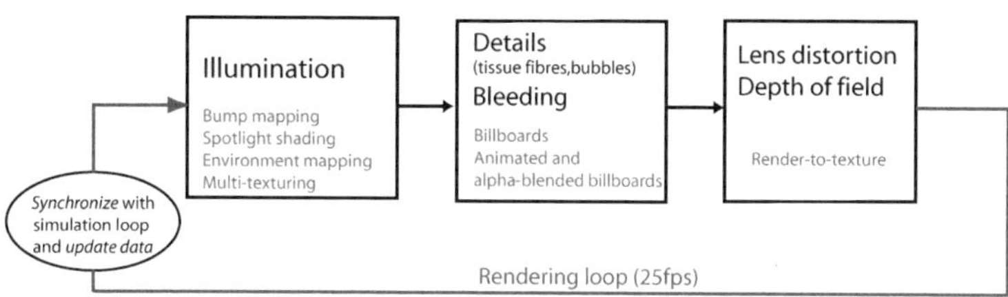

Figure 1. Pipeline of the rendering steps

3. Individual rendering components

3.1. Illumination model

The first element of the illumination model is a bump mapping pass [8]. Here we create a rough looking surface by using a texture map that contains a set of surface normals in its rgb-information (Figure 2). To convert the surface normals from the map into world-space, the normal and the tangents of the mapped texture must be transformed from texture-space to world-space for each vertex. Due to our special situation with deformable geometry, this step must be repeated in every frame.

In a second pass, the scene is drawn as a blank white object, illuminated by the standard OpenGL lighting (Figure 3). This pass is used to achieve the white spotlight effect by modulating the result of this pass with the bump mapping pass. Thus, the illuminated area of the bump mapped scene stays visible, while the area outside the spotlight is blind out.

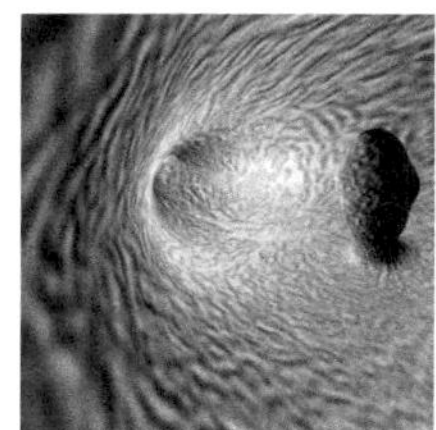
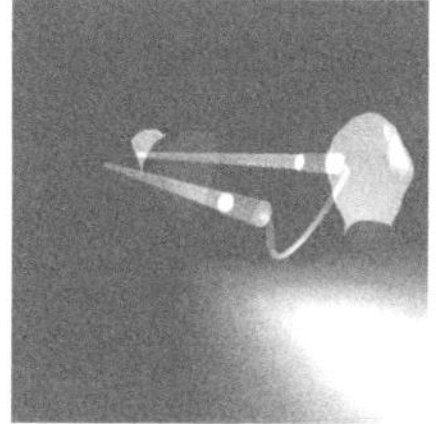
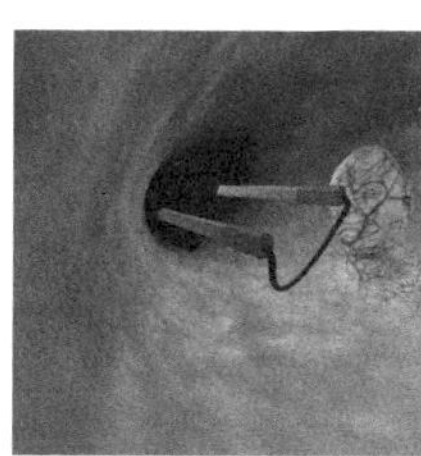
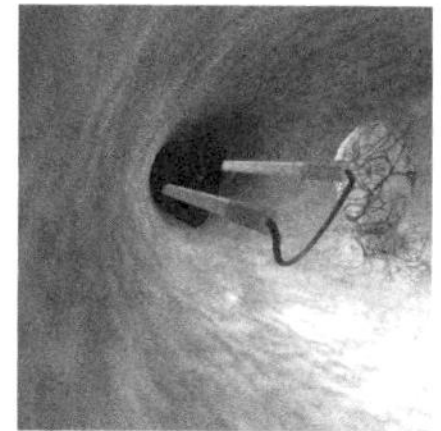

Figure 2. Pass 1 Bump mapping

Figure 3. Pass 2 Spotlight

Figure 4. Pass 3 Texture mapping

Figure 5. Combination of pass 1-3

This combination of bump map and spotlight is then fed into the main rendering pass, which contains textures and environment maps (Figure 4). The resulting image (Figure 5) contains in addition to the regular scene all necessary components, a rough surface around the spotlight area, a strong white spotlight and environment mapping for shiny materials.

3.2. Additional visual details

In order to further increase the fidelity of the scene, the graphics engine incorporates floating endometrial material, tissue fibres, debris, bubbles and bleeding into the scene (Figure 6, 7 and 8). All these features have to adapt their behavior to the actual geometry and to the flow of the distension liquid, which is adjusted by the surgeon via the valves on the hysteroscope.

Instead of modeling and rendering these objects in 3D, which would be a waste of resources of the graphics engine, we make use of the billboarding technique. Billboarding is an efficient approach in computer graphics, that adjusts the orientation of a simple object so that it faces the camera and as such it makes possible to give the illusion of a 3D object without having modeled it by large number of polygons. In our case the tissue fibres, debris and air bubbles are represented as properly textured quads always oriented towards the camera and they are moved around in the scene according to the flow field. The flow is computed in real-time according to the actual boundary conditions [9].

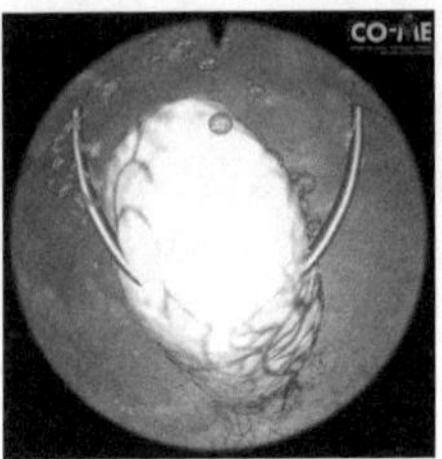

Figure 6. Bubbles and tissue fibres during cutting

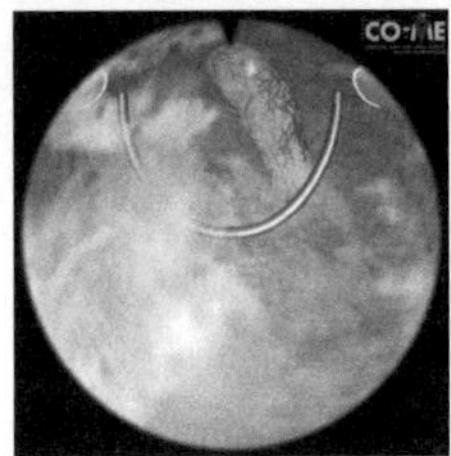

Figure 7. Tissue fibres on uterus

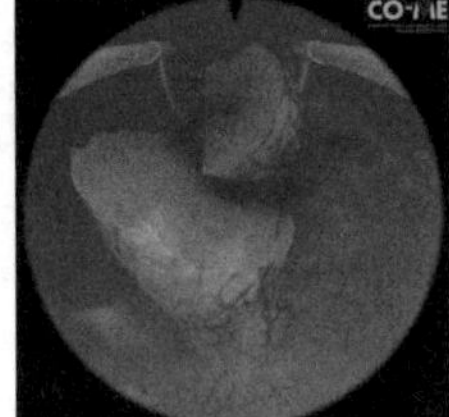

Figure 8. Heavy bleeding after a cut

All freely floating objects are included in the collision detection. Thus, e.g. bubbles, which are created during cutting or enter at the tip of the tool, can stick to object surfaces.

During cutting or strong collisions with the uterine wall, vessels can be damaged, which causes bleeding depending on the size of the vessel. We developed a bleeding model which enables us to simulate versatile bleeding from oozing to fast spurts, and from focal to diffuse types in different levels depending on the information coming from the vascular structure of the scene. As a solution we have chosen to use particles with animated billboards. The particles allow for the realistic movement and the interaction with the environment, while the billboards with changing texture ensure an efficient rendering performance with configurable and versatile visual appearance. A bleeding source is considered as an emitter, producing non-interacting particles during the period of a bleeding. The size of the quads attached to the particles and the texture applied is continuously altered according to the type and phase of the bleeding. In the final rendering stage the textured billboards are alpha-blended. This results in a realistic volumetric effect, with relatively low cost of rendering performance.

3.3. Lens distortion and depth of field effect

Although endoscopic cameras with almost no lens distortion are available today, they are not widely used in the clinical practice due to their higher price. Thus, we need to simulate the lens distortion of the endoscopic camera in order to get as close to reality as possible. In addition, the lens causes a depth of field effect, which blurs the scene when the camera is out of focus.

The general idea behind emulating lens distortion with OpenGL is a two pass rendering strategy [7]. The scene is rendered in a first step, but not yet displayed. In the second step the framebuffer is copied into a texture, and this texture is mapped onto a screen-sized rectangle that is tessellated into small 20×20 pixels quads. The texture coordinates of these quads are distorted according to the properties of the camera. To eliminate an undesirable staircase effect around the optical axis due to excessive distortion, the scene can be rendered into a higher resolution buffer instead of the framebuffer. By using a higher resolution image for the distortion pass, the final image quality can be improved. Unfortunately, such a pixel buffer is not yet supported by all graphics card drivers. Thus, we simply use anti-aliasing to eliminate this staircase effect, which works well for small distortions.

The other property of a camera lens is the depth of field. Simulating this effect in 3D computer graphics is a difficult and expensive task. A possible solution is to use a programmable vertex- and pixel-shader to blur the unfocused area [6]. However, this solution is expensive and needs top of the line graphics hardware with vertex- and pixel-shader support. Fortunately, the depth of field effect is difficult to detect for very short object camera distances as usual in hysteroscopy. Accordingly, all we have to simulate is a general blur if the whole scene is out of focus. This solution is much cheaper than applying a real depth of field effect. As we already have a texture map with the rendered scene as a result of the lens distortion simulation, we simply draw this texture several times with a small offset and linearly combine the results.

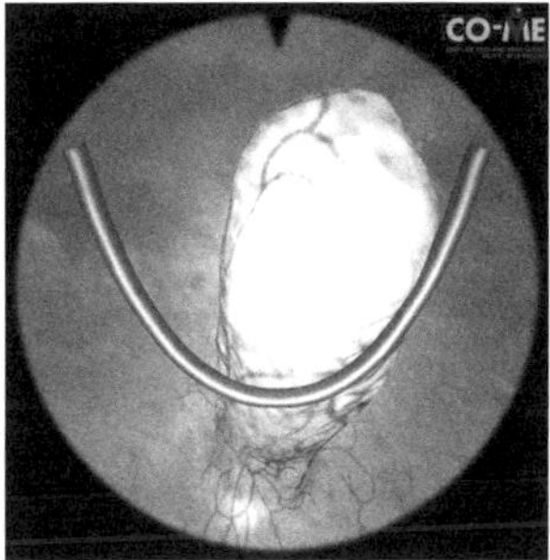

Figure 9. Camera view without lens distortion

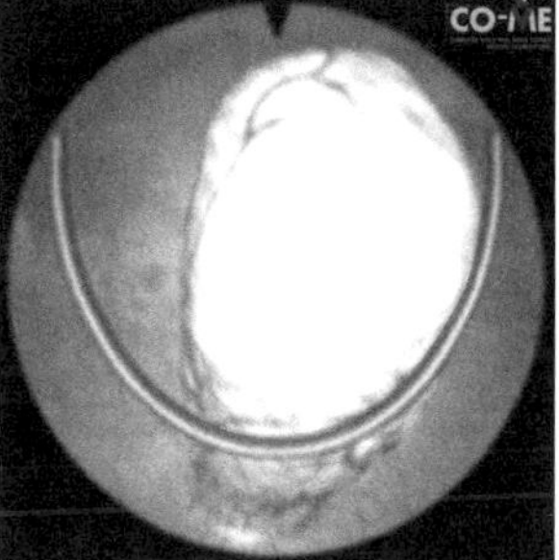

Figure 10. Camera view with lens distortion and depth of field effect

Figure 9 shows a scene without any distortion, while the same view corrupted by lens distortion and depth of field effect is presented in Figure 10.

4. Summary and conclusions

A number of visual cues exist in the uterine cavity, which have to be included in a realistic simulation. They contribute to the visual realism of the scene and should exhibit plausible physical behavior. We presented a graphics engine, which meets these requirements and runs on standard hardware with 3D graphics capabilities. If specific functionality is not supported by a graphics accelerator in a configuration, the respective effect is automatically disabled. The graphics engine is stand-alone with well defined interfaces, and can easily be adapted to different surgical training applications. A view of a simulated intervention using our engine is shown in Figure 12.

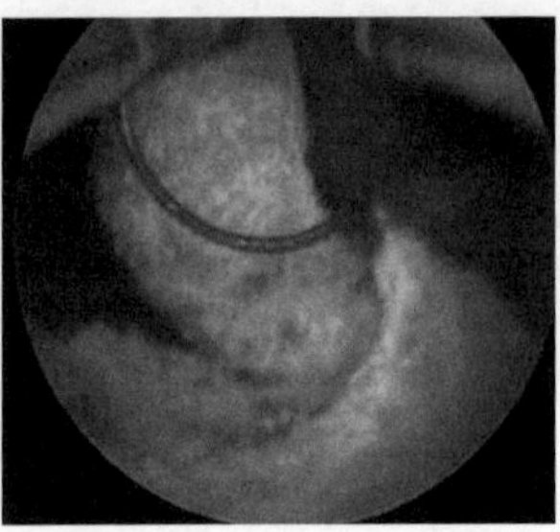

Figure 11. Real view of uterine cavity during intervention

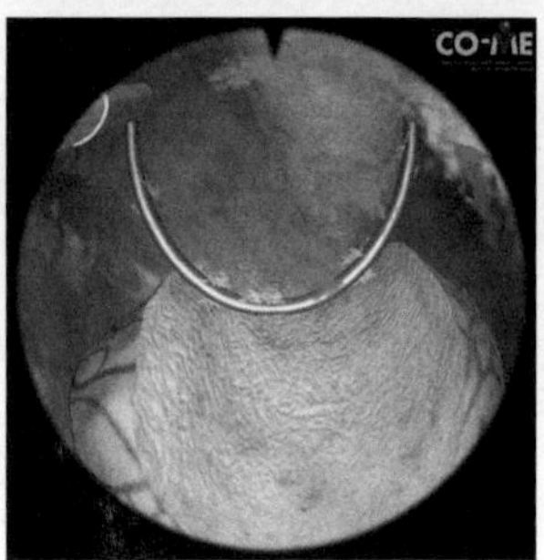

Figure 12. Simulated view of hysteroscopic intervention

Acknowledgment

This research has been supported by the NCCR Co-Me of the Swiss National Science Foundation. The authors would like to thank all developers of the hysteroscopy simulator project.

References

[1] J.S. Levy. Virtual reality hysteroscopy. *J Am Assoc Gyn. Laparosc.*, 3, 1996.
[2] Immersion Medical. AccuTouch system. Company webpage (visited Mar 2005).
[3] K. Montgomery, L. Heinrichs, C. Bruyns, S. Wildermuth , C. Hasser, S. Ozenne and D. Bailey. Surgical simulator for hysteroscopy: A case study of visualization in surgical training. In *IEEE Visualization*, 449-452, 2001.
[4] W.K. Muller-Wittig, A. Bisler, U. Bockholt, J.L. Los Arcos, P. Oppelt and J. Stahler. LAHYSTOTRAIN - development and evaluation of a complex training system for hysteroscopy. In *MMVR Proceedings*,81:336-340, 2001.
[5] R. Sierra, M. Bajka, C. Karadogan, G. Szekely and M. Harders. Coherent Scene Generation for Surgical Simulators. Medical Simulation Symposium ISMS, 221 - 229, 2004..
[6] J. Demers, NVIDIA. Depth of Field: A Survey of Techniques. In *GPU Gems I*, 375-389, 2004.
[7] Paul Bourke. Nonlinear Lens Distortion. http://astronomy.swin.edu.au/~pbourke/projection, 2000.
[8] Bump mapping tutorial. http://www.paulsprojects.net/, December 2002.
[9] R. Sierra,J. Zátonyi,M. Bajka,G. Székely,M. Harders. Hydrometra Simulation for VR-Based Hysteroscopy Training. In *Proceedings of Miccai 2005*, 575-582, Springer Verlag, 2005

Medicine Meets Virtual Reality 14
J.D. Westwood et al. (Eds.)
IOS Press, 2006

The Surgical Simulation and Training Markup Language (SSTML): An XML-Based Language for Medical Simulation

James BACON[a1], Neil TARDELLA[a], Janey PRATT[b], John HU[a] and James ENGLISH[a]
[a]*Energid Technologies Corporation*
[b]*Massachusetts General Hospital*

Abstract. Under contract with the Telemedicine & Advanced Technology Research Center (TATRC), Energid Technologies is developing a new XML-based language for describing surgical training exercises, the Surgical Simulation and Training Markup Language (SSTML). SSTML must represent everything from organ models (including tissue properties) to surgical procedures. SSTML is an open language (i.e., freely downloadable) that defines surgical training data through an XML schema. This article focuses on the data representation of the surgical procedures and organ modeling, as they highlight the need for a standard language and illustrate the features of SSTML. Integration of SSTML with software is also discussed.

Keywords. Surgery, XML, simulation, interoperability, training, standard language

Introduction

To address the high computational cost and heterogeneous nature of military simulations, the U.S. Department of Defense for more than a decade has mandated the use of protocols that allow networked simulations to work together. The first of these protocols was the Distributed Interactive Simulation (DIS), which was later replaced by the High Level Architecture (HLA) [1]. An opportunity is now present to create common protocols specifically for medical simulation. The new protocols should leverage the knowledge learned from DIS and HLA, yet embrace new commercial standards and state-of-the-art software architectures. This article discusses a potential contribution to a new standard protocol.

Under contract with TATRC, Energid Technologies is developing a new language for describing surgical training exercises—The Surgical Simulation and Training Markup Language (SSTML). SSTML is based on the Extensible Markup Language (XML), a popular commercial standard. XML allows multiple languages to be created and combined, thereby allowing multiple language-development efforts to contribute to a common standard. SSTML is part of a larger project to develop a novel untethered open surgery training system [2], and this article also describes how this new language is integrated with simulation software.

---

[1] Corresponding Author: Principal Engineer, Energid Technologies Corporation, 124 Mount Auburn Street, Suite 200 North, Cambridge, MA 02138; E-mail: jab@energid.com.

1. Description of SSTML

XML is a recent, general standard for describing information [3]. It uses tags to describe data that is organized in a hierarchical fashion. It is flexible, commercially accepted, human readable, secure, and compressible. XML is used to create application-specific configuration languages that are easy to modify and understand. SSTML, an XML application, was designed as part of a larger effort to create an open-surgical (as opposed to laparoscopic) simulation language.

The open-surgical simulation being developed contains interchangeable modules, as shown in Figure 1. Each container can optionally operate on a single thread on one computer or on several threads using several computers. SSTML is used in two ways as it regards these containers. It is used to configure the containers when the trainer starts, and it is used to communicate between containers during execution. Each container has its own XML namespace. This prevents naming conflicts between existing containers, and it allows new containers to be added without concern for naming conflicts. The namespaces also trigger loading new DLLs to support specific surgical procedures and upgrades.

XML's often-discussed drawback is that it is verbose. Every data tag—a string—is repeated (occurring at the beginning and ending of each hierarchy), string values are used for every type of data, and whitespace is typically used to indent tags. This leads to large files and messages. To have both the flexibility of XML and the conciseness of a binary format, messages are compressed in the open-surgical simulation. GZIP is (optionally) used on all configuration files and messages resulting in size reductions of 10 to 20 times. GZIP is free software that can be integrated into any application [4].

1.1. SSTML Schema

The standard provides two approaches for defining an XML language: schemas and document type definitions (DTDs). Schemas have more features and provide a more thorough approach to data validation. For example, DTDs have no awareness of namespaces. SSTML utilizes many of the features provided by schemas, which made definition through a schema a natural choice.

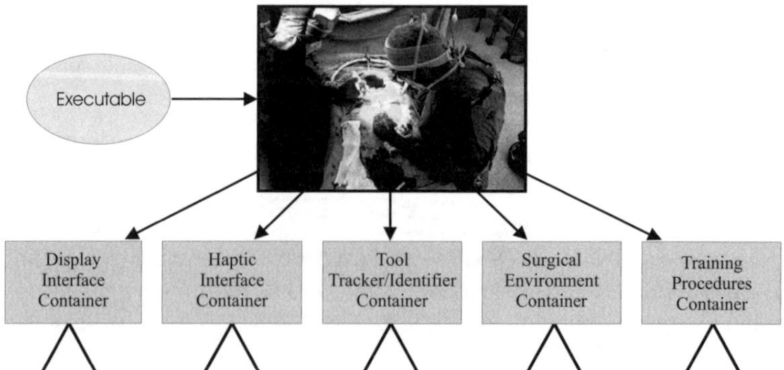

Figure 1. Top level architecture for the open-surgical simulation. The containers are fully configurable through SSTML .

All of the data necessary for configuring the containers illustrated in Figure 1 are defined in SSTML, and all of the open surgery XML content, including network messages, can be validated against the SSTML schema using commercial tools. As users modify the configuration files, they can check the integrity of these changes using the schema.

SSTML contains built-in versioning. The root tag of each XML file contains a version attribute. This was originally used to verify version compatibility between the code base and the XML file—the open-surgery simulation warns users of incompatibilities as it loads the XML. But the attribute has also proven useful for warning the user of version incompatibility during validation.

1.2. Software Architecture for Surgical Simulation

When configuring each container (as in Figure 1) through XML, the simulation software determines which C++ object (essentially a bundle of executable algorithms and data) to load based on the XML element name in the configuration file. This is illustrated in Figure 2. For simple configurations, each container's intrinsic software implementation can define the element names it expects to encounter, and the corresponding objects. For complex configurations, if a new element is encountered (i.e., not listed in the container), the element can signal the loading of a new DLL to define the object to load. SSTML allows the user to put in a list of DLL names which are loaded prior to the new element.

The SSTML schema is composed of several files (one for each namespace) with each file containing hundreds to thousands of lines. The namespace architecture parallels the simulation architecture shown in Figure 1.

1.3. Surgical Procedures

The open-surgical simulation provides a generic framework for simulating many different procedures. Procedures can have multiple, XML-configurable paths leading to successful surgery, with each path scoring the trainee. This is implemented through a tree structure, as illustrated in Figure 3.

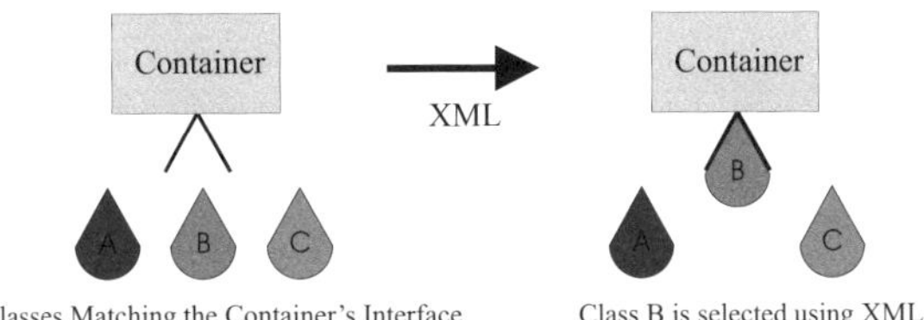

Figure 2. Each of the containers in Figure 1 provides a software interface which is configured through SSTML. There may be multiple sets of code, or classes, that meet this interface—illustrated here as A, B, and C.

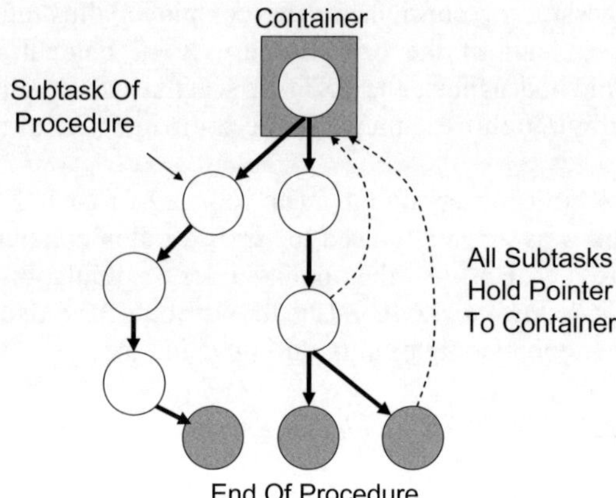

Figure 3. Example procedure tree configurable through SSTML. Each procedure has multiple paths to completion, each composed of multiple subtasks.

For example, Energid is currently implementing a splenectomy procedure. It is divided into seven segments, as shown in Table 1. There are classes and descriptions available for each subtask. For example, "Open Abdomen" is the third step in the splenectomy procedure and SSTML contains a tag describing this subtask. Each subtask in turn can hold a branch in the tree. As the XML configuration file is loaded, the container vector for each subtask is defined to hold a list of sub-tasks that reflect instruction sets. This provides the flexibility to train and test different judgment paths. It also supports randomization for realistic simulation—surgery always involves the unexpected. For example, the simulation may induce more bleeding due to random variation, which may cause the trainee to take measures to stop the bleeding at different times for each exercise. Each of these extra measures takes the trainee down a different path in the tree.

Table 1. Surgical skills tested for splenectomy procedure

Segment	Skills Tested
Initial Trauma Bay Assessment	Understanding of initial exterior survey, patient interview and diagnosis.
OR Prep	Understanding of steps required to prep patient for surgery.
Open Abdomen	Understanding of the proper geometry and location of incision. Proper tool selection. Dexterous manipulation.
Initial Survey Of Abdomen	Exploration of abdomen. Use of retractor.
Control of Splenic Blood Supply and Mobilization	Spleen anatomy. Identification of splenic artery and vein. Knot tying. Blunt dissection of ligaments.
Preparation For Closure	Closing preparation. Counting sponges, surveying the abdomen, etc.
Closure of Abdomen	Choice of suture material. Skill at forceps and needle holder manipulation.

From a general perspective, every procedure may have more than one instruction set, each leading to success. Though many paths may lead to a "successful" outcome, only one will be optimal from a clinical standpoint [5]. As such, a metric-based scoring methodology, configurable through SSTML, weights each path and computes an aggregate score. This score is combined with other metrics to arrive at an overall assessment of the operation.

New surgical training procedures can be easily added to the trainer using SSTML. Energid is currently developing three surgical scenarios (splenectomy, burr hole placement, and sentinel node biopsy), but plans to eventually develop a complete suite of procedures. These XML-based descriptions will be downloadable through the Internet.

2. Results

The SSTML snippet shown in Figure 4 gives a representative *question and answer* block used as part of the Initial Trauma Bay Assessment for the splenectomy procedure described in Table 1. Note SSTML is just text, with tokens not unlike those found in HTML.

All content, including images to display, what questions to ask, and what answers to expect, is encapsulated by SSTML. The Surgical Simulation GUI will automatically switch between description mode, questions and answer mode, and simulation mode based on the XML data.

The SSTML listing left of Figure 5 shows a small portion of the XML used to define how a surgical tool interacts with an organ. In this case, the interaction is between a scalpel and a kidney. The XML defines what type of processing should be performed when an interaction between the two objects occurs.

All objects in the environment are described through surface properties that assign myriad physical and visual attributes. As in Figure 5, they can even define the best choice of tissue-deformation algorithm (in this case the radius of influence method) [6].

```
<hk:questionAndAnswerSubtask answerMode="choice">
<hk:subtaskName>Initial Trauma Bay
Assessment</hk:subtaskName>
  <hk:answer>1 2 3 4 5 6 7</hk:answer>
  <hk:answerSelection size="7">
  <hk:element>Perform primary survey</hk:element>
  <hk:element>Obtain Heart Rate and
Pressure</hk:element>
                :
  <hk:element>Start Oxygen</hk:element>
  </hk:answerSelection>
<hk:imageFile>\images\traumaBay.JPG</hk:imageFile>
<hk:question>
  You begin your initial trauma bay assessment.
  In what order should the following sequence be
performed?
</hk:question>
```

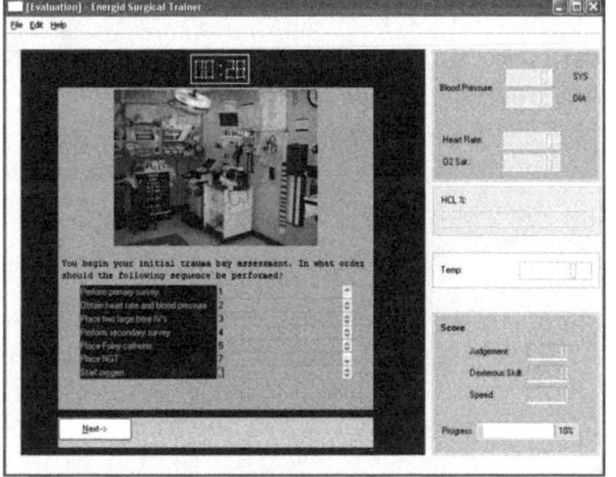

Figure 4. Left: SSTML for a portion of the Q&A sequence. Right: The corresponding GUI display.

```
<surfacePropertyDeformationProcessorMap>
 <element>
  <key>kidney-surface</key>
    :
    <key>scalpel-surface</key>
    <value>
     <radiusOfInfluenceDeformationProcessor>
     <defaultRadiusOfInfluence>0.05
     </defaultRadiusOfInfluence>
     </radiusOfInfluenceDeformationProcessor>
    :
 </surfacePropertyDeformationProcessorMap>
```

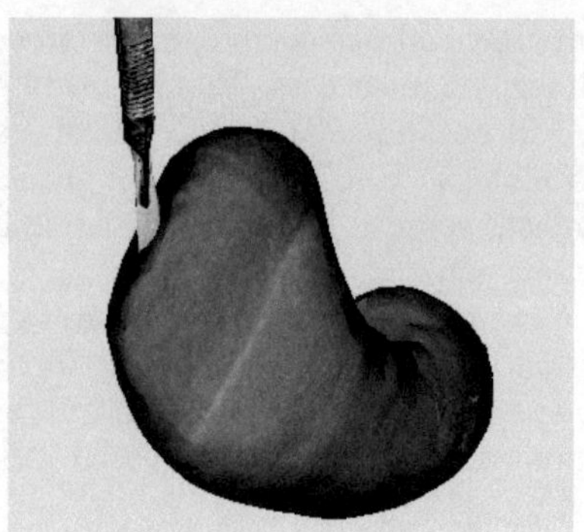

Figure 5. Left: SSTML data describing a deformation algorithm. Right: A kidney being deformed as prescribed. The best algorithm in all cases can be specified through SSTML-based surface properties.

3. Conclusion and Future Work

SSTML makes it easy to represent many aspects of surgical simulation and training in a hierarchical, text-based form that is compressible, human readable, and network transferable. In the system Energid is implementing, surgeons will be able to download and practice new procedures from anywhere in the world, upon their need and convenience. Procedures will be updated through a central server as surgical methods evolve and new tool and anatomy models become available. The SSTML schema is necessary to validate the integrity of these configuration files, and is the key to making this effort tractable.

Energid's long term plan is to develop an authoring tool that will allow doctors and healthcare professionals to create new training scenarios. The tool will be a network application loadable from a web browser, and it will have a simple, easy-to-use interface for creating Q&A modules, metrics definitions, and dynamic-simulation modules.

Currently the SSTML schema is in development. We plan to offer the schema and detailed specifications from the website www.sstml.com. We also encourage feedback from the medical simulation community while we are in the early stages of development.

References

[1]   P.K. Davis, Distributed interactive simulation in the evolution of DoD warfare modeling and simulation, *Proceedings of the IEEE*, volume 83, issue 8, 1995.

[2]   J. English, C. Chang, N. Tardella, and J. Hu, A vision-based surgical tool tracking approach for untethered surgery simulations and training, *MMVR 13*, San Diego, IOS Press, 2005.

[3]   B. Bos, *XML in 10 points*, Revised 13 Nov. 2001, W3C Communications, http://www.w3.org/XML/1999/XML-in-10-points.

[4]   J. Gailly and M. Adler. *GZIP*, http://www.gzip.org.

[5]   J. Watts and W. Feldman, Assessment of technical skills, *Assessing clinical competence*, V. Neufeld and G. Norman eds., New York, Springer, 1985.

[6]   C. Basdogan, M. Srinivasan, S. Small and S. Dawson, Force Interactions on Laparoscopic Simulations: Haptic Rendering of Soft Tissues, *MMVR 6*, San Diego, IOS Press, 1998.

Medicine Meets Virtual Reality 14
J.D. Westwood et al. (Eds.)
IOS Press, 2006

Online Robust Model Estimation During In Vivo Needle Insertions

Laurent Barbé [a,1], Bernard Bayle [a] and Michel de Mathelin [a]

[a] *LSIIT, UMR CNRS 7005, University of Strasbourg,*
Bld Sébastien Brant BP 10413,
F-67412, Illkirch Cedex, France

Abstract. Soft tissue modeling is of key importance in medical robotics and simulation. In the case of percutaneous operations, a fine model of layers transitions and target tissues is required. However, the nature and the variety of these tissues is such that this problem is extremely complex. In this article, we propose a method to estimate the interaction between in vivo tissues and a surgical needle. The online robust estimation of a varying parameters model is achieved during an insertion in standard operating conditions.

Keywords. Soft tissue modeling, online robust estimation, in vivo needle insertion

Introduction

Percutaneous needle insertions are among the most common procedures in medicine. They probably represent the least invasive way to directly access internal zones of a body. So, additionally to the classical subcutaneous injections, percutaneous procedures have also developed in surgery and interventional radiology. The corresponding medical treatments range from simple biopsies to radiofrequency ablation of cancers, typically in the liver. However, the influence of the needle tip position on the success of the treatments and the exposition of the physician to X rays radiations in the case of CT scan guided interventions have led to the development of different robotized needle insertion systems [1,2]. The positioning platform we have already developed [2] will be equipped with a teleoperated insertion device. The present work is a preliminary contribution to the development of an innovative teleoperation system.

1. Modeling and Estimation of Needle Insertion Forces

In the context of interactions with soft tissues, modeling is of key importance. In the case of percutaneous interventions, a precise haptic perception of layers transitions and target tissues is determining. It allows to convey realist haptic feelings in the case of teleopera-

---

[1] Correspondence to: L. Barbé, LSIIT, BP10413, 67412 Illkirch, France. E-mail: barbe@eavr.u-strasbg.fr
The authors would like to thank the IRCAD/EITS staff for arranging ideal surgical facilities. This work is supported by the Alsace Regional Council and the French National Center for Scientific Research (CNRS).

tion or to control the interactions of a robotic system with organic tissues. Unfortunately, it is established that the nature and the variety of the tissues involved in a needle insertion is such that the modeling of this type of interaction is extremely complex. To take into account variability in the patients, the parameters of the corresponding models have to be identified. On the one hand different biomechanical viscoelastic models can be identified online [3]. Nevertheless, they all apply to artificial materials and viscoelastic stimuli, *i.e.* without cutting. On the other hand, the methodologies proposed in the case of needle insertions [4] are based on specific tests that require experimental methodologies which are not compatible with real operations conditions.

We thus decided to identify a varying parameters model that is not necessarily physically consistent, but that allows to reconstruct and characterize the force evolution. When the needle is inserted, the considered model writes: $f(t) = -K(p,\ t)p(t) - B(p,\ t)v(t)$, where f is the force along the needle shaft, p and v represent the needle position and velocity, and K and B are coefficients that correspond to stiffness and damping if viscoelastic stimuli are applied. The position $p = 0$ corresponds to the initial position of the tissue. The estimation is carried out by a recursive least mean square with covariance resetting. Additionally to the standard algorithm we use a dead-zone function so that the estimation may remain robust. Though this method is generally adapted to slowly varying parameters, we will see in the next section that the estimated force accurately match the measured force even during transition phases.

2. In vivo Experiments

To evaluate the estimation procedure we built the following setup. We use a PHANToM 1.5/6DOF haptic device from Sensable Technologies as an instrumented passive needle holder. Its end effector is equipped with an ATI Nano17 force sensor. The PHANToM encoders are used to measure the motions of the needle during the insertions, with a precision of 30 μm. Measurements are acquired at 1 kHz frequency rate, under real-time constraints imposed by the software implemented for Linux RTAI operating system.

The experiments were performed in standard operating conditions. Needle insertions in the liver of anesthetized pigs were adopted as benchmarks for two main reasons: 1) the liver and the tissues (skin, fat, muscles, liver) of a young pig are rather similar to human ones, 2) the properties of the tissues and the exerted force are much more realistic under clinical conditions, in particular because blood irrigation and breathing are maintained.

Direct Needle Insertion into the liver   In this first procedure, a surgeon opened the abdomen of the pig to directly access the liver as in classical surgery. This procedure is used to identify the mechanical properties of the liver. Figure 1 presents the measured and estimated forces and the absolute estimation error. Figure 2 gives the evolution of the estimated parameters. The ruptures of the hepatic membrane can be observed on both figures.

Needle Insertion into the liver through the skin   In this second procedure, the insertion was done through small incisions on the epidermis, as usually done in interventional radiology. The insertion was then performed through the dermis, the fat and the muscle to finally access the liver. Figure 3 presents the measured and estimated forces and the absolute estimation error. Figure 4 gives the evolution of the estimated parameters. The

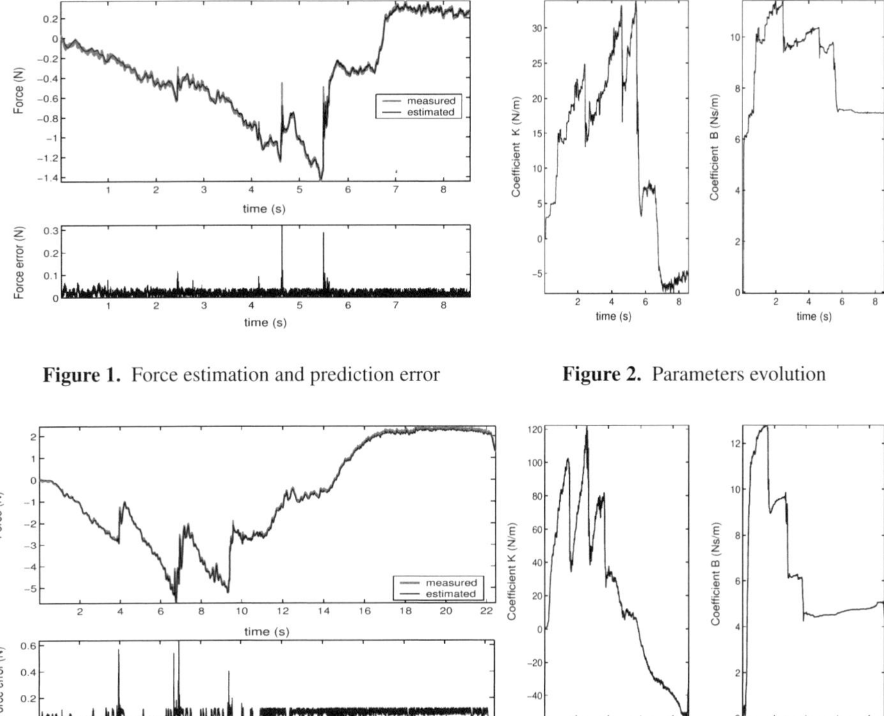

Figure 1. Force estimation and prediction error　　　　　**Figure 2.** Parameters evolution

Figure 3. Force estimation and prediction error　　　　　**Figure 4.** Parameters evolution

successive ruptures of the anatomical layers can be observed. Greater force values and greater discontinuities are observed compared to direct insertions in the liver. This is due to the greater stiffness of the skin and the muscles. It suggests that the detection of the hepatic membrane rupture during a percutaneous operation from force measurements only is a difficult task.

References

[1] D. Stoianovici, J. A. Cadeddu, R. D. Demaree, H. A. Basile, R. H. Taylor, L. L. Whitcomb, and L. R. Kavoussi. A novel mechanical transmission applied to percutaneous renal access.*ASME Dynamic Systems and Control Division*, 61:401–406, 1997.

[2] B. Maurin, J. Gangloff, B. Bayle, M. de Mathelin, O. Piccin, P. Zanne, C. Doignon, L. Soler, and A. Gangi. A parallel robotic system with force sensors for percutaneous procedures under CT-guidance. In *Medical Image Computing and Computer Assisted Intervention*, pp. 176–183, 2004.

[3] N. Diolaiti, C. Melchiorri, and S. Stramigioli. Contact impedance estimation for robotic systems. In *International Conference on Intelligent Robots and Systems*, pp. 2538–2543, 2004.

[4] A. Okamura, C. Simone, and M. O'Leary. Force modeling for needle insertion into soft tissue. *IEEE Transaction on Biomedical Engineering*, 51(10):1707–1716, 2004.

Medicine Meets Virtual Reality 14
J.D. Westwood et al. (Eds.)
IOS Press, 2006

A Software Framework for Surgical Simulation Virtual Environments

Lee A. Belfore II [a,1], Jessica R. Crouch [a] Yuzhong Shen [a] Sylva Girtelschmid [a] and Emre Baydogan [a]

[a] *Old Dominion University*

Abstract. Surgical simulators are an integration of many models, capabilities, and functions. Development of a working simulator requires the flexibility to integrate various software models, to support interoperability, and facilitate performance optimizations. An object oriented framework is devised to support multithreaded integration of simulation, deformation, and interaction. A demonstration application has been implemented in Java, leveraging the features that are built into the language including multithreading, synchronization, and serialization. Future work includes expanding the capabilities of the framework with a broader range of model and interactive capabilities.

Keywords. Surgical simulation, Framework, Java

Introduction

Surgical simulators are interactive systems that model surgical procedures on simulated biological tissues along with other processes relevant to surgical procedures. The simulation process is complicated by several scientific and technological limitations. Scientific limitations include an incomplete understanding of the properties of biological tissues and processes as well as identifying those aspects of a simulated procedure most amenable to training transfer. Technological limitations include the inability to provide real time performance for models at the desired fidelity. In addition, input devices may not provide a satisfying surrogate that is consistent with the manipulations required in a surgical procedure. In order to provide grounding to manage these issues and facilitate research, a flexible software architecture is necessary to support simulator system development. In light of these issues, an object-oriented framework is proposed to support straightforward integration of the various functional components composing a surgical simulator. The work described here is part of a larger project [1]. This paper is organized in five sections including an introduction, a summary of related works, an overview of the software framework, presentation of a demonstration, and finally a summary and future work.

---

[1] Correspondence to: Lee A. Belfore, Dept. ECE, Old Dominion University. Tel.: 757-683-3746; Fax: 757-683-3220; E-mail: lbelfore@odu.edu.

1. Related Work

Surgical simulation holds the promise of giving medical practitioners the ability to perform some of their training on simulators, raising the expertise of practitioners when they first interact with patients. In Reference [2], a technology independent language CAML is introduced as a foundation for medical simulation systems. Specific to the work here, Spring [3] offers a framework for surgical simulation that includes many models for surgical intervention, a mass-spring model for soft tissue modeling, and distributive collaborative functionality. Finally, the GiPSi system [4] provides a framework with broad capabilities that organ level simulations of physical, functional, and spatial modeling.

2. An Overview of the Software Framework

The software framework is built upon an abstract class structure that holds the relevant parameters and references to support communication and interaction among the respective objects. The abstract classes are then extended to provide a specific functionality. All objects fundamentally share a common link in the form of the basic geometry which each act upon and update. Communicating this information among the objects and synchronizing the updates enables all to receive the most current information in a consistent fashion. Further, having different objects in separate threads limits the interactions among objects to the pure geometry information and provides a pathway to a coarse granularity parallel implementation through the use of threads. Among the geometry linked objects can include the tissue simulation, dynamic texturing, collision detection, remeshing, visual rendering, and haptics rendering. Each of these can function autonomously, updating and responding at its necessary inherent update rate, provided up-to-date geometry is available. Figure 1 provides a generic perspective on the interaction among these threads. The wound debridement simulation companion paper [1] describes an application where this software framework could be used.

3. Demonstration Implementation

A prototype implementation of this framework has been developed in Java using the Java3D API. This platform was selected for convenience as it includes all of the powerful features of Java, i.e. object oriented class structure, multithreading, serialization, and synchronization. Furthermore, the Java platform provides some inherent capabilities that can be leveraged in collaborative applications. Among the features of the implementation, abstract classes are defined to hold information that must be synchronized among threads. Abstract classes define the generic features for each major thread and are extended to provide the functional implementations desired. Furthermore, different functionalities, i.e. model enhancements, model evaluation, can be easily replaced and evaluated without disrupting the rest of the application. Figure 2 shows an example screen capture of the demonstration application.

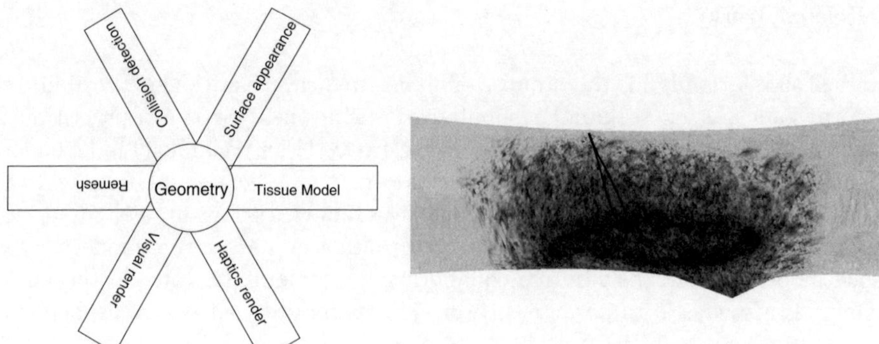

Figure 1. Software Architecture   **Figure 2.** Example Image

4. Summary and Future Work

In this paper, we have presented a software framework that can be used in the development of surgical simulation virtual environments. We plan to continue to develop the framework, to investigate its operation on a C++ platform for enhanced performance, and work towards simpler integration with other libraries and commercial products.

Acknowledgements

This project was a collaborative effort between the Virginia Modeling, Analysis and Simulation Center (VMASC) at Old Dominion University and the Eastern Virginia Medical School. Partial funding was provided by the Naval Health Research Center through NAVAIR Orlando TSD under contract N61339-03-C-0157, and the Office of Naval Research under contract N00014-04-1-0697, entitled "The National Center for Collaboration in Medical Modeling and Simulation". The ideas and opinions presented in this paper represent the views of the authors and do not necessarily represent the views of the Department of Defense.

References

[1] J. Seevinck, M.W. Scerbo, L.A. Belfore, L.J. Weireter, J.R. Crouch, Y. Shen, F.D. McKenzie, H.M. Garcia, S. Girtelschmid, E. Baydogan, and E.A. Schmidt, A simulation-based training system for surgical wound debridement, *Proceedings of the Medicine Meets Virtual Reality 14*, Long Beach, CA, January 24-27, 2006.

[2] S. Cotin, D.W. Shaffer, D. Meglan, M. Ottensmeyer, P. Berry, and S.L. Dawson, CAML: A general framework for the development of medical simulations. In H. Pien (Ed.), *Digitization of the Battlespace V and Battlefield Biomedical Technologies II, Proceedings of SPIE*, Vol. 4037, 2000, pp. 294-300.

[3] K. Montgomery, C. Bruyns, J. Brown, G. Thonier, A. Tellier, J.C. Latombe, Spring: A general framework for collaborative, real-time surgical simulation, *Proceedings of Medicine Meets Virtual Reality 9*, Newport Beach, CA, January 23-26,2001.

[4] M.C. Cavusoglu, T.G. Goktekin, F. Tendick, and S. Sastry, GiPSi: An open source/open architecture software development framework for surgical simulation, *Proceedings of the Medicine Meets Virtual Reality 12*, Newport Beach, CA, January 14-17, 2004, pp. 46-48.

Medicine Meets Virtual Reality 14
J.D. Westwood et al. (Eds.)
IOS Press, 2006

Augmented Assessment as a Means to Augmented Reality

Bryan Bergeron, MD
HST Division of Harvard Medical School & MIT

Abstract. Rigorous scientific assessment of educational technologies typically lags behind the availability of the technologies by years because of the lack of validated instruments and benchmarks. Even when the appropriate assessment instruments are available, they may not be applied because of time and monetary constraints. Work in augmented reality, instrumented mannequins, serious gaming, and similar promising educational technologies that haven't undergone timely, rigorous evaluation, highlights the need for assessment methodologies that address the limitations of traditional approaches. The most promising augmented assessment solutions incorporate elements of rapid prototyping used in the software industry, simulation-based assessment techniques modeled after methods used in bioinformatics, and object-oriented analysis methods borrowed from object oriented programming.

Keywords. Augmented reality, simulation, assessment, intelligent tutoring systems

Introduction

The rate of technological change in medical education has followed the traditional s-shaped technology adoption curve since the introduction of the digital computer [1]. Many computer technology companies, developers, and educators have focused on shortening the time required for technology-based educational products to progress from early adopter to early majority user status [2]. Several models have been advanced to describe the impediments to rapid technological change in medical education and training. The most insightful, such as the appropriation/disappropriation model, focus on user behavior change and are concerned more with the transformation of the user than with the evolution of technology [3].

Whether the models focus on behavior change or pure technology to explain user adoption rates, they are incomplete unless they consider assessment, often the largest gap in the development pipeline of innovative and disruptive educational technologies. For example, thanks to off-the-shelf computer based training development tools, given content and a motivated educator, a computer-based training (CBT) course can be developed in days instead of weeks or months. Similarly, commercial game development shells, which can be used to create 3D augmented reality environments and various forms of serious games, are commodity items. Content and the comfort of educators and developers with the technology, are rate-limiting factors. Another, often ignored factor in the acceptance of new educational technology is assessment. Unfortunately, assessment has evolved little since the era of timesharing-based CBT.

1. Traditional Assessment

The commercial marketing press is filled with stories of human simulators, serious games, and similar technologies that have been developed and sold to hospitals, clinics, and military training facilities. However, the academic literature is lacking information on long-term studies on the effectiveness of these educational systems in increasing the quality of care provide by clinicians. One hurdle to obtaining effectiveness and return on investment data is the cost of a traditional summative assessment, which can overshadow the initial investment in technology. Someone or some entity has to provide the funding for the studies. The other hurdle the duration of a rigorous assessment, which often extends past the effective lifespan of the technologies in question. For example, Compact Disc – Interactive (CD-I) technology was on the consumer market for only a few years during the early 1990s. By the time a few prototype systems in medical education had been developed, the technology had been replaced.

While the medical education community is focused on innovative, effective uses of technology, it is largely ignoring the challenge of keeping the assessment component of development in step with the technology. For example, the US Military, academic medical centers, and medical schools worldwide are installing mannequin-based patient simulators for training nursing students, medical students, residents, and practicing physicians. However, there is no compelling scientific evidence that this technology produces medic and clinicians with better clinical outcomes five and ten years out.

Conservative educators abide by the strategy of sidelining promising technologies until assessment either supports or refutes the sometimes over-enthusiastic claims. For example, many educators are hesitant to use serious computer games in the classroom or study areas until studies prove the effectiveness of games-based education relative to other computer-based instruction modalities and didactic lectures. Given the fate of CD-I, interactive laserdiscs, edutainment software, and other evolutionary dead-ends, this conservative stance is understandable. However, the lost opportunity cost for not working with promising educational technologies before they are proven by lengthy and expensive summative evaluations can be significant.

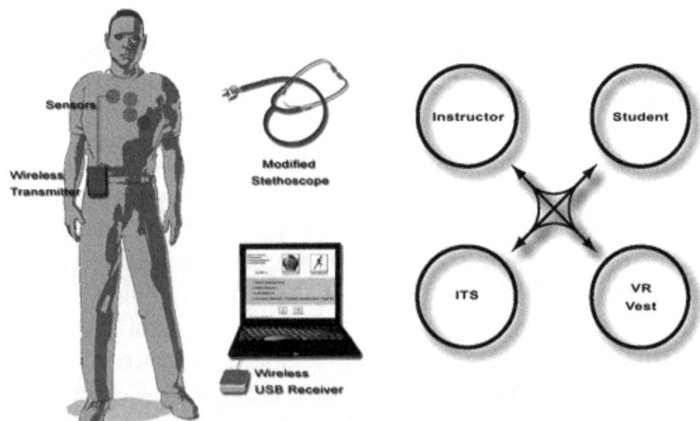

Figure 1. Augmented reality system (left) and associated interactions (right).

2. Challenges

Clearly, technology-enabled education would benefit from better assessment methodologies. These would ideally provide developers with a calculus that not only obviates the practical limitations of traditional assessment, but that empowers developers and educators to evaluate the technologies from complex behavioral and cognitive perspectives. As an example of the complexity that must be addressed by these improved assessment methodologies, consider our application of augmented-reality to standardized patients, shown in Figure 1. Wireless, computer-controlled sensor vests provide the cardiac, pulmonary, and abdominal sounds appropriate for the patients supposed medical condition and clinical maneuvers. Furthermore, an intelligent tutoring system (ITS) directs the wearer and the student through a progression of patient cases appropriate for the student's demonstrated skill level.

Assessing the educational effectiveness of a system of this complexity by traditional means is problematic because of the multi-dimensional dialogue supported by the system. There is communications from instructor to student, from the ITS to instructor and student, and the student's interaction with the vest. In this scenario, there can be uncertainty in the student's mind over whether the computer or the instructor is the ultimate authority. Furthermore, because a good instructor can overcome the deficiencies in the ITS, the effectiveness of the system can be difficult to reproduce – a cornerstone of the scientific method.

3. Potential Solutions

We have identified several technologies, components of which can address modern assessment needs. These include rapid prototyping, system simulation, and object-oriented analysis (OOA). In rapid prototyping, assessment is a relatively brief, focused activity during development. System simulation, which is being applied to the bioinformatics domain, has the potential to compresses years of analysis into days or weeks. The most significant augmented assessment approach is a derivative of the OOA methodology used in object-oriented programming, in which software requirements and specifications are expressed in an object model composed of interacting objects as opposed to a data or functional view [4]. The major upside of using OOA is that reusable, pre-assessed components of educational technology can be used to simplify the assessment of an educational system. A remaining challenge is developing standards for encapsulation and for methods of communicating assessment findings among disparate educational systems.

References

[1]   G. Moore, *Crossing the Chasm: Marketing and Selling High-Tech Products to Mainstream Customers*, HarperBusiness, 1999.
[2]   B. Bergeron, J. Blander, *Business Expectations: Are You Using Technology to its Fullest?* John Wiley & Sons, 2002.
[3]   J. Blander, B. Bergeron, *Clinical Management Systems: A Guide for Deployment,* HIMSS, 2004.
[4]   C. Baudoin, G. Hollowell, *Realizing the Object-Oriented Lifecycle*, Prentice Hall, 1996.

Medicine Meets Virtual Reality 14
J.D. Westwood et al. (Eds.)
IOS Press, 2006

A Holographic Collaborative Medical Visualization System

Fabio BETTIO[a], Francesca FREXIA[a], Andrea GIACHETTI[a], Enrico GOBBETTI[a], Gianni PINTORE[a], Gianlugi ZANETTI[a], Tibor BALOGH[b], Tamás FORGÁCS[b], Tibor AGOCS[b], Eric BOUVIER[c]
[a] *CRS4, Pula,Italy – www.crs4.it/vic/*
[b] *Holografika, Budapest, Hungary – www.holografika.com*
[c] *C-S, Paris, France – www.c-s.fr*

Abstract. We report on our work on the development of a novel holographic display technology, capable of targeting multiple freely moving naked eye viewers, and of a demonstrator, exploiting this technology to provide medical specialists with a truly interactive collaborative 3D environment for diagnostic discussions and/or pre-operative planning.

Keywords. 3D displays, holography, collaborative work, medical data visualization.

1. Background and Motivation

The collaborative, multi-disciplinary, analysis of 3D datasets derived from medical imaging is gradually becoming an important tool for the modern clinical practice decision process. Fully 3D immersive visualization could dramatically improve this process, since decisions depend on the deep understanding of complex three-dimensional shapes. The currently available display solutions capable of feeding the human brain with all the visual cues needed to reconstruct three-dimensional scenes are, however, limited to single user configurations. Here, we report on the development of a novel holographic display technology that supports multiple freely moving naked eye viewers and on a prototype application – a tool for the planning of Abdominal Aortic Aneurysm (AAA) treatment – that exploits this technology to provide medical specialists with a truly interactive 3D collaborative environment for diagnostic discussions and/or pre-operative planning and acts as a driving force for display development.

2. Display technology

Our display uses a specially arranged array of micro-projectors to generate an array of pixels at controlled intensity and color onto a custom designed holographic screen. Each point of the latter then transmits different colored light beams into different directions. The display is thus capable of generating light fields appropriate to faithfully reproducing natural scenes. Each micro-projector forms the image on a micro

LCD display and projects it through special aspheric optics with a 50 degrees horizontal field-of-view. A high-pressure discharge lamp illuminates all the displays, leading to a brightness comparable to the brightness of a normal CRT display. In the current prototype, 96 optical modules project 240 pixels horizontally and 320 vertically. Each pixel on the screen is illuminated by 60 different LCDs. Since 60 independent light beams originate from each pixel in the 50 degrees field of view, the angular resolution of the display is 0.8 degrees. With proper software control, the light beams leaving the various pixels can be made to propagate in specific directions, as if they were emitted from physical objects at fixed spatial locations. In our prototype, a custom parallel implementation of OpenGL generates the module images required for holographic viewing by appropriately reinterpreting the standard OpenGL stream. More information on our display technology is available elsewhere [1][2].

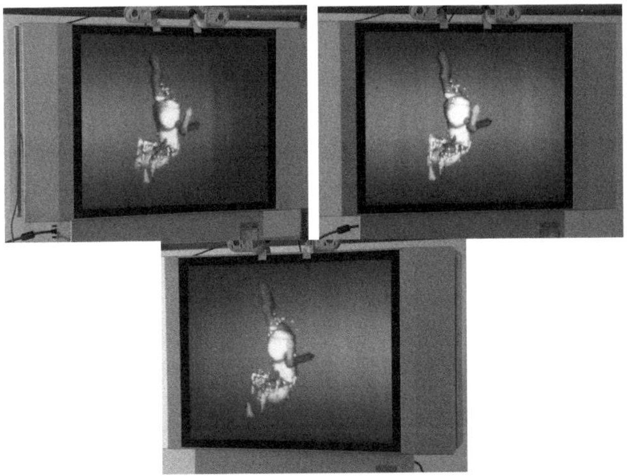

Figure 1. Selected frames of a video recorded using a hand-held video camera. Note the parallax effects.

3. Collaborative Medical Data Analysis Prototype

The current display prototype is already sufficient to develop compelling prototype 3D applications that exploit its truly multi-user aspects. We are currently developing a few domain specific demonstrators, which act as driving forces for the development of the display. In the medical domain, we are focusing on a system for supporting diagnostic discussions and/or pre-operative planning of Abdominal Aortic Aneurisms. The overall application is distributed using a client-server approach, with a Data Grid layer for archiving/serving the data, 2D clients for medical data reporting (textual/2D image browsing), and 3D clients for interacting with 3D reconstructions. The 2D user interface for model measurement and reporting has been developed as a web application that can be executed on a tablet PC or a palmtop computer. The 3D application renders reconstructed object on the holographic display, and interacts with the SRB [3] archive for data loading, and with the measurement interface for communicating anatomical measures. Since objects rendered on the holographic display appear floating in fixed positions, it is possible to naturally interact with them with a 3D user interface that supports direct manipulation in the display space. This is achieved by using tracked 3D cursors manipulated by users. Multiple cursor control interfaces have been developed, using both commercial 3D trackers (Logitech 3D mouse) and custom-made wireless solutions (camera based tracking of pointers, using a wireless USB interface for buttons).

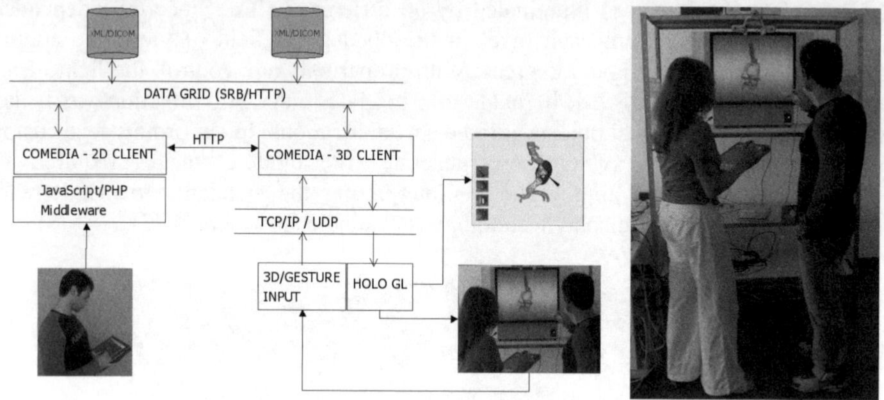

Figure 2. Left: Structure of the distributed application prototype. Right: Multi-user discussion

4. Conclusions

We presented a design and prototype implementation of a scalable holographic system, that targets multi-user interactive computer graphics applications. The current display prototype is already sufficient for developing compelling prototype 3D applications that exploit its truly multi-user aspects. On a single GeForce6800 system, the currently achieved frame-rate is about 10Hz, which proved sufficient to provide the illusion of continuous motion in animation and 3D interaction tasks. We described a particular application, targeting Abdominal Aaortic Aneurisms, that uses starndard 2D displays for accessing medical data records and the holographic display to present and directly interact with reconstructed 3D models. The application is in the early stages of development, but already demonstrates the possibility of sharing a fully 3D synthetic workspace in a local multiuser setting. Our current work focuses on improving the display drivers, completing the application prototype, and assessing its benefits and limitations.

Acknowledgments. This research is partially supported by the COHERENT project (EU-FP6-510166), funded under the European FP6/IST program.

References

[1]   Tibor Balogh, Tamás Forgács, Tibor Agocs, Olivier Balet, Eric Bouvier, Fabio Bettio, Enrico Gobbetti, and Gianluigi Zanetti. A Scalable Hardware and Software System for the Holographic Display of Interactive Graphics Applications. In EUROGRAPHICS 2005 Short Papers Proceedings, 2005.

[2]   Tibor Balogh, Tamás Forgács, Olivier Balet, Eric Bouvier, Fabio Bettio, Enrico Gobbetti, and Gianluigi Zanetti. A Scalable Holographic Display for Interactive Graphics Applications. In Proc. IEEE VR 2005 Workshop on Emerging Display Technologies, 2005. CD ROM Proceedings.

[3]   Storage Resource Broker, Version 3.1, SDSC   (http://www.npaci.edu/dice/srb).

Medicine Meets Virtual Reality 14
J.D. Westwood et al. (Eds.)
IOS Press, 2006

55

Bounds for Damping that Guarantee Stability in Mass-Spring Systems

Yogendra BHASIN [a] and Alan LIU [a,1]

[a] *The Surgical Simulation Laboratory*
National Capital Area Medical Simulation Center
Uniformed Services University
http://simcen.usuhs.mil

Abstract. Mass-spring systems are often used to model anatomical structures in medical simulation. They can produce plausible deformations in soft tissue, and are computationally efficient. Determining damping values for a stable mass-spring system can be difficult. Previously stable models can become unstable with topology changes, such as during cutting. In this paper, we derive bounds for the damping coefficient in a mass-spring system. Our formulation can be used to evaluate the stability for user specified damping values, or to compute values that are unconditionally stable.

Keywords. Mass-spring, stability bounds, Deformable models, Medical simulation,

1. Introduction

Mass-springs [1,2] are a common method for modeling deformable objects [3]. Mass-spring models are characterized by a network of point masses connected to its neighbors by massless springs. Individual masses may optionally be acted upon by external forces. A mass-spring system with n nodes can be described by the following equation,

$$m_i\, a_i^t = [\sum_{j \in N(i)} \kappa_{ij}\, \hat{d}_{ij}^t\, (l_{ij}^t - l_{ij}^0)\,] - \gamma_i\, v_i^t + f_{exti}^t \tag{1}$$

a_i^t is the acceleration of the mass m_i at time t. N(i) are all the neighbors of m_i, where a spring is connected between m_i and each neighbor. κ_{ij} is the stiffness coefficient of the spring connecting m_i and m_j. $\hat{d}_{ij}^t$ is the unit vector between m_i and m_j at time t. l_{ij}^t is the spring length between m_i and m_j at time t. l_{ij}^0 is the spring length between m_i and m_j at rest. γ_i is the viscous damping coefficient. v_i^t is the velocity of m_i at time t. f_{exti}^t is the external force acting on m_i at time t.

The first term in equation 1 denotes the internal force due to the tension of the springs connecting m_i with its neighbors. Viscous damping represents resistance due to air or

---

[1] Correspondence to: Alan Liu, http://simcen.org/surgery.

any other medium in the system, and acts in the opposite direction of the velocity of the mass.

For a set of N points in 3D space, let X be a $3 N \times 1$ column of position vectors at the current time. Then the mass-spring system can be expressed as, $M \ddot{X} = K X - Y \dot{X} + F_{ext}$ where, M and Y are $3N \times 3N$ diagonal mass and damping matrices respectively, F_{ext} is a $3 N \times 1$ column of vectors representing external forces, K is a $3N \times 3N$ banded matrix of stiffness coefficients. This equation can be rewritten as a set of first order differential equations, and solved using standard numerical integration methods [4].

Mass-spring models are readily understood. Fast, efficient methods exist for solving them. Mass-spring models can be fairly large and complex without sacrificing real-time response to user interactions. For surgical simulation, the Explicit Euler scheme is widely used [5,6,7,8]. Explicit Euler integration has the benefits of simplicity and computational efficiency [9]. It can be used to update models used for both haptic and visual rendering [10].

Mass-spring models have disadvantages. Finding an appropriate set of parameters that is realistic can require considerable trial and error. Once a solution is found, a small time step may be necessary to maintain stability.

Previous work has addressed instability issues in various ways. Delingette [11] described a condition that can lead to numerical instability. For a dynamic mass-spring model with n nodes and total mass m_{total}, $k_c \approx \frac{m_{total}}{n \; \pi^2 \; (\Delta t)^2}$, where Δt is the time step and k_c is the critical stiffness beyond which the system of equations is divergent. Provot [2] described a similar stability condition where the maximum allowed time step should be smaller than the natural period T_0 of the system, $T_0 \approx \pi \sqrt{\frac{m_i}{\kappa_i}}$. While these equations provide a better understanding of the relationship between mass-spring parameters and stability, it does not provide an accurate means of determining when instability occurs. Kacic-Alesic [12] described a stability condition for the Verlet integration method as, $\Delta t \leq 2 \sqrt{\frac{m}{K}}$, where K is the combined spring coefficient of all the springs. However, the condition provided an excessively conservative bound.

In these attempts, stability was achieved at the cost of a smaller timestep, increasing computational complexity. In this paper, we approach the stability problem from a different perspective. Instead of changing the time parameter, we derive a relationship between the damping coefficient of a mass-spring system and its other three parameters (mass, stiffness coefficient, and time step). The bounds unconditionally guarantee a stable system. Section (2) describes the derivation, sections (3) and (4) outline our experiments and their results respectively. Sections (5) will show how these bounds can be used to preserve stability with minimal impact to the overall simulation. Section (6) summarizes our contribution.

2. Derivation

In this section, we motivate the rational behind our derivation, and provide the details of our formulation.Our derivation is based on Explicit Euler integration because it is widely used in medical simulation and other fields. The principal is not limited to this method however and can be easily extended to other numerical integration methods.

To simplify the discussion, we assume that the mass-spring system is unforced, and that the spring coefficient is the same for all springs, i.e., $\kappa_i = \kappa$ for $i \in [1..n]$. Equation (1) can then be rewritten as a standard second-order differential equation, i.e.,

$$m_i \, a_i^t + \gamma_i \, v_i^t - \kappa \, p_i^t = 0 \tag{2}$$

where, $p_i^t = \sum_{j \in N(i)} \hat{d}_{ij}^t \, (l_{ij}^t - l_{ij}^0)$. Using the Explicit Euler method, the position $x_i^{t+\Delta t}$ and velocity $v_i^{t+\Delta t}$ of the mass m_i at time $t + \Delta t$ is computed as,

$$v_i^{t+\Delta t} = v_i^t + (a_i^t)\Delta t \tag{3}$$

$$x_i^{t+\Delta t} = x_i^t + (v_i^{t+\Delta t})\Delta t \tag{4}$$

Lower bound for damping. Consider a mass-spring system with two nodes, m_0 and m_1. Let m_0 be fixed. Then equation (2) describes an unforced, damped system. The form of the solution to the characteristic equation (2) depends on the quantity $\gamma_1^2 - 4 \, m_1 \, \kappa$ [13].

When $\gamma_1^2 - 4 \, m_1 \, \kappa < 0$ the system is underdamped. An underdamped system is characterized by oscillatory motion. When $\gamma_1^2 - 4 \, m_1 \, \kappa \geq 0$, the system does not oscillate. However, the time to reach equilibrium increases as γ_1 increases. [13]. When $\gamma_1^2 - 4 \, m_1 \, \kappa = 0$, the system reaches equilibrium in the shortest time, and without oscillation.

In summary, underdamped systems oscillate. For large mass-spring systems, local oscillations are visually displeasing and should be avoided. Local oscillations can also produce cumulative errors that cause instability. By applying the constraint,

$$\gamma_i \geq 2\sqrt{m_i \kappa} \tag{5}$$

for $i \in [1, n]$, this situation is avoided. As will be shown in section 4, mass-spring systems that violate this constraint can also become unstable. Thus, equation (5) provides a lower bound for stability.

Upper bound for damping. When Explicit Euler integration is applied to solving the mass-spring equations, the physical properties of the system can be violated for large time steps. An explicit formulation of these constraints forms the basis for a derivation of an upper bound on the damping coefficient γ_i as a function of m_i, Δt, v_i^t and κ.

Substituting the value for acceleration from equation (2) into equation (3) and re-arranging the terms yield $v_i^{t+\Delta t} = v_i^t + (\frac{\kappa \, p_i^t - \gamma_i \, v_i^t}{m_i})\Delta t$. Let $v_{s\,i}^t = \frac{\kappa \, p_i^t}{m_i} \Delta t$ and $v_{d\,i}^t = \frac{\gamma_i \, v_i^t}{m_i} \Delta t$. Then $v_{s\,i}^t$ is the difference in velocity between time t and $t + \Delta t$ due to spring forces. Similarly, $v_{d\,i}^t$ is the velocity difference due to damping between t and $t + \Delta t$. Damping dissipates energy from a mass-spring system. The nodes slow down as a result. Thus, between t and $t + \Delta t$, $v_{d\,i}^t$ can at most bring the node to a halt, it cannot cause the node to move faster. That is, $v_{d\,i}^t$ cannot be the dominant term. Expressing this mathematically, we get $|v_i^t + v_{s\,i}^t| \geq |v_{d\,i}^t|$. Expanding $v_{s\,i}^t$ and $v_{d\,i}^t$ yields, $|v_i^t + F_i^t \frac{\Delta t}{m_i}| \geq \frac{\gamma_i \Delta t}{m_i}|v_i^t|$, where $F_i^t = \kappa p_i^t$, is the internal spring force. So,

$$\gamma_i \leq \frac{|v_i^t \frac{m_i}{\Delta t} + F_i^t|}{|v_i^t|} \; for \; |v_i^t| \neq 0 \tag{6}$$

When $|v_i^t| = 0$, the damping coefficient has no effect on the system.

3. Experiments

Experiments were conducted to validate our theoretical development. A 20 x 20 cm planar mesh with 1300 nodes and 3750 edges was used. The mesh was aligned along the xz plane. The distance between the adjacent nodes was 0.57 cm. An additional spring was attached from each mass to its rest position so that the system always returned to its initial configuration. For all experiments, one or more nodes were perturbed by a specified amount, then the system was allowed to run until the initial configuration was restored. The model was assumed to be restored to its original configuration when all nodes were within 1% of the initial perturbation value. For each trial, all the spring coefficient and mass values were set to the same κ and m values repectively, i.e., $\kappa_i = \kappa$ and $m_i = m$ for $i \in [1..n]$.

Validating the lower bound. To validate the lower bound, an arbitrary node near the model's center was displaced by 5 cm from its rest position along the y-axis. Spring-meshes with a wide range of different parameters were tested. The spring coefficient and mass values were varied between 0.0001 to 0.1 in steps of 0.0001. For each combination of mass and spring coefficient, the damping coefficient was varied between 0 and the optimum damping value $(2\sqrt{m\kappa})$ in increments of 0.0001. The time step was set to 50 msec. In total, 1 million combinations of mass and spring coefficient values were tested. Each trial was allowed to run until either the model returned to the initial configuration, or until 1000 iterations were performed.

Validating the upper bound. We performed two set of experiments to validate the upper bound. In the first set, the damping was varied according to the upper bound value described by equation (6). In the second set, the damping was set to a value 5% larger than the upper bound. For each set of experiments, the spring coefficient and mass values were varied between 0.0001 to 0.1 in steps of 0.0001, resulting in 1 million trials. The time step was set to 50 msec. Again an arbitrary node was displaced by 5 cm from its rest position. Overdamped systems take a longer time to reach steady state. So, each trial was allowed to run for 10,000 Euler iterations, or until the initial configuration was restored.

4. Results

Validating the lower bound. This experiment evaluated a mesh with $m \in [0.0001, 0.1]$, $\kappa \in [0.0001, 0.1]$, $\gamma_i = \gamma \in [0, 2\sqrt{m\,\kappa}]$ for $i \in [1,n]$ and $\Delta t = 50$ msec. For all cases (1 million trials), the mesh behaved as predicted. When $\gamma \leq 2\sqrt{m\,\kappa}$, the mesh failed to return to its initial configuration and kept oscillating. Fig. 1 illustrates a typical case over time for $\kappa = 0.001$, $m = 0.001$ and $\gamma = 0.0005$, 0.001 and 0.002. The graph plots the absolute distances of the initially displaced node from its rest position during the simulation.

Validating the upper bound. The adaptive damping experiment examined a mesh with $m \in [0.0001, 0.1]$, $\kappa \in [0.0001, 0.1]$ and $\Delta t = 50$ msec. All one million trials produced similar results. Fig. 2 shows a typical case. The absolute distance of the initially displaced node from its rest position is plotted on a logarithmic (Base 10) scale when $\kappa = 0.1$ and $m = 0.005$. It is evident from the graph that the system with damping greater than the upper bound was unstable. Some nodes in the mesh did converge initially but ultimately became unstable. However, the system with the damping equal to the upper bound value achieved stability within 652 iterations and remained stable thereafter.

5. Discussion

In applications such as medical simulation, surgical procedures such as cutting and tearing can dynamically change the characteristics of a mass-spring model. Finding a set of parameters suitable for all situations can be challenging. The bounds we have derived can ensure system stability while reducing the effort required to formulate plausible soft-tissue models. In this section, we discuss the significance of our results. While our discussion is made in the context of medical simulation, the implications are generalizable to other application areas.

Dynamic stability checks. Our results can be used to determine if a mass-spring system has become unstable during runtime. From equations (5) and (6), at time t, if $2\sqrt{m_i\kappa} > \frac{|v_i^t \frac{m_i}{\Delta t} + F_i^t|}{|v_i^t|}$, then no real value of damping exists that make the system stable. The ability to dynamically evaluate stability is especially useful if the model changes during runtime. A statically tuned model may exhibit different properties if its topology changes. To our knowledge, no comparable work exists that provides a closed-form solution to evaluating stability in this fashion.

Dynamic damping. The ability to evaluate stability at runtime is important. However, it may not be possible to tune a mass-spring model to exhibit the desired behavior and still be stable under all conditions. Accommodating all situations may require a sub-optimal set of parameters that decreases realism. Equations (5) and (6) can be used in an adaptive damping scheme that permits the model to use user-specified damping values but when instability is detected, damping is clamped to either bound.

Limitations. Presently, our derivation describes bounds only for damping. The results cannot be used to derive practical bounds for other mass-spring parameters, such as time step. Work is ongoing to address this aspect.

6. Conclusion

This paper established a stability criterion for an unforced, damped mass-spring system using the Explicit Euler integration method as,

$$2\sqrt{m_i\kappa} \leq \gamma_i \leq \frac{|v_i^t \frac{m_i}{\Delta t} + F_i^t|}{|v_i^t|}$$

We conducted a series of experiments to validate our findings. For each case, validation was performed using one million different spring-mass configurations, with the smallest and largest values for each parameter differing by three orders of magnitude. In every case, the system behaved exactly as predicted by our equations. While it is impossible to evaluate all possible combinations of mass-spring parameters, these experiments lend greater confidence to the validity of our theoretical development.

Determining a suitable set of parameters for mass-springs can be difficult. Our results can reduce the efforts required to tune mass-springs and can be used to model any changes during runtime. The adaptive damping scheme can be used to restore stability when instability occurs.

The implications of our results were briefly discussed. Using our findings, it is possible to perform run-time instability detection, implement an adaptive damping-correction scheme to ensure system stability, and simplify the creation of realistic mass-spring models.

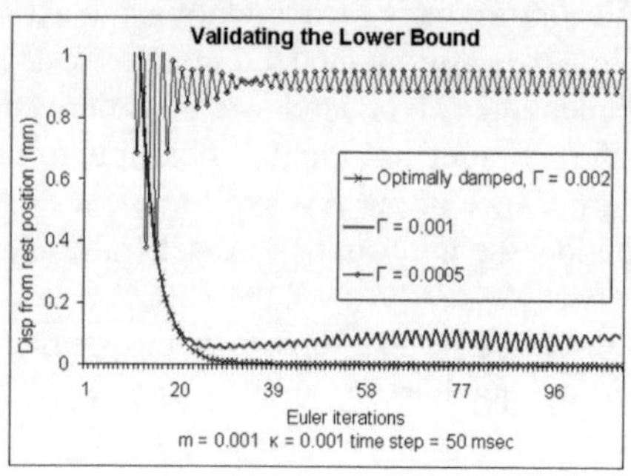

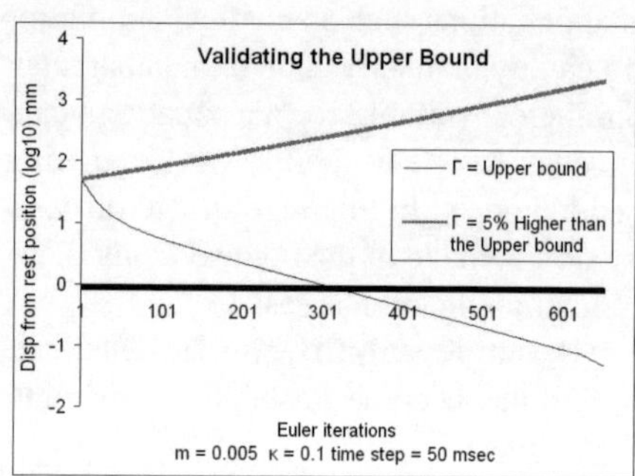

Figure 1. The behavior of a mesh with $\kappa = 0.001$, $m = 0.001$ and $\gamma = 0.0005$, 0.001 and 0.002 after a single initial impulse. γ below the lower bound (0.002) caused the mesh to oscillate indefinitely. At the computed lower bound, the mesh reached steady state after 34 iterations

Figure 2. Validating the upper bound. The distances of the displaced node are in logarithmic (Base 10) scale

References

[1] D. Baraff and A. Witkin. Large steps in cloth simulation. In *Computer Graphics Proceedings, Annual Conference Series, SIGGRAPH, ACM Press*, pages 43–54, 1998.

[2] Xavier Provot. Deformation constraints in a mass-spring model to describe rigid cloth behavior. In *Graphics Interface*, pages 147–154, 1995.

[3] Sarah Gibson and Brian Mirtich. A survey of deformable modeling in computer graphics. Technical Report TR-97-19, Mitsubishi Electric Research Lab, Cambridge MA, USA, 1997.

[4] D. Kincaid and W. Cheney. *Numerical Analysis: Mathematics of Scientific Computing*. 3rd edition, 2002.

[5] U. Kühnapfel, H. K. Çakmak, and H. Maaß. Endoscopic surgery training using virtual reality and deformable tissue simulation. *Computer Graphics*, 24:671–682, 2000.

[6] M. Bro-Nielsen, D. Helfrick, B. Glass, X. Zeng, and H. Connacher. Vr simulation of abdominal trauma surgery. In *Medicine Meets Virtual Reality: Art, Science, and Technology*, pages 117–123. IOS Press, 1998.

[7] M.H. Choi M.H. Kim Y.J. Choi, M. Hong. Adaptive mass-spring simulation using surface wavelet. In *Proceedings of International Conference on Virtual Systems and MultiMedia*, pages 25–33, 2002.

[8] Y. Lee, D. Terzopoulos, and K. Waters. Realistic modeling for facial animation. In *Proceedings of ACM SIGGRAPH*, volume 2, pages 55–62, 1995.

[9] A. Witkin. Physically based modeling. ACM SIGGRAPH Course Notes, 2001.

[10] L. P. Nedel and D. Thalmann. Real time muscle deformations using mass-spring systems. In *Proceedings of Computer Graphics International*, pages 156–165, Hannover, Germany, 1998.

[11] Hervé Delingette. Towards realistic soft tissue modeling in medical simulation. Technical Report RR-3506, INRIA, Sophia Antipolis, France, 2000.

[12] Z. Kacic-Alesic, M. Nordenstam, and D. Bullock. A practical dynamics system. In *Eurographics Symposium on Computer Animation*, pages 7–16, 2003.

[13] Leonard Meirovitch. *Elements of Vibration Analysis*. McGraw-Hill, 2nd edition, 1986.

Medicine Meets Virtual Reality 14
J.D. Westwood et al. (Eds.)
IOS Press, 2006

Bootstrapped Ultrasound Calibration

Emad M. Boctor[a], Iulian Iordachita[a], Michael A. Choti[b],
Gregory Hager[a], and Gabor Fichtinger[a]
[a] *Engineering Research Center, Johns Hopkins University*
[b] *Department of Surgery, Johns Hopkins University*

Abstract. This paper introduces an enhanced (bootstrapped) method for tracked ultrasound probe calibration. Prior to calibration, a position sensor is used to track an ultrasound probe in 3D space, while the US image is used to determine calibration target locations within the image. From this information, an estimate of the transformation matrix of the scan plane with respect to the position sensor is computed. While all prior calibration methods terminate at this phase, we use this initial calibration estimate to bootstrap an additional optimization of the transformation matrix on independent data to yield the minimum reconstruction error on calibration targets. The bootstrapped workflow makes use of a closed-form calibration solver and associated sensitivity analysis, allowing for rapid and robust convergence to an optimal calibration matrix. Bootstrapping demonstrates superior reconstruction accuracy.

Keywords. Ultrasound calibration, Tracked ultrasound, Bootstrapped calibration

1. Background and Significance

Ultrasound (US) imaging has emerged as a popular guidance modality for medical interventions, since it is real-time, safe, and inexpensive compared to other modalities. Quantitative ultrasound originates from interventional applications and recently it also has become useful in external beam radiation therapy (EBRT) guidance [1]. EBRT is expected to grow to the largest market for tracked ultrasound. With prostate cancer alone 65,000 patients are treated with EBRT in the United States each year. Significant research has been dedicated to quantitative tracked ultrasound. Typically, tracking is achieved by rigidly attaching 3D localizers to the US probe. The missing link, however, is the spatial transformation between the US image and the tracking body attached to the US probe, which requires calibration. Hence, calibration is ubiquitously present in all systems where ultrasound is used for quantitative image guidance. Calibration accuracy is the most significant factor in tracked US systems and therefore it is a logical imperative to minimize calibration error.

In all current calibration methods, as explained in Fig. 1, a set of objects (phantoms) of known geometrical properties is scanned by the tracked US probe, and then various mathematical procedures are applied to discern the unknown transformation that maximizes the similarity between the US images and the objects. Typically, point [2-6] and planar [3] features are used. The relative locations of the features are determined by precise machining [2-5], or by digitization [6]. Typical calibration methods [2-4,6] use non-linear optimization, in contrast to the methods in [5] where a closed-form formulation was applied. There is error associated with each stage of the calibration process: phantom fabrication, digitization, image acquisition, tracking, et cetera. These errors may aggregate to a prohibitively large final error in the calibration. In order to evaluate the overall accuracy of calibrated system, usually an object (typically cross-wire) is scanned from multiple directions and reconstructed in 3D space, and then the standard deviation of registration accuracy is reported as the measure of the quality of calibration. All current calibration methods, however, terminate at this point and fail to optimize the calibration toward minimum target reconstruction error. In this paper, we propose to close the loop on reconstruction accuracy and use it for minimizing the calibration error. We refer to this iterative process as bootstrapped calibration.

2. Materials and Methods

Concept of Bootstrapping

In order to improve target calibration accuracy, conventional methods simply increase the amount of input data and average the result of several calibration procedures. This brute force approach

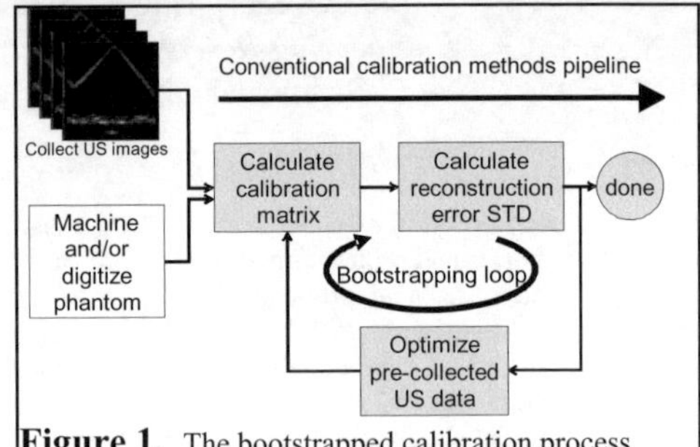

Figure 1. The bootstrapped calibration process

tends to improve on the precision of calibration, i.e. the expected uncertainty in a single calibration. In addition to using this versatile tool, we also propose bootstrapping the conventional calibration process by adding an iterative feedback loop to minimize the reconstruction error. There are two basic approaches to bootstrapping. The first is to acquire new relevant US calibration data to enhance parameters estimation. The second approach (Fig 1), which was implemented for this paper, is based on correcting the already acquired tracked US data that we use to calculate the calibration matrix. In contrast to the first approach, here we do not take new US images during the bootstrapping process. Instead, we iteratively reduce the error and noise in the tracked ultrasound data that was collected before running the calibration process.

Probe calibration accuracy traditionally has been very difficult to assess. A common approach is to measure how closely a point in 3D reconstruction coincides with its true 3D position, also known as reconstruction (or navigation) accuracy. Another approach called distance reconstruction accuracy is to check how well distances measured in the 3D reconstruction correspond to true lengths. In this paper, we recalculate the calibration matrix in the bootstrapping loop until minimum standard deviation of the reconstruction accuracy metric is achieved. But if the residual reconstruction error remains high, then additional US data need to be collected. Our bootstrapped calibration provides superior reconstruction accuracy, precisely because we obtain the optimal calibration through minimizing reconstruction accuracy.

Closed-Form Solver

In US probe calibration, arrays of wires are traditionally used to establish the relationship between the coordinate systems of the US and the tracking device. This approach typically involves laborious manual segmentation to extract the wire points in the US images and then relate these points to the tracking device coordinate system. We take a different approach by using the closed-form solver introduced in [5] that allows for calibration in real-time from as few as only three poses. Fig. 2 presents the coordinate systems for mathematical formulation in the closed form solver. A is the relative transformation between the US image frame at pose $k+1$ and k. Note that A can be recovered using a calibration phantom or recovered directly by matching the 2D ultrasound images acquired in these poses to a prior 3D model of the phantom object. B_k, B_{k+1} are the tracking device readings for the sensor frame with respect to tracker reference frame at poses k and $k+1$, respectively. The relative pose between sensor frame at pose k and $k+1$ is given by $B = (B_k)^{-1}B_{k+1}$. This yields the following homogeneous matrix equation $AX=XB$, where A is estimated from images of a simple phantom, B is assumed to be known from the external tracking device, and X is the unknown transformation between the US image coordinate system and the sensor frame. Detailed description of the $AX=XB$ solver is available in [5].

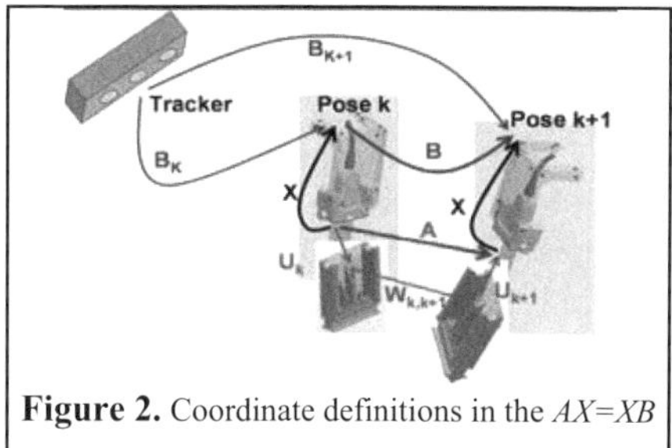

Figure 2. Coordinate definitions in the $AX=XB$

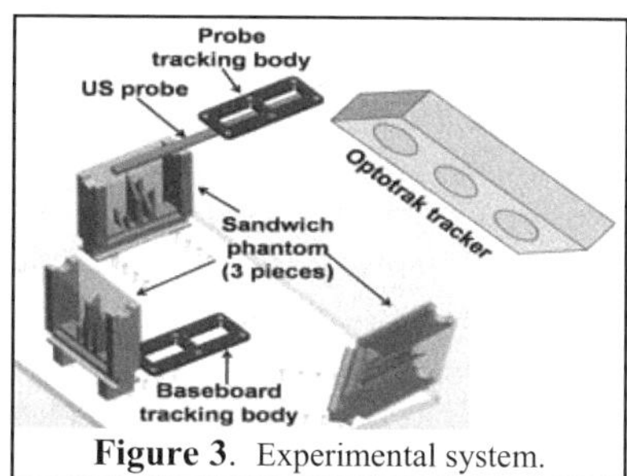

Figure 3. Experimental system.

The significance of the closed form $AX=XB$ solver is manifold. First, it allows us to initiate a non-linear optimization loop over the reconstruction accuracy, which the accepted metric of calibration accuracy. Another benefit of the $AX=XB$ solver is that it requires only few US images, compared to all previous methods that require massive amount of input data. For example, a set of 5 images yields to 120 (5*4*3) independent calibration scenarios, thereby increasing the precision of calibration significantly. Moreover, moving between poses in the $AX=XB$ solver is mathematically different. It is because the poses in the $AX=XB$ solver belong to an $SE(3)$ motion group for which probability distribution is non-commutative. Without providing a detailed sensitivity analysis here, we can intuitively accept that a few but favorable poses can provide a fairly precise calibration; a claim that previous experiments have corroborated [5].

Experimental System Design
In the embodiment shown in Fig.3, we used an Aloka US system (Aloka Ultrasound Inc.) with a laparoscopic probe. Multiple optical markers were attached to the probe holder, which then were tracked by an Optotrak device (Northern Digital Inc.). We used a three-piece phantom described in the next section. A rigid body marker is attached to the base plate of the phantom, to serve as the common frame of reference set rigidly with respect to the phantom. We chose to demonstrate the bootstrapped calibration on tracked laparoscopic ultrasound that has been known as the most challenging type of calibration, due to the relatively large distance between the probe tracking markers and the US crystal, while there is relatively little separation between the individual probe tracking markers.

A novel three-piece phantom was designed to take full advantage of the $AX=XB$ closed form formulation. We built three identical sandwich pieces and arranged them on an acrylic board in known relative poses, as shown in Fig 3. The relative pose among the sandwiches is such that it provides the widest possible angular separation between the required three US poses. The US probe is brought to contact with a sandwich as seen in Fig. 4 (left). We liberally apply coupling gel and twist US probe on the edge of the sandwich, to collect a chunk of fan beams. Each sandwich contains three pairs of wedges, inspired by the earlier work of Prager et al. [7]. The wedges are arranged in line as shown in Fig. 4 (center) and are covered with Agar gel. The gel is held in place between two plates like a sandwich. As seen in Fig. 4 (right), the wedges provide sharp features in the US image that are easy to segment, and then using simple rules of descriptive geometry, the pose of the US image can be determined with respect to the sandwich. We can easily estimate the relative pose between the US probe and a sandwich, thereby discerning the *A* matrix for the *AX=XB* equation, as explained earlier in relation to Fig. 2.

$$A = U_k W_{k,k+1} U_{k+1}^{-1} \tag{1}$$

Where U_k is the relative transformation between the US image frame and the double-wedge frame at pose k. $W_{k,k+1}$ is the transformation between the double-wedge phantoms at poses k and $k+1$. Note that $W_{k,k+1}$ can be estimated from a precise machining or using calibrated digitizing pointer, with an uncertainty below 100μm. The uncertainty of the U matrices, however, is significantly higher. The accuracy of the calibration is predominately controlled by how well we can estimate the U matrices.

The approach of our bootstrapped calibration is to perturb the out-of-plane motion parameters of the U matrices to compute a more accurate calibration.

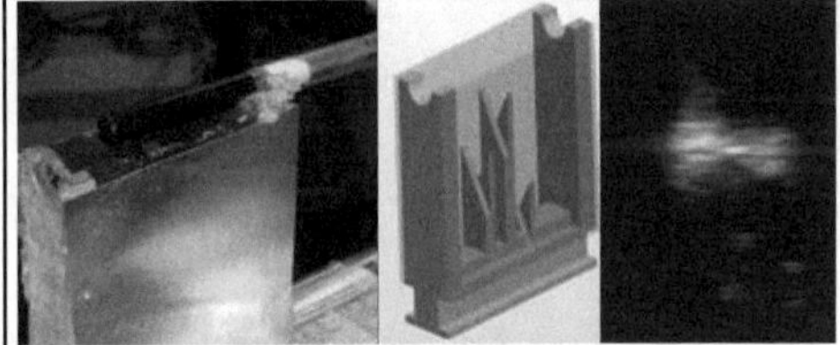

Figure 4. Sandwich phantom piece: w/ US probe (left), CAD model (center), US image (right)

3. The Bootstrapped Workflow

Our bootstrapped calibration protocol is simple to execute. The double-wedge sandwich phantom and US probe are brought the field of the Optotrak. The phantom is prepared by applying coupling gel on the edge of each sandwich. An image is collected from each sandwich, in the pose shown in Fig 4 (left). The probe and center plane of the sandwich being in the same plane forms a constraint. In the k_{th} sandwich, we assume that the U_k transformation matrix is the relative transformation between sandwich and the US image. U_k has an in-plane offset and rotation that can be calculated from the pixel coordinates of the wedges in the US image. U_k also has an out-of-plane motion component, which is supposed to be near to identity, when the probe is in the central plane of the sandwich. The US probe is rotated over the wedge till the left and right sides of the US image match. This can be achieved with freehand motion of the probe, owing to the sharp features of the double-wedges in the US image. (Note that could as well collect a fan beam of US images, process them numerically, and select the one closest to the center plane of the sandwich.) When the desired image is found to be coincident with the center plane of the sandwich (when U_k has practically no out-of-plane components), we record the picture and the reading from the tracker. We determine the wedge points from the images, either by mouse click or image processing. Thus we can compute the *A* and *B* matrices and then run the *AX=XB* module to estimate the full calibration matrix. (Also note that while 3 images are sufficient to recover the calibration matrix with acceptable accuracy, 2 additional images can generate 120 calibration datasets, and thus ensure significantly higher precision.) Having obtained a reasonable estimate of the calibration matrix, we can bootstrap the process, i.e. refine the calibration. With the tracked ultrasound probe we image a target from different directions. We reconstruct the expected target location in each image, with the use of the calibration matrix provided earlier by the *AX=XB* solver. Finally, we calculate the standard deviation between the observed and reconstructed target points, denoted as *R-STD*. The value of *R-STD* is a good measure of the quality of calibration and it can be used to drive a non-linear optimization loop. We apply such a nonlinear optimization to change parameters in the *AX=XB* equation until *R-STD* settles in a minimum. In our experimental system, we used a common cross-wire target made of nylon filaments, submerged in a water tank at room temperature. In our prototype system, we can trust the result of the closed form solver (X matrix), the Optotrak readings (B matrix), the machining of the phantom, the processing of US images of the sandwiches, and the segmentation of the cross-wire. The least trusted element of the calibration is our free-hand maneuvering ability to bring the US image into the center plane of the sandwich, i.e. the out-of-plane component of the U_k and $(U_{k+1})^{-1}$ in Eq 1. In each cycle, we modify these and then once we have a new *A*, we recalculate *X* using the original *B*, and finally recalculate *R-STD* for the pre-segmented cross-wire images.

4. Results and Discussion

Table 1 shows the standard deviation of position reconstruction accuracy in mm, for three calibration methods: a pointer-based approach by Galloway et al. [6], the original *AX=XB* closed form calculation [5], and our bootstrapped calibration. The original *AX=XB* is more favorable than the pointer-based method, while the bootstrapped method is superior to both. The largest contributor to the residual *R-STD* that remains after bootstrapping is incorrect segmentation of the cross-wire targets and temporal calibration. Ultrasound velocity also appears to be a significant factor. The calibration was performed on a gel phantom in which the speed of sound is 1,540 m/sec, but the cross-wire was placed in room temperature water in which the speed of sound is only 1,420 m/sec. From this problem alone we can suffer as much as 0.4 mm error at 10 cm penetration depth. One fundamental problem with reconstruction error based accuracy analysis is that it cannot separate calibration error from other factors of error. One could, however, obtain an estimate based on the uncertainties of the independent variables feeding into the closed-form solver, which can be accomplished by propagating input uncertainties or by Monte-Carlo simulation.

In the pointer-based method, the increased deviation along the elevation direction (x) is associated with the beam width problem. While the *AX=XB*

Pointer [10]			AX=XB [8,9]			Bootstrapped		
x	y	z	x	y	z	x	y	z
3.6	2.8	2.1	2.5	3.3	2.2	2.5	2.5	2.0

Table 1: Standard deviation of position reconstruction accuracy (R-STD) in mm, for three calibration methods

provided a better estimate, bootstrapping did not improve *R-STD* along that axis. The reason for that appears to be that the cross-wire target tended to fall in the center of the US images, roughly in the gravity center of the double-wedges. When bootstrapping fixes the out-of-plane rotation of the image with respect to the sandwich, it leads to relatively little out-of-plane motion in the image center where the cross-wire resided. Had we placed the cross-wire farther from the image center, bootstrapping would have shown more significant enhancement over the *AX=XB* method, in terms of residual *R-STD*. A cross-wire target placed farther away from the gravity center of the three wedges would drive bootstrapping more aggressively. In our system embodiment, perturbing the *A* matrix alone drives the overall calibration optimization effectively, but there is still residual *R-STD* that could be further reduced. In other words, some parameters that we had trusted could also be perturbed to achieve a smaller *R-STD*. The next obvious candidate is segmentation of the cross-wire targets. We performed this task manually, but the process could be aided by advanced image processing. Indeed, a significant advantage of bootstrapping is that the previously manual segmentation and correspondence process can be easily automated using the initial calibration estimate. Nevertheless, a simpler target structure, such as single wall [3], may be more favorable. In our system, processing the US images of the sandwich phantom (i.e. in-plane portion of *A*) and the readings from the tracker (i.e. *B* matrix) are very reliable and perturbing these does not promise further improvement on *R-STD*.

We have also developed an image-based method to estimate the out-of-plane motion of the US probe by maximizing the similarity between the US image and the descriptive geometrical model of the sandwich. The calculated out-of-plane motion is in a good agreement with the out-of-plane correction provided by the bootstrapping. Apparently, we can derive an estimate of the out-of-plane motion based on image processing alone, but this takes time and is also prone to human error. On the other hand, we always need some form of accuracy assessment and once *R-STD* is calculated, bootstrapping is essentially free. Because the *AX=XB* closed form solver works in real-time and the bootstrapping needs only a few iterations, the computational time required for a full calibration is negligible. In addition, we only need to use few images, the acquisition and processing of which is quick and easy. A further unique feature of the sandwich phantom is that, unlike all other phantoms, it does not reside in a water tank. The phantom could be covered with sterile plastic drape in the operating room, allowing for in-situ calibration. The cross-wire (or a single wall) target could also be packaged with the sandwich phantom, thereby eliminating the earlier mentioned discrepancy in speed of sound between the sandwich and target phantom images.

Because conventional calibration methods relied on image information from an US machine, registration accuracy, to a large extent, also depended on the resolution of the US imaging system and the accuracy of feature extraction. These factors practically disappear with bootstrapped calibration that can minimize *R-STD* effectively even if the segmentation of features is somewhat incorrect. Thus the remaining significant sources of error left in the calibration matrix are the inaccuracy of the tracking and temporal synchronization; the ultimate limit for any calibration.

References

1. Langen KM, Pouliot J, et al. Evaluation of ultrasound-based prostate localization for image-guided radiotherapy. *Int J Radiat Oncol Biol Phys. 57(3):635-44.*
2. P. R. Detmer, G. Bashein, et al. 3D Ultrasonic Image Feature Localization based on Magnetic Scanhead Tracking: In Vitro Calibration and Validation. *US in Med. Biol., 23(4):597-609, 1996.*
3. R.W. Prager, Rohling R. N., et al. Rapid Calibration for 3-D Freehand Ultrasound, *US in Med. Biol., 24(6):855-869, 1998.*
4. N. Pagoulatos, D. R. Haynor, et al. A Fast Calibration Method for 3-D Tracking of Ultrasound Images Using a Spatial Localizer. *US in Med.Biol., 27(9):1219-1229, 2001.*
5. E.M. Boctor, A. Viswanathan, et al. A Novel Closed Form Solution for Ultrasound Calibration, *In IEEE Int Symp. On Biomedical Imaging, 2004.*
6. Muratore DM, Galloway RL. Beam calibration without a phantom for creating a 3-D freehand ultrasound system. *Ultrasound Med Biol. 2001 Nov;27(11):1557-66.*
7. A. H. Gee, N. E. Houghton, G.M. Treece and R.W. Prager. 3D Ultrasound Probe Calibration Without a Position Sensor. *CUED/F-INFENG/TR-488, September 2004.*

Combining High-Fidelity Human Patient Simulators with a Standardized Family Member: A Novel Approach to Teaching Breaking Bad News

Mark W. BOWYER, Lisa RAWN, Janice HANSON, Elisabeth A. PIMENTEL,
Amy FLANAGAN, E. Matthew RITTER , Anne RIZZO, Joseph O. LOPREIATO
*National Capital Area Medical Simulation Center of the Uniformed Services
University of the Health Sciences, Bethesda, Maryland*
e-mail: mbowyer@usuhs.mil

Abstract. Our novel approach to teaching Breaking Bad News (BBN) involves having students actively participate in an unsuccessful resuscitation (mannequin) followed immediately by BBN to a standardized patient wife (SPW) portrayed by an actress. Thirty-nine 3rd year medical students completed a questionnaire and then were divided as follows: Group 1 (n=21) received little to no training prior to speaking with the SPW. Group 2 (n =18) received a lecture and practiced for 1 hour in small groups prior to the resuscitation and BBN. Both groups self assessed ability to BBN ($p<.0002$ & $p<.00001$), and ability to have a plan ($p<.0004$ & $p <.0003$) improved significantly over base line with greater improvement in group 2. Group 2 (pre-trained) students were rated superior by SPW's in several key areas. This novel approach to teaching BBN to 3rd year medical students was well received by the students and resulted in marked improvement of self assessed skills over baseline.

1. Introduction

One of the most challenging instances in the doctor-patient relationship is when the physician informs the patient of adverse news. Bad news can mean anything from the obvious, a diagnosis of incurable cancer or the death of a loved one, to the more mundane, the need for eye-glasses or a cavity to be filled. How this encounter proceeds can greatly impact the patient and the physician, and impact the level of confidence that the patient places in the hospital and physician. [1, 2] While some doctors may be considered innately good at this part of their job, others are notorious for the brusque manner in which they perform this duty. [3] Few, if any, physicians are trained for this important communication with their patients and their families. The current standard is to observe a peer or supervisor when he or she must deliver bad news to a patient or the family members.[2] That method of training is "catch as catch can", being only as good as the physician being observed.

In 1999, the American Council of Graduate Medical Education (ACGME) endorsed six general competencies as the foundation of all graduate medical education. Among these general competencies is that of Patient Care which includes the ability to communicate effectively and demonstrate caring and respectful behaviors when interacting with patients and their families. Another general competency is that of Interpersonal and Communication skills. A third of these general competencies are Professionalism, which includes the ability to demonstrate sensitivity and responsiveness to the patients' culture, age, gender, disabilities and emotional state. It is clear that the ability to BBN to a patient or family member requires integration of at least three of the core competencies, and is therefore essential to all health care professionals and should be taught as early as possible.

With the availability of Simulation Based Training there is a safe and realistic learning environment in which to teach the skills necessary to inform a patient of bad news. It also allows the student to receive instant feedback from staff physicians and standardized patients on the effectiveness of his/her interaction as well as objective metrics of performance. This particular kind of communication can have a significant impact on a patient's life and physicians are duty bound to make it the best it can be given the circumstances. This has particular military relevance at this time, given the increase in and type of patients returning from armed conflicts. These patients' lives have been significantly and irrevocably altered. In this environment, the military physician must be especially able to effectively and compassionately deliver bad news. In reality it is the first step in healing. An important first step, that when carried out appropriately can make all of the difference.

It is generally agreed upon that delivering bad news to patients is a difficult, but important undertaking. There have been studies that investigate medical students' opinions on the subject before and after a course, as well as studies on the level of residents' notification skills. [4, 5] While the subject of breaking bad news has been explored and evaluated by physicians and educators for a number of years, few have investigated how best to teach medical students and residents this important skill. [1, 6, 7] Additionally, there is practically no evidence that anyone has determined what constitutes an effective evaluation tool to ensure that students have integrated these skills once taught. Of the papers that investigate these strategies, none has quantitatively measured the effectiveness of breaking bad news teaching methods against a baseline. This study addresses the need for validation studies to demonstrate that the teaching methods are effective by performing a comparative evaluation of training methods used to teach medical students how to delivery bad news to patients.

2. Methods

As part of the normal third-year Surgery Clerkship curriculum, thirty-nine 3rd year medical students participated in a formative clinical skills laboratory that introduced them to the skills they need on the surgical wards. Each student went through a series of skills stations. One of those stations was a trauma resuscitation simulation in which the student was asked to treat a patient arriving in the trauma ER. The patient in this case is a high-fidelity human simulator mannequin made up to portray a multiple gunshot victim. The students were asked to evaluate and treat this patient but despite their best efforts the patient died. After completing the trauma ER scenario, the students' next skills station was informing the patient's wife of her husband's death. These students typically have had little experience dealing with the death of a patient and no practical experience informing the deceased patient's family of the bad news. Prior to the encounter all students completed a pre-encounter questionnaire (5 point Likert scale) about their preparedness for delivering bad news to patients. Group 1 (n=21) received little to no training prior to performing the resuscitation and speaking with the patient's wife. Group 2 (n =18) received training in the form of a didactic lecture about how to deliver bad news to a patient, followed by small group sessions that allowed the students to practice these skills and receive feedback (Figure 1). [8, 9] The instruction was based on the SPIKES model developed to teach these communication skills (Table 1). Both groups then participated in the unsuccessful resuscitation scenario in which the patient died (Figure 2). The student was then informed that the patient's wife (portrayed by a standardized patient wife (SPW) actress) was in the waiting room and that they must deliver the news to her (Figure 3).

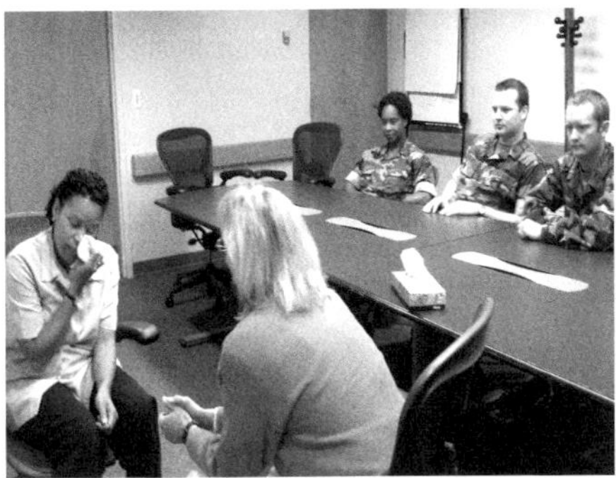

Figure 1. Group 2 students receive training in BBN prior to the interaction with the SPW. They receive a didactic lecture and a small group training session.

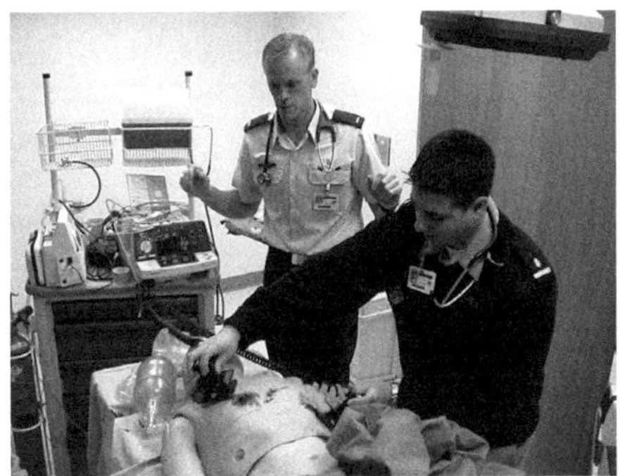

Figure 2. Both groups of students participate in an unsuccessful resuscitation of a penetrating trauma scenario using a high-fidelity human patient simulator.

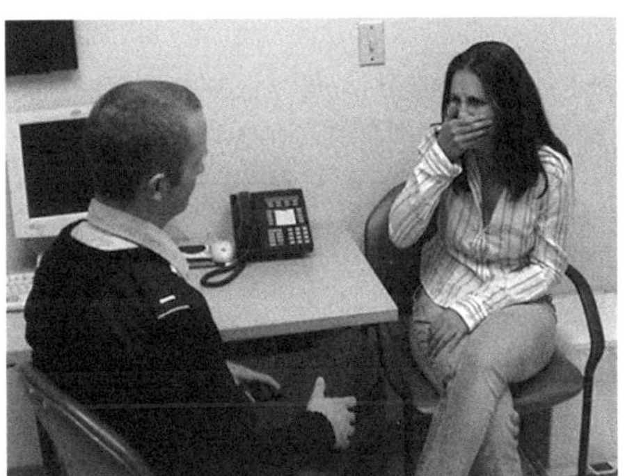

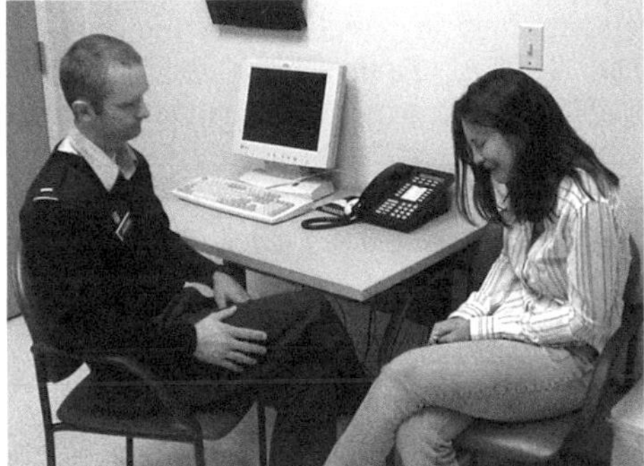

Figure 3. Students must break the bad news to the patient's wife that despite their best efforts her husband has died. The standardized patient wife (SPW), who has been trained specifically for this scenario, displays a range of appropriate and realistic emotions to include shock (left) and grief (right) as depicted above.

After the encounter, the students all completed a post-encounter questionnaire (5 point Likert scale) that self-assessed their ability to have a plan and to break bad news. Each student was additionally evaluated by the SPW on a 5 point Likert scale on 21 items related to the student's appearance, communication skills, and emotional affect. Group 1 students received cross-over training after the encounter.

                    M.W. Bowyer et al. / A Novel Approach to Teaching Breaking Bad News

Table 1. The SPIKES Protocol for Delivering Bad News to Patients*

Step	Description of Task
Setting	Establish patient rapport by creating an appropriate setting that provides for privacy, patient comfort, uninterrupted time, setting at eye level, and inviting significant other(s) (if desired).
Perception	Elicit the Patient's perception of his or her problem.
Invitation	Obtain the patient's invitation to disclose the details of the medical condition
Knowledge	Provide knowledge and information to the patient. Give information in small chunks, check for understanding, and frequently avoid medical jargon.
Empathize	Empathize and explore emotions expressed by the patient.
Summary and strategy	Provide a summary of what you said and negotiate a strategy for treatment of follow-up.

*From [4] Baile WF, Kudelka AP, Beale EA, et al. Communication skills training in oncology: description and preliminary outcomes of workshops on breaking bad news and managing patient reactions to illness. Cancer. 1999;86:887-97.

3. Results

Groups 1 and 2 were equal in terms of their previous breaking bad news training (2.0 vs. 2.11 hrs) and in belief that learning this skill was very important (avg. 4.2 on Likert scale of 1-5). Both groups' self-assessed ability to break bad news ($p<.0002$ & $p<.00001$) (Figure 4), and ability to have a plan to break bad news ($p<.0004$ & $p <.0003$) improved significantly over base line with greater improvement in group 2 (Figure 5). Both rated the experience as extremely valuable (avg 4.7) and very realistic (avg 4.6 on a 5 point scale). Group 2 (pre-trained) students were rated superior by SPW's in terms of their comfort level ($p <.02$); whether they had a plan ($p <.04$); assessment of information the SPW already knew ($P<.0008$), preparation of the SPW to receive news ($p <.02$); ability to provide guidance ($p <.02$), and whether the student inspired trust ($p<.03$) (Figure 6).

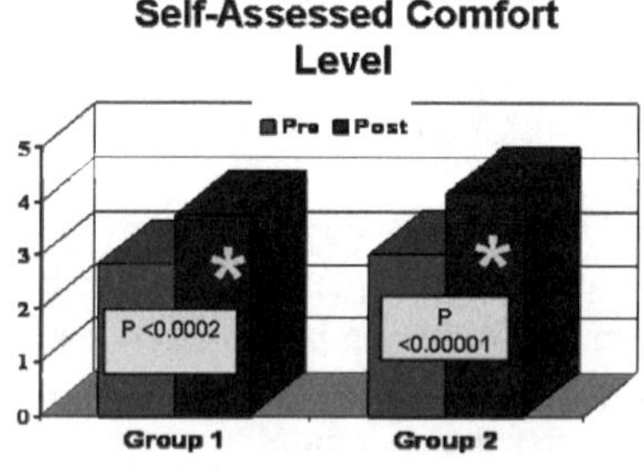

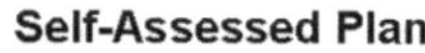
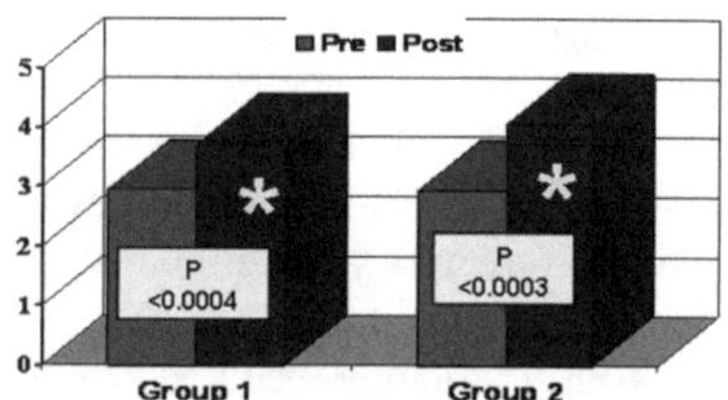

Figure 4. The students' self-assessed comfort level with BBN improved significantly over baseline in both groups.

Figure 5. The students self-assessed ability to have a plan for BBN improved significantly over baseline in both groups.

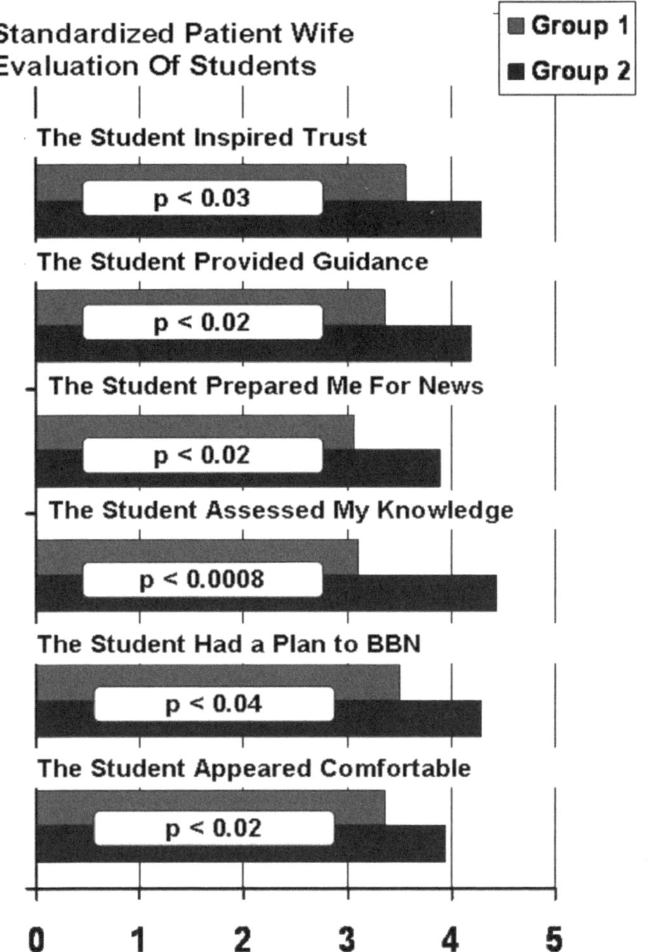

Figure 6. The students were rated by the standardized patient wives who were blinded to group, on twenty-one items related to the student's appearance, communication skills, and emotional affect. Group two (pre-trained) students were rated significantly higher on the six factors depicted. Values are depicted on a 5-pt Likert scale in which 1 = strongly disagree and 5 = strongly agree.

4. Conclusions

This novel approach to teaching BBN to 3rd year medical students was well received by the students and resulted in marked improvement of self-assessed skills over baseline. Coupling the resuscitation experience with a didactic lecture and small group practice sessions greatly enhanced the performance of student's ability to BBN. This approach to Breaking Bad News merits further evaluation for inclusion in future adverse news curricula.

Acknowledgements

The authors wish to thank Ms. Jennifer Fellows for her support in operating the high-fidelity human patient simulators. The authors also wish to thank Mr. Eric Singdahlsen and Ms. Mary Donovan for their support in standardized patient training and editorial review.

This work was conducted at the National Capital Area Medical Simulation Center of the Uniformed Services University, a Department of Defense Facility. The views, opinions and/or findings contained in this report are those of the authors and should not be construed as an official Department of Defense position, policy or decision unless so designated by other documentation.

References

[1] Ptacek, J. T. PhD; Eberhardt, Tara L. Breaking Bad News: A Review of the Literature. JAMA. 1996;276:496-502.

[2] Vaidya, V. U. MD, et. Al. Teaching Physicians How to Break Bad News. Arch Pediatr Adolesc Med. 1999;153:419-422

[3] Dias, Lauren, Chabner, Bruce A., Lynch, Thomas J., Penson, Richard T. Breaking Bad News: A Patient's Perspective. The Oncologist. 2003; 8:587-596

[4] Benenson, R. S. MD, Pollack, M. L. MD, PhD. Evaluation of Emergency Medicine Resident Death Notification Skills by Direct Observation. Acad Emerg Med. 2003; 10:219-223.

[5] Greenberg L. W. et al. Communicating Bad News: A Pediatric Department's Evaluation of a Simulated Intervention. Pediatrics. 1999;103:1210-1217.

[6] Rosenbaum, M. E. PhD, Ferguson, K. J. PhD, Lobas, J. G. MD. Teaching Medical Students and Residents Skills for Delivering Bad News: A Review of Strategies. Acad Med. 2004;79:107-117.

[7] Parker, P. A. et al. Breaking Bad News About Cancer: Patients' Preferences for Communication. J Clin Onc. 2001; 19:2049-56.

[8] Baile, W. F., Buckman, R., Lenzia, R., Glober, G., Beale, E. A., Kudelka, A. P. SPIKES—A Six-Step Protocol for Delivering Bad News: Application to the Patient with Cancer. The Oncologist. 2000; 5:302-311.

[9] Garg, A. MD, Buckman, R. MB, PhD, Kason, Y. MD, Med. Teaching medical students to break bad news. Can Med Assoc J. 1997;156:1159-1164.

Medicine Meets Virtual Reality 14
J.D. Westwood et al. (Eds.)
IOS Press, 2006

Virtual Environment-Based Training Simulator for Endoscopic Third Ventriculostomy

Nathan BROWN[a], Suriya NATSUPAKPONG[a], Svend JOHANNSEN[a],
Sunil MANJILA[b], Qingbo CAI[a], Vincenzo LIBERATORE[a], Alan R. COHEN[b],
M. Cenk CAVUSOGLU[a,1]

[a]*Dept. of Electrical Eng. and Computer Sc., Case Western Reserve University*
[b]*Dept. of Neurosurgery, Rainbow Babies' and Children's Hospital*

Abstract. A virtual environment-based endoscopic third ventriculostomy simulator is being developed for training neurosurgeons as a standardized method for evaluating competency. Magnetic resonance (MR) images of a patient's brain are used to construct the geometry model, realistic behavior in the surgical area is simulated by using physical modeling and surgical instrument handling is replicate by a haptic interface. The completion of the proposed virtual training simulator will help the surgeon to practice the techniques repeatedly and effectively, serving as a powerful educational tool.

Introduction

Endoscopic neurosurgery has gained widespread popularity because of the ability to perform invasive therapy with little disruption of neural structures, giving rise to the term, minimally invasive neurosurgery. Third ventriculostomy is the most commonly employed endoscopic procedure at any neurosurgical center in the world and a fundamental step in training. Despite the widespread popularity of neuroendoscopy, the instruction and evaluation of surgeons in this technique continues to be difficult because of the limited field of view, amount of instrument handling, and access by the surgeon, and also the intricacies of the tight operating volume surrounded by critical structures. This, however, lends itself nicely to a virtual environment-based endoscopic simulation. This paper describes the current state of our ongoing project of developing a virtual environment-based training simulator for endoscopic third ventriculostomy.

1. Objective

The broad objective of the research is to develop a neuroendoscopy simulation, initially of endoscopic third ventriculostomy for obstructive hydrocephalus. The specific goals of the project are to construct patient specific models of the ventricular geometry starting from MR images of patients, create a visually and dynamically realistic virtual

---

[1]Corresponding Author: M. Cenk Cavusoglu, Case Western Reserve University, 10900 Euclid Avenue, Cleveland, OH 44106, U.S.A.; E-mail: cavusoglu@case.edu

environment using these models, and construct a training simulator using this virtual environment to teach and validate the steps of the endoscopic procedure.

The GiPSi/GiPSiNet open source/open architecture framework for surgical simulation [1, 2] is used as the software system to build the simulator. GiPSiNet is the network middleware module, to allow remote display and haptics functionalities.

2. Methods

In construction of the surface models of the third ventricular geometry from MR images, the key concern is the visibility of the floor of the third ventricle – how to distinguish it from the ventricular cerebrospinal fluid. This is especially pertinent for the endoscopic third ventriculostomy, which involves puncturing the floor of the third ventricle using the tip of a catheter. Another concern in the construction of geometric models of ventricular anatomy from MR images is the dimension of the third ventricle and the resolution of the geometrical models that can be constructed from the images. The basic prototype constructed from MR images of normal anatomy with voxel sizes of 0.37x0.37x0.80mm demonstrated that the resolution was sufficient to differentiate the bodies, and there was enough contrast between the membrane and the other surrounding tissues for effective segmentation of the ventricles. The results reveal that the thin sliced T1 MR images yield resolution and contrast high enough to construct a geometrical model of the ventricular anatomy.

A nonlinear plastic lumped element model is used to simulate the physical behavior of the membranes on which the surgeon operates. Use of heterogeneous physical models, i.e. using different type of physical models for different parts of the virtual environment, is at the core of our approach to address the computational complexity of the dynamical models. Developing a simulator with heterogeneous physical models is not trivial. However, unlike other simulation frameworks, our GiPSi framework has been specifically designed for creating simulations that incorporate these heterogeneous physical models, with well defined APIs and mechanisms for interfacing them.

Computer renderings of ventricular anatomy (using a third party geometric model) created with the new visualization engine of GiPSi are shown in Figure 1. The images shown are generated in real-time at an interactive rate of more than 30 fps, on a single processor PC workstation dedicated to graphics display. The newly added programmable shader support of the GiPSi visualization engine allows the use of custom vertex and fragment shaders created with the OpenGL Shading Language. A tissue shader developed in-house employs a Phong illumination model together with texture and bump mapping, superimposing capillaries and other visual details onto the gross geometry, extended to include the effects of glossiness and multi-layered nature of the tissue. The tissue shader produces a photo-realistic view of the third ventricle's semi-transparent floor, exposing the mamillary bodies below it, which during the real ventriculostomy helps the surgeon select the site of puncture and avoid inadvertent damage to the basilar artery.

We have designed a prototype haptic interface specific for endoscopic neurosurgery, based on a modification of the PHANTOM® Omni™ Haptic Device. Motion of the neuroendoscopic haptic instrument has four degrees of freedom (DOF) constrained by the fulcrum at the burr hole site, and an additional DOF for the relative rotation of the camera with respect to the trocar. To produce a four DOF interface with proper kinematics and force feedback, we adopted the design developed by Tendick et al. [3] for a laparoscopic surgery simulator. The major extensions over the four DOF design of Tendick et al. are the addition of the extra DOFs for the motion of the endoscope relative to the trocar and the motions and actions of the catheters used during the surgery. The multirate simulation method [4] is used to achieve high quality haptic interaction with the deformable models.

As part of the project, the steps of the endoscopic third ventriculostomy have been described and analyzed to categorize the stages of the operation.

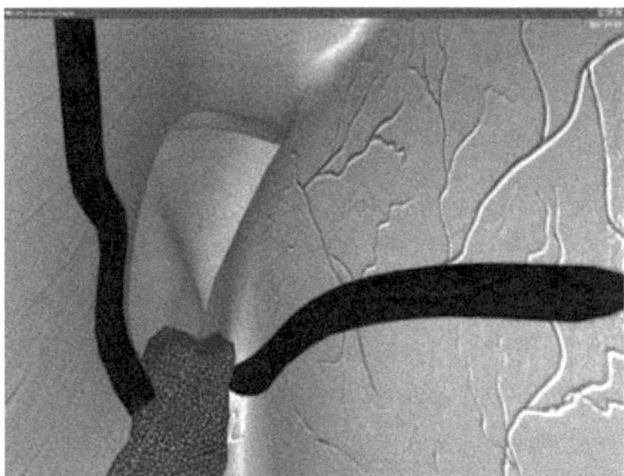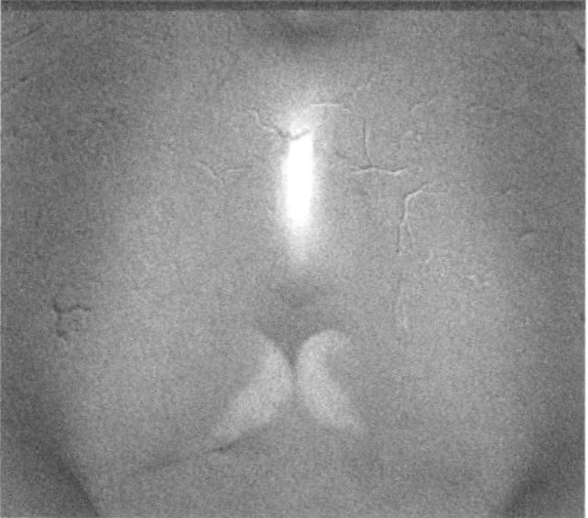

Figure 1. Computer renderings of the ventricular anatomy from a simulation created using GiPSi. (a) The view from the lateral ventricle, looking towards the third ventricle through foramen of Monro. (b) The floor of the third ventricle as seen from inside of the third ventricle. The basilar artery and the mamillary bodies are visible through the semi-transparent membrane at the floor of the third ventricle.

3. Future Work

In this paper, we have reported the current state of our ongoing project of developing a virtual environment-based training simulator for endoscopic third ventriculostomy.

Construct validity of a simulator is an indicator of the usefulness of the simulator as a teaching and evaluation tool. The construct validity of the simulator will be established through a randomized double-blind study based on the successful completion of the operation stages. The construct validity is the key to verify the skill transfer from the virtual environment-based training simulator to real surgery, and is crucial for adoption of the simulator as a training tool and inclusion as part of the surgical curriculum.

References

[1] M.C. Cavusoglu, T.G. Goktekin, and F. Tendick. "GiPSi: A Framework for Open Source/Open Architecture Software Development for Organ Level Surgical Simulation." In *IEEE Transaction on Information Technology in Biomedicine*, 2005. *(In press)*
[2] V. Liberatore, M.C. Cavusoglu, and Q. Cai. "GiPSiNet: a middleware for networked surgical simulations." In IASTED Telehealth 2005, Banff, Canada, July 2005, pp. 35-40.
[3] F. Tendick, M. Downes, T. Goktekin, M.C. Cavusoglu, D. Feygin, X. Wu, R. Eyal, M. Hegarty, and L.W. Way. "A Virtual Environment Testbed for Training Laparoscopic Surgical Skills." In Presence, Vol. 9, No. 3, June 2000, pp. 236-255.
[4] M.C. Cavusoglu, F. Tendick. "Multirate Simulation for High Fidelity Haptic Interaction with Deformable Objects in Virtual Environments." In Proc. of the IEEE International Conference on Robotics and Automation (ICRA 2000), San Francisco, CA, April 24-28, 2000, pp. 2458-2465.

Medicine Meets Virtual Reality 14
J.D. Westwood et al. (Eds.)
IOS Press, 2006

Evaluation Methods of a Middleware for Networked Surgical Simulations

Qingbo Cai [1], Vincenzo Liberatore, M. Cenk Çavuşoğlu and Youngjin Yoo
Case Western Reserve University

Abstract. Distributed surgical virtual environments are desirable since they substantially extend the accessibility of computational resources by network communication. However, network conditions critically affects the quality of a networked surgical simulation in terms of bandwidth limit, delays, and packet losses, etc. A solution to this problem is to introduce a middleware between the simulation application and the network so that it can take actions to enhance the user-perceived simulation performance. To comprehensively assess the effectiveness of such a middleware, we propose several evaluation methods in this paper, i.e., semi-automatic evaluation, middleware overhead measurement, and usability test.

Keywords. Surgical simulation, Virtual environment, Network, Middleware, Usability test

1. Introduction

Distributed surgical virtual environments are desirable since they substantially extend the accessibility of computational resources by network communication. However, network conditions critically affects the quality (fidelity and realism) of a networked surgical simulation in terms of bandwidth, delays, packet losses, etc. A solution to this problem is to introduce an intermediary (middleware) between the surgical simulation application and the network so that it can take actions to remediate for the lack of network QoS (Quality of Service) [1].

Systematic evaluation methods are needed to comprehensively assess the effectiveness of such a middleware, i.e., to measure the performance enhancement the middleware brings and the overheads it incurs. In this paper, we propose three methods to achieve this: semi-automatic evaluation, overhead measurement, and usability test.

2. Evaluation methods

2.1. A semi-automatic evaluation framework

In order to evaluate a middleware's performance on different network configurations, we can execute a standard task suite remotely and measure the task performance with an

---

[1]Correspondence to: Vincenzo Liberatore or M. Cenk Çavuşoğlu, Department of Electrical Engineering and Computer Science, Case Western Reserve University, 10900 Euclid Avenue, Cleveland, OH 44106, U.S.A. Tel.: +1 216 368 4088; E-mail: vxl11@case.edu or cavusoglu@case.edu.

automatic procedure. Specifically, we can implement an automatic controller to execute each task. For example, we may build an automatic controller, which moves the scalpel using compliant control to perform the Fitts' task [2,3] and uses the Fitts' index of performance as performance metrics, to observe the controller performance under various network conditions.

A semi-automatic evaluation framework consists of a benchmark suite of representative surgical tasks and the infrastructure for network emulations of a middleware. The benchmark tasks should be i) simple so that they can be programmed with control techniques of general knowledge; and ii) representative of a human user's simple operations. One example is the standard Fitts' task. Alternative benchmark task can be general tasks performed in typical surgery, including tasks that require tracking of simple trajectories using surgical tools and maintaining constant contact force between the surgical tool and tissue, with appropriate performance metrics such as task completion time and error in trajectory tracking, and the amount of simulated damage that a controller inflicts under poor network conditions for constant force application tasks.

2.2. Overhead measurement

An ideal middleware should have minimal latency and throughput overhead, and moderate computational requirement. Unfortunately, this is not always the case. The overhead imposed by a middleware can be evaluated by comparing the packet delay and throughput of a middleware with point-to-point plain socket communication. To assess the computational requirements and running time of the individual modules within a middleware or the middleware as a whole, a middleware should include instrumentation software that can be selectively turned on or off at run-time.

2.3. Usability test

The ultimate goal of the middleware is to enhance the user-perceived performance of a networked surgical simulation. Consequently, user experiences should also be included in a comprehensive evaluation. From the middleware perspective of view, our concerns are the issues related to the network influences on user experiences, such as the responsiveness of haptic devices, the stability of haptic feedback, the smoothness of remote visualization, etc.

A usability test of virtual environments (VE) differs from traditional one in that it introduces factors such as presence, physiological effects, locating and manipulating objects, etc. Although intensive research has been done in VE and usability, few examples exist to apply usability in VE. An overview of usability evaluation in virtual environments is given in [4]. A popular and effective technique to collect qualitative data during usability tests is the "think-aloud" protocol [5], where a participant vocalizes his feelings and thoughts regarding the interfaces while performing a task. Comparative evaluation may also be conducted by asking subjects to operate the benchmark tasks on several programs representing different configurations of the middleware. Then, a statistical analysis is performed to validate the techniques applied in the middleware. There are several factors that can affect the result of a usability test, for example, the subjects' prior experience with VE and surgical tasks, the model of learning (individual or pair work), the learning curve, etc. Therefore, we should consider the influences of these factors during the usability evaluation planning and analyzing so that the test can carry more meaningful results.

3. Conclusions and future work

In this paper, we described the methods to evaluate a middleware for networked surgical simulations. In our ongoing project, we will develop a middleware *GiPSiNet* [6] to extend *GiPSi* (General Interactive Physical Simulation Interface) [7,8], our open source/open architecture framework for developing surgical simulations, to a network environment. We will apply the evaluation methods presented to assess the effectiveness of GiPSiNet.

Acknowledgements

The authors acknowledge Technology Opportunities Program (TOP) of Department of Commerce, NASA NNC05CB20C, NSF CCR-039910, NSF IIS-0222743, NSF EIA-0329811, NSF CNS-0423253, and the Virtual Worlds Laboratory at Case Western Reserve University.

References

[1] J. Smed, T. Kaukoranta, H. Hakonen: Aspects of networking in multiplayer computer games, *Proceedings of the International Conference on Applications and Development of Computer Games in the 21st Century* 2001, 74–81.

[2] P. M. Fitts: The information capacity of the human motor system in controlling the amplitude of movement, *Journal of Experimental Psychology* **47**, 1954, 381–391.

[3] P. M. Fitts, J. R. Peterson: Information capacity of discrete motor responses, *Journal of Experimental Psychology* **67**, 1964, 103–113.

[4] D. A. Bowman, J. L. Gabbard, D. Hix: A Survey of Usability Evaluation in Virtual Environments: Classification and Comparison of Methods", *Presence: Teleoperators and Virtual Environments* **11**(4), 2002, 404–424.

[5] D. Hix, H. R. Hartson: *Developing user interfaces: Ensuring usability through product and process*, John Wisley and Sons, 1993.

[6] V. Liberatore, M. C. Cavusoglu, Q. Cai: GiPSiNet: An Open Source/Open Architecture Network Middleware for Surgical Simulations, *Medicine Meets Virtual Reality 14 (MMVR 2006)*, 2006.

[7] M. C. Cavusoglu, T. G. Goktekin, F. Tendick, S. S. Sastry: GiPSi: An Open Source/Open Architecture Software Development Framework for Surgical Simulation, *Medicine Meets Virtual Reality XII (MMVR 2004)*, 2004, 46–48.

[8] M. C. Cavusoglu, T. G. Goktekin, F. Tendick: GiPSi: A Framework for Open Source/Open Architecture Software Development for Organ Level Surgical Simulation, *IEEE Transactions on Information Technology in Biomedicine*, 2005 (In Press).

Medicine Meets Virtual Reality 14
J.D. Westwood et al. (Eds.)
IOS Press, 2006

79

A Biomechanical Analysis of Surgeon's Gesture in a Laparoscopic Virtual Scenario

Filippo CAVALLO [1], Giuseppe MEGALI, Stefano SINIGAGLIA, Oliver TONET,
and Paolo DARIO
CRIM Lab – Scuola Superiore Sant'Anna, Pisa, Italy

Abstract. Minimally invasive surgery (MIS) has become very common in recent years thanks to many advantages that patients can get. However, due to the difficulties surgeons encounter to learn and manage this technique, several training methods and metrics have been proposed in order to, respectively, improve surgeon's abilities and assess his/her surgical skills. In this context, this paper presents a biomechanical analysis method of the surgeon's movements, during exercise involving instrument tip positioning and depth perception in a laparoscopic virtual environment. Estimation of some biomechanical parameters enables us to assess the abilities of surgeons and to distinguish an expert surgeon from a novice. A segmentation algorithm has been defined to deeply investigate the surgeon's movements and to divide them into many sub-movements.

Keywords. Gesture analysis, surgical training, laparoscopy, biomechanics metric, segmentation.

Introduction

MIS has assumed, in the medical scenario, a dominant role as a consequence to the remarkable social and economic improvement that it involves. While on one hand MIS procedures ensure many advantages to patients, on the other hand they require surgeons to undergo a long and difficult training in order to manage and master these techniques. Mainly, surgeons encounter perceptual limitations (lack of stereoscopic view, limited field of view, and reduced force and tactile sensing), and motor limitations (reversed motion, movement scaling and limited degrees-of-freedom) [6]. In this context, a biomechanical analysis is crucial to establish efficient training exercises for enhancing surgeons' dexterity and to define objective metrics for assessing the surgeons' experience and performance.

Most previous works in the field of surgical training in virtual environments revolve around the definition of metrics for an objective evaluation of the surgical performances. One of the main scope is to assess the abilities of surgeons and also to measure the skill level of experts and novices. Many kinematic parameters and various index have been proposed and also segmentation procedures have been employed to characterize different phases of movement [1]-[5]. The segmentation procedure is a more chance to deeply investigate the surgeon's gesture. It allows to split the surgeon's

---

[1] Corresponding author: Filippo Cavallo, CRIM Lab - Scuola Superiore S.Anna, Pisa, Italy; E-mail: f.cavallo@crim.sssup.it

gesture into basic sub-movements: typical procedures include videotape review [3]-[4]. Unfortunately, even if a videotaped segmentation gives the opportunity to annotate the time-line of the entire exercise and identifies sub-movements, however it remains rather subjective and not rigorous.

In this paper the biomechanical parameters, computed from the motion of tip instruments during a typical Laparoscopic procedures, are presented. The scope of this work is, firstly, to investigate the relationship among several parameters, computed on the data concerning a whole exercise. Secondly, to asses the properties of single sub-movements, obtained by means of a segmentation procedure, based only on the tip coordinates. Our aim is to define parameters that allow us to deeply characterize the surgeon's movement during a surgical procedure, and also to distinguish expert surgeons from less experienced surgeons such as residents and novices. A careful consideration is done about the improvement of subjects during the session and their position on the learning curve.

1. Methods

We used the commercial laparoscopic simulator LapSim Basic Skills 2.2 (Surgical Science AB, Göteborg, Sweden) which allows to perform exercises in a virtual environment and easily acquire data concerning instrument positions. This feature gives different subjects the possibility to execute identical exercises, allowing to elaborate generic and objective metrics independent from external variations, and gives the same subject the possibility to perform the same exercise at different times, allowing the monitoring of his/her learning curve.

A group of four novices and a group of two expert surgeons were asked to complete an experimental session of four consecutive trials. Each exercise consisted of reaching, alternatively with the right and left instruments, ten balls (spheres with radius of 15mm) which appeared one at a time in the virtual scenario. These exercises allow to train the surgeon's ability in the bi-manual movement coordination of surgical instruments and in depth perception using laparoscopic view.

1.1. Data processing and parameters

The tip positions of the two instruments, measured by the three encoders of the hardware interface, has been sampled at a frequency of 60 Hz, high enough to describe human gesture [7]. Components of both tips were off-line processed and the parameters listed below were computed. Only low-frequency components are present in surgeon's movements. However due to artefacts and some error of instruments, 3D position data is also contaminated by high-frequency noise. Since our data analysis involves first, second and third derivative, the acquired data are off-line filtered using a numerical fourth-order low-pass Butterworth filter, with cut-off frequency of 25 Hz.

Further a segmentation procedure is used to split the whole exercise in different sub-movements, which correspond to each ball to be reached in the exercise. The first sub-movement (right hand) starts at the beginning of the exercise and finishes as soon as the right tip touches the first ball. Next sub-movements start at the end of the previous ones and finish as soon as the tip touches the next ball. By knowing the position of the ten spheres in the coordinate framework of the virtual scenario, it is possible to detect the time when a tip touches a ball. The algorithm procedure, used for segmentation, evaluates the distance between the centre of the ball and the position of the tip. When it is equal to the ball radius, then the task is completed.

- *Duration (T)*: that is the total time spent by subjects to complete the exercise (measured in seconds).
- *Path length (D)*: that is the length of the trajectory carried out by the tip of instrument during the trial. It is expressed in cm and is defined as:

$$D = \int_0^T \sqrt{\left(\frac{dx}{dt}\right)^2 + \left(\frac{dy}{dt}\right)^2 + \left(\frac{dz}{dt}\right)^2}\, dt \tag{1}$$

- *Mean speed (Vm)*: that is the speed of the tip, calculated with the finite-difference formula and averaged on the entire exercise (measured in cm/s).
- *Maximum speed (Vmax)*: that is the maximum value of the instrument speed during the whole session (cm/s).
- *Mean acceleration (Am)*: that is the acceleration of the tip, calculated with the finite-differences formula and averaged on the entire exercise (m/s^2).
- *Maximum acceleration (Amax)*: that is the maximum value of the instrument acceleration during the whole session (m/s^2).
- *Normalized jerk*: that is a measure of the motion smoothness during each trial and it is a rate of change in acceleration. It is normalized for different task durations and path lengths.

$$\text{Jerk}_{norm} = \sqrt{\frac{T^5}{2D^2} \int_0^T \left[\left(\frac{d^3x}{dt^3}\right)^2 + \left(\frac{d^3y}{dt^3}\right)^2 + \left(\frac{d^3z}{dt^3}\right)^2\right] dt} \tag{2}$$

- *Straightness*: that is the ratio of the straight line, connecting the start and end of the task, and the actual tip path (total distance of the hand travel).
- *Path Deviation*: that is the maximum of perpendicular distance of the tip from the straight line connecting the start and end of the task (measured in cm).
- *IAV*: that is the integral of magnitude of the total acceleration vector (measured in m/s^2) and it represents a value correlated to the energy expenditure during the movement [12].

$$IAV = \int_0^T \sqrt{\left(\frac{d^2x}{dt^2}\right)^2 + \left(\frac{d^2y}{dt^2}\right)^2 + \left(\frac{d^2z}{dt^2}\right)^2}\, dt \tag{3}$$

2. Results

The time spent by subjects in each trials was useful to evaluate improvements in doing the task (Figure 1). Duration of whole experiments in novices was greatly inconstant and the duration trend from the first to the last trial was usually decreasing. In expert surgeons, the duration trend during the session was quite constant, with a mean value less than for the novices. This confirms the fact that experts' improvements usually are less than in the novices. However one of the novices had a constant trend, similar to experts, but with a duration mean value bigger then experts.

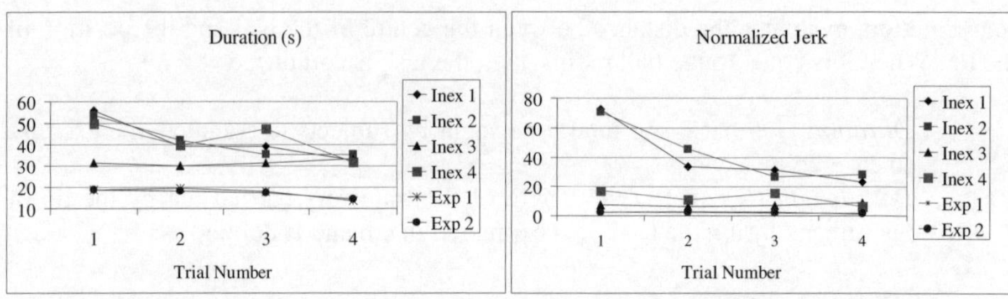

Figure 1. Durations of trial and normalized jerk (scaled by 10^6) for all subjects and trials.

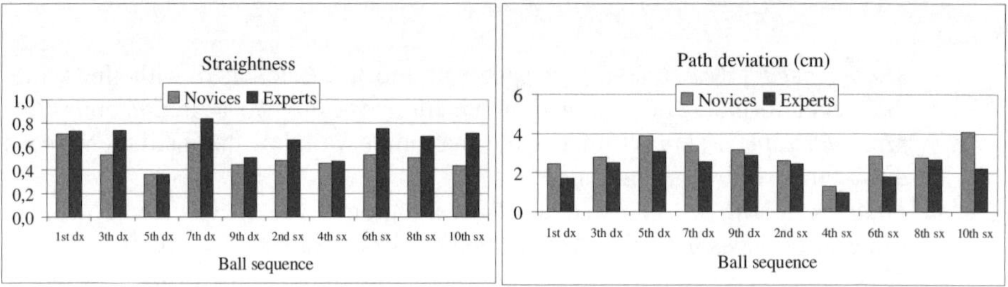

Figure 2. Straightness and path deviation for each single sub-movement.

In all subjects jerk values for both hands were quite similar. In Figure 1 normalized jerk, averaged for right and left hands, is shown for all subjects and trials. Expert surgeon movements appeared to be smoother than those of novices. In fact jerk values in experts were firmly low and constant, and are overlapping and difficult to distinguish in figure. Novices usually had high values, even if in some cases, when they are particularly able, their jerk values were similar to experts.

In Table 1 the mean value of path length, speed (Vm) and acceleration (Am) and the maximum of speed (Vmax) and acceleration (Amax) on the whole session are presented. The path length, on average, was greater in novices and also the differences between right and left hand appeared to be higher. The mean speed was higher for experts and lower for novices, especially for those considered more able by seeing the previous parameters. The mean value of acceleration and maximum speed value for experts were in the middle between the more and less able novices. Furthermore maximum acceleration value typically was low for experts and able novices.

In Figure 2, the straightness and the path deviation, calculated on the single sub-movement and averaged on both groups, are respectively shown. They appeared to be quite inconstant, depending on the single sub-task. On average, the straightness was higher in the expert group, while the path deviation was higher in the novice group.

Table 1. Kinematics parameters for both hands.

	Inex1		inex2		inex3		inex4		exp1		exp2	
	dx	sx	dx	Sx	dx	sx	dx	sx	dx	sx	dx	sx
Path (cm)	92.1	100.9	105.9	113.2	84.2	90.6	144.6	106.0	87.1	92.2	87.5	87.9
Vm (cm/s)	3.5	4.0	4.0	4.3	2.7	2.9	3.4	2.6	5.1	5.3	5.1	5.2
Vmax (cm/s)	52.8	67.7	103.3	70.3	26.2	35.1	32.4	43.0	48.8	43.9	51.1	42.2
Am (m/s^2)	2.4	2.6	2.7	2.9	1.0	1.1	1.2	0.9	1.8	1.9	1.8	1.8
Amax (m/s^2)	39.1	41.9	100.5	56.8	13.6	20.5	15.6	15.1	28.7	14.7	20.7	15.9

The IAV is a value greatly correlated to the energy expenditure of subject during the exercise [9]. In Figure 3, the level of energy expenditure in right and left-task, i.e.

when respectively the right and left hand is used to touch the balls and the other one is not used, are presented. On averaged, the energy expenditure is higher for the hand directly involved in the task, and for both hands it is higher in novices, even if best novices have a level consumption quite similar to experts. In Figure 3 the whole consumption is shown as a sum of consumption of each single sub-task.

3. Discussions

The proposed movement analysis in virtual laparoscopic scenario showed that it is complicated to find a distinctive threshold in the learning curve that permits to easily distinguish an expert from a novice. In fact, in the proposed exercise some inexpert subjects appear to be particularly able with respect to other novices and some of their estimated biomechanical parameters appear to be quite similar to those of experts. Consequently an adequate set of different biomechanical parameters has to be considered in order to estimate the skill level of expert and inexpert subjects.

In the inexpert group we found firstly different levels of ability, according to the personal skill and training experience, and secondly inexpert subjects faster than others to improve their abilities and capabilities during a whole session. Improvement of abilities reflects an high variability, i.e. standard deviation, of estimated parameters during all the trials included in the session. In the expert group, instead, the variability of estimated parameters during the whole session of experiments is low, according to the fact that, after a complete training procedure or a practise made, the level of ability for experts is more uniform.

High standard deviation and a decreasing trend of duration and jerk over the whole session suggests us that a subject is improving his performance and therefore that he is an inexpert surgeon. However subjects belonging to inexpert group with good abilities have shown a low standard deviation and a constant trend, showing a behaviour very similar to the experts, so that they can be confused as experts. This suggests the consideration that each parameter alone is not enough to evaluate the surgeon performances and that different parameters must necessarily be combined together. For example, if the estimation of duration and jerk standard deviation does not permit to assess that the third subject is an inexpert, because of that values are very similar to the expert subjects, however the averaged speed demonstrated how the third subject is actually the slowest one. As well, also the fourth subject has a jerk profile similar to the experts, but the averaged speed is lower and the duration is pretty long.

The mean speed appears to be higher in experts. In the inexpert group, instead, the mean speed is higher for the less able novices: this is due to the fact that more able novices are more circumspect in using instruments (lowest Amax and Vmax) and less able novices are characterized by possible unexpected and non-smooth movements (highest Amax and Vmax), typical of inexpert subjects. For the same reason, the mean acceleration is higher for less able novices and lower for more able.

Jerk values for experts has a low variability and lower mean value respect to the others. However some case of inexpert with a low variability and a similar mean value can be detect. Figure 1 seems to suggest us that there are four experts and two novices, but this is consequence of being very circumspect for novices that actually spent about ten seconds more than experts in completing task and have a little bit low mean speed.

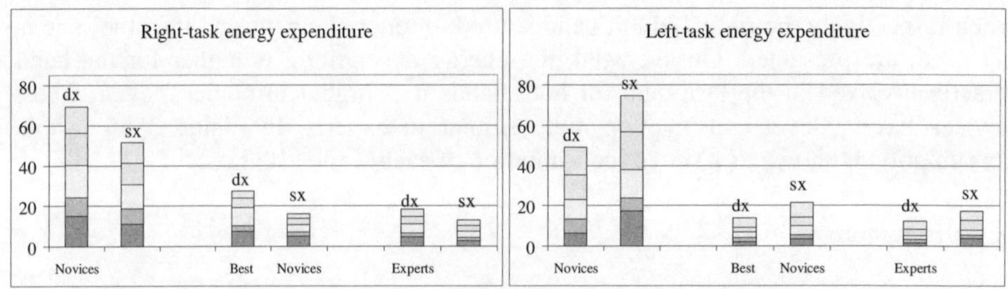

Figure 3. Energy expenditure for whole exercise and single sub-task in both hands.

The higher straightness and lower path deviation for experts denote that their path, covered during the trial, is more straight toward the task to be reached. Interestingly, straightness and path deviation appear to be very heterogeneous on all ten sub-tasks. We believe that it is due, firstly, to different depth perception of the balls in the virtual scenario framework, which in some case lead to more limited perception. Secondly, because of the constraint of trocars, subjects encounter more difficult in performing a direct path from one task to another.

4.   Conclusions

In this article a biomechanical analysis of the surgeon's gesture was performed and some parameters, calculated only using the coordinate of instrument tips, were defined to, firstly, assess the abilities of surgeons in the bi-manual movement of surgical instruments and in depth perception and, secondly, to find a criterion to distinguish experts from novices. Further a segmentation procedure, based on tip coordinates, was used to deeply investigate each single sub-movements of the gesture. This work shows that an adequate and substantial set of parameters is necessary to investigate and analyze the surgeon's performance. Actually this work is still in progress and our future commitment in this field is to analyze more complex surgical procedures with other sensor systems.

References

[1] S. Cotin, N. Stylopoulos, M. Ottensmeyer, P. Neumann, D. Rattner, and S. Dawson, "Metrics for laparoscopic skills trainers: the weakest link!", LNCS 2488 (Berlin Heidelberg) (T. Dohi and R. Kikinis, eds.), MICCAI 2002, Springer Verlag, 2002, pp. 35–43.

[2] D.Risucci, J.A. Cohen, J.E. Garbus, M. Goldestein, and M.G. Cohen, "The effects of practise and instruction on speed and accuracy during resident acquisition of simulated laparoscopic skills", Current Surgery, 2001.

[3] S. Payandeh, A.J Lomax, J. Dill, C.L. Mackenzie, and C.G.L. Cao, "On defining metrics for assessing laparoscopic surgical skills in a virtual training environment", MMVR, 2002.

[4] C.G.L. Cao, C.L. Mackenzie, and S. Payandeh, "Task and motion analyses in endoscopic surgery", ASME IMECE Conf. Proceedings, 1996, pp. 583-590.

[5] L.Verner, D. Oleynikov, S. Holtmann, H. Haider, and L. Zhukov, "Measurements of the level of surgical expertise using flight path analysis from da Vinci^{TM} robotic surgical system", MMVR 11, 2003. 373-78.

[6] J. Shah, and A. Darzi, "The impact of inherent and environmental factors on surgical performance in laparoscopy: a review", Min Invas Ther & Allied Tecnholo, 12, 69-75, 2003.

[7] G.C. Burdea, "Force and touch feedback for virtual reality", Wiley Interscience Publication, July 1996.

[8] G. Megali, S. Sinigaglia, O. Tonet, and P. Dario, "Modelling and Evaluation of Surgical Performance using Hidden Markov Model", IEEE Trans Biomed Eng, 2005, submitted.

[9] K. Tsurumi, T. Itani, N. Tachi, T. Takanishi, H. Suzumura, and H. Takeyama, "Estimation of energy expenditure during sedentary work with upper limb movement", J. Occup. Health, 2002, 44, 408-413.

Smart Tool for Force Measurements During Knee Arthroscopy: In Vivo Human Study

G. Chami*[1], J. Ward[1], D. Wills[1], R. Phillips[1], K. Sherman[2]
[1]Department of Computer Science, University of Hull, Hull, UK, HU6 7RX.
[2]Hull and East Yorkshire Hospitals NHS Trust.
**Email: g.chami@hull.ac.uk*

Abstract. This paper describes the magnitude and patterns of forces obtained by using a probe, equipped with a six-axis force torque sensor, in knee arthroscopy. The probe was used by orthopaedic surgeons and trainees, who performed 11 different tasks in 10 standard knee arthroscopies. The force magnitude and patterns generated are presented; which can support the development of virtual arthroscopy systems with realistic haptic feedback. The results were compared across both groups of surgeons. A difference in the force patterns generated by senior versus junior surgeons was noted which can aid in the development of an objective assessment system for arthroscopy skills. The results could potentially be useful to assess future performance in real arthroscopy.

1. Background

Arthroscopic skills are essential for orthopaedic surgeons and form a standard part of their training. These skills are hard to acquire and they need a long learning curve to master [1]. Virtual arthroscopy provides risk-free and cost-effective training material [2]. It aims to mimic real arthroscopy by providing similar visualisation and haptic force feedback. The visual realism of virtual arthroscopy can be easily compared to video recording of real arthroscopy which is ready available. However there is little published data of the haptic feedback forces that occur in real arthroscopy, which is certainly useful when for the development and validation of Virtual Arthroscopy systems.

The scope of the study presented in this paper was to measure the forces applied through the arthroscopic probe handle during standard tasks of knee arthroscopy. An additional purpose of the study was to analyse the force patterns generated by arthroscopically skilled surgeons versus orthopaedic trainees, which could then be used to inform an automated and objective assessment of surgeons performance during both real and virtual arthroscopies.

2. Methodology

A smart arthroscopic tool was built using a standard arthroscopic probe fitted with a six degree of freedom force torque sensor FT [3] with necessary modifications to meet safety and sterility requirements (Figure 1). The FT sensor is capable of measuring up to a maximum of 50 N force and 500 mNm torque, with a resolution of 50 mN and 0.25 mNm, respectively. All six FT parameters (Fx, Fy, Fz, Tx, Ty, Tz) were recorded at a sample rate of 170 Hz. Each sample was also time-stamped (1ms resolution clock). The tool was tested for electrical safety HEI 95 as per Medical Devices Agency Guidelines. Ethical Committee approval was obtained for its use during standard knee arthroscopy procedures.

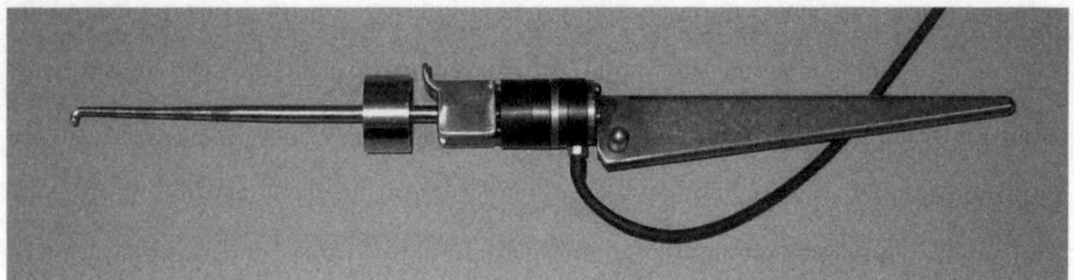

Figure 1. Probe equipped with 6-axis force torque

Four surgeons, with differing levels of experience in the operation, were asked to perform 11 separate tasks as shown in Table 1 during knee arthroscopy procedure for two patients. The sensor was zeroed outside the knee at the start of each task. The procedure was video recorded along with an audio signal from the computer to allow synchronization with the force data. The FT signal graph was later superimposed on the video (Figure 2). It is then possible to view the force profile associated with any given task.

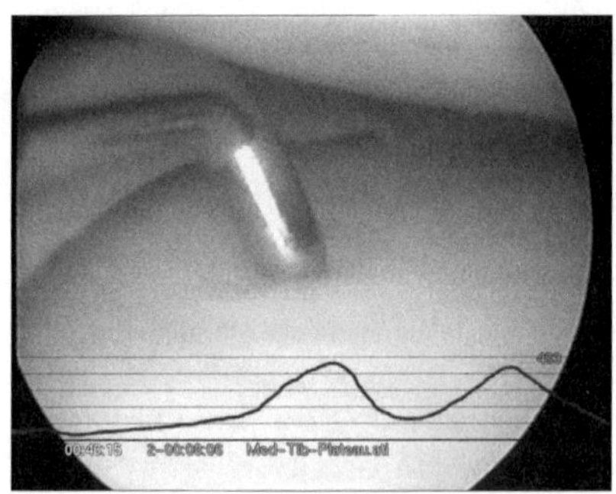

Figure 2. F/T graph overlaid on video The graph scrolls right-to-left in time with the video, and shows peak values.

Table 1. Tasks performed during a knee arthroscopy session

No.	Task Description
T01	Probing medial femoral condyle at three points: Superior, Middle and Inferior. Press each twice.
T02	Probing medial tibial plateau at three points: Posterior, Middle and Anterior. Press each twice.
T03	Probing medial meniscus. Continuous run once, then three points: Posterior, Middle and Anterior. Press each twice.
T04	Probing under surface of medial meniscus. Continuous run once, lift at Posterior middle and Anterior margin twice.
T05	Probing anterior cruciate ligament. Continuous run once, then two pulls.
T06	Probing lateral femoral condyle. Three points: Superior, Middle, Inferior. Pressing each twice.

T07	Probing lateral tibial plateau. Three points: Posterior, Middle, Anterior. Press each twice.
T08	Probing lateral meniscus. Continuous run once, then press at three points: Anterior, Middle, Posterior. Press each twice.
T09	Probing popliteal hiatus, two pulls.
T10	Probing under surface of lateral meniscus. Continuous run once, lift at posterior middle and anterior margin twice.
T12	Probing under surface of patella. Three points: Medial, Middle, Lateral. Press each twice.

The trials demonstrated that forces can be broadly categorized into two force groups: 1) navigation forces which are likely to be generated from the soft tissue around the entry port, 2) procedure force features such as probing the meniscus which are manifested as peaks. For each case, the FT data was analysed in terms of these two categories.

To support comparison between experienced and less experienced arthroscopists, the procedure was repeated with two skilled surgeons (more than 500 procedures) and two trainees (less than 20 procedures). Ten knee arthroscopies were performed and the forces applied by each group were compared.

3. Results

The force magnitude *Fm* was calculated as the length of the vector (Fx, Fy, Fz) for the navigation force in the three compartments of the knee. The mean and standard deviation of the force magnitude Fm and torque magnitude Tm for all users are shown in Figure 3. It is noted that there was generally more resistance to the movement of the instrument in the lateral compartment. This was reflected in an increase of the mean force magnitude from 1102.9 to 1273.4mN, and from 95.7 to 110.6mNm in the torque magnitude. This could be due to the placement of the probe entry point in the medial compartment which forces the probe to push onto the anterior cruciate ligament or the fat pad in order to reach the lateral compartment.

Although navigation forces in the patella femoral joint are generally lower than those observed in the medial compartment with a mean of 803.4mN versus 1102.9mN, an increase in the mean torque magnitude from 95.7 to 103mNm was measured, as the surgeon had to apply greater twisting forces in order to probe the chondral surface of the patella.

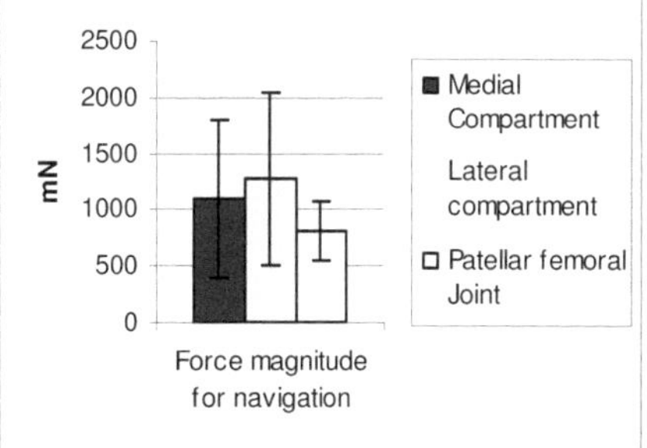

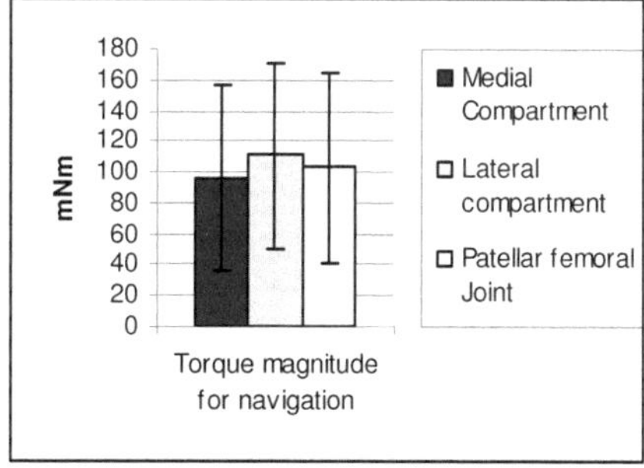

Figure 3. Navigation forces

The procedural features for each task were identified. The changes in torque magnitude measured at the sensor are quite large, as would be expected given the long lever arm of the instrument, and correspond well with the procedural features that were used in this study. The average magnitude of the torques for each feature in each task was calculated as the mean length of the vector (Tx, Ty, Tz). The navigation torque magnitude which is located on both sides of each feature was identified by the lowest magnitude that occurs after the end of the peak within 0.1 second.   The mean magnitude for the area either side of the feature peaks was calculated, then subtracted that from the peak. This is intended to reduce the effect of the torques generated from either soft tissue pressure or pivoting of the probe arm on the feature. The results are shown in Figure 4 and Table 2.

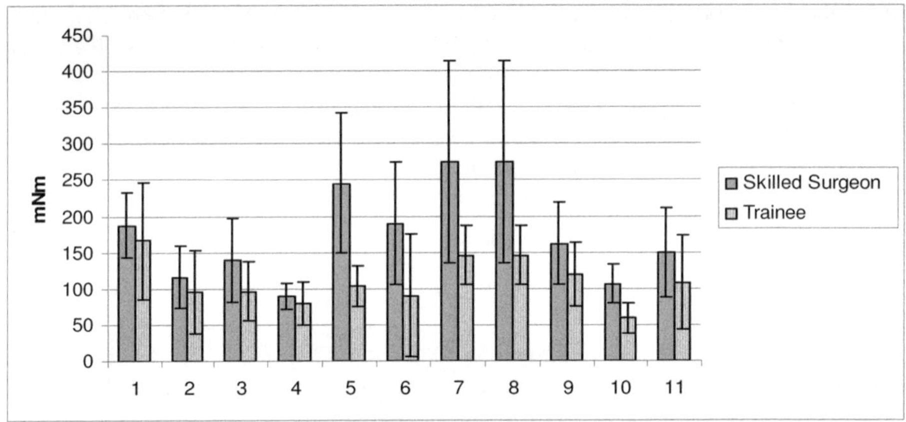

Figure 4. Torque magnitude for each procedural feature by tasks

Table 2. Torque magnitude for each procedure feature in tasks.

Task No.	T01	T02	T03	T04	T05	T06	T07	T08	T09	T10	T11
Skilled Surgeon (mNm)	187	116	139	89	245	189	275	275	162	106	150
Trainee (mNm)	166	95	96	80	104	90	146	146	120	59	108

It is noted that the mean procedural features produced by the skilled surgeons are more pronounced when compared with features produced by trainees. This is clearly reflected in the increase in the magnitude of the feature for the skilled surgeon as shown in Figure 4 and it is observable in all tasks. The difference is larger in more difficult tasks such as probing the lateral meniscus as shown in Figure 4. Furthermore, the standard deviation in feature magnitude per-surgeon is lower for the skilled surgeon, which suggests that they are more consistent. The average duration of the forces for probing a chondral surface was 0.85 seconds, while 0.89 seconds was observed when probing the meniscus and 1.2 seconds when pulling on the anterior cruciate ligament.

Less noise was observed in the force patterns generated by skilled surgeons versus trainees as shown in Figure 5; this indicates that skilled surgeons were more economical in terms of movement.

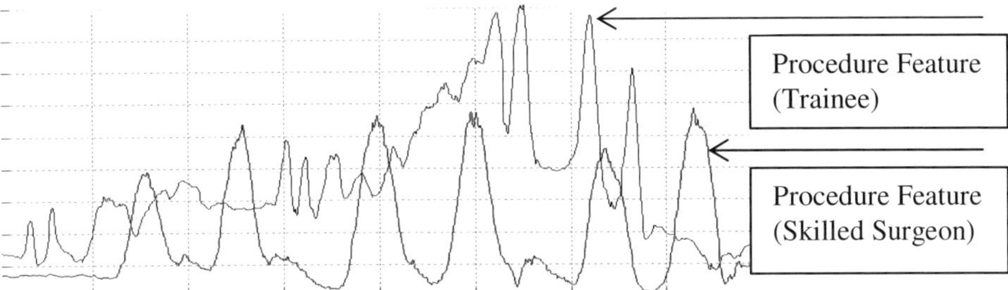

Figure 5. Torque magnitude generated by a skilled surgeon and trainee for the same task (T06). The skilled surgeon generates more pronounced features and better matches the number of required probes in the task. There was also less noise between features.

It was noted that using the probe over an irregular surface such as cartilage fibrillation generated high frequency noise that has the potential to be used in diagnosis of pathologies.

4. Conclusion

Tactile sensing in knee arthroscopy differs according to the surgeon, procedure, and the probe position and incision site. Measuring and recording these forces using smart tools adds important information to the procedure, which has many beneficial aspects.

This study yielded useful information about the range and distribution of forces that is relevant to the design of force feedback devices, in terms of peak and continuous operating force requirements. The data is also useful as a standard of comparison, so that simulated tasks with force feedback can be evaluated against pre-recorded tasks from this study.

Parameters for comparison between junior and senior arthroscopists were also investigated. Although the feature magnitudes and standard deviation was consistently higher for skilled surgeons versus trainees, it will require a larger study to reliably demonstrate the effect of experience levels on the force pattern generated by the surgeon. The study also suggests that the force pattern can be used to assess certain pathology such as cartilage fibrillation and osteoarthritis.

References

1. Miller, W.E., Learning arthroscopy. South Med J, 1985. 78(8): p. 935-7.
2. Sherman, K.P., et al., A portable virtual environment knee arthroscopy training system with objective scoring. Stud Health Technol Inform, 1999. 62: p. 335-6.
3. Ward JW,. et al, The Acquisition of Force Feedback Data for a Virtual Environment Knee Arthroscopy Training System. in Virtual Reality and 3D Modelling Symposium, Advanced Simulation Technologies Conference (ASTC '99). 1999. San Diego CA.

Medicine Meets Virtual Reality 14
J.D. Westwood et al. (Eds.)
IOS Press, 2006

Factors Affecting Targeting Using the Computer Assisted Orthopaedic Surgery System (CAOSS)

G. Chami*[1], R. Phillips[1], J.W. Ward[1], M.S. Bielby[1], A.M.M.A. Mohsen[2]
[1]Department of Computer Science, University of Hull, Hull, UK, HU6 7RX.
[2]Hull and East Yorkshire Hospitals NHS Trust.
**Email: g.chami@hull.ac.uk*

Abstract: An advantage of CAOS over traditional surgery is improved precision of implant position and trajectories in 3D space. However, the implementation of these trajectories often adds an extra step to the operation that increases operative time and requires extra training. This paper reports a study of variation in time-to-task and learning curve in performing a standard task of targeting in 3D space using Hull's CAOSS . It shows that time-to-task can be reduced by replacing a 3D targeting task with multiple independent 2D targeting tasks whilst potentially reducing targeting error. Based on this better understanding of targeting a novel jig was developed for performing dynamic hip Screw (DHS) insertion using CAOSS that would provide improved targeting performance by the surgeon.

1. Background.

Over the past ten years or so CAOS has been applied to most fields of orthopaedic surgery such as joint replacement [1] and osteotomy. This new technology has failed to be widely used in hospitals despite published literature clearly showing that CAOS improves the accuracy of implant position [2]. Some of the main reasons seem to be the increase in the operative time [3] and additional training. The aim of the study presented here is to address these issues by analysing factors affecting time-to-procedure and learning curves of a standard task in CAOS, namely, positioning a wire on a planned trajectory in 3D space..

2. Methods.

The Computer Assisted Orthopaedic Surgical System (CAOSS) [4] developed by Hull University and the Hull NHS Trust hospitals was used for the study. CAOSS comprises of a standard C-arm image intensifier, a computer and an optical tracking system that tracks an end-effector attached to a hand lockable passive arm. The position of the x-ray cone of the image intensifier is achieved using a tracked registration phantom. CAOSS typically creates a 3D surgical plan for an operations by reconstructing information from a pair of 2D fluoroscopic images of the targeted bone. The positional accuracy of CAOSS has been shown to be within 0.7 mm with angular accuracy within 0.2 degrees. The computer guides the surgeon to a planned trajectory by a quantitative graphical display of a targeting screen with one cross indicating the entry point of the end-effector whilst the another cross indicates the alignment position. Also displayed is the positioning error from the target in terms of spatial position and angle.

The study involved six users. Each performed a standard task of positioning a K-wire, using a planned trajectory for a dynamic hip screw operation (DHS). This involved three sub-tasks, namely: 1) reaching an entry point position for a guiding cannula held in the end-effector; 2) obtaining accurate alignment of the end-effector; 3) maintaining the position of the end-effector by locking the mechanical arm. Times were recorded for six different conditions, namely: a) achieving a position with an error of less than 1 mm; b) achieving a position with an error of less than 2 mm; c) changing the position of the display screen; d) performing the three sub-tasks in sequence but allowing the tip of the guiding cannula to be placed on the bone which helps preserve position (as in CAOSS); e) performing the sub-tasks in sequence but without contact with the bone; f) performing the sub-tasks in sequence and independently, i.e. without having to maintain position of the previous sub-tasks . Each user repeated a task nine times in order to evaluate the learning curve of the task.

3. Results.

Training reduced targeting task time from an average of 180 seconds (s) to 59 s with the most reduction being for locking the arm. The standard deviation between users reduced from 65s to 13s. The best improvements were observed when performing the sub-tasks independently, or when the error margin was increased (see Fig. 1).

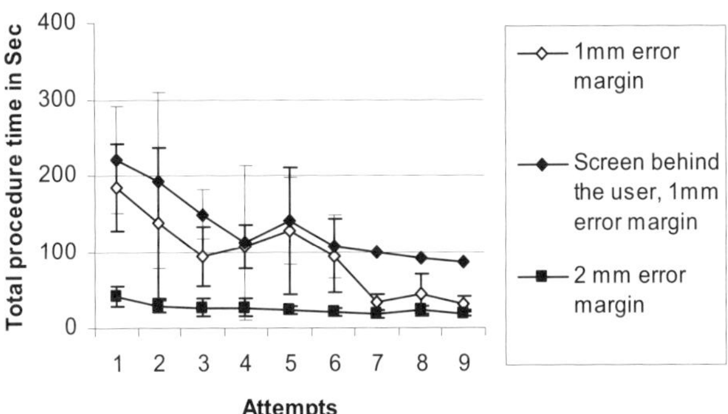

Figure 1: Learning curve of the task for the different conditions.

Increasing the error margin from 1 mm to 2 mm had two beneficial effects; it reduced the standard deviation in task time between users from 38 s to 8 s and it reduced the task time from an average of 59 s to 20 s.

In the operating theatre it is not always possible to position the display in front of the surgeon, which may impair performance. This was verified experimentally by positioning the display screen behind the user. The task time in this case increased from an average of 59 s to 113 s and it had minimal effect on the learning curve.

When the 3D targeting task was broken down into multiple independent 2D targeting sub-tasks (i.e. condition f), the total time averaged 13 s, with a shorter learning curve. However, when the same sub-tasks were performed in sequence and allowing the instrument tip to be placed on the bone (i.e. condition d), the average time was 59 s. However, when no such assistance for instrument positioning was allowed (i.e. condition e), task time increased to an average of 371 s with a large standard deviation between users of 114 s (see Fig. 2).

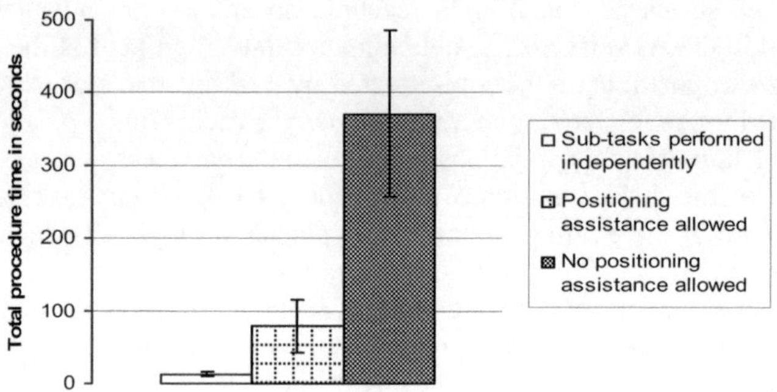

Figure 2: The effect on targeting time with different constraints between sub-tasks.

4. Discussion and conclusions.

Ideally CAOS should be easy to use, fast to learn, and a change in the precision of the procedure having minimal effect on task performance. The results of the study indicate that the present targeting system of CAOSS is less than ideal. They suggest that targeting performance of a sureon can be improved, in terms of training and procedure time, by replacing the 3D targeting task with multiple independent 2D targeting tasks.

To improve targeting in CAOSS for the DHS operation a novel jig has been devised. This has multiple, parallel drilling canals, arranged at an angle of 135 degrees to a base plane and attached to tracking frame.. The jig's base acts as a fulcrum to rotate the jig over the proximal femoral shaft so as to assist targeting of the anteversion angle of the femoral neck. From a planned trajectory, CAOSS indicates the optimal canal to drill through. Thus the new jig breaks down the 3D targeting task into separate independent 2D targeting tasks. The built-in 135 degree angle effectively removes one of the 2D targeting tasks. The entry point position is targeted by indicating to the surgeon the position of the nearest drilling canal in columns and rows. The only targeting task left to the surgeon is the 2D targeting task of aligning the drilling canal trajectory with the anteversion angle of the femoral neck.

References

.1.   Keppler, P., et al., *Computer aided high tibial open wedge osteotomy.* Injury, 2004. 35 Suppl 1: p. S-A68-78.

2.   Jolles, B.M., P. Genoud, and P. Hoffmeyer, *Computer-assisted cup placement techniques in total hip arthroplasty improve accuracy of placement.* Clin Orthop Relat Res, 2004(426): p. 174-9.

3.   Langlotz, F., *Potential pitfalls of computer aided orthopedic surgery.* Injury, 2004. 35 Suppl 1: p. S-A17-23.

4.   Phillips, R., et al., *A phantom based approach to fluoroscopic navigation for orthopaedic surgery.* in *Medical Image Computing and Computer Assisted Intervention, MICCAI.* 2004. Rennes St-Malo.

Medicine Meets Virtual Reality 14
J.D. Westwood et al. (Eds.)
IOS Press, 2006

Contouring in 2D While Viewing Stereoscopic 3D Volumes

W.K. Chia and Luis Serra
Volume Interactions Pte. Ltd.

Abstract: The ability to manually specify contours in a volumetric data is often required in situations when automatic algorithms are unable to accurately extract the desire volume. Conventionally, the contours are drawn over a slice, working on plane-by-plane basis usually constrained to orthogonal planes. In defining the contour on a 2D image, the user faces the problem of loosing 3D context (does the tissue belong to inside the contour or outside?). This requires the constant back and forth movement from a plane view where the interaction takes place (usually with the mouse) to the 3D volumetric view that provides the contextual information. We present an interactive environment that allows for efficient contouring while providing contextual 3D information to the user.

Keywords: contours; semi-automatic segmentation, integrated virtual environment

1. Introduction

One of the shortcomings of automatic segmentation is that while it is always desirable, it might not always yield the accurate or desired results required by the user. The ability to manually define contours and perform segmentation using the contours provides a viable alternative to automatic segmentation in certain situations. However, the use of contours as a mean of segmentation has its own set of challenges. Defining contours can be time consuming, especially if there is a need to define a lot of contours to achieve the desired segmentation result. The contours are also drawn on a 2D image and hence there is a loss in its equivalent 3D context.

Most current approaches use a window-based approach and require the user to work in either 2D or 3D context at any one time. Users define the contours in one window and switch to another window to view the position of the contours in the 3D context. The 3D view is important in the proper understanding of relation of the contours with reference to the volume object so as to effectively perform accurate segmentation. This involves multiple switching between the 2D and 3D views, hence making contours definition tedious and inefficient.

In this paper, we present a novel interaction paradigm of integrating a 2D interface for contour definition within a 3D virtual environment. This integrated virtual environment provides users with the ability to work comfortably in 2D and at the same time showing a clear and stereoscopic representation of the 3D object where the contours are being drawn, making it easy and efficient to accurately define contours.

2. Method

2.1. Configuration

The interaction paradigm for the above mentioned contouring is based on the Dextroscope®, a two-handed stereoscopic 3D virtual reality environment for working with medical images [1]. The user interacts with the 3D volume through 3D tracking devices on each hand: the right hand holds a pen-like stylus, while the left holds a joystick-like 6-DOF controller. Precise 3D interaction is ensured through a combination of comfortable arm resting and pivoting of the hands around the wrist. Intuitive 2D interaction is achieved by providing passive haptic feedback by means of a *virtual control panel* whose position coincides with the physical surfaces encasing the system [2]. The stylus interacts with the widgets as though it was a mouse, in a similar fashion to [3].

We have taken advantage of the virtual control panel to provide an efficient 2D contour-editing environment. We use the stylus to manually draw the contours over the virtual control panel as though it was a 'tablet'. Simultaneously, the user sees in the 3D space above the control panel the results of the 2D work inserted into the volume rendered data set. This setup results in a single integrated environment in which users can simultaneously benefit from comfortable 2D contouring over an image slice while visualizing stereoscopically the relation of the contours with the volume object in 3D. Figure 1 shows the integrated virtual environment

2.2. Extension

Our proposed paradigm also includes the implementation of a range of tools that, whenever possible, provide automation for the definition of the contours. Examples include active contours [4] and Livewire [5]. Once defined, the contours can be used to create either a closed polygonal surface or to extract the volume within, allowing volume segmentation and subsequently volumetric calculations. The virtual environment also allows for the visualization of automatically generated 4D (in space-time domain) contours of the heart [6], making it valuable for visualizing contours like contours of cardiac walls, etc. The implementation of a range of semi-automatic tools, with the tight integration of the 3D virtual environment has provided greater efficiency and flexibility in the contours definition process, compared with just implementing these tools within a pure 2D environment.

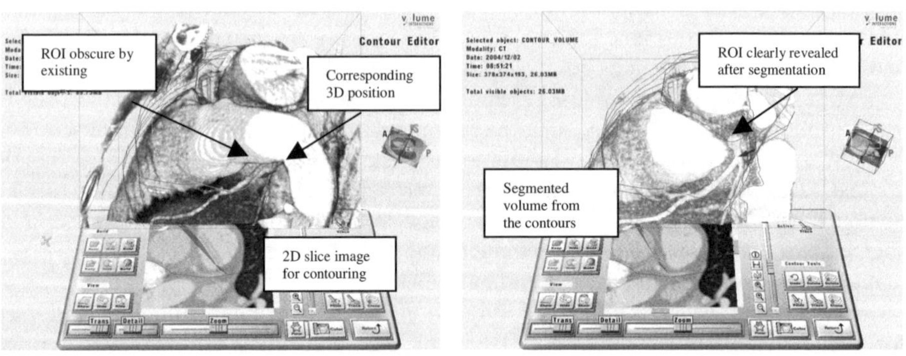

Figure 1: Left shows the contouring on 2D slice with position reflected by the arrow in the 3D. Right shows the segmented volume base on the contours with ROI clearly revealed.

3. Results

Neurosurgeons routinely use the Contour Editor on the Dextroscope to segment difficult tumors in the brain as part of their surgical planning. It has also been used in two occasions to segment the brains of conjoined twins to plan their separation. Radiologists use the editor as part of their diagnostic process to extract the heart from the rib-cage, and to isolate the liver from the surrounding structures. In addition, the Contour Editor is also used to facilitate the use of other automatic algorithms. The user first roughly defines key regions of interest and performs a first level segmentation. This result is then fed as an input into our existing automatic segmentation algorithms. This has yielded better results because in the initial stage, the user is able to apply his domain knowledge to remove the "noise" from the initial data and provide the automatic algorithms with a better-defined dataset for automatic segmentation. Contours defined in one volume object can also be mapped to another co-registered volume object of another modality to give users a better perspective of the spatial relationship of the contours with other objects. 4D contours generated automatically from existing cardiac software are also loaded into the editor in which users can visualize and refine the auto-generated contours.

4. Conclusion

While automatic segmentation is a desired feature, semi-automatic segmentation using contours still has an important role due to its flexibility and its ability to directly include the user input. The challenge is to make the process more effective for the user. The proposed interaction paradigm provides a novel way of integrating a 2D interface for contour definition within a 3D virtual environment. It provides users with a clearer representation of the contours and their spatial relationship with the volume object. This provides for fast and accurate tracing of the contours, resulting in an efficient workflow in performing segmentation. As the user is able to provide the inputs interactively, this allows greater control and flexibility in the volume segmentation workflow. This paradigm effectively bridges the functional gap between manual, semi-automatic and fully automatic segmentation procedures.

5. References

[1]　Kockro RA et al. Planning and Simulation of Neurosurgery in a Virtual Reality Environment, Neurosurgery, 46 (1), pp. 118-137.

[2]　Serra et al. An Interface For Precise And Comfortable 3D Work With Volumetric Medical Datasets, in MMVR7, pp. 328-334.

[3]　Sowizral, H.A., (1994) Interacting with virtual environments using augmented virtual tools, In Proc. Stereoscopic Displays and Virtual Reality Systems 94, SPIE, 2177, pp. 409-416.

[4]　M. Kass, A. Witkin, and D. Terzopoulos. Snakes: active contour models. International Journal of Computer Vision 1(4), pp. 321-331, 1988.

[5]　E.N.Mortensen, W.A.Barrett, Intelligent Scissors for Image Composition, Computer Graphics (SIGGRAPH '95), pp. 191-198, Los Angeles, CA, Aug. 1995

[6]　Magnetic Resonance Ventricular Analysis, http://www.piecaas.com

Medicine Meets Virtual Reality 14
J.D. Westwood et al. (Eds.)
IOS Press, 2006

Integrative Haptic and Visual Interaction for Simulation of PMMA Injection During Vertebroplasty

Chee-Kong Chui[a, 1], Jeremy Teo[a], Zhenlan Wang[a], Jackson Ong[a], Jing Zhang[b], Kuan-Ming Si-hoe[a], Sim-Heng Ong[b, c], Chye-Hwang Yan[b], Shih-Chang Wang[d], Hee-Kit Wong[d], James H. Anderson[e], and Swee-Hin Teoh[a]

[a] *Department of Mechanical Engineering*
[b] *Department of Electrical & Computer Engineering*
[c] *Division of Bioengineering*
[d] *Faculty of Medicine, National University of Singapore, Singapore*
[e] *Johns Hopkins University School of Medicine, Baltimore, USA*

Abstract. In vertebroplasty, physician relies on both sight and feel to properly place the bone needle through various tissue types and densities, and to help monitor the injection of PMMA or cement into the vertebra. Incorrect injecting and reflux of the PMMA into areas where it should not go can result in detrimental clinical complication. This paper focuses on the human-computer interaction for simulating PMMA injection in our virtual spine workstation. Fluoroscopic images are generated from the CT patient volume data and simulated volumetric flow using a time varying 4D volume rendering algorithm. The user's finger movement is captured by a data glove. Immersion CyberGrasp is used to provide the variable resistance felt during injection by constraining the user's thumb. Based on our preliminary experiments with our interfacing system comprising simulated fluoroscopic imaging and haptic interaction, we found that the former has a larger impact on the user's control during injection.

Keywords. Haptic rendering, PMMA injection, virtual reality, human-machine interface

1. Introduction

In vertebroplasty, physician relies on both sight and feel to properly place the bone needle through various tissue types and densities, and to help monitor the injection of polymethylmethacrylate(PMMA) or cement into the vertebra. Over injecting and reflux of the PMMA into areas where it should not go can result in detrimental clinical complication. Apart from the visual cues from real time fluoroscopic imaging, the physician uses his haptic senses to regulate the rate and amount of injection. This paper focuses on the human-computer interaction for simulating PMMA injection in our virtual spine workstation.

---

[1] Corresponding Author: Chee-Kong Chui, Centre for Biomedical Materials Applications & Technology, E3-05-23, Engineering Drive 3, S(119260), Singapore. Email: mpecck@nus.edu.sg

Many interactive simulation systems for needle placement surgeries have been reported, and many of these systems include haptic interactions for needle placement [1]. In comparison, there are few works on simulation of realistic injection [2]. PMMA injection is a complex image guided procedure that requires a high degree of hand-eye coordination skills on the physician. For realistic training, real surgical devices should be used, and haptic interaction should be implemented in combination with simulated fluoroscopic views. It is interesting to study the relative importance of fluoroscopic imaging and haptic feedback to physician during PMMA injection.

2. Materials and Methods

The amount of force feedback during injection is calculated based on the rate, location, rheological parameters of PMMA and volume of injection over time using finite element method. We start with a needle already inserted, and assume that the flow will follow a defined path in the vertebral body from the needle tip. The path shaped like a tree with multiple branches, each modeled as a rigid generalized cylinder with uniform wall thickness. Excessive injection will cause PMMA to flow out from the path. The flow is stored as a volume data with voxel value indicating the intensity of flow. The computational model and biomechanical simulation serves as the linkage between haptic and visual renderings.

The physician relies heavily on the fluoroscopic view as well as the haptic sense in controlling the amount of force he is to use in pushing the PMMA through the syringe with his thumb, and hence, controlling the rate and volume of injection. Resultant volume data from the computation and the original CT patient data are input to a 4D volume rendering algorithm [3] with maximum intensive projection to generate the fluoroscopic image. The user's finger movement is captured by an Immersion CyberGlove data glove. The CyberGrasp is used to provide the variable resistance felt during injection by pulling the user's thumb at various levels. Figure 1 illustrates the control flow between the various components in this integrative haptics and visual approach. The simulation is driven by the biomechanical models.

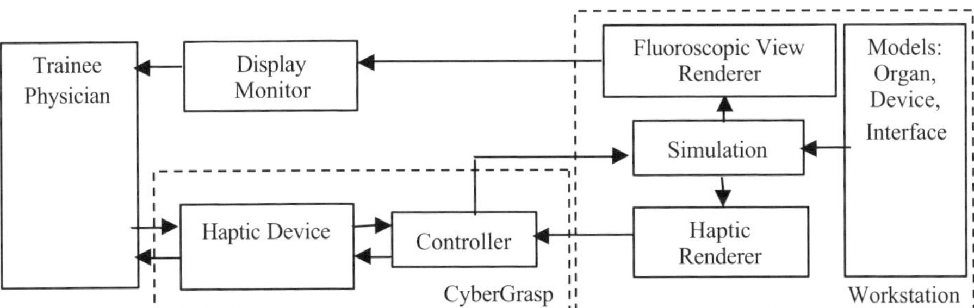

Figure 1. Integrative haptic and visual control

3. Results

Figure 2(a), (b), (c) are snapshot of the implementation, clinical syringe for injection, and force feedback glove respectively. We can achieve real time interaction (15Hz of graphics, and approximately 500Hz for haptic rendering) on an Intel P4-based workstation. The maximum variable force component felt on the thumb is 12N. Our preliminary experience indicates that real time fluoroscopic imaging is the main source of influence. We hope to conduct experiments involving a large pool of diverse users for better assessment.

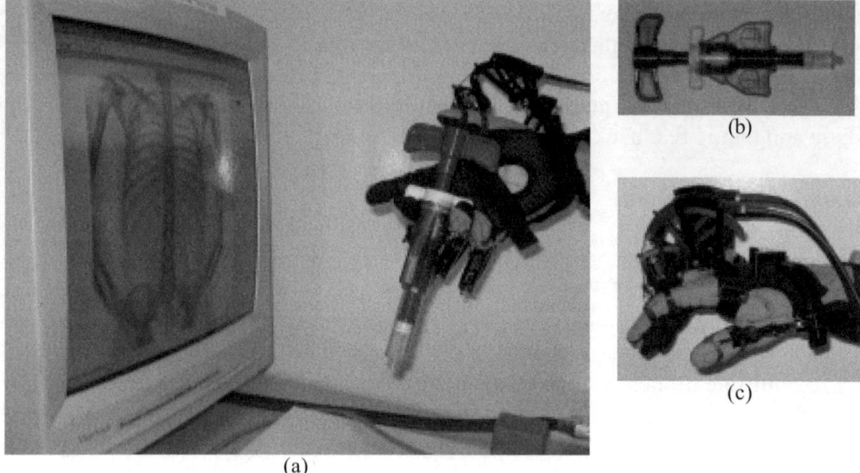

Figure 2. Overview of haptic and visual interaction for simulation of PMMA injection

4. Discussion and Conclusions

Our interfacing system with simulated fluoroscopic imaging and haptic interaction using real surgical syringe is applicable to training of other image guided injection process. This setup is efficient and effective by focusing on the essential components - the haptic feedback is on the thumb, and computation and resultant visual update occurs around the needle path. There is no need to model the whole vertebra. We are also exploring the possibility of using lower cost lower resolution gaming gloves to replace the CyberGrasp system for a less expensive solution.

For realistic surgical planning, a more complex computational model that is patient specific in both geometrical and biomechanical senses is desired. In bone, pathology such as tissue destruction or tumor present a different resistance to the force needed to inject PMMA into the vertebra. More quantitative validation will be planned for this clinically viable computational model and simulation.

Acknowledgement

The authors wish to thank Singapore's Agency of Science and Technology (A-STAR) for support of this research.

References

[1]   Ra, JB et al. A visually guided spine biopsy simulator with force feedback, SPIE Medical Imaging, pp 36-45, 2001

[2]   Dang, T. et al. Development and evaluation of an epidural injection simulator with force feedback for medical training, Studies in Health Technology and Informatics, vol 25, pp 564-579, 1996.

[3]   Wang, Z et al. DLLO-based volume rendering algorithms for interactive microsurgical simulation, International Journal Imaging & Graphics, 2005. accepted

Medicine Meets Virtual Reality 14
J.D. Westwood et al. (Eds.)
IOS Press, 2006

Flow Visualization for Interactive Simulation of Drugs Injection During Chemoembolization

Chee-Kong Chui[a, b, 1], Yiyu Cai[c], Zhenlan Wang[a], Xiuzi Ye[d], James H. Anderson[e],
Swee-Hin Teoh[a] and Ichiro Sakuma[b]

[a] *Department of Mechanical Engineering, National University of Singapore, Singapore*
[b] *Graduate School of Frontier Sciences, University of Tokyo, Tokyo, Japan*
[c] *School of Mechanical Engineering, Nanyang Technological University, Singapore*
[d] *The State Key Laboratory of Computer Aided Design and Computer Graphics,
Zhejiang University, China*
[e] *Johns Hopkins University School of Medicine, Baltimore, USA*

Abstract. Chemoembolization is an important therapeutic procedure. A catheter
was navigated to the artery that feeds the tumor, and chemotherapy drugs and
embolus are injected directly into the tumor. There is a risk that embolus may
lodge incorrectly and deprive normal tissue of its blood supply. This paper focuses
on visualization of the flow particles in simulation of chemotherapy drugs
injection for training of hand-eye coordination skills. We assume that the flow
follows a defined path in the hepatic vascular system from the catheter tip. The
vascular model is constructed using sweeping and blending operations.
Quadrilaterals which are aligned to face the viewer are drawn for the trail of each
particle. The quadrilateral in the trail is determined using bilinear interpolation. On
simulated fluoroscopic image, the flow is rendered as overlaying and semi-
transparent quadrilaterals representing the particles' trails. This visualization model
achieves a good visual approximation of the flow of particles inside the vessels
under fluoroscopic imaging.

Keywords. Visualization, physical-based modeling, liver, human-machine
interface

1. Introduction

Chemoembolization – an interventional approach is an important therapeutic procedure.
Studies have shown that 70 percent or more liver cancer patients experience
improvement. The patients who go through chemoembolization may live longer
depending on the type of cancer [1]. In the procedure, interventional radiologists gain
access to the site of internal lesions and pathology within the liver organ using
catheters that are inserted into a blood vessel through a puncture in the skin at the groin.
The catheter is used as conduit to pass a combination of chemotherapy drugs and tiny
particles (embolus) to treat the diseased condition. Real-time X-ray fluoroscopy is used
to monitor the passage of catheter through the artery that feeds the tumor, as well as

---

[1] Corresponding Author: Chee-Kong Chui, Centre for Biomedical Materials Applications & Technology,
E3-05-23, Engineering Drive 3, S(119260), Singapore. Email: mpecck@nus.edu.sg

direct injection of drugs into the tumor. The focus of this paper is on visualization of the flow particles in interactive simulation of chemotherapy drugs injection during chemoembolization.

Several groups have been working on interactive simulation systems on catheter navigation for training and surgical planning [2][3]. Chemotherapy drugs injection is just as important compared to manipulation of catheter in chemoembolization. The embolus can lodge in the wrong place and deprive normal tissue of its blood supply. Injection is a complex image guided procedure that requires a high degree of hand-eye coordination skills on the physician. The visualization model should achieve a good visual approximation of the flow of particles inside the vessels, and computational efficient so as to provide the physician an effective training on chemotherapy drugs injection.

2. Materials and Methods

In the simulation for drugs injection, we start with a catheter already inserted and navigated to the artery that feeds the tumor, and assume that the flow comprising many particles will follow a defined path in the hepatic vascular system from the catheter tip. The vascular segments in the hepatic vascular system are modeled using sweeping operations while vascular bifurcations are modeled using blending (sweeping plus hole filling) operations [4]. The hepatic vascular model defines the trajectories of the particles or drugs. A tumor is a terminal vessel with spherical shape.

The conservation of mass applies to steady flow results in $\rho A v = $ constant, where ρ is the fluid density, A is the cross sectional area of the blood vessel, and v is the velocity. This is the equation of continuity. Assuming that the flow is compressible, $Av = $ constant. The flow velocity can hence, be determined since cross sectional area of each segment of vessel is given.

There are a variety of methods for three-dimensional flow visualization. Our implementation is similar to the "Virtual Tubelet". Readers are to refer to [5] for details on virtual tubelet. Instead of drawing many polygons, quadrilaterals which are aligned to face the viewer are drawn, and shaded appropriately. The head of list of quadrilaterals is positioned at the current position of the corresponding particle with its tails passing through the particle's recent positions. To depict the washing out effect during injection, the quadrilaterals are drawn in decreasing grayness from the head to the last quadrilateral. Bilinear interpolation is used to determine the grayness. The "flow" stays at the targeted tumor for several instances before diminishing. A flow at the tumor with size larger than the spherical tumor implies an overflow. Figure 1 illustrates the flow of one injection over a single vessel leading to a tumor.

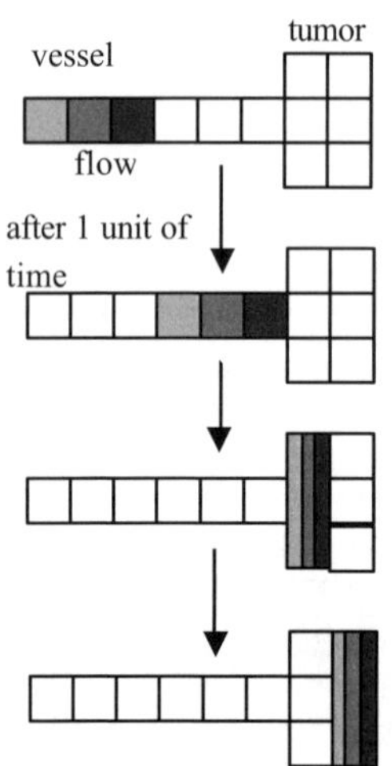

Figure 1. Illustration of flow simulation

3. Results

Figure 2(a) shows the model of a human liver and its hepatic vascular system. Figure 2(b) is snapshot of the implementation over a fluoroscopic view. The flow is rendered as overlaying and semi-transparent quadrilaterals representing the particles' trails. The tumor is not shown. This visualization method is applicable to render flow particle within the tumor. We can achieve real time interaction on an Intel P4-based 1GHz workstation with graphics acceleration board.

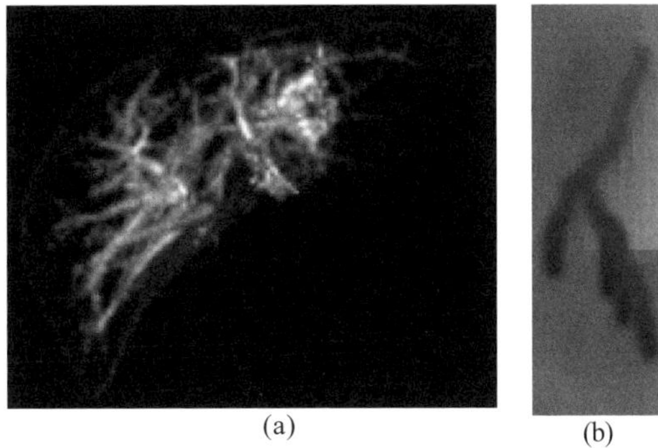

(a)   (b)

Figure 2. Liver model and visualization of drugs injection

4. Discussion and Conclusions

The focus of this paper is on flow visualization in interactive simulation of drugs injection for the purpose of surgical training, particularly on the hand-eye coordination skills. Flow in blood vessel is very complex. At the start of drugs flow in a relatively large artery, the blood flow is a balance between pressure forces, inertia forces, and forces of tissue and muscle. The vessel diameter decreases with each division of artery. Beyond the terminal arteries and in the capillaries, the flow is determined by the balance of viscous stresses and pressure gradient. For our purposes, we made assumptions and significantly simplified the flow biomechanics. We are in the process of implementing a more accurate flow dynamic model which is essential for a clinically viable solution. More quantitative validation will be planned with this new model.

For realistic interactive surgical training, the varying shape and size of tumor will present a different resistance to the force needed to inject drugs which is important to provide a more complete solution to hand-eye coordination training. A computational model that is patient specific in both geometrical and biomechanical senses is desired.

Acknowledgement

The authors wish to thank Singapore's Agency of Science and Technology (A*STAR) for support of this research.

References

[1]   Society of Interventional Radiology: http://www.sirweb.org
[2]   Chui et al: Training and pretreatment planning of interventional neuroradiology procedures - initial clinical validation, *Studies in Health Technology and Informatics* 85, 2002, pp 96-102.
[3]   Alderliesten et al: Simulation of minimally invasive vascular interventions for training purposes. *Computer Aided Surgery*, 9(1/2):3-15, 2004.
[4]   Ye et al: Constructive modeling of G1 bifurcation, *Computer Aided Geometric Design*, 19(7), 2002, pp 513-531.
[5]   Schirski et al: Efficient visualization of large amounts of particle trajectories in virtual environments using virtual tubelets, Proc. ACM SIGGRAPH Virtual Reality Continuum and its Applications in Industry, 141-147, 2004.

Medicine Meets Virtual Reality 14
J.D. Westwood et al. (Eds.)
IOS Press, 2006

The Use of a Computer Aided Design (CAD) Environment in 3D Reconstruction of Anatomic Surfaces

Octavian CIOBANU
The "Gr. T. Popa" University of Medicine and Pharmacy, Medical Bioengineering
Faculty, Iasi, Romania (oct@as.ro)

Abstract: Paper presents an evaluation and comparison of two different types of software for generating a 3D model from medical imaging data: first, a dedicated 3D reconstruction Mimics interface, by Materialise and second, an engineering CAD (a Solid Works and AutoCAD) interface. Advantages and limitations of both software types are outlined and there some observations for 3D reconstruction of anatomic surfaces are presented.

Keywords: 3D reconstruction, software, CAD, comparison

Introduction

CAD has been traditionally used to assist in engineering design and modeling for representation, analysis and industrial manufacturing. Advances in computing technologies in terms of hardware and software and in Bioengineering have helped in the advancement of CAD in applications beyond that of traditional design and analysis. CAD is now being used extensively in biomedical engineering in applications ranging from clinical medicine and 3D reconstruction [1, 2] to customized medical implant design and tissue engineering, with many novel and important medical applications.

In 3D reconstruction of anatomic surfaces there are now two main software types: dedicated 3D reconstruction software and CAD software.

Dedicated software permits image processing and measurements for MRI, CT, PET, microscopy etc. and supports both grayscale and color images stored in DICOM, TIFF, Interfile, GIF, JPEG, PNG, BMP, PGM, RAW or other image file formats. They can create 3D surface models and volume rendering from 2D cross-section images in real time which can be exported to STL, DXF, IGES, 3DS, OBJ, VRML, XYZ and other formats for different applications [3, 4].

3D reconstructions of anatomic surfaces by dedicated software have advantages but also limitations compared to CAD software. Here we try to show our results in a comparison between reconstructions performed with these types of software.

1. Method

In order to achieve a comparison, a 3D reconstruction was performed using two types of software: Mimics (a 3D reconstruction dedicated software) and Solid Works and AutoCAD (CAD software).

A portion of a skull was reconstructed starting from prepared slices obtained by CT scans. Some slices in jpeg format are presented in Fig.1.

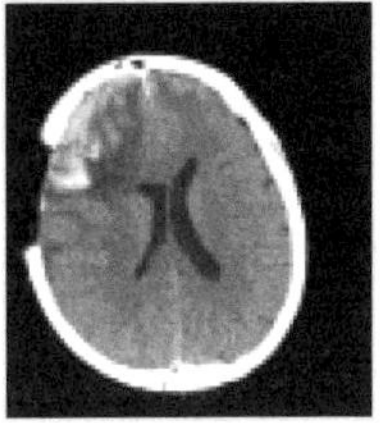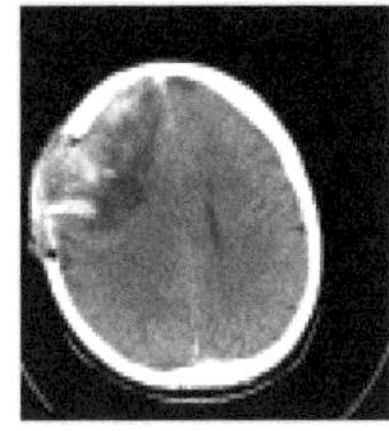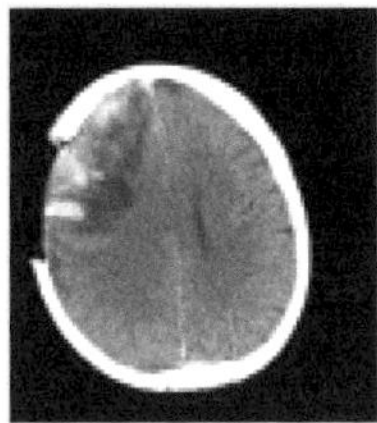

Fig.1 Samples of slices used in 3D reconstruction

2. Results

Figure 2 shows an example of 3D reconstructions of the same anatomic surface created by different software: dedicated software (Mimics) and CAD software (Solid Works and AutoCAD).

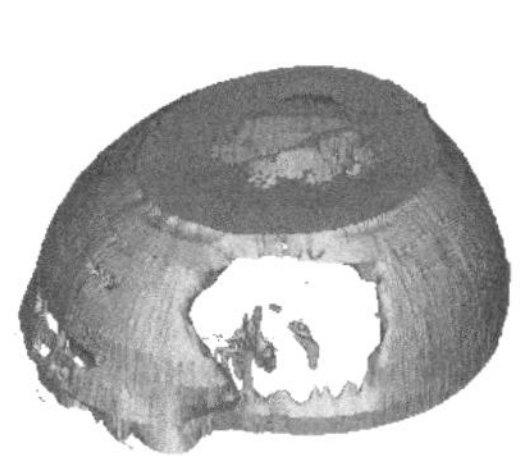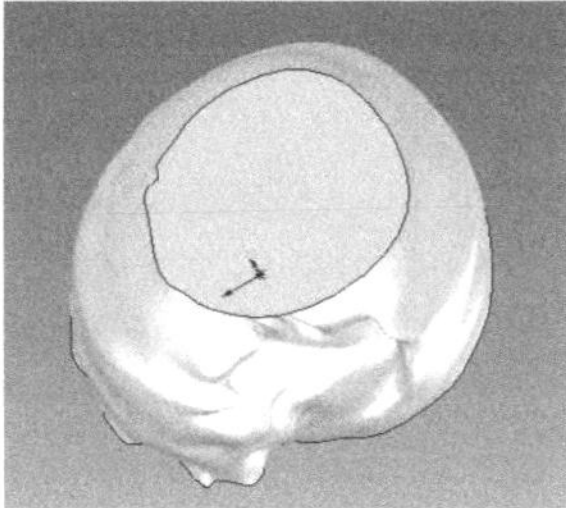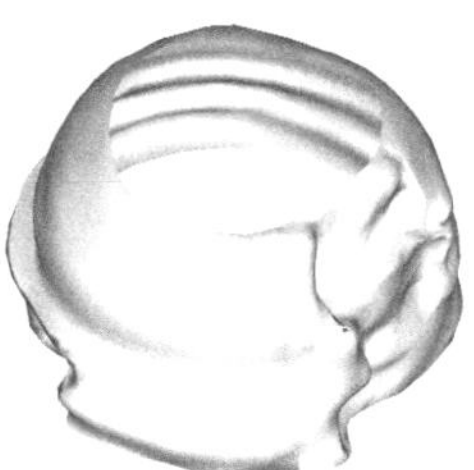

Fig.2 Reconstructions using Mimics (left), Solid Works (center) and AutoCAD (right)

3. Discussion

A short comparison between 3D reconstruction of anatomic surfaces with dedicated and CAD software is made in table 1. Discussion has as object the reconstructions of 3D anatomic surfaces from figure 2, using three different software for the same object.

Table 1. Comparison of 3D reconstruction software

Software	Price	Quality of reconstruction	Type of segmentation	Speed of reconstruction	Implant design
Mimics	high	high	automatic	high	partially
Solid Works	low	high	manual	slow	allowed
AutoCAD	low	high	manual	slow	allowed

The most important advantage for CAD software is the price and it can be between 10 to 20 times smaller than dedicated reconstruction software for educational licenses. Due to its low price and versatility, CAD software has spread throughout schools, universities and image processing laboratories. Another advantage is the possibility of CAD software for creating the design of implants (2D and 3D) and augmenting anatomic reconstructions.

The most important limitation of a CAD software is the low speed of reconstruction because of manual segmentation. In 3D reconstruction, each slice is processed independently leading to the detection of the contours of the living tissue. The contours are assembled, also manually, to create a solid model.

In connection to these observations, an international project on 3D reconstruction started on November 2005 at the Center of Human Simulation, University of Colorado, in order to construct a database of anatomic surfaces exploiting only advantages of CAD software. Author of paper is involved in this project, supported by a Fulbright grant

4. Conclusion

None of above interfaces has been widely adopted by the biomedical engineering community due to the inherent complexity of the anatomic structures. Effective methods for the conversion of CT or MRI data into solid models still need to be developed [5,6,7].

CAD environments have the great advantage of being very cheap and well spread but the reconstruction speed is still slow.

References

[1] O. Ciobanu, 3D reconstruction of anatomic surfaces. Proceedings of Third European Conference on Intelligent Systems and Technologies ECIT, ISBN 973-7994-78-7, Iasi, July 21-23, 2004

[2] O. Ciobanu, Reconstructia grafica a suprafetelor anatomice (Romanian) *Revista medico-chirurgicala*, vol. 108, Nr.4, 2004, ISSN 0048-7848, pp.920-923

[3] W. Sun, B. Starly, J. Nam, A. Darling, Bio-CAD modeling and its applications in computer-aided tissue engineering, Computer-Aided Design 37, 2005, pp 1097–1114

[4] C. Soussen, A.Mohammad-Djafari, Multiresolution approach to the estimation of the shape of a 3D compact object from its radiographic data, Proceedings of SPIE, Denver, CO,USA, 1999, pp 150-160

[5] V. Elangovan A direct method for segmenting tomographic data. Master's thesis, University of Utah, School of Computer Science, 2001

[6] D. Moody, and S. Lozanoff,. SURFdriver: A practical computer program for generating three-dimensional models of anatomical structures. The 14th Annual Meeting of the American Association of Clinical Anatomists, Honolulu, Hawai'I, July 8-11, 1997.

[7] J. Lotjonen, E. Magnin, J. Nenonen, T. Katila Reconstruction of 3D geometry using 2D profiles and a geometric prior model. IEEE Trans.Medical Imaging, 18(10), 1999, pp 992-1002

Medicine Meets Virtual Reality 14
J.D. Westwood et al. (Eds.)
IOS Press, 2006

Simulating the Domain of Medical Modeling and Simulation: The Medical Modeling and Simulation Database

C. Donald Combs, Ph.D., Kara Friend, M.S.,
Melissa Mannion and Robert J. Alpino, M.I.A.
*National Center for Collaboration in Medical Modeling and Simulation
and Office of the Vice President for Planning and Program Development,
Eastern Virginia Medical School, Norfolk, Virginia, U.S.A.*
Email: combscd@evms.edu, friendke@evms.edu, mannioml@evms.edu,
alpinorj@evms.edu

Abstract. Over the past year the National Center for Collaboration in Medical Modeling and Simulation's (NCCMMS) Medical Modeling and Simulation Database (MMSD) has grown dramatically. There are now over 170,000 entries including current articles and upcoming conference listings. In addition, in the near future, the scope of the NCCMMS website will expand to include an evaluation section where NCCMMS researchers will compile data describing the efficacy and cost efficiency of many commercially available simulators. The NCCMMS also plans to create a new collaborative forum on the website. This message board area will provide a single location for researchers to discuss new simulation techniques and programs. It will help to facilitate communication between companies and researchers in the field by creating a comprehensive forum for medical modeling and simulation discussions. The newly expanded MMSD and NCCMMS websites are designed to create a simple way for researchers and companies to work together to facilitate the sharing of information and to spur advancement of the medical modeling and simulation discipline.

Keywords. Database, NCCMMS, MMSD, collaboration, evaluation

Introduction

The rapid expansion of the Medical Modeling and Simulation domain has left many in the field at a loss as to the best method to survey the domain. Researchers generally work in isolated labs with discrete simulated sections of the human body or with a very limited set of simulations. If it were possible for researchers across the globe to work together in an easy fashion, the efficacy of research in the medical modeling and simulation field could be increased by avoiding redundant research efforts and by promoting cooperative research initiatives. The National Center for Collaboration in Medical Modeling and Simulation (NCCMMS) was created to encourage such collaborative research. The NCCMMS (http://www.evms.edu/nccmms) has created a prototype Medical Modeling and Simulation Database (MMSD) to help foster awareness of the work being performed in other labs worldwide. The MMSD contains bibliographic information about articles published in the field as well as contact and product information for companies involved in simulation research. The database has grown from the 15,000 entries noted last year to over 115,000 entries today (http://mmsd.evms.edu). This figure includes the addition of over 200 new conference and company entries and thousands of new articles. The articles included range from those on simulator evaluation and simulator development to those on mathematical models of microscopic movement. The MMSD has been designed to be inclusive of any simulator that has medical relevance. The MMSD has been welcomed by those in the field as there previously was no single place for researchers to obtain such comprehensive coverage of the field. With the establishment of the database now complete, NCCMMS researchers have improved the information available for researchers by conducting a meta-analysis of the data.

Simulator Analysis

NCCMMS researchers are currently developing a new feature for the MMSD database that is designed to further its usefulness and to assist researchers contemplating new medical simulator development. They are developing an analytic tool that will identify those areas of medicine that have not been adequately covered by the recent increase in medical simulator development. Unfortunately, with the medical modeling and simulation field being as disjointed as it is, it is often difficult to determine what types of simulators various labs are developing. This new feature of the MMSD database will be able to group research both by topic and by the number of database entries in a given topic field, and will provide the reader with guidance on the relative number of active researchers in the topic field. Should researchers post information about their ongoing work to this website, other interested parties will then have the opportunity to contact them to explore possible collaborative efforts.

On the horizon is an even more advanced section of the database where NCCMMS researchers will evaluate those medical and surgical simulators currently on the market for their efficacy based on a set of relevant criteria for the type of simulator being evaluated. Through this effort, the leadership of the NCCMMS seeks to assist various types of educational institutions and those other organizations that acquire medical and surgical simulators, e.g., the U.S. military, in acquiring the most appropriate simulator for achieving their educational objectives within the budget parameters of the organization. NCCMMS researchers also plan to examine the latest medical and surgical simulators available as they are introduced at various conferences and trade shows to maintain familiarity with the newest products on the market. NCCMMS researchers will work closely with institution or company representatives and examine brochures and specifications at these various events to develop an informed assessment about the new simulators that can be included in the MMSD. Should insufficient information be initially available to develop such an assessment, the medical or surgical simulator will be added to the MMSD Companies and Projects section and the institution or company will be contacted by NCCMMS researchers for further information.

Additions to the NCCMMS Website

In addition to the improvements to the MMSD outlined above, the NCCMMS website will be expanded to include several on-line research message forums that will consist of message boards for various topic areas of medical modeling and simulation research.

The goal of these research forums is to expand the usefulness of the NCCMMS website for researchers by promoting collaborative research efforts. If, for example, there was a research team working on a skeletal simulator of the foot, it is entirely conceivable that they may be unaware of another research team working on a muscle/soft tissue simulator of the foot at another company or institution. If both teams had access to the MMSD research forum for simulator development and learned of each others efforts, they may be more likely to collaborate together to develop a more complete simulator product. Such forums would also be places where researchers could meet on-line to discuss challenges they have encountered in their research and development efforts to determine if other labs were either encountering the same problems or if they perhaps developed a novel solution.

The NCCMMS is also exploring the migration of the MMSD database to another database program that would provide a more user-friendly site. Ideally, the new program would offer better mapping capability and help the user link keywords in a more functional manner. It would also export data to a wider variety of programs to facilitate data analysis.

Conclusions

The medical modeling and simulation field urgently needs to become more unified in a manner that allows researchers to interact in a meaningful way to facilitate the rapid and effective transfer of information in the domain. The NCCMMS, through its MMSD product and its other initiatives, is working hard to establish objective criteria for the evaluation of medical and surgical simulators and a working model through which the science of simulation can be rapidly advanced. The new NCCMMS website and MMSD database additions will make collaboration between researchers simple and effective while allowing each company and laboratory to maintain its autonomy. Furthermore, the independent and objective evaluations and rankings of simulators will be indispensable to organizations contemplating purchasing a simulator; for such purchases are critical ones for these organizations as such simulators are often quite costly and very often one-time only purchases. The expanded MMSD database and newly updated NCCMMS website will bring researchers and organizations from across the globe together for more meaningful and expedited research while creating a more user-friendly resource for simulator purchasers. The newly expanded MMSD will provide the most comprehensive review of the literature available as well as providing a virtual forum for those interested in collaboration while simplifying the research process for anyone involved in the medical modeling and simulation field.

ACKNOWLEDGEMENT

This study was a collaborative project between the Virginia Modeling, Analysis and Simulation Center (VMASC) at Old Dominion University and the Eastern Virginia Medical School. Partial funding was provided by the Naval Health Research Center through NAVAIR Orlando TSD under contract N61339-03-C-0157, and by the Office of Naval Research under contract N00014-04-1-0697, entitled "The National Center for Collaboration in Medical Modeling and Simulation". The ideas and opinions presented in this paper represent the views of the authors and do not necessarily represent the views of the Department of Defense.

Medicine Meets Virtual Reality 14
J.D. Westwood et al. (Eds.)
IOS Press, 2006

Assessing Cognitive & Motor Performance in Minimally Invasive Surgery (MIS) for Training & Tool Design

Sayra M. CRISTANCHO[a,c,1], Antony J. HODGSON[a], George PACHEV[b],
Alex NAGY[b], Neely PANTON[b], Karim QAYUMI[b]
[a]*Dept. of Mechanical Engineering, The University of British Columbia, Canada*
[b]*Faculty of Medicine, The University of British Columbia, Canada*
[c]*Facultad de Ingeniería Electrónica, Universidad Pontificia Bolivariana*
Bucaramanga, Colombia

Abstract. The objective of this paper is to present the development of a new modelling diagram (MCMD) to represent MIS procedures in terms of both motor and cognitive actions. Through observation and analysis of several laparoscopic cholecystectomy procedures and based on task analysis techniques, we created a diagram language composed of six primary symbols: processes, decisions, interrupt service routines (ISRs), options points and AND and OR gates. We then tested and refined them during 10 new cases until no further changes seemed necessary, we have since applied this approach to 6 laparoscopic colorectal surgeries and have found that no further symbols were necessary though the procedural representation was naturally different. This modelling diagram allowed us to represent both cognitive and motor performance aspects of surgical procedures in a unified framework and will in future allow us to assess motor performance on particular surgical tasks at particular points in the procedure (i.e., the *surgical context*).

Keywords. Surgical training, Motor and Cognitive Modelling Diagram (MCMD), Minimally Invasive Surgery

INTRODUCTION

Surgical training is a long, involved process that is currently based mainly on an apprenticeship model. Residents are assessed by more experienced surgeons, but many of the specific assessment techniques normally used have been shown to be unreliable, especially when performed in the operating room where patient variability has a significant effect on the assessment [1]. If we are to develop more objective assessment techniques that can be reliably applied in the OR, then we need to develop assessment techniques that take procedural variability into account.

Cao [2] provided an analytical framework based on a hierarchical decomposition (i.e., a context-free decomposition into fundamental motor actions) for studying differences in motor task performance among surgeons performing laparoscopic

---

[1] Corresponding Author: Department of Mechanical Engineering, The University of British Columbia, 2054-6250 Applied Science Lane, Vancouver, BC, V6T 1Z4

procedures. McBeth [3] extended her work and performed a quantitative analysis of motor performance during selected standard surgical tasks.

Since surgery involves both cognitive and motor skills, we also need to model the cognitive aspects of surgery. This means that we need to track the task sequences during a procedure, which, in turn, will enable us to evaluate motor tasks in their surgical context. As described below, task analysis methods from psychology and education theory seem to be best suited to represent in a single model both motor skills and cognitive operations, as well as the decisions necessary to accomplish a task [4].

Task analysis is an important tool for assessing learning environments. Its purpose is to provide a representation of task components. The following parameters need to be identified to understand and design a particular training and evaluation process: who the learners are, what they need to know, how they should perform, what skills they need to develop, and how the context may affect their decisions [4].

The aim of this work, therefore, is to extend the application of task analysis methods to summarize both motor and cognitive actions in a single diagram, which we call an MCMD (Motor and Cognitive Modelling Diagram) and to demonstrate the application of the MCMD to both a common surgical procedure (laparoscopic cholecystectomy) and a more advanced procedure (laparoscopic colorectal surgery), through which we could prove its general applicability.

1. Task Analysis in MIS

Task analysis is appropriate to use in identifying key components of complex activities such as surgery that need to be analyzed when designing training and evaluation systems.

With regard to the issue of instrument design, [5] argued that we need to know how an instrument is actually used in context (i.e., at particular points in a surgery) and what impact its use has on the flow or dynamics of the procedure (i.e., which tasks are associated with certain patterns, and how the flow of the procedure, in terms of the route taken by the surgeon, affects the use of instruments). This argument suggests that we need an alternative to the hierarchical decomposition in order to explicitly describe all the flow and progress of a surgery. Although hierarchical decomposition offers a good description of the low level actions, it does not explicitly represent the flow of a procedure.

This lack has led to the development of structured methods as in [3] to provide a standard framework for objectively describing the flow of the procedure in a way that allows comparison to be made between surgeons while taking proper account of normal surgical variability (i.e., a low-level action early in surgery may bear little relation to the same kind of action performed later; therefore, we must have some consistent way to describe the context of particular surgical actions)

1.1. Purpose of Task Analysis

Although task analyses are commonly carried out, there is no unique definition of what is involved. Different kinds of analyses are used depending on the purpose of the analysis, the context in which it is applied, and the type of performers involved. From the educational perspective, task analysis could be defined as a process to determine statements of learning goals, to describe and prioritize tasks and subtasks that the learner will perform, and to develop assessment methods to determine what actually gets taught or trained while performing a particular activity [4].

Since learning is a human-centered activity, all learning situations will differ according to their different contexts; therefore, there are many different task analysis methods. According to [4], however there are 5 main kinds of task analyses: Job analysis, Cognitive task analysis, Activity analysis, Content matter analysis, and Learning analysis.

From this wide variety of task analysis techniques, we focused our approach on two learning analysis methods: Hierarchical Analysis (for intellectual skills) and Information-Processing Analysis (for procedural and cognitive tasks) because together they allow us to represent both the surgeon's motor actions and decision-making processes. Other methods such as cognitive task and activity analyses that seem to be also applicable were discarded since they focus more on the identification of knowledge than on the description of a subject's performance [4].

1.2. Task Analysis Methods

We implemented two types of task analysis to determine the operational components of a minimally invasive surgery procedure (i.e. laparoscopic cholecystectomy) and to describe in an event sequence diagram the activities that surgeons perform, how they accomplish tasks and how they reason about the surgery.

We decided to use both Hierarchical Analysis (to represent the broad flow of the procedure) and Information-Processing Analysis (to represent decision-making and motor processes at a more detailed level) because of the power of having two complementary representations of the tasks and the steps needed to accomplish them (see Table 1). Accounting for both types of considerations required us to pay attention both to the surgeons' motor actions and to their decision-making processes.

Table 1. Comparative table: Hierarchical Analysis Vs Information-Processing Analysis

Hierarchical	Information-processing
Solve the question: "What must the learner know in order to achieve this task?"	Solve the question: "What are the mental and/or physical steps that the learner must go through in order to complete this task?"
Developed from general to specific	Developed step-by-step (It has a start and an end)
Represented in terms of levels of tasks	Represented as a flowchart or an outline
Based on learning taxonomies (from most to least complex)	It is procedural in nature

2. Protocol

Our main goal was to develop a method to describe Laparoscopic Cholecystectomies and other MIS procedures that integrates descriptions of both motor and cognitive actions in a unified framework so that we can analyze these actions in relation to their *surgical context* – understood as the current state of the surgery.

Based on *task knowledge structures* proposed by [4], we modified and implemented the following steps:

Phase I: Collected information about the surgical procedure

Observation: We videotaped 10 laparoscopic cholecystectomy procedures performed by two expert surgeons and manually divided the procedure into various tasks. These observations allowed us to identify typical surgical tasks and alternatives.

Think-aloud: We asked the surgeons to describe during the surgery what tasks they were performing and what decisions they were making.

Interviews: We developed preliminary diagrams prior to the interviews based on textbook descriptions of the surgical procedure and updated them following the operating room (OR) observations. We then interviewed the surgeons as a follow-up to the intraoperative think-aloud process.

Phase II: Constructed procedure model. We designed a new hierarchical Motor and Cognitive Modelling Diagram (MCMD – a kind of flowchart) to capture the task sequences of laparoscopic cholecystectomies based both on our observations and on elements of two different types of task analyses (i.e., Hierarchical Analysis and Information-Processing Analysis). We found that we had to add a new symbol to appropriately represent certain kinds of actions (e.g., surgeons will interrupt tasks to deal with critical issues such as the appearance of a bleeder – we refer to this as an Interrupt Service Routine (ISR) by analogy to microprocessor behaviour). Our final diagram was the result of eight iterations of interviews with the surgeons. We did not acquire motor performance measures during these procedures, but the process nodes are designed to contain these measures.

3. Results

MCMD is composed of a hierarchical set of diagrams that allows to represent a surgical procedure at various levels of detail: phase, stage, task, sub-task, and action levels. The higher levels are generally uncontroversial in terms of order and sequence, but variations in order and decision-making processes generally come into play at the task level and below. As an example, Figure 1 presents the corresponding diagram for the task named *12. Isolate CD/CA (CD: cystic duct; CA: cystic artery).*

The operational components of the 10 laparoscopic cholecystectomies we observed could be represented in a relatively simple event sequence diagram composed of six primary symbols (see Figure 2): processes, decisions, ISRs, option points and AND and OR gates. These symbols (or diagram language) were formulated in advance through the observation of several procedures; we then refined the conventions and tested them on subsequent laparoscopic cholecystectomy procedures until no further changes seemed necessary. We have since applied this approach to 6 laparoscopic colorectal surgeries, a more advanced procedure, and found that no further symbols were necessary even though the procedural representation itself was naturally different.

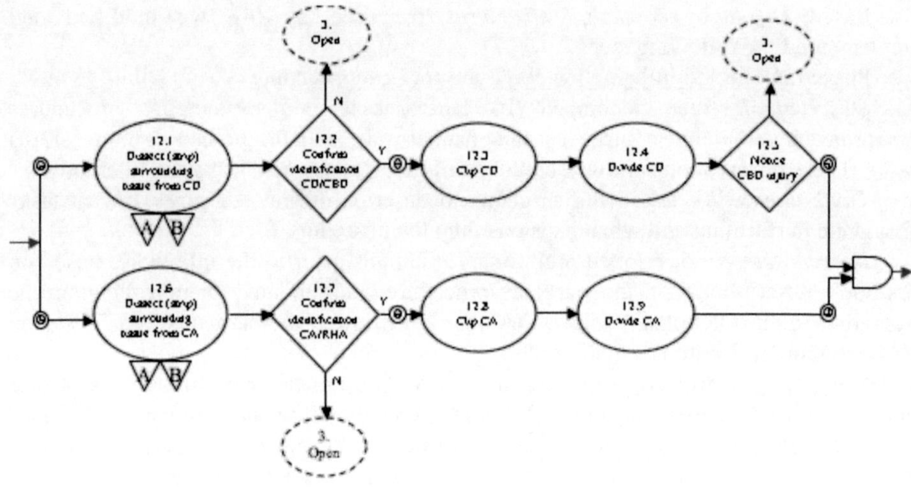

Figure 1: MCMD diagram for *12. Isolate CD/CA* task in Lap Chole

(CD: cystic duct; CA: cystic artery; CBD: common bile duct; RHA: right hepatic artery)

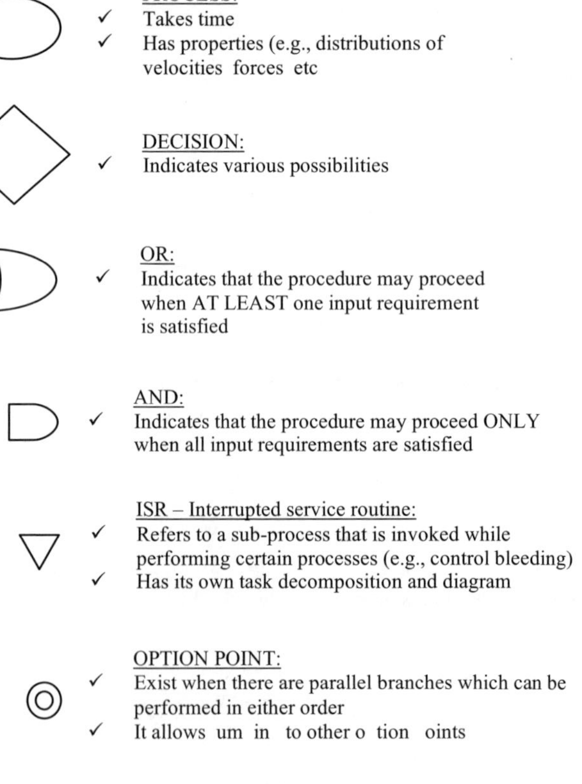

Figure 2: MCMD symbology

4. Conclusions

We have shown that a relatively straightforward extension of task-modelling methods known in the cognitive sciences literature can be used to describe the event sequences observed in minimally invasive surgical procedures. This modelling diagram allows us to represent both cognitive and motor performance aspects of surgical procedures in a unified framework and will in future allow us to assess motor performance on particular surgical tasks at particular points in the procedure (i.e., the *surgical context*). We added a novel notion – that of the interrupt service routine – that seemed to be lacking in the standard task representations. In general, our notation allows us to represent motor actions, decision points, transitions, conditions to proceed, and independent routines. The final diagram is a left-to-right step-by-step graphical representation of the flow of the procedure, which illustrates the possible routes that might be followed to achieve the overall objective. Since each step of the MCMD represents a collection of motor actions, we plan to augment the educationally most important steps using state diagrams to model transition probabilities and measures of kinematic and force variables to assess motor performance.

In this paper we have concentrated on Laparoscopic Cholecystectomy since it is the most widely practiced MIS procedure. However, to prove the generality of our modelling approach, we also successfully modelled the more complex Laparoscopic Colorectal procedure.

5. References

[1] Rosser J., Rosser L., Savalgi R (1998). Objective Evaluation of a Laparoscopic Surgical Skill Program for Residents and Senior Surgeons. *Arch Surg*; 133(6): 657-661
[2] Cao CGL, Mackenzie CL, Ibbotson JA, Turner LJ, Blair NP, Nagy AG (1999) Hierarchical decomposition of laparoscopic procedures. MMVR, IOSPress, pp 83–89
[3] McBeth P (2002). A Methodology for Quantitative Performance Evaluation in Minimally Invasive Surgery. UBC M.Sc. Thesis
[4] Jonassen D., Tessmer M., Hannum W (1999). Task Analysis Methods for Instructional Design. Lawrence Erlbaum Associates, Publishers. London
[5] Mehta N., Haluck R., Frecker M., Snyder A (2002). Sequence and task analysis of instrument use in common laparoscopic procedures. Surg Endosc 16: 280–285

Medicine Meets Virtual Reality 14
J.D. Westwood et al. (Eds.)
IOS Press, 2006

Virtual Patients: Assessment of Synthesized Versus Recorded Speech

Robert Dickerson[1], Kyle Johnsen[1], Andrew Raij[1], Benjamin Lok[1],
Amy Stevens[2], Thomas Bernard[3], D. Scott Lind[3]
[1]Department of Computer Information Science Engineering, University of Florida
[2]College of Medicine, University of Florida
[3]Medical College of Georgia

Abstract.   Virtual patients have great potential for training patient-doctor communication skills.   There are two approaches to producing the virtual human speech: synthesized speech or recorded speech. The tradeoffs in flexibility, fidelity, and cost raise an interesting development decision: which speech approach is most appropriate for virtual patients? Two groups of medical students participated in a user study interviewing a virtual patient under each condition. We found no significant differences in the overall impression, speech intelligibility, and task performance. Our conclusion is that if the goal is to train students of which questions to ask, synthesized speech is just as effective as recorded speech. However, if the goal is to teach the student how to ask the correct questions, a high level of expressiveness in the virtual patient is needed.   This in turn necessitates the higher cost – even with the lower flexibility – of recorded speech.

Keywords. Synthesized speech, Virtual Patients, Medical Education

1. Introduction

Virtual patients are receiving serious attention as a powerful tool for educating medical students. Through repeated experiences with virtual patients, medical students can be exposed to, and evaluated on, many more situations then through traditional methods. To better the training potential of virtual patients, we must study in-depth the components necessary to create compelling social experiences. Each of the core components: graphics rendering, speech recognition, speech processing, and speech synthesis play a part in the overall impression of a virtual human. Medical textbooks frequently detail the value of verbal cues as a critical source of patient information[1]. When designing virtual patient systems, developers are presented with two approaches to generate speech: pre-recorded or synthesized speech.

Recorded Speech – speech of the virtual patient is recorded using voice talent. While monetarily costly, time consuming, and inflexible, recorded speech has very high fidelity and can be extremely emotive.

Synthesized Speech - given a text string, software libraries generate audio output. While the fidelity can range from 'robotic' to passable, the low cost (time and money) and dynamic nature of synthesized speech makes it an attractive approach.

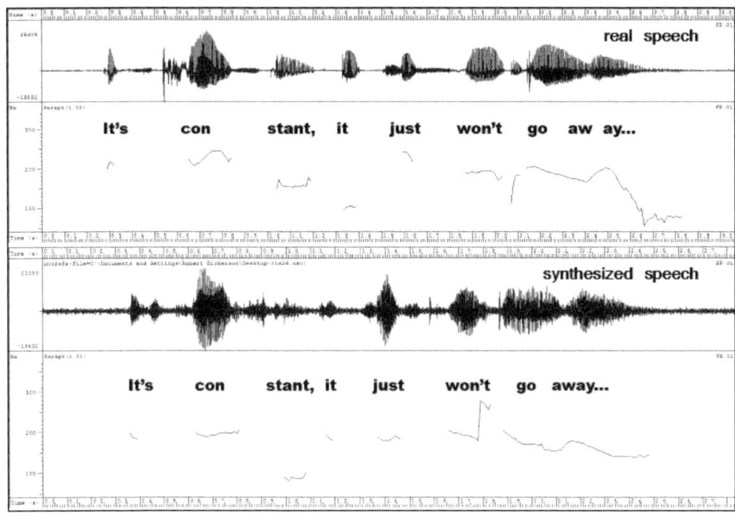

Figure 1. Comparison of intonation contours from a fundamental-frequency analysis for the VP's emotive expression "It's constant, it just won't go away", generated with Speech Filing System.

Spoken dialogue systems (such as telephony applications) typically use recorded speech whenever possible. When user interfaces employ synthetic speech, they typically use messages with simple structure to reduce the cognitive and memory demands on the user. Table 1 shows the tradeoffs from using either synthesize or recorded speech. Using recorded speech is time consuming since a voice talent is required to pre-record all the virtual standardized patient's responses. Synthesized speech makes it easy to update the script quickly and easily. Pre-recorded speech makes it difficult to use dynamic data, (such using names after introductions, or dynamically generating new responses). Systems using AI such as natural language generation would require the use of synthesized voice. However NLP seems unnecessary for closed domain scenarios such as the acute-abdominal pain, because of the predictability of the set of questions [2].

Table 1. Trade-off matrix for recorded speech vs. synthesized speech

Recorded speech	Synthesized Speech
Inflexible (non-dynamic)	Flexible (dynamic)
High fidelity (emotive)	Low fidelity (non-emotive)
Costly (time consuming)	Inexpensive (quick)

The tradeoffs in the three dimensions (flexibility, fidelity, and cost) raise an interesting development decision: which speech approach is most appropriate for virtual patients?

To investigate this question, we employ the high fidelity virtual interactive patient system (VIPS). In VIPS, medical students naturally interact with a virtual patient, DIANA (DIgital ANimated Avatar). DIANA is projected onto the wall of a mock examination room (she's 5'6") and talks and gestures with the student [Figure 2]. Modeled after a standardized patient experience, DIANA is scripted with an abdominal pain condition, and the student's goal in the 10-minute experience is to explore the history of present illness (with no physical exam). Previous work has presented the system [2-4], the student-virtual patient interaction [5], and the students' responses [4].

Would experiencing DIANA with synthesized speech (Group SS) cause the student to perform differently than recorded speech (Group RS)? We conducted an experiment with medical students to explore how the virtual patient's speech type (RS or SS) impacted the experience.

The study result provides insight into the advantages and disadvantages of using synthesized speech and evaluates the necessary fidelity for communication skills training. Our approach was to empirically compare the two speech modes and weigh each against a human standardized patient. Could a lower fidelity system still be acceptable if it preserves the accuracy of simulation and training?

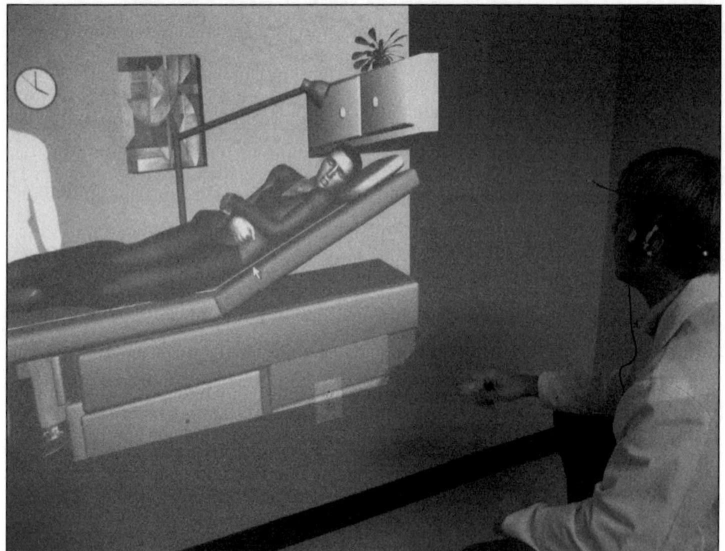

Figure 2. Medical student practices the AAP scenario with a virtual patient

2. TOOLS AND METHODS

2.1. Study Description

A user study was run with seventeen medical students at the Medical College of Georgia in their second or third year of study. All had several prior experiences with standardized patients. Participants were divided randomly into two groups with a system running with recorded speech (N=9) or synthesized speech (N=8).

Each participant filled out a background survey. Then they entered the exam room and spent 10 minutes interviewing with a virtual patient, took a history of present illness, and stated their differential diagnosis to a virtual instructor. After the interview, the participants completed a set of questionnaires then a recorded debriefing interview.

We used the "Crystal" 16K voice from the AT&T Labs Natural Voices SDK for synthesized speech. The recorded speech came from a female adult voice talent.

2.2. Measures

1. *Speech Quality Questionnaire.* The quality judgments were made by using an adapted questionnaire developed for evaluating telephone dialogue systems [6], targeting intelligibility, naturalness, pleasantness, comprehension, and overall acceptance of the voice.

2. *Maastricht Assessment of the Simulated Patient* [7]. The questionnaire is the standard method for assessing a standardized patient.

3. *Expert Evaluation.* Experts evaluated the tapes of the interactions and determined student task performance by identifying which core pieces of information, such as symptoms and signs, the student was able to elicit from DIANA including sections from chief complaint, history of present illness, sexual history, etc. Examples include: "I've been nauseous", "I have a fever", and "I am sexually active".

3. RESULTS

3.1. Learning objectives were met in both cases - no effect on task performance

Table 2. Expert Evaluation

	Synthesized	Real Speech	p
Evaluation Rating (score out of 12)	$\mu = 4.37$ $\sigma = 1.59$	$\mu = 5.00$ $\sigma = 1.85$	0.45

No differences were found in the task performance ratings assigned by experts [Table 2]. The ratings reflect the number of core questions asked during the interview. The SS condition presents lower fidelity audio than with RS, and may impact the effectiveness and believability of the simulation especially under more emotive scenarios. Synthesized speech allows the student to still meet educational objectives, and students scored DIANA was equally under each condition for teaching (RS μ 5.6, SS μ 5.6, p=0.46) and training (RS μ 5.1 μ SS 5.1, p=0.49) value.

3.2. No differences were identified in how participants' rating of the intelligibility, naturalness, pleasantness, comprehension, and overall acceptance of the voice

Based from questionnaire results, there was no reported difference in the intelligibility (RS μ 4.9, SS μ 4.6, p<0.28), naturalness (RS μ 4.3, SS μ 4.2, p<0.47), and clarity (RS μ 5.2, SS μ 5.0, p<0.46) of the voice.

In the post-experience debriefing, SS participants had varied impressions. One responded that *"[The VP's voice] was clear"* another said, *"I had expectation that she wasn't going to sound exactly like a real person. She sounded like a telephone operator."* Most RS participants were very satisfied with the quality of the voice. One said, *"I felt like they were really realistic as far as their voice intonation."*

3.3. Some SS participants noted the synthetic speech sounded unnatural at first, yet they adapted to it.

During interactions, there is often readjustment period that occurs when adapting to the speech recognition and being exposed to synthesized speech. Quickly the participants stopped paying attention to the lack of prosody, and accepted the flow of conversation that the interface presented them. The following are debriefing comments received by participants in the synthesized speech condition:

"For some people I can see how [the voice] would get confusing because [I heard the speech] just one word at a time, but it was ok for me because I had heard it many times before. Synthetic speech is clearly not a human being."

"If she's in that much pain she should be making more sounds."

"[VP's] voice could have been improved. I had difficulty hearing [the VP] at first".

In the questionnaire, the participants responded whether "this encounter is similar to other standardized patient encounters that I've experienced", there is some indication that recorded speech is more familiar to students than synthesized (RS: μ 2.8, SS: μ 2.0 $p<0.06$).

3.4. Lack of prosody was not detrimental for the basic skills teaching

The role of prosody (non-verbal cues) is used to identify grammatical structure, convey attitude and emotion, and convey personal or social identity [8]. However, these cues seemed to minimally impact this relatively simple scenario.

Stress and intonation can help identify grammatical structure. Stress is used to highlight or give emphasis to word, and can help with clarification. Intonation is used differentiate a question (yes/no, either or) from a simple declaration. The SS participants did not find SS limiting due to the simplicity of the VP's responses, the assumption that every response was a statement, and the simplicity of the conversation flow. Ambiguity did occur once in the scenario when the VP spontaneously asks the participant "can you help me!?" some SS participants were thrown off and had difficulty registering it as a question.

Speech can show attitude and emotion, personality and social identity, however much of this information is visually presented. There may be a synergy of graphics and audio, and DIANA's expressive animation might have filled in what the audio had missing. Prosody appears more important for speech-only systems.

4. Conclusion

The results indicate no significant difference in performance between Group SS and Group RS in many of the task performance measures, such as the asking the correct questions.

One important external validity measure is to identify the similarities and differences between experiencing a virtual patient and standardized patient – as clearly they are not equal. Upon closer inspection, there exist subtle – yet important – differences between virtual patients and standardized patients, primarily relating to *conversation flow* and the significant difference in level of *expressiveness*. Part of the lowered expressiveness is auditory, and thus SS's lower level of emotive expression impacts the overall experience. Recorded speech appears to be required to explore higher order communication skills. Our conclusions are as follows:

For lower level learning of communication skills, (knowledge on Bloom's Taxonomy of Learning), there appears to be little difference between RS and SS. Thus if the goal is to teach the student *which questions to ask*, SS provides a compelling dynamic approach with minimal loss of educational objectives.

However, if the goal is to teach the student *how to ask the correct questions*, (analysis and application) a high level of expressiveness in the virtual patient is needed. Essential information of the patient's condition could be lost from using synthesized speech. This in turn necessitates the higher cost – even with the lower flexibility – of recorded speech.

5. Future Work

In order to build more effective virtual patient applications we intend to explore other system design decisions, such as graphics, immersion, and speech understanding and how they affect overall system impressions.

6. References

1.	Coulehan, J. and M. Block, *The Medical Interview: Mastering the Skills for Clinical Practice.* 1997.
2.	Dickerson, R., K. Johnsen, A. Raij, B. Lok, J. Hernandez, A. Stevens. *Evaluating a Script-Based Approach for Simulating Patient-Doctor Interaction.* in *International Conference on Human-Computer Interface Advances for Modeling and Simulation (SIMCHI).* 2005. New Orleans, LA.
3.	Johnsen, K., et al., *Using Immersive Virtual Characters to Educate Medical Communication Skills.* Presence: Teleoperators and Virtual Environments, 2005.
4.	Stevens, A., et al., *The Use of Virtual Patients to Teach Medical Students Communication Skills.* American Journal of Surgery, 2005.
5.	Raij, A., et al. *Interpersonal Scenarios: Virtual ≈ Real?* in *VR 2006.* 2006.
6.	Möller, S., *Quality of Telephone-Based Spoken Dialogue Systems.* 2005: Springer.
7.	Wind, L., et al. *Assessing Simulated Patients in an Educational Setting: The Maastricht Assessment of Simulated Patients.* in *Medical Education.* 2004.
8.	Cohen, M., J. Giangola, and J. Balogh, *Voice User Interface Design.* 2004: Addison-Wesley.

Medicine Meets Virtual Reality 14
J.D. Westwood et al. (Eds.)
IOS Press, 2006

Needle Artifact Localization in 3T MR Images [1]

S.P. DiMaio [a,2], D.F. Kacher [a], R.E. Ellis [a], G. Fichtinger [b], N. Hata [a],
G.P. Zientara [a], L.P. Panych [a], R. Kikinis [a], F.A. Jolesz [a]

[a] *Brigham and Women's Hospital, Harvard Medical School*
[b] *Johns Hopkins University*

Abstract. This work explores an image-based approach for localizing needles during MRI-guided interventions, for the purpose of tracking and navigation. Susceptibility artifacts for several needles of varying thickness were imaged, in phantoms, using a 3 tesla MRI system, under a variety of conditions. The relationship between the true needle positions and the locations of artifacts within the images, determined both by manual and automatic segmentation methods, have been quantified and are presented here.

Keywords. needle tracking, magnetic resonance imaging, susceptibility artifact

1. Introduction

This study explores the feasibility of localizing standard MRI-compatible needles by detecting their susceptibility artifacts directly from images, for the purpose of tracking and navigation during MRI-guided interventions. A variety of approaches for tracking instruments in MRI have been presented in the past [1–4]. Although typically fast and accurate, such approaches can have drawbacks such as line-of-sight limitations, heating, sensitive tuning, calibration and expense. Passive tracking approaches, in which the needle position is detected directly from the images, provide an alternative solution. Paramagnetic needles produce field distortions that appear as local regions of signal loss [5] when imaged. The advantages of an image-based passive tracking approach are that needles and devices do not require expensive instrumentation, and that both the interventional device and the patient's anatomy are observed together in the same image space. There is, however, a compromise between imaging speed and quality that can degrade needle localization accuracy and reliability. The visual appearance of susceptibility artifacts produced by needles in 0.2, 0.5, 1.0 and 1.5 Tesla MRI images has been

---

[1] This work was partially funded by NSF ERC 9731748, NIH 5-P01-CA067165-07 and 1-U41-RR019703.
[2] Correspondence to: Simon DiMaio, Brigham and Women's Hospital, 75 Francis Street, Boston, 02115. E-mail: simond@bwh.harvard.edu

characterized in [6–9], while techniques for optimizing visualization of artifacts are described in [10].

The paper is organized as follows: Section 2 describes a set of needle artifact imaging experiments performed in a 3T MRI system, as well as the methods used to localize and compare needle and needle artifact positions computed from images. Section 3 presents a summary of results quantifying the location of needle artifact in the images. Finally, Section 4 concludes with an interpretation of the results and scope for future work.

2. Materials and Methods

We localized needles by automatically detecting image artifacts using fast imaging sequences that are useful for interventional guidance and navigation. Three needles of varying thickness (18G×10cm, 20G×10cm and 22G×10cm MRI histology needles, E-Z-EM Inc.) were clamped horizontally in an acrylic needle holder, as shown in Figures 1(a) and (b). The needle holder was attached to the bottom of a plastic container, but was free to rotate in the horizontal plane, with gradations marked at $10°$ intervals for accurate orientation. For imaging, we used

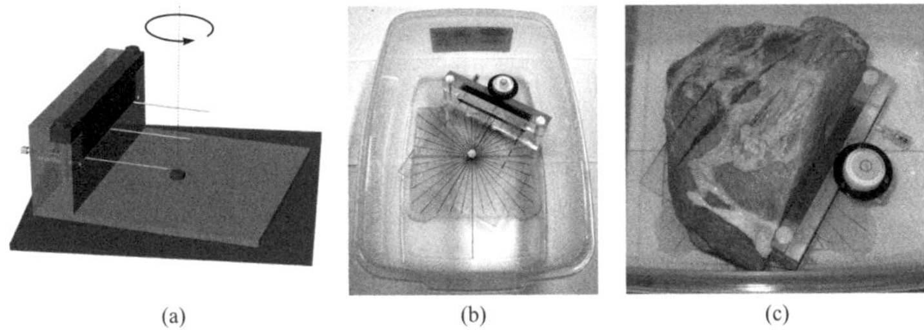

(a)   (b)   (c)

Figure 1. Experiment apparatus: (a,b) rotating acrylic needle holder, (c) needles embedded in an ex vivo tissue sample.

a 3-tesla MRI scanner (GE Healthcare, Milwaukee, WI). The plastic container was placed into a standard head imaging coil (GE quadrature birdcage) and filled with a Nickel Chloride solution ($< 1\%$ NiCl). The needle holder included two cylindrical fiducials precisely machined in the same plane as the needles, for scan plane alignment, and to determine the true needle positions within the images. All combinations of the imaging protocols, needle orientations, image orientations and phase/frequency-encoding directions, listed below, were imaged.

Imaging Protocol:	*Single-Shot Fast Spin Echo* (SSFSE) and *Fast Gradient Recalled Echo* (FGRE).
Needle Orientation:	Needle axis horizontal, $0 - 90°$ with respect to B_0 in $10°$ increments.
Slice Orientation:	Single image with needles in plane, and a set of images taken transversely through the needle shafts, from base to tip (to be called axial images).
Frequency Direction:	Parallel and perpendicular to the needle shaft for in-plane images.

Standard half-Fourier single-shot fast spin echo (SSFSE) and fast gradient recalled echo (FGRE) imaging protocols were used: **2D SSFSE** (TR=2500ms, TE=65.832ms, flip angle=$90°$, 62.5kHz bandwidth, 24cm FOV, 0.9375 pixel spacing, 4mm slice, 256×256 matrix, 0.5 NEX); **2D FGRE** (TR=29ms, TE= 5.5ms, flip angle=30°, 15.63kHz bandwidth, 24cm FOV, 0.9375 pixel spacing, 4mm slice, 256×128 matrix, 1 NEX). Scan time per image was less than four seconds for the SSFSE and less than one second for the FGRE.

The experiments were repeated with the needles inserted into an ex vivo tissue sample, as shown in Figure 1(c). Needles were rotated axially while being inserted into the tissue, and symmetrical bevels were used to minimize needle deflection.

2.1. Artifact Detection

In this preliminary study, we used a primitive artifact-detection algorithm to illustrate the feasibility of image-based needle localization. Each in-plane needle image was processed in order to determine: 1) the true needle positions, 2) the centroid and tip of each artifact by manual segmentation, and 3) the automatically detected centroid and tip of each artifact. The true needle positions were determined by detecting the needle holder fiducials which have a known relationship to the needles. Each image is divided into three regions of interest, each containing just one needle artifact. Automatic detection of each artifact is computed using an algorithm based on the linear Hough transform, as shown in Figure 2. The detection algorithm operates on both the raw image regions and their

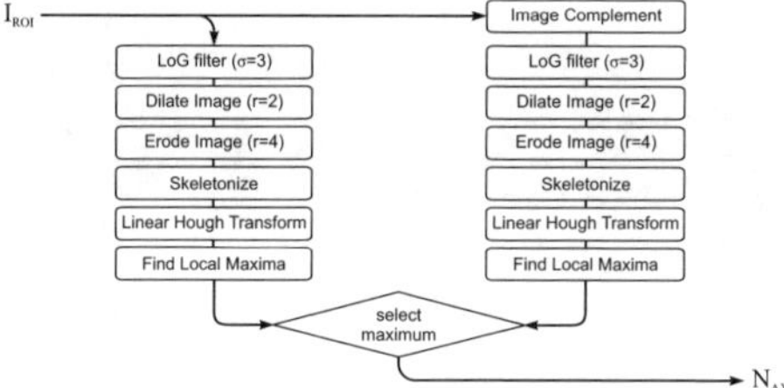

Figure 2. Flowchart illustrating the artifact detection algorithm.

complements (grayscale intensities inverted), in order to detect both enhancing and non-enhancing needle artifacts. Occasional manual intervention was required to correct a poor decision in the final step of the algorithm; otherwise, all other parameters remained constant for all images. The tip of each artifact was computed by finding the peak image intensity gradient along the detected artifact axis N_{AXIS}.

3. Results

Examples of needle artifacts are shown in Figure 3. The FGRE artifacts are significantly larger than the SSFSE artifacts when perpendicular to B_0. Artifacts are shifted along the frequency-encoding direction in both SSFSE and FGRE sequences, and become better defined when this direction is perpendicular to the needle shaft. The quantitative relationship between the artifact location and true needle position is illustrated in Figure 4, where both the difference in tip depths and shaft positions are shown. Here, the artifact location is based on a manual

(a) SSFSE

(b) FGRE

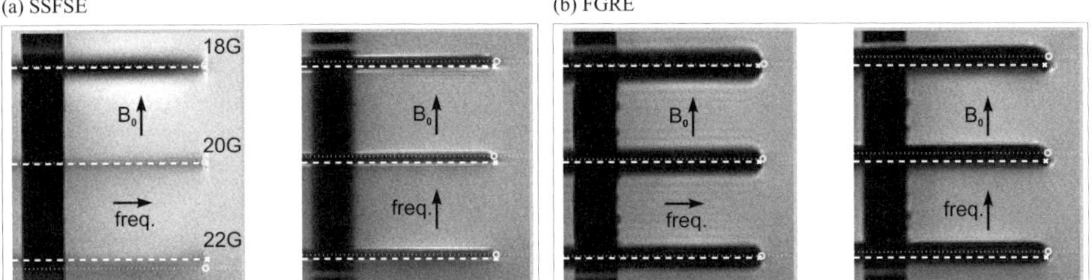

Figure 3. Artifacts with needles perpendicular to B_0, imaged with (a) SSFSE, and (b) FGRE, with needles emersed in a NiCl solution. Frequency-encoding directions both parallel and perpendicular to the needle shaft are shown. Dashed lines and crosses are actual needle shaft and tip, while dotted lines and circles indicate detected artifact.

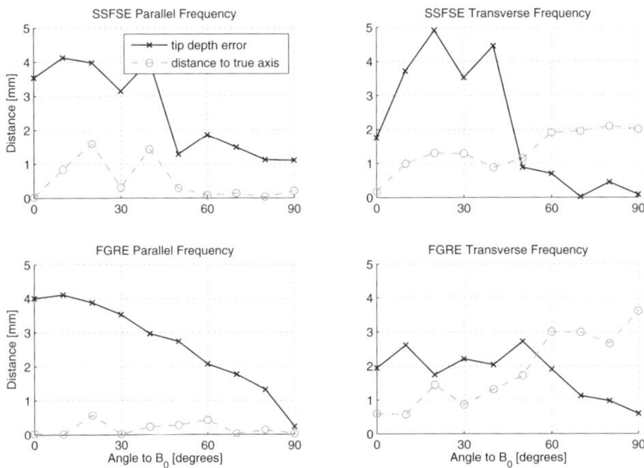

Figure 4. Comparison of manually segmented artifact to true needle position. Results for the 20G needle are shown.

segmentation for which the centroid and tip of the artifact were determined visually. When the needle is parallel to B_0, the visible SSFSE artifacts tend to under-represent the tip depth by up to 5mm and the FGRE artifacts tend to over-represent the tip depth by up to 4mm; however, these discrepancies decrease to below 1mm by the time the needle is perpendicular. The centroid of the artifact is very close to the true needle axis (<1mm) when the frequency-encoding direction runs parallel to the needle; however, when the frequency direction is perpendicular, the artifact is increasingly shifted away from the needle axis as the needle is rotated to 90° from B_0. For SSFSE images, this shift reaches 2mm, while the FGRE images exhibit a maximum shift of 3.6mm—this is visible in Figure 3. These results are shown for the 20G needle, while similar behaviour is observed for the 18G and 22G needles.

The automatic artifact detection algorithm was compared against both the true needle position and the manually segmented artifact location. In Figure 5 the distance between the detected artifact axis, and the true axis, evaluated at the needle tip, is plotted with respect to the needle orientation angle. The distance to the manually specified artifact centroid is also shown. For all combinations of the

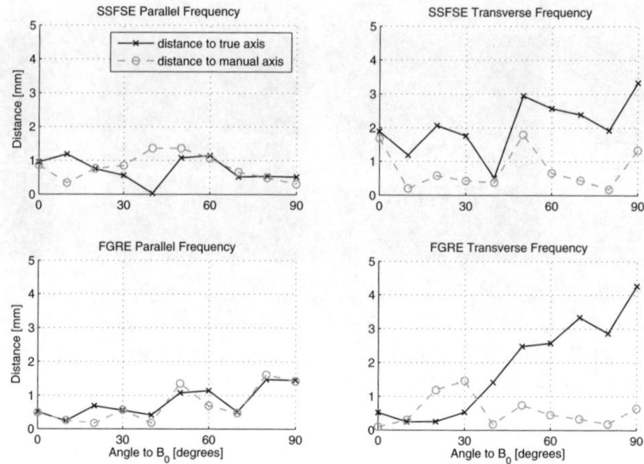

Figure 5. Comparison of automatically segmented artifact to true needle positions and manually segmented artifact. Results for the 20G needle are shown.

imaging sequence and frequency-encoding direction, the automatically detected artifact axis lies well within 2mm of the visible artifact (manually segmented artifact centroid). However, when the frequency-encoding direction is perpendicular to the needle, the detected artifact is shifted with respect to the true needle, increasing with B_0 angle. In the SSFSE and FGRE images, this shift reaches 3.4mm and 4.4mm, respectively, in a manner similar to that observed in Figure 4. Similar results were obtained for 18G and 22G needles. Transverse images of the needle shafts exhibit similar characteristics as in-plane images. Artifact size and shift increase with B_0 angle, particularly when using the FGRE sequence. All of the abovementioned imaging was repeated using an ex vivo tissue sample. Similar needle detection results were obtained from these images, as shown in Figure 6.

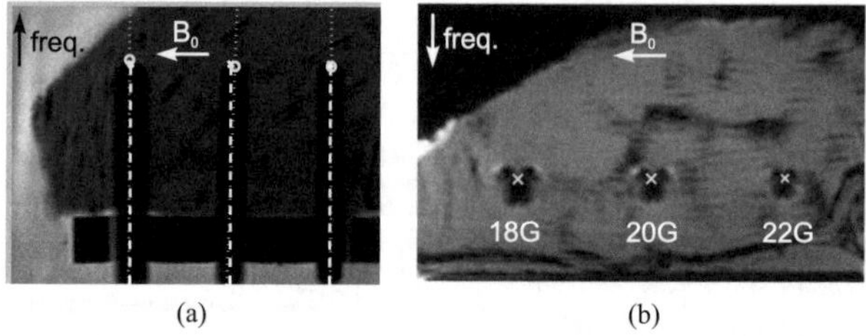

(a)   (b)

Figure 6. Needle artifact in a tissue sample: (a) in-plane images indicating true needle (dashed line and cross) and detected artifact (dotted line and circle); (b) axial image with true needle axes marked.

4. Conclusions

Artifact characteristics appear to vary systematically with respect to the B0 angle and frequency-encoding direction, which implies three opportunities for future work. First, from knowledge of these critical parameters, it may be possible to correct for the spatial shifts of the artifacts from a single image; this might be possible with a combination of a physics-based approach (e.g., based on dipole field models) and empirically determined corrections. Second, multiple orthogonal images may be useful in correcting for the spatial shift. Finally, from the angle of the artifact with respect to the B0 and frequency-encoding directions, it may be possible to optimize the frequency direction from image to image and to adapt echo time and bandwidth to perform real-time control of the MRI sequences to optimally image a needle during an interventional procedure.

This work is significant because robust and reliable needle and device tracking will be required for tracking and navigation of needle placement inside the 3T magnet bore, using either manual or robot-assisted positioning. A localization approach that does not rely upon additional instrumentation, and that is intrinsically registered to the targeting plan is highly desirable. This study indicates the feasibility of such an approach.

References

[1] S. G. Silverman, B. D. Collick, M. R. Figueira, R. Khorasani, D. F. Adams, R. W. Newman, G. P. Topulos, and F. A. Jolesz, "Interactive MR-guided biopsy in an open-configuration MR imaging system," in *Radiology*, vol. 197(1), pp. 175–181, 1995.

[2] C. L. Dumoulin, S. P. Souza, and R. D. Darrow, "Real-time position monitoring of invasive devices using magnetic resonance," in *Magnetic Resonance in Medicine*, vol. 29, pp. 411–415, 1993.

[3] J. A. Derbyshire, G. A. Wright, R. M. Henkelman, and R. S. Hinks, "Dynamic scan-plane tracking using MRI position monitoring," in *J. Mag. Res. Imag.*, vol. 8(4), pp. 924–932, 1998.

[4] S. G. Hushek, B. Fetics, R. M. Moser, N. F. Hoerter, L. J. Russell, A. Roth, D. Polenur, and E. Nevo, "Initial Clinical Experience with a Passive Electromagnetic 3D Locator System," in $5^t h$ *Interventional MRI Symp., Boston MA*, pp. 73–74, 2004.

[5] J. F. Schenck, "The role of magnetic susceptibility in magnetic resonance imaging: MRI magnetic compatibility of the first and second kinds," in *Medical Physics*, vol. 23(6), pp. 815–850, 1996.

[6] C. Frahm, H. Gehl, U. H. Melchert, and H. Weiss, "Visualization of Magnetic Resonance-Compatible Needles at 1.5 and 0.2 Tesla," in *Cardiovascular Interventional Radiology*, vol. 19, pp. 335–340, 1996.

[7] M. E. Ladd, P. Erhart, J. F. Debatin, B. J. Romanowski, P. Boesiger, and G. C. McKinnon, "Biopsy Needle Susceptibility Artifacts," in *Magnetic Resonance in Medicine*, vol. 36, pp. 646–651, 1996.

[8] J. S. Lewin, J. L. Duerk, V. R. Jain, C. A. Petersilge, C. P. Chao, and J. R. Haaga, "Needle Localization in MR-Guided Biopsy and Aspiration," in *American Journal of Radiology*, vol. 166, pp. 1337–1345, 1996.

[9] H. J. Langen, H. Kugel, W. Heindel, T. Krahe, J. Gieseke, and K. Lackner, "Localization of puncture needles in MRI: experimental studies on precision using spin-echo sequences at 1.0 T," in *Rofo Fortschr Geb Rontgenstr Neuen Bildgeb Verfahr*, vol. 167(5), pp. 501–508, 1997.

[10] K. Butts, J. M. Pauly, B. Daniel, S. Kee, and A. Norbash, "Management of Biopsy Needle Artifacts: Techniques for RF-Refocused MRI," in *Magnetic Resonance Imaging*, vol. 9, pp. 586–595, 1999.

Medicine Meets Virtual Reality 14
J.D. Westwood et al. (Eds.)
IOS Press, 2006

Robot-Assisted Needle Placement in Open-MRI: System Architecture, Integration and Validation

S.P. DiMaio [a,1], S. Pieper [b], K. Chinzei [c], N. Hata [a], E. Balogh [d],
G. Fichtinger [d], C.M. Tempany [a], R. Kikinis [a],

[a] *Brigham and Women's Hospital, Harvard Medical School*
[b] *Isomics Inc.*
[c] *National Institute of Advanced Industrial Science and Technology, Japan*
[d] *Johns Hopkins University*

Abstract. This work describes an integrated system for planning and performing percutaneous procedures—such as prostate biopsy—with robotic assistance under MRI-guidance. The physician interacts with a planning interface in order to specify the set of desired needle trajectories, based on anatomical structures and lesions observed in the patient's MR images. All image-space coordinates are automatically computed, and used to position a needle guide by means of an MRI-compatible robotic manipulator, thus avoiding the limitations of the traditional fixed needle template. Direct control of real-time imaging aids visualization of the needle as it is manually inserted through the guide. Results from in-scanner phantom experiments are provided.

Keywords. robot-assisted needle biopsy, MR-compatible robot, prostate cancer

1. Introduction

Accurate navigation of surgical instruments (e.g., biopsy and therapy needles), based on pre-operative trajectory plans and intra-operative guidance, is a challenging problem in image-guided therapy. Stereotactic frames and needle template guides are typically used to calibrate and constrain instrument motion, but often lead to inflexible guidance mechanisms and workflows. In this work, we focus on prostate biopsy and brachytherapy procedures that are currently performed under MRI guidance at the Brigham and Women's Hospital [1]. Similarly to the standard transrectal-ultrasound-guided approaches, these procedures rely on a fixed needle template guide that constrains trajectory resolution and orientation.

MRI is an attractive choice for image-guidance, due to its excellent soft tissue contrast, multi-parametric imaging protocols, high spatial resolution, and mul-

---

[1]Correspondence to: Simon DiMaio, Brigham and Women's Hospital, 75 Francis Street, Boston, 02115. E-mail: simond@bwh.harvard.edu

tiplanar volumetric imaging capabilities. The peripheral zone (PZ) can be seen in T2-weighted images, and used to identify suspicious nodules in the peripheral zone. A multi-year clinical trial of MRI-guided prostate biopsy is described in [2], and uses an intra-operative open 0.5 tesla MR imager (GEMS Signa SP). While the use of MRI imaging in prostate cancer biopsy and therapy appears to have helped improve outcomes, the manual method of needle placement has remained unchanged. The use of a fixed needle guide template, with holes spaced at least 5mm apart, limits needle trajectory position and orientation. In addition, template registration and the manual computation and transcription of coordinates are prone to human error. *This paper introduces a system that integrates an interactive planning system and real-time imaging control interface with an MR-compatible robotic assistant that acts as a dynamic needle guide for precise, yet flexible targeted needle placement. The system has been validated for a prostate biopsy procedure, and approved for a first clinical trial. It is based on an a modular and extensible architecture.*

Robotic assistance has been investigated for guiding instrument placement in MRI, beginning with neurosurgery [3] and later percutaneous interventions [4,5]. Chinzei et al. developed a general-purpose robotic assistant for open MRI [6] that was subsequently adapted for transperineal intra-prostatic needle placement [7]. Krieger et al. presented a 2-DOF passive, un-encoded and manually manipulated mechanical linkage to aim a needle guide for transrectal prostate biopsy with MRI guidance [8]. With three active tracking coils, the device is visually servoed into position and then the patient was moved out of the scanner for needle insertion. Other recent developments in MRI-compatible mechanisms include haptic interfaces for fMRI [9] and multi-modality actuators and robotics [10].

This paper is organized as follows: Section 2 describes the architecture of the robot-assisted system that includes a planning interface and an MRI-compatible needle positioning device (Section 3). Preliminary results from in-scanner phantom tests are given in Section 4. Concluding remarks are provided in Section 5.

2. System Architecture

The architecture of the MR-guided, robot-assisted percutaneous intervention system is shown in Figure 1. The three major subsystems, namely the planning environment, the MR scanner (GE Signa SP, Milwaukee WI), and the motion controlled robotic manipulator, are integrated as shown. The workflow is as follows:

1. Visualize pre-procedural MR images I_{MRI} to specify a set of biopsy targets. Image visualization and target planning are performed using the 3D Slicer [11]. For each biopsy plan, the physician specifies two points along the needle trajectory, namely a target and an entry point, by clicking on coordinates on T2-weighted images viewed in the Slicer.
2. The robot is visualized in conjunction with the images and the biopsy plan, and positioning motions can be simulated and rendered on-screen for trajectory verification.
3. Calibrate robot to image space using a Flashpoint® optical tracking system.
4. Execute robot joint-space motion commands $(q,\ \dot{q},\ \ddot{q})$ via an ethernet connection with the robot controller.
5. Robot motion proceeds and is continuously monitored and compared against a simulated robot motion model; any significant trajectory deviation halts motion.

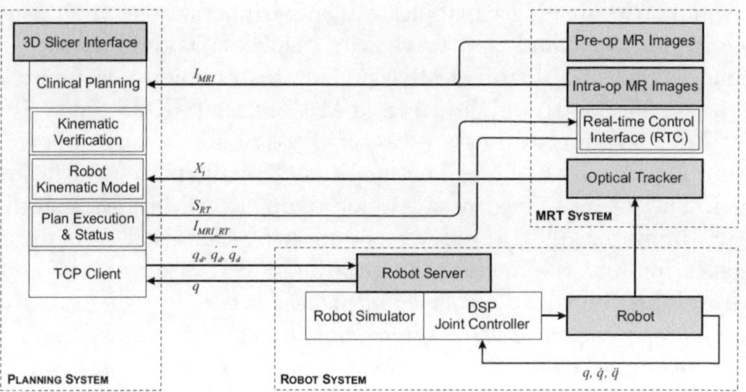

Figure 1. The percutaneous intervention system, comprised of a planning sub-system, the MRT, and an MR-compatible robot.

6. Verify robot position by comparing the optically tracked needle guide position (X_t) with the biopsy plan. Steps 4-6 are repeated until the positioning error is satisfactorily compensated.
7. Imaging plane coordinates (S_{RT}) corresponding to the plane of the needle are sent from the 3D Slicer to the scanner's Real Time Control interface, and real-time images (I_{MRI_RT}) are aquired and displayed.
8. The needle is manually inserted through the needle guide, under real-time MR guidance (3-6s image update), and a biopsy sample is taken. Steps 4-8 are repeated until all target sites have been sampled.

3. MRI-compatible Needle Positioning Device

For this work, we use a first-generation MRI-compatible robotic assistant developed by [12–14] for use in a Magnetic Resonance Therapy operating room (MRT) equipped with a GE SIGNA SP open-MRI scanner. The robotic device consists of five linear motion stages arranged to form a 2-DOF orienting mechanism attached to a 3-DOF Cartesian positioning mechanism. The base of the robot is mounted above the surgeon's head in the open MRI magnet and two rigid arms reach down into the surgical field. The ends of the arms are linked to form a tool holder, which in this case is a linear needle guide (Figure 2(b)). There is a Flashpoint® optical marker attached to the needle guide, providing independent redundant encoding of end-effector pose, as shown in Figure 2(b-inset). The mechanism is constructed almost entirely from non-ferrous, MR-compatible materials. The gantry frame is composed of aluminum and titanium elements, and each linear motion stage comprises plastic, titanium, stainless steel (YHD50) and beryllium-copper (Be-Cu) components. All sensors are optical and signals are transferred to and from the magnet room via fiber-optics. Linear optical encoders measure the displacement of each motion stage with 20μm resolution (Encoder Technology, Cottonwood, AZ). The actuators are ultrasonic motors (Shinsei travelling-wave USR60 USM) that contain no magnetic or ferrous components. The MRI compatibility of the robotic mechanism was evaluated in the open-MR scanner and found to produce no adverse effects. In fact, the robot created less field distortion than the body of the patient, as measured by [13].

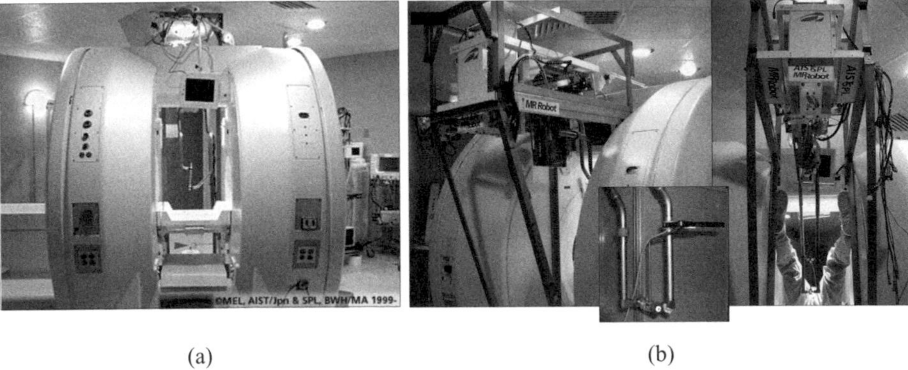

(a)　　　　　　　　　　　　　　　　　(b)

Figure 2. (a) GE Signa SP open-MRI scanner, with (b) integrated 5-DOF MR-compatible robot. The robot end-effector is equipped with an optical tracking marker (inset).

4. Phantom Experiments

Needle placement has been verified using a polyvinyl chloride (PVC) tissue phantom measuring $9 \times 9 \times 11$cm. The phantom incorporates a prostate model, as well as several acrylic beads that serve as targets. The beads have a hole diameter of 3mm, and are embedded at depths up to 9cm from the inferior surface of the phantom. The tissue phantom was placed into a patient leg model, as shown in Figure 3(a), and transferred into the MRI scanner in order to mimick the clinical procedure. Sterile draping is applied to both the patient model and the robot manipulator arms, as shown in Figure 3(b). The phantom was scanned and the image volume imported into the 3D Slicer for planning and placement, as described in Section 2, and shown in Figure 3(c). In this study, we attempted to

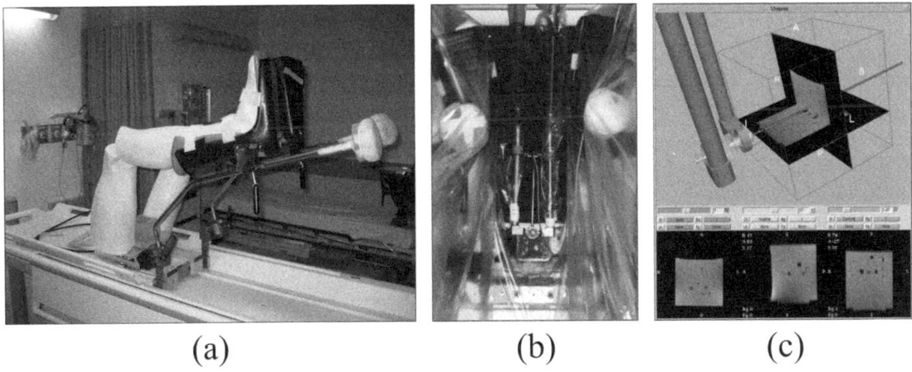

(a)　　　　　　　　　　(b)　　　　　　　　　　(c)

Figure 3. Phantom experiments: (a) scale models of legs and PVC prostate phantom with embedded targets, (b) patient model and robot placement inside the scanner, with sterile draping, (c)needle trajectories are interactively specified in the planning environment.

place 10 needles (E-Z-EM Inc., MRI Histology) into the centres of the beads from a variety of different trajectory angles. 7 needles were placed into centres of the beads, while 2 needles hit the sides of their target beads. One needle, which was targeted along an elevated oblique angle, was placed adjacent to its target bead.

Examples of images, showing needle placement in the phantoms, are provided in Figure 4.

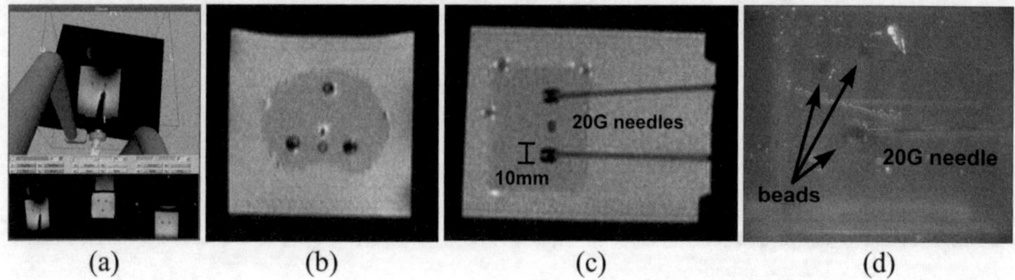

(a)   (b)   (c)   (d)

Figure 4. (a) Real-time image visualization in the Slicer interface during needle insertion; (b,c) MRI images of needle placement in the phantom; and (d) the target phantom.

In experiments, the system consistently placed needles to within 2mm of their intended targets in a tissue phantom. Increased placement error was found for severely oblique needle trajectories, largely due to calibration errors between the optical tracker and the needle holder. This has subsequently been ameliorated through improved calibration. In general, system performance is dependent on accurate calibration between the optical tracker and the image coordinate space, as is also the case for all clinical cases undertaken in the MRT. An image-based registration and tracking approach would be preferable, and can be incorporated into our present system architecture. The advantage of such a visual servo approach is that the image and device coordinate systems are explicitly registered, as opposed to a "register and shoot" approach that is dependent on calibrated external sensors.

5. Conclusion

We have developed an integrated planning system and a robotic assistant that acts as a dynamic needle guide. This approach helps to simplify workflow by providing an interactive "point and click" trajectory planning interface and an MRI-compatible robotic mechanism for precise, yet flexible needle placement. In-scanner phantom tests have been performed in order to validate system performance and needle placement, and preparations are underway for clinical trial. The system is based on a modular and extensible architecture that will be used as a testbed for the development of novel image-based navigation and visual servo techniques in open- and closed-bore MRI scanners, in order to be extended to other applications of MRI-guided percutaneous therapy in the future.

Acknowledgements

This work was partially funded by NSF ERC 9731748, NIH 5-P01-CA067165-07 and 1-U41-RR019703. We would like to thank Dan Kacher and Janice Fairhurst for scanning assistance, and Mike McKenna for assistance with Slicer programming.

References

[1] A. V. D'Amico, C. M. Tempany, R. A. Cormack, N. Hata, M. Jinzaki, K. Tuncali, M. Weinstein, and J. P. Richie, "Transperineal magnetic resonance image guided prostate biopsy," in *Journal of Urology*, vol. 164(2), pp. 385–387, Aug. 2000.

[2] A. V. D'Amico, R. A. Cormack, and C. M. Tempany, "MRI-guided diagnosis and treatment of prostate cancer," in *New England Journal of Medicine*, vol. 344(10), pp. 776–777, Mar. 2001.

[3] K. Masamune, E. Kobayashi, Y. Masutani, M. Suzuki, T. Dohi, H. Iseki, and K. Takakura, "Development of an MRI-compatible needle insertion manipulator for stereotactic neurosurgery," in *Journal of Image Guided Surgery*, vol. 1(4), pp. 242–248, 1995.

[4] A. Felden, J. Vagner, A. Hinz, H. Fischer, S. O. Pfleiderer, J. R. Reichenbach, and W. A. Kaiser, "ROBITOM-robot for biopsy and therapy of the mamma," in *Biomedical Technology*, vol. 47, pp. 2–5, 2002.

[5] E. Hempel, H. Fischer, L. Gumb, T. Hohn, H. Krause, U. Voges, H. Breitwieser, B. Gutmann, J. Durke, M. Bock, and A. Melzer, "An MRI-compatible surgical robot for precise radiological interventions," in *Computer Aided Surgery*, pp. 180–191, Apr. 2003.

[6] K. Chinzei, N. Hata, F. A. Jolesz, and R. Kikinis, "MR compatible surgical assist robot: system integration and preliminary feasibility study," in *Medical Image Computing and Computer Assisted Intervention*, vol. 1935, pp. 921–933, Oct. 2000.

[7] S. P. DiMaio, S. Pieper, K. Chinzei, G. Fichtinger, C. Tempany, and R. Kikinis, "Robot assisted percutaneous intervention in open-MRI," in 5th *Interventional MRI Symposium*, p. 155, 2004.

[8] A. Krieger, R. C. Susil, C. Menard, J. A. Coleman, G. Fichtinger, E. Atalar, and L. L. Whitcomb, "Design of a novel MRI compatible manipulator for image guided prostate interventions," in *IEEE Trans. on Biomedical Engineering*, vol. 52, pp. 306–313, Feb. 2005.

[9] G. Ganesh, R. Gassert, E. Burdet, and H. Bleule, "Dynamics and control of an MRI compatible master-slave system with hydrostatic transmission," in *International Confennee on Robotics and Automation*, pp. 1288–1294, Apr. 2004.

[10] D. Stoianovici, "Multi-imager compatible actuation principles in surgical robotics," in *International Journal of Medical Robotics and Computer Assisted Surgery*, vol. 1, pp. 86–100, 2005.

[11] N. Hata, M. Jinzaki, D. Kacher, R. Cormak, D. Gering, A. Nabavi, S. G. Silverman, A. V. D'Amico, R. Kikinis, F. A. Jolesz, and C. M. Tempany, "MRI imaging-guided prostate biopsy with surgical navigation software: device validation and feasibility," in *Radiology*, vol. 220(1), July 2001.

[12] K. Chinzei, R. Kikinis, and F. A. Jolesz, "MRI Compatibility of Mechatronic Devices: Design Criteria," in *International Conference on Medical Image Computing and Computer-Assisted Intervention (MICCAI)*.

[13] K. Chinzei, N. Hata, F. A. Jolesz, and K. Kikinis, "MRI Compatible Surgical Assist Robot: System Integration and Preliminary Feasibility Study," in *International Conference on Medical Image Computing and Computer-Assisted Intervention (MICCAI)*.

[14] K. Chinzei, N. Hata, F. Jolesz, and R. Kikinis, "Surgical Assist Robot for the Active Navigation in the Intraoperative MRI: Hardware Design Issues," in *Proceedings of the IEEE/RSJ IROS*, pp. 727–732, 2000.

Medicine Meets Virtual Reality 14
J.D. Westwood et al. (Eds.)
IOS Press, 2006

Polymer Film Based Sensor Networks for Non-Invasive Medical Monitoring

Martin DUDZIAK, PhD[1]
TETRAD Technologies Group, Inc., USA

Abstract. An instrumentation system based upon laminate polymer film composition with embedded ultra-flat imaging sensors has been designed for application to both external and internal monitoring during medical procedures or post-operative care.   This technology is based upon a common architecture employing PET (polyethelene terephthalate) film substrates laminated with conductive printed circuit logic and the inclusion of discrete ultra-flat imaging sensors which are based upon the principle of compound eye vision. The system enables the construction of variable-size, variable-geometry sheets that can be applied physically to different locations including objects in an environment that requires frequent monitoring.

Keywords. Polymer film, compound eye, artificial vision, sensor fusion, monitor

Patient safety and survival as well as the ability to record and review procedures ranging from drug administration to surgical procedures and post-operative monitoring are problem issues in crisis environments. The experiences of medical personnel in two well-known settings – the Iraq warfront and the post-Katrina flooding and destruction in New Orleans – exemplify the contexts for which new forms of assistance in visual and other means of real-time situation awareness are needed. We set out to design a multi-purpose solution for situation awareness when there inadequate resources or exacerbating conditions; e.g., staff shortage, requirements for sharing critical care equipment, power outages, hose leaks, shifting of patients and equipment or furnishings. Our principal focus has been upon the exacerbated and disadvantaged operational environment, the cases where organizational and supervisory infrastructure also may have collapsed or been stretched to the limits of effective attention and awareness by responders and providers. In particular we have been motivated by cases where there is no reliable information flow for tracking procedures and events such as the sequence and dosage of drug administration to patients being treated in a "field setting."

The concept of compound eyes is not new to artificial vision systems [1] and has been principally studied with a view toward engineering visual sensors that can replicate the functions and behaviors of an insect eye for obstacle avoidance or navigation [2]. Our approach has been to take the general model of the compound eye, as well as some specific sensing technology that has been developed following that model for providing vision capabilities in extremely flat and small electro-optics, and to experiment with ways in which this technology can be adapted to high-stress, high-noise, low-resource operational environments and in particularly to situations where it cannot be predicted in

---

[1] Corresponding author: TETRAD Technologies Group, Inc., 28 Chase Gayton Circle, Suite 736, Richmond VA 23238 USA   Email: <u>martin@forteplan.com</u>

advance of need where all the visual sensors should be placed and how they should communicate with one another. Paramount in our architectural design work has been the need to develop solutions that can be used in a diversity of physical locations, power constraints, and interfaces but to also provide a means for adding future capabilities beyond the visual optical spectrum.

The architecture, referred to as the SenseNet, is based upon four components: (1) individual sensor elements (currently considering only visual sensors, described in Section 2) that are embedded (one or more) in Patches, wireless-accessible flexible units. Each Patch consists of a laminate polymer construction involving (2) industry-standard PET (polyethelene terephthalate) film as the primary substrate bonded to a standard neoprene or PVC base layer for additional strength and (3) a OLED (organic light-emitting diode) multilayer with specific HIL (hole injection layer) technology [3] that is laminated to the PET, plus (4) industry-standard wireless communication electronics drawn from conventional 802.11 wireless internet products. SenseNet components are illustrated in Figure 1 and Figure 2 below.

SenseNet Patch units are each linked to a standard 802.11 access point and thereby into the local intranet or internet that has been established for the operational space. Data communications from Patches are input to a server which in turn maps the image data (or in the case of non-visual sensor data in the form of text) directly into a resident archiving database and a dynamic web management application for interactive display via standard browsers on PC, PDA or other internet accessible devices. In this manner, SenseNet data is real-time provided to the following communities of users:

- Individuals working in the actual operating space
- Observers working remotely or requiring real-time knowledge of various conditions in the operating space (patient medical observables, status of equipment under visual observation, status of physical lines, cables, tubing, or structures, and historical recording of events such as administration of drugs, movement of patient(s) or equipment, surgical procedure sequences, etc.
- Post-facto viewers and reviewers who have need for a transcript of events that have occurred, such as in the case of caregivers for a patient who has been moved.

From the standpoint of system integration we have developed software that is designed as an intelligent agent-enabled content management system [4] using C++, Java and PHP-based components, treating the data as a stream of information handled in a conventional extract-transfer-load (ETL) scenario that is common in the management of very large databases and data warehouses. Agents in the ETL pipeline react to both direct demands and inferred associations and pattern recognition events and thereby route sensor (image) data to particular defined dynamic web pages or through notifications sent as email or SMS packets to pre-identified individuals. Thus a wide and extensible variety of people connected with the procedures at hand can be notified real-time of events and relationships (detected patterns) that merit attention and/or intervention. Within the limits of the present paper it is not possible to describe further the content management or fault-tolerance logic used for communications processing.
The visual units are critical to the utility of the SenseNet. We have selected for our study and experimentation the two different methods, one an artificial apposition eye and the other a cluster eye design, developed by Duparre et al [5,6]. The designs derive from insect eyes and the Gabor-Superlens. The apposition eye unit has been tested

experimentally and returns images that are of high quality at 17cm with a horizontal FOV of 63° achievable for a system employing a 2mm thin imaging system with 21x3 channels, 70° x10° field of view and 4.5mm x 0.5mm image size. This is a promising start for the type of applications discussed in Section 1.

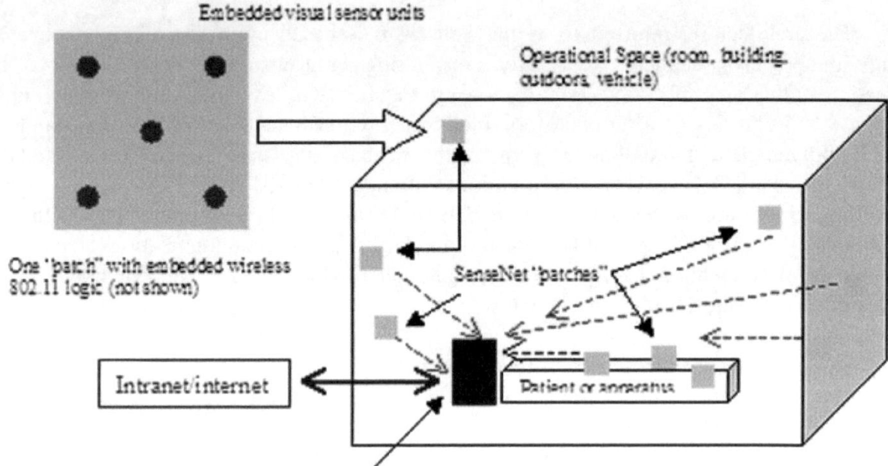

Figure 1 – SenseNet Configuration Schematic

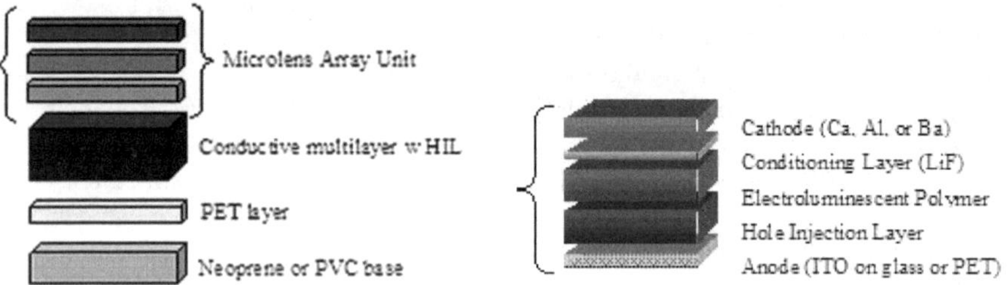

Figure 2 – SenseNet Layering Schematic   Figure 3 – Conductive Multilayer (shown as OLED) [3]

References

[1] Hoshino, K., Mura, F., Morii, H., Suematsu, K. and Shimoyama, I., A Small-Sized Panoramic Scanning Compound Eye Inspired by the Fly's Eye, *1998 IEEE Int'l Conference on Robotics and Automation*, IEEE Press (1998)

[2] *Conference on Neurotechnology for Biomimetic Robots*, Northeastern University, May 14-16, 2000, http://www.neurotechnology.neu.edu/ConferenceProgram.pdf

[3] see www.plextronics.com

[4] *AdaM Active Data Mover* and *Nomad Eyes Network* [www.tetradgroup.com]

[5] Duparré, J., Schreiber, P., Dannberg, P., Scharf, T., Pelli, P., Völkel, R., Herzig, H.-P., Brauer, A., Artificial compound eyes – different concepts and their application to ultra flat image acquisition sensors, *MOEMS and Miniaturized Systems IV*, A. El–Fatatry, ed., Proc. SPIE **5346**, 89–100 (2004)

[6] Völkel, R., Eisner, M., Weibel, K. J., Miniaturized Imaging Systems, *Microelectronic Engineering* 67–68, 461–472 (2003)

Medicine Meets Virtual Reality 14
J.D. Westwood et al. (Eds.)
IOS Press, 2006

135

Detecting Trigger Points and Irreversibility Thresholds in Shock and Trauma

Martin DUDZIAK, PhD[1]
TETRAD Technologies Group, Inc., USA

Abstract. We investigate the model of unstable recurrent patterns within chaotic and highly turbulent systems as a possible avenue for linking shifts in parameters that can be indicators of nonlinear and irreversible transitions leading to mortality. The argument presented is that in the case of mass injury and trauma events from natural or intentional causes, large numbers of people may be in situations where clinical testing infrastructures have been disabled or destroyed, further reducing the ability of medical caregivers to accurately notice indicators and signals of impending critical and irreversible conditions. Identification of a reduced set of observables that can be linked with unstable yet recurrent patterns may provide a means for improved monitoring and life support under such adverse conditions.

Keywords. shock, trauma, chaos, turbulence, dissipation, emergency preparedness

Introduction

Anomaly and intrusion detection methods may enable the examination of unstable and semi-stable recurrent patterns in dissipative extended systems and provide a set of advance-warning indicators that can be associated with impending critical life support conditions. The target situation occurs when there are hundreds or even thousands of persons subjected, within a comparatively short period of time (minutes or hours) by exposure or ingestion to toxic agents or impact events. Our goal has been to set the stage for identifying if the abstract model that results can find a match with known observable parameters from the critical care world, working abductively and intuitively toward defining a dataset that can be tested with both the turbulence characteristics and the existence of unstable and semi-stable recurrent patterns (hereafter referred to as λ-recurrence) fitting the initial abstract model. Automatically we must rule out any testing that requires remote and time-intensive laboratory testing that cannot be performed in an emergency room "on the spot." We prefer to focus upon those parameters that can be collected in a field setting such as that of a combat area field hospital or onboard a medivac helicopter. Certainly in the space of possible parameters are those employed in the Glasgow Scale but from the outset we do not know if we should consider one particular parameter p (e.g., SpO2/SaO2) or a set S = {p, q, r}, for which the relationship between 2+ members of S is the critical meta-parameter; i.e, where we find chaotic behavior of the "interesting" sort (meaning, with λ-recurrence).

---

[1] Corresponding author: TETRAD Technologies Group, Inc., 28 Chase Gayton Circle, Suite 736, Richmond VA 23238 USA   Email: <u>martin@forteplan.com</u>

We are automatically limited in the range of clinical tests that can be considered. Parameter sets useful for tracking λ-recurrence may emerge including quantities that are relatively stable on scales of minutes or even hours but for which modest changes coupled with other set members can serve as triggers of a λ-recurrence. Measures of pro- and anti-inflammatory cytokine and adhesion molecule patterns [1] are already employed on a 2 to 4 hour basis for indications of septic shock onset or susceptibility. Within our investigations, the In-Check microfluidic diagnostic chip and platform[2] offers the possibility of such new classes of tests through highly-automated PCR-based analysis in a portable lightweight and low-power configuration capable of performing multiple tests in parallel.

Recurrent Patterns in Dissipative Turbulence - the Kuramoto-Sivashinsky Model

Our goal is to find behaviors similar to the basic Kuramoto-Sivashinsky (KS) system,

$$u_t = (u^2)_x - u_{xx} - \nu u_{xxxx} \tag{1}$$

representing, for example, the general case for amplitudes of interfacial instabilities such as flame fields, nonlinear through term $(u^2)_x$, ν a damping parameter. The solution $u(x,t) = u(x+L, t)$ is periodic and can be expanded into a discrete spatial Fourier series

$$u(x,t) = \sum_{k=-\infty}^{+\infty} a_k(t)e^{ikx} \tag{2}$$

It is possible to extend periodic orbit theory to spatiotemporal chaotic systems and the KS system [2] and reduce a high-demensional system (from 16 to 64 dimensions) down to one, namely a return map. Following Cvitanovi_ and others [3] we postulate that a predictive system for non-equilibrium turbulence of the type that may exist in breathing irregularities, cardiac beat-to-beat chaos and other chaotic-like behavior measured through electrocardiograms, or in molecular patterns[3] such as cytokine levels, may require only $10^2 - 10^4$ recurrent pattern instances as opposed to classical expectations ($\approx 10^{10}$) from Monte Carlo and other PDE simulations. This means fewer cycles of per-patient monitoring and possibly a manageable cycle of acquire-search-compare-evaluate computations to perform (returning to our clinical focus) for large populations when situations impose sparser data collection intervals and less robust computational resources.

Dynamical behavior such as 3-D Navier-Stokes turbulence in many different media often exhibits a variety of unstable recurrent patterns that can in turn be applied to provide indicators of general characteristics or imminent phase shifts. The challenge is how to find such patterns since by definition they are themselves unstable and not the same in amplitude or other dynamical characteristics in each recurrence. Why they may be indicators of trigger-like conditions, including irreversible conditions leading to

---

[2] http://www.st.com/stonline/prodpres/dedicate/labchip/labchip.htm
[3] Recurrent patterns of interest are not necessarily chaotic and the absence or decrease of chaos in certain bioparameters may be indicate onset of a disabling or life-threatening condition (Poon and Merrill, regarding congestive heart failure [4])

death, in the case of individuals experiencing a variety of trauma conditions is not at all obvious. However, on the one hand there is the evidence of sudden death linked with a larger variety of CNS and cardiovascular conditions for which there are no externally observable nor commonly measureable indicators but which have may have increases or decreases in chaotic patterns such as EKG.

How to find and associate recurrent patterns with biomedical conditions

Finding periodic orbits may be enhanced by algorithms but it is still somewhat "trial and error." Cvitanovi_ and Lan apply an iterative approach to begin with a calculated guess and then to monitor the attraction of the solution towards or away from this target. This in turns builds an approach using Newton-Raphson or alternatively by minimizing a cost function. These and other methods like them will not tell which patterns are recurrent nor how "near" everything is in the interpolative process. Here additional heuristics and probabilistic data can be used to reduce the iterative cycle. There are known techniques within the study of anomaly detection and tracking, such as multivariate statistics and neural network classification. At a higher scale probabilistic (Bayesian) networks can be employed with specific rules drawn from the operations domain. Periodic orbit theory [5] proposes that the greater the unstability, the more accurate will be the predictions that are based upon a small number of the shortest recurrent patterns. In turn, once a sufficient number of individual unique patterns can be discriminated, then these can be use together to predict global averages. Average is considered as a sum over all possible patterns which are grouped hierarchically according to the likelihood of each pattern's occrrence in the system.

$$\langle a \rangle = \lim_{t \to \infty} \frac{1}{t} \langle A^t \rangle, \quad A^t(x) = \int_0^t d\tau a(x(\tau)) \tag{3}$$

where the dynamical trajectory x(t) is some point in a high-dimension state space and the object is for short cycles, short patterns, to contribute information collectively as an aggregate to information on the invariant set, the long-term cycle. This offers a logical step from simple observable patterns that can be captured relatively easily, through pulse oxymetry, temperature, pressure, pulse, and other means, to information about impending, imminent shifts in the long-term cycle, the "big picture" of systemic changes that could be the difference between death and life.

References

[1] V von Dossow, K Rotard, U Redlich, O V Hein and CD Spies, Circulating immune parameters predicting the progression from hospital-acquired pneumonia to septic shock in surgical patients, *Critical Care* 2005, **9:**R662-R669

[2] P Cvitanovi_ and T Lan, Turbulent fields and their recurrences, in N Antoniou, ed., *Proc. Of 10th Int'l Workshop on Multiparticle Production: Correlations and Fluctuations in QCD*, World Scientific, Singapore 2003

[3] P Holmes, JL Lumley and G Berkooz, Turbulence, Coherent Structures, Dynamical Systems and Symmetry, *Cambridge Univ. Press*, Cambridge 1996

[4] CS Poon and CK Merrill, Decrease of cardiac chaos in congestive heart failure, *Nature* 1997 Oct 2;389(6650):492-5

[5] P Cvitanovi_ et al, Chaos: Quantum and Classical, *Niels Bohr Institute*, 2003

Medicine Meets Virtual Reality 14
J.D. Westwood et al. (Eds.)
IOS Press, 2006

A Haptic VR Milling Surgery Simulator – Using High-Resolution CT-Data

Magnus ERIKSSON [a], Mark DIXON [b] and Jan WIKANDER [a]
[a] The Mechatronics Lab/Machine Design, KTH, Stockholm, Sweden
[b] SenseGraphics AB, Stockholm, Sweden

Abstract. A haptic virtual reality milling simulator using high resolution volumetric data is presented in this paper. We discuss the graphical rendering performed from an iso-surface generated using marching cubes with a hierarchical storage method to optimize for fast dynamic changes to the data during the milling process. We also present a stable proxy-based haptic algorithm used to maintain a tip position on the surface avoiding haptic fall-through.

Introduction

The work presented here describes the use of a surgical training simulator for temporal bone milling that has been developed by the authors. This system will be used to educate and train surgeons for milling operations, e.g. complicated temporal bone operations such as removal of brain tumors. In such an operation the surgeon mills a path through the skull with a small hand held mill so that the tumor can be reached easily and with minimal damage to surrounding tissue. The milling phase of an operation of this type is difficult, critical and very time consuming. Reduction of operation duration time by only a few percent has potential for large savings in health costs.

Haptic and virtual reality simulation of the bone milling process is a new and largely unexplored research topic. However, some research groups are dealing with this problem [1], [2], [3]. All these groups are at an early stage in their research, the solutions are deficient and much more development must be done in this field to find adequate solutions. Our simulator differs from the ones mentioned above in that we are using high-resolution data sets, which give us very realistic 3D visualization of the milling process. Our haptic rendering algorithm also improves on previous work giving greater stability and reducing fall-through issues.

Our approach handles the challenging problem of rendering dynamic volume data in real-time and fulfills the given requirements for haptic and VR applications.

1. Graphical rendering

Skull bone is represented using data acquired from a CT-scan which offers high quality imaging of bone structures. Our simulator supports importing patient specific DICOM format volume data which makes it possible to use the simulator for surgeons wanting to practice a particular patient-specific operation.

There are several different methods for graphical rendering of volumetric data. The most common are; Ray-Casting [4], 3D texture mapping [5] and Marching cubes [6].

As in [7], our simulator uses the Marching Cubes algorithm because it meets our requirements for image quality and speed. The simulator performs stereographic rendering of the surface with a minimum update rate of 30Hz and a latency of less than 300ms [8] for dynamic updates to volume data from the milling process.

An optimized variation of the marching cubes algorithm has been implemented that allows real-time updating of a restricted area of the volume data using the method described herein:

1. Read in volume data and generate voxel gradients based on density. Create an octree structure with a user specified tree depth, applying marching cubes to each leaf node in the octree.
2. Check for milling, updating volume density and gradient data if necessary.
3. Apply a localized marching cubes algorithm on any modified octree leaf nodes.
4. Render octree leaf nodes using OpenGL display lists for optimized rendering of unchanged nodes.
5. Repeat from 2.

These steps are described in detail below.

1.1. Read in and store the volumetric data

For volumetric data an Octree-based structure [9] is well suited for visualization of the bone milling process. The Octree-based structure uses a hierarchical representation of the data to efficiently detect and update localized changes to the data. Each node in the octree represents a fixed axis-aligned sub-region of the data. Various optimizations can be implemented that take advantage of this hierarchical structure.

Maintaining minimum and maximum density information for each node allows our marching cubes algorithm to trivially reject any node in the octree with all density values either higher or lower than the iso-surface density value [10].

OpenGL display list caching has also been optimized by taking advantage of the octree structure. Each node in the octree has a display list cache that caches the rendering of a particular node. Leaf node display lists cache triangle rendering of a sub-region of the iso-surface. Non-leaf nodes use display lists to cache sub-regions of the octree. In this approach, any changes to a single leaf node only breaks the caches of that leaf and all of its ancestors, minimizing the number of display list caches that need to be regenerated.

Octree depth is a trade-off between having too many and too few voxels in each leaf node. If there are too few voxels in each leaf node then the overhead of the octree outweighs the benefits. Too many voxels in each leaf node means that the localized updates need to update an unnecessarily large area and are thus inefficient. Experiments show that an octree depth of three or four is optimal depending on the size of the volume data.

1.2. Check for milling

The haptic device has two buttons, one for removal of material and one for adding material. When either button is pressed a milling algorithm for updating voxel density is applied and a localized update of the marching cubes algorithm is performed. The tip of the mill is represented as a sphere with a radius r and an axis-aligned bounding box is used to quickly find the voxels located inside the sphere as described in figure 1.

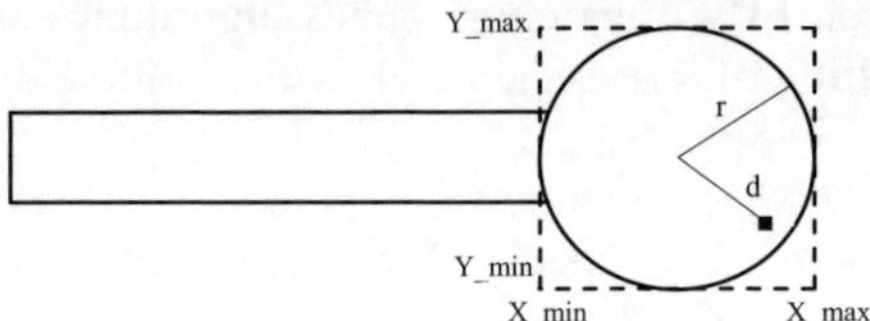

Figure 1. 2D representation of the axis-aligned bounding box region.

Only voxels that fall inside the axis-aligned bounding box are checked for collision with the tool. Voxels located inside the bounding box with a distance, d, less than the radius, r, are affected by the milling tip. Adding or removing material is simulated by increasing or decreasing voxel density as a function of time and distance from the tool surface.

Changes in voxel density will result in an update of the voxel gradients used to determine surface normals for the isosurface rendering.

Updating the voxel density of any voxel in a particular leaf node will thus break the display list caching for that leaf node and its ancestors.

1.3 Apply the Marching cubes algorithm on the updated tree nodes

After checking for changes to voxel density as a result of haptic milling, the graphical rendering algorithm will check for any octree leaf nodes that need regenerating. If an octree leaf node is *out-of-date,* the current iso-surface vertex and normal data is deleted and the marching cubes algorithm is applied locally to compute new vertex and normal geometry.

1.4 Isosurface rendering.

The iso-surface is rendered by performing a depth-first traversal of the octree structure, checking for invalid display list caches.

On the first rendering traversal all leaf-nodes will need to be rendered and a display list cache generated for them. The subsequent n-1 graphic updates (where n is the tree depth) of unchanged data will result in display list caches being generated for the parents of leaf-nodes, grand-parents, etc, until the root node is cached in a display list. Changes to voxel density as a result of haptic milling break the cache of one or more leaf-nodes resulting in one or more branches of the octree having invalid caches which will be rebuilt over the next n graphic updates. Figure 2 shows three objects that have been graphically rendered using our optimized octree approach described above. The tooth is a CT scan in DICOM format with a resolution of 256 x 256 x 176, the skull is also a DICOM CT data file with a resolution of 512 x 512 x 176 and the sphere is a dynamically generated data set with a resolution of 256 x 256 x 256.

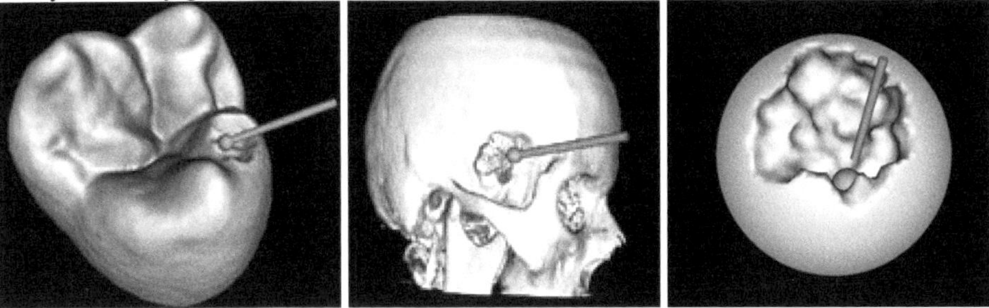

Figure 2. Graphical rendering of a tooth, a skull and a free-form object.

2. Haptic rendering

Our haptic rendering algorithm presented here is a proxy-based rendering technique [11] that will render an arbitrary density value as a haptic surface. For high-quality haptic rendering, the haptic process needs to be run in a separate thread from the graphical updates at an update rate of 1000Hz. The haptic algorithm is as follows:

1. Calculate the density value at the position of the proxy using trilinear interpolation.
2. If the density value ≥ the iso-value ⇒ collision, update proxy position. Else ⇒ no collision and the proxy position remains the position of the probe.
3. Calculate the force = k*(proxy_position – probe_position).
4. If milling ⇒ add vibration force.
5. Return the total force to the haptic device.

The haptic rendering algorithm maintains a proxy at a position where voxel density is less than the density value used for iso-surface generation. If the density value at the position of the haptic device is lower than the density value of the isosurface then we update the proxy position to be that of the haptic device. Otherwise we need to update the proxy to minimize the distance between the haptic device and the proxy whilst maintaining the requirement that the proxy remain at a position with a lower density than that of the isosurface. This is performed using an algorithm that is a variant of those described in [2, 12].

The general approach of our algorithm is to update the proxy position with a two-step movement. First we move the proxy in a direction tangential to the surface. We then compute the voxel gradient at this new location to compute a normal vector. Finally the proxy is moved along this normal vector towards the surface. The algorithm is computed with the following variables:

1. Normalized gradient, $\hat{n}_1$, at $\overline{P}_{proxy}$ trilinear interpolation.
2. Distance $\overline{a} = \overline{P}_{probe} - \overline{P}_{proxy}$ between haptic device and proxy.
3. Projection of $\overline{a}$ on $\hat{n}_1$, $a_1 = \overline{a} \cdot \hat{n}_1$.
4. Tangential direction, $\overline{n}_2 = \overline{a} - (a_1 \cdot \hat{n}_1) \Rightarrow a_2 = n_2$ and $\Rightarrow \hat{n}_2$.
5. Friction $\mu \cdot |a_1| \Rightarrow$ Magnitude of proxy movement $a_3 = \max(a_2 - \mu \cdot |a_1|, 0)$.

6.   New proxy position, $\bar{p}_{proxy\_tng} = \bar{p}_{proxy} + a_3 \cdot \hat{n}_2$.

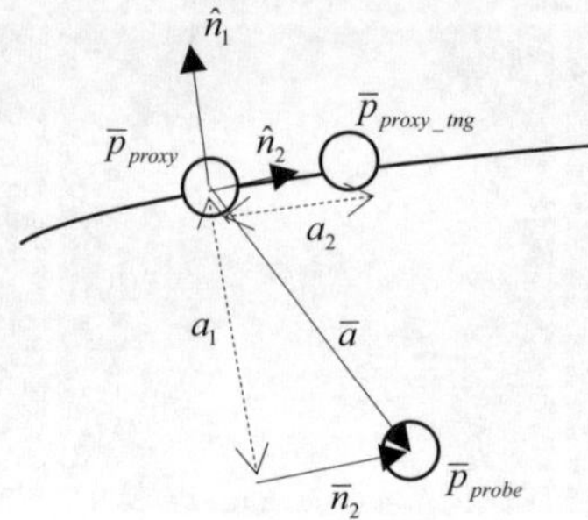

Figure 3. The algorithm for the tangential movement of the proxy.

When the new tangential proxy position has been found, the intersection point with the "surface" is derived based on the following computations:

7.   The normalized gradient, $\hat{n}_3$, and the density value v_{proxy_tng} at $\bar{p}_{proxy\_tng}$

8.   If $v_{proxy\_tng} \geq$ iso-value $\Rightarrow$ inside the object $\Rightarrow$ set the step direction $\hat{d} = \hat{n}_3$,

else $\Rightarrow$ outside the object $\Rightarrow$ set $\hat{d} = -\hat{n}_3$

9.   New proxy position $\bar{p}_{proxy\_new} = \bar{p}_{proxy\_tng} + \bar{s}$, where $\bar{s} = step\_size \cdot \hat{d}$

10. The density value v_{proxy_new} at $\bar{p}_{proxy\_new}$

Steps 9 and 10 are performed iteratively until either a point outside (or inside) the surface is found or a maximum number of iterations is reached. Linear interpolation between the last two points used in step 9 will give an approximation to a point that intersects the surface, $\bar{p}_{proxy\_intersection}$. By computing the gradient at $\bar{p}_{proxy\_intersection}$ we can finally move the proxy away from the surface by the radius of the proxy to ensure that the proxy is located entirely outside of the surface.

The haptic force is computed using a spring function between the haptic device and the proxy, $\bar{F} = k \cdot (\bar{p}_{proxy\_surface} - \bar{p}_{probe})$. If the user has activated the milling mode then we add a small random variation to the final force to simulate the vibration of the drill.

3. Equipment and implementation

Our application uses the SenseGraphics H3D API to manage graphical and haptic rendering and the synchronization between the two processes. Haptic rendering is performed using a PHANToM Omni haptic device. The workspace of the Omni is sufficient to realistically mimic a real surgery situation. One limitation with using this device is that it cannot render torque forces. Another limitation is the poor stiffness of the device, which is very important for a realistic feeling when interacting with stiff materials such as bone. The application is designed to be run in a SenseGraphics 3D Immersive Workbench, a co-located hapto-visual display system that incorporates stereographic image rendering. This places an extra burden on the graphical rendering since objects must be rendered twice to form a stereo pair.

4. Conclusion and future work

Our simulator can import patient specific DICOM data from a high-resolution CT or MRI scan to be used for both graphical and haptic rendering. The graphical rendering is performed using an iso-surface generated using an optimized marching trees algorithm that uses a hierarchical storage method to optimize for dynamic changes to the data. A proxy-based haptic rendering method is used to maintain a tip position on the surface and to avoid fall-through problems. The density values of the voxels inside the sphere are reduced during milling to simulate the removal of bone material.

This simulator can also be used in other areas such as dental simulation, simulation of craniofacial surgery and freeform design/sculpting of high-resolution volumetric data sets. The skull shown in this paper has a resolution of 512*512*174 generating 2420458 triangles, rendered at a frame rate of 30 Hz. The haptic rendering loop is updated at 1000 Hz. The simulation has been tested on a Pentium 4 3.2GHz processor PC with a Quadro FX1400 graphics card.

Additional features of our application include the use of cutting-planes and zoom and rotation to explore interesting regions of the data. Milling sound effects are also simulated to give a more realistic feeling to the milling process. Future work will look at improvements to the haptic rendering algorithm and stability issues that occur where two stiff materials are intersecting. We will also perform more tests to establish if the PHANToM Omni device can generate sufficient forces for simulation of the milling process. A simple particle simulation is also planned to visualize dust generated during material removal for more realistic visual rendering. The performance of the simulator will be tested and validated by surgeons.

References

[1]   Agus M. et al, *Real-time Haptic and Visual Simulation of Bone Dissection*, IEEE Virtual Reality Conference, pages 209-216, IEEE Computer Society Press, 2002.
[2]   Pflesser B., *Volume Cutting for Virtual Petrous Bone Surgery*, Comp. Aid. Surgery 7, pages 74-83, 2002.
[3]   Sewell C., Morris D. et al., *Quantifying Risky Behavior in Surgical Simulation*, Medicine Meets Virtual Reality Conference, January 27-29 2005, pp. 451-457.
[4]   Levoy M., *Display of surfaces from volume data*, Computer Graphic Applications, May 1988, pp.29-37.
[5]   Cabral B., Cam N., Foran J., *Accelerated volume rendering and tomographic reconstruction using texture mapping hardware*, 1994 Symposium on Volume Visualization , 1994, pp. 91-98.
[6]   Lorensen W.E., Cline H.E., *Marching cubes: a high resulotion 3D surface construction algorithm*, Computer Graphics, 21(4), July 1987, pp. 163-169.
[7]   Peng X., Chi X., Ochoa J.A., Leu M.C., *Bone surgery simulation with virtual reality*, ASME DETC2003/CIE, Chicago USA, September 2-6 2003.
[8]   Mark W.R., Randolph S.C., Finch M., Verth J., *Adding force feedback to graphics system: issues and solutions*, 23rd Conference on Computer Graphics, 1996, pp. 447-452.
[9]   Foley et al, *Computer Graphics: Principles and practice*, 2nd edition, 1996.
[10] Wilhelms J., Van Gelder A., *Octrees for Faster Isosurface Generation*, ACM Trans. Graphics, vol. 11, no. 3, 1992, pp. 201-227.
[11] Zilles, C.B., Salisbury, J.K., *A Constraint-based God-object Method for Haptic Display*, Proceedings of the 1995 IEEE Conference on Intelligent Robots and Systems, Vol. 3, PA, 1995, pp. 146-151.
[12] Vidholm E., Agmund J., *Fast surface rendering for interactive medical image segmentation with haptic feedback,* SIGRAD 2004.

Medicine Meets Virtual Reality 14
J.D. Westwood et al. (Eds.)
IOS Press, 2006

Virtual Reality Thread Simulation for Laparoscopic Suturing Training

Pablo J. FIGUERAS SOLA[a], Samuel RODRIGUEZ BESCÓS[a], Pablo LAMATA[a],
J. Blas PAGADOR[b], Francisco M. SÁNCHEZ-MARGALLO[b], Enrique J. GÓMEZ[a]

[a] *Grupo de Bioingeniería y Telemedicina, UPM, Madrid, Spain {figueras, srodrigu, lamata, egomez @gbt.tfo.upm.es}*
[b] *Minimally Invasive Surgery Centre, Cáceres, Spain {jbpagador, msanchez @ccmi.es}*

Abstract: The level of realism in virtual reality trainers might not be proportional to its didactic value. As an example, three exercises to train suturing skills are proposed in this article. They use a discrete thread model with a simple but good enough behaviour, and constitute a training means for three laparoscopic skills: (1) **Accurate grasping**, which trains grasping a precise point in the thread. (2) **Coordinated Pulling**, which trains tightening the thread co-ordinately and in different space orientations; and (3) **Knotting**, which allow the surgeon to practice this manoeuvre. These three exercises, found interesting among experts in surgical training, are now being validated in MIS workshops at the Minimally Invasive Surgery Centre of Cáceres (Spain).

Keywords: laparoscopic surgery, virtual reality, thread simulation, level of realism.

1. Introduction

Laparoscopic suturing is one of the most difficult skills to be acquired by surgeons. Learning processes are long and require several basic skills previously trained (eye-hand co-ordination, grasping and manipulation of little objects, etc.). One possible way of learning these tasks is using a physic simulator that provides a box with direct or indirect vision of the scene where the surgeon practices. Trainees with this means of training require a tutor behind them to guide exercises and provide some kind of skill assessment. As an alternative, virtual reality simulators offer surgeons an autonomous tool for practicing tasks, in a controlled and reproducible environment, as many times as needed to develop laparoscopic skills effectively [1]. Moreover, these systems might offer a system of objective evaluation, contrasted by experienced surgeons.

Nowadays there are some commercial solutions in surgery simulators: among them SEP (Simsurgery, Oslo, Norway)[2], MIST (Mentice, Göteborg, Sweden)[3], LapMentor (Simbionix, Lod, Israel) [4] or LapSim (Surgical Science, Göteborg, Sweden) [5]. Although these systems provide a great level of graphic realism, its better effectiveness over traditional box trainers is still not clear. [6].

Some times, the level of realism in a VR simulator is not necessarily proportional to its didactic value [7]. In this paper, the design of the VR training tool for suturing is faced in the frame of the Spanish Collaborative Network SINERGIA (G03/135).

2. Tools and Methods

Three didactic exercises have been implemented, using a simple but effective model of thread described in [8]. The thread of length L is modelled as a set of n cylindrical segments of length $L_{seg}=L/n$ and radius $R=L_{seg}/2$, which join a pair of consecutive nodes (see Figure 1).

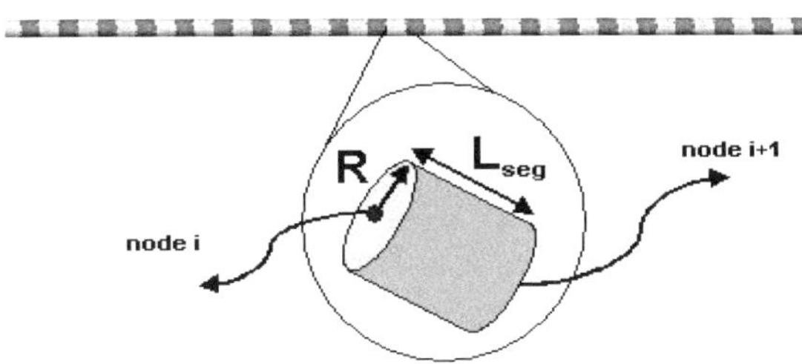

Figure 1: Detailed configuration of the thread

Those n+1 nodes propagate the movement by means of the algorithm FTL (Follow the Leader), which translates into the new positions the restrictions originated by (1) the collisions in the previous cycle of simulation and (2) the nodes that the user grasped. A scheme is shown in Figure 2.

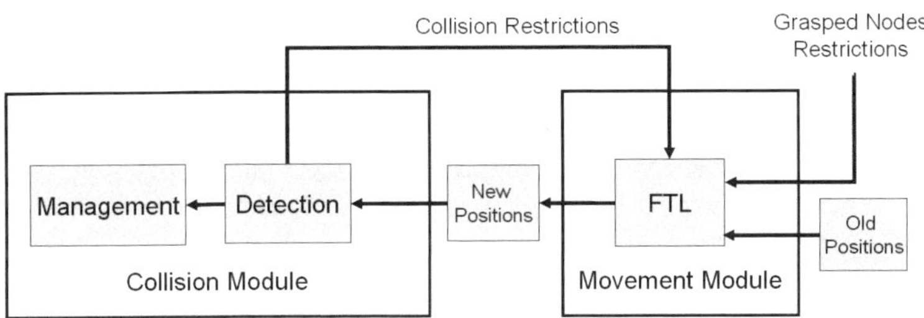

Figure 2: FTL Scheme. The old positions and both restrictions (grasped nodes and collision) are the inputs to the FTL algorithm so that the outputs are the new positions of the thread

2.1. Suturing Simulator

The three simulation exercises have been defined and implemented in the frame of a suturing simulator with the following architecture (figure 2):

1. Haptic server: Manages the information supplied by the haptics and suits it to the simulator.
2. Movement module: receives and manages the information provided by the input devices (haptics, mouse and keyboard) and propagates the movement through the thread.
3. Collision module: calculates the collisions between the virtual tools and the thread, as well as its self-collisions.
4. Drawing module: shows the scene on the screen using Open GL.

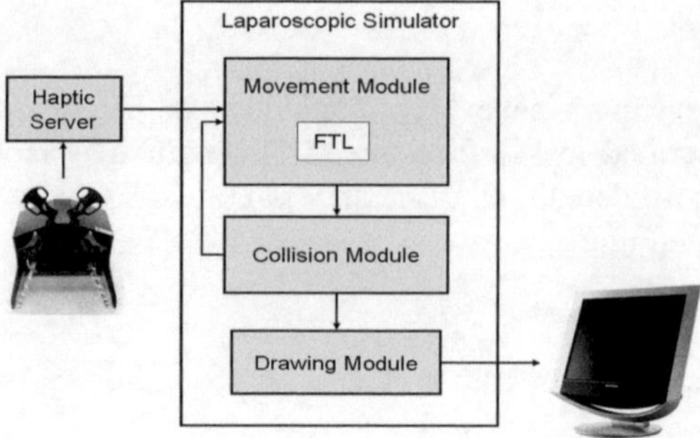

Figure 3: Suturing Simulator Arquitecture

2.2. Exercises

The three exercises offer, as an additional cue, vertical projections as shadows of the scene tools in the easiest level of difficulty. This helps novice trainees to perceive deepness. In a higher level, this shadow is removed making the scene equal to a real laparoscopic scene.

2.2.1. Accurate Grasping

The main objective of this task is to exercise accurate grasping, the ability to grasp tissues lightly without harming the structures of the organ which wraps. In this direction, we approach the problem with an exercise in which the user has to grasp certain points of the thread in a precise way and without causing noticeable deformation to it.

The exercise disposes a thread placed horizontally and inside a training box. Every five seconds, a pair of spheres appears in two nodes of the thread indicating the segment where the user has to grasp. If the spheres are light/dark blue, the manoeuvre must be done with the left /right tool.

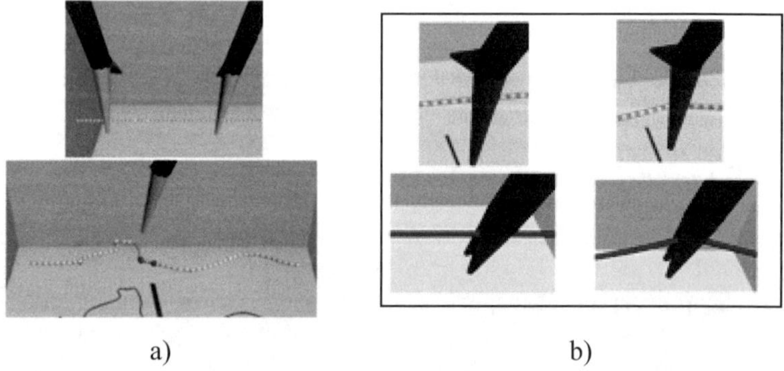

a)   b)

Figure 4: "Accurate grasping" exercise. a) Two levels of difficulty: *fixed ends mode* (left) and *free ends mode* (right). b) A good (left) and a bad (right) grasp.

Different levels of difficulty can be determined by the space between the two spheres. In addition another level of difficulty is established if the thread is fixed or not by its ends. If "*fixed ends mode*" is selected the thread will come back to its rest position gradually after being deformed. In the other mode (*"free ends mode"*) the thread will fold as the user makes mistakes, making the task more difficult (figure 4.a)

In this scenario, the skill of the surgeon is evaluated by the measure of different metrics: time, distance covered by each tool, mistakes when grasping the thread (the user grasps a non-selected area, the user grasp with the wrong tool) and delicateness assessed as the deformation caused to the thread when grasping. If the user grasps the thread in the line of the tool, it is a good grasp, but if it is grasped out of place is a worse grasp (see figure 4.b).

2.2.2. Coordinate Pulling

The formative objective in this exercise is to train the surgeon to pull the ends of the suturing thread coordinately and in opposite ways. That action is performed at the end of the intracorporeal knot task.

In the scenario of this exercise, the thread is placed in a "U" position with its two ends horizontally. Trainees have to grasp the thread by the two spheres located at both ends and separate them until reaching a pair of lateral spheres following the shortest way, which is indicated by a white path (see figure 5).

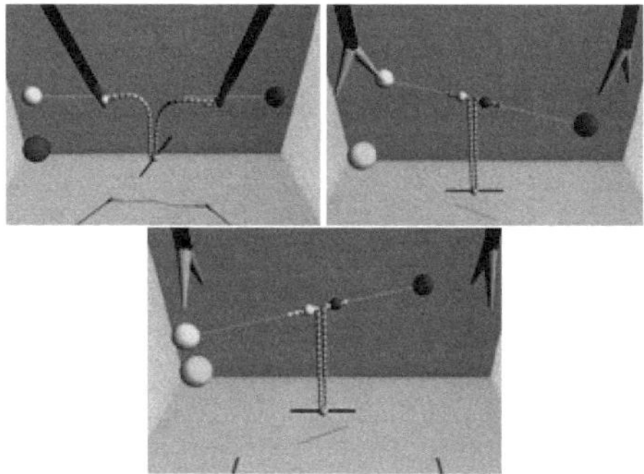

Figure 5: "Coordinate pulling" exercise: the three different orientations of the thread.

Due to the property of the FTL algorithm, when the spheres at both ends are separated, the central node will be displaced towards the end that suffers the mayor displacement. Therefore, if the user moves away the two ends in a symmetric way, the central node will stay in the bounds of the Z axis respect to its initial position (figure 6).

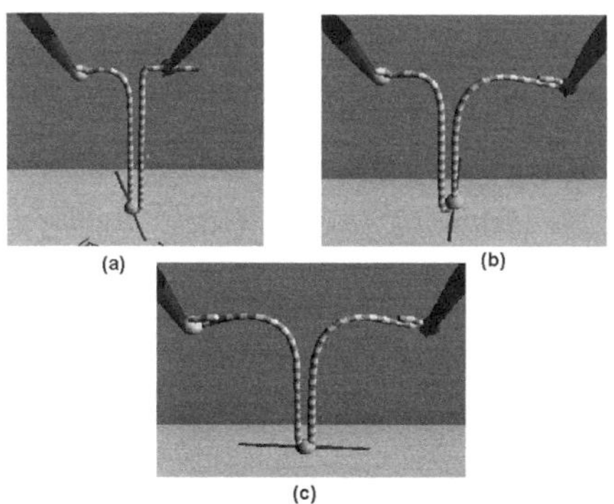

Figure 6: "Coordinate pulling" exercise: behaviour of the red control bar. a) Left end displaced and right fixed. b) Left end fixed and right displaced. c) Both ends displaced symmetrically.

A bar has been added to the thread giving a visual feedback to the user in order to keep the movement symmetry. In addition, three different orientations are included, so the user can practice in three different angles (figure 5).

Skill assessment metrics for this exercise are time, the distance travelled by each tool and the times the bar's inclination is greater than a given angle. The latest combined with the analysis of the path followed by the tools provides information about the symmetry of the movement.

2.2.3. Knotting

This exercise allows the user to practice the first suturing knots (supposed the previous manoeuvre of stitching done). In the first of two difficulty levels, the simulation begins with the suturing knot disposed in the middle of a training box, with the central node fixed on the base. This simulates the suturing task after the first knot is done. In the second, the thread is not fixed on any point so that the thread has a slippery behaviour through the sphere - wound. This second level, emulates the first knot, just after the stitching of the needle.

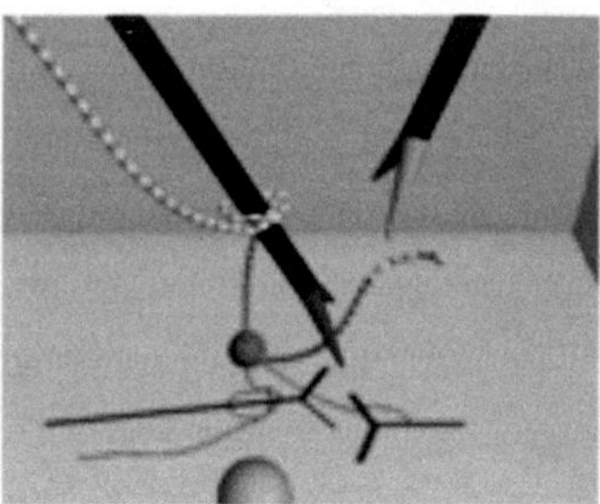

Figure 7: "Suturing" exercise: The grey sphere simulates the wound area where the knot is performed.

This exercise allows the user to perform the manoeuvre as many times as needed. To end the exercise the user must place the closed tool tip in a sphere located in the lower part of the box. Assessment metrics collected in this task are time and the distance covered by each tool.

3. Results and discussion

Thread has been simulated for its incorporation in a VR simulator. Simulation reaches an update rate of 25 frames/second with a Windows workstation (Pentium IV 2.8MHz micro and 512Mb RAM)..

Simulation is not just emulating reality. Virtual objects are a suitable way to offer metaphors for training skills. Implemented thread model is an example: it lacks of a high realism, but allows the design of useful didactic exercises. Moreover, this model is quite robust beside other complex and more realistic models [9], and requires little computational cost.

Moreover, virtual reality is something more than just emulating reality. Different aids and cues can be delivered to guide and help the trainee. As an example, shadows have been added artificially to facilitate deepness perception in the easier levels of difficulty. As the user improves, this cue is removed in order to not introduce vices in the trainee .

The three presented exercises have found a good acceptance among experts in surgical training. They are now being validated in MIS workshops at the Minimally Invasive Surgery Centre of Cáceres (Spain).

4. Conclusion

Three didactic exercises for laparoscopic training based on the simulation of a suturing thread are presented. This work has shown how VR can be useful for training surgical skills without requiring high levels of realism.

Acknowledgements

This research has been partially funded by the SINERGIA Thematic Research Collaborative Network (G03/135) of the Spanish Ministry of Health & Education. Authors would like to express their gratitude to all members of the SINERGIA consortium. Our special thanks to Oscar López (MediCLab, Polytechnic University of Valencia).

References

[1]   R. Aggarwal, K. Moorthy and A. Darzi. "Laparoscopic skills training and assessment", Br J Surg, 91:1549-1558, 2004.

[2]   Simsurgery simulation company and its simulator SEP. http://www.simsurgery.no/. (Last referenced Septiembre 2005).

[3]   Mentice simulation company and its simulator MIST. http://www.mentice.com/sch/mentice.nsf/. (Last referenced Septiembre 2005).

[4]   Simbionix simulation company and its simulator Lapmentor. http://www.simbionix.com/. (Last referenced Septiembre 2005).

[5]   Immersion simulation company and its simulator Lapsim. http://www.immersion.com/medical/products/laparoscopy/modules/?m=nav_2_5_1. (Last referenced Septiembre 2005).

[6]   Munz Y., Kumar B.D., Moorthy K., Bann S. y Darzi A.. Laparoscopic virtual reality and box trainers: is one superior to the other? Surg Endosc, vol. 18, no. 3, pp. 485-494, 2004.

[7]   Grober E.D., Hamstra S.J., Wanzel K.R., Reznick R.K., Matsumoto E.D., Sidhu R.S. y Jarvi K.A.. The educational impact of bench model fidelity on the acquisition of technical skill: the use of clinically relevant outcome measures. Ann. Surg, vol. 240, no. 2, pp. 374-381, 2004.

[8]   J. Brown, S. Sorkin, J.C. Latombe, K. Montgomery and M. Stephanides. "Algorithmic tools for real-time microsurgery simulation". Medical Image Analysis, 6:289–300,2002.

[9]   J. Lenoir, P. Meseure, L. Grisoni. and Ch. Chaillou. "Suture Model for Surgical Simulation". Lecture Notes in Computer Science 3078:105-113, 2004.

[10] Aggarwal R., Moorthy K., Darzi A., Laparoscopic skills training and assessment, Br J Surg, 91 (2004) 1549-1558.

Medicine Meets Virtual Reality 14
J.D. Westwood et al. (Eds.)
IOS Press, 2006

MRI Image Overlay: Applications to Arthrography Needle Insertion

Gregory S. Fischer [a,1], Anton Deguet [a] Daniel Schlattman [a] Russell Taylor [a]
Laura Fayad [b] S. James Zinreich [b] and Gabor Fichtinger [a]

[a] *Engineering Research Center, Johns Hopkins University, Baltimore, MD*
[b] *Johns Hopkins Hospital, Baltimore, MD*

Abstract.

Magnetic Resonance Imaging (MRI) has unmatched potential for planning, guiding, monitoring and controlling interventions. MR arthrography (MRA) is the imaging gold standard to assess small ligament and fibrocartilage injury in joints. In contemporary practice, MRA consists of two consecutive sessions: 1) an interventional session where a needle is driven to the joint space and gadolinium contrast is injected under fluoroscopy or CT guidance. 2) A diagnostic MRI imaging session to visualize the distribution of contrast inside the joint space and evaluate the condition of the joint. Our approach to MRA is to eliminate the separate radiologically guided needle insertion and contrast injection procedure by performing those tasks on conventional high-field closed MRI scanners. We propose a 2D augmented reality image overlay device to guide needle insertion procedures. This approach makes diagnostic high-field magnets available for interventions without a complex and expensive engineering entourage.

Keywords. MRI, Image Overlay, Augmented Reality, Arthrography, Percutaneous Therapy

1. Introduction

Magnetic Resonance Imaging (MRI) is superior to all other imaging modalities in detecting diseases and pathologic tissue in the human body. Thus MRI has an unmatched potential for guiding, monitoring and controlling therapy [1]. In needle biopsies, the high sensitivity of MRI in detecting lesions allows good visualization of the pathology, and its superior soft tissue contrast helps to avoid sensitive structures in the puncture route [2]. Advances in magnet design and magnetic resonance (MR) system technology have contributed to increased interest in interventional MRI; minimally invasive diagnostic and therapeutic image-based interventions can now be performed under near real-time MRI guidance [3].

At the same time, MRI presents challenges; perhaps the most daunting problem is access to the patient inside the magnet. Open magnets offer good access, but they are built with a decrease in field strength and homogeneity, thereby offering a lesser image quality. Short magnets may provide access in certain procedures, but performing an intervention inside the bore remains inconvenient. Specially designed robots can work in the bore of closed [4] and open [5] magnets, but are unlikely to be practical in the foreseeable future.

---

[1] Correspondence to: Gregory Fischer, 3400 N. Charles Street, NEB-B26, Baltimore, MD 21218, USA. Tel.: +1 410 467 1124; Fax: +1 410 516 3332; E-mail: gfisch@jhu.edu.

We propose a 2D augmented reality image overlay device similar to those in [6,8] to guide needle insertion procedures. This approach can make diagnostic high-field magnets available for interventions without involving prohibitively complex and expensive engineering entourage. The prime objective of our research is providing clinically sufficient accuracy while limiting faulty needle insertion attempts.

While routine noncontrast MRI has a high sensitivity and specificity for most ligamentous and tendon injuries, MR arthrography (MRA) is the imaging gold standard to assess small ligament and fibrocartilage injury in joints, particularly if there has been prior surgery, in the assessment of re-injuries to these intra-articular structures. Direct MRA (DMRA), where contrast is directly injected into the joint, is excellently tolerated and in efficacy is comparable to joint arthroscopy, the absolute gold standard in the evaluation of joints [9]. In contemporary practice, DMRA consists of two consecutive sessions. First a needle is driven to the joint space and gadolinium contrast is injected into the joint. This session is usually performed with radiological image guidance, typically under fluoroscopy or sometimes under CT guidance [10]; attempts at using a functionally equivalent CT Image Overlay device for arthrography needle guidance have been successful [6], and are shown in Fig. 1. Following contrast injection, a diagnostic MRI session is scheduled to visualize the distribution of contrast inside the joint space and evaluate the condition of the joint. Thus current direct MRA comprises two distinct procedures: a needle injection intervention and a diagnostic MRI session before the contrast washes out. Such a tightly sequenced double-procedure makes contemporary DMRA exceedingly expensive, resource intensive, and difficult to schedule, which together make this procedure unavailable in many non-specialized centers. To address this problem, [11] reports the use of an open MRI scanner configuration where needle insertion and contrast injection are performed directly inside scanner.

Our approach to direct MRA is to eliminate the separate radiologically guided needle insertion and contrast injection procedure from the procedure by performing those tasks right on conventional high-field closed MRI scanner with the MR Image Overlay technique. This promises to reduce the inconvenience for the patient and logistical difficulties associated with current direct MRA of large joints, in a manner that is practical and affordable for average care facilities that own conventional MRI scanners.

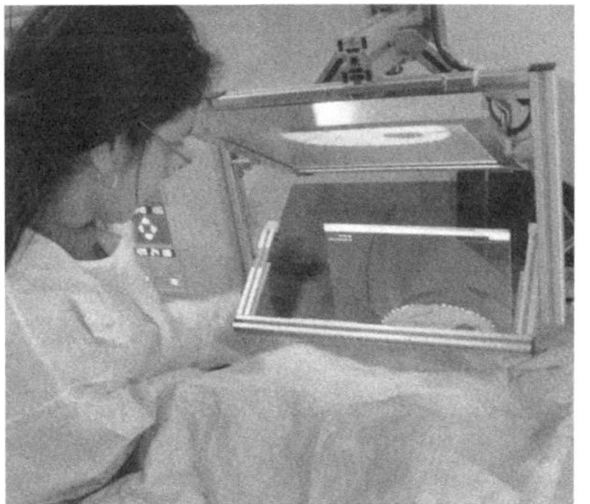
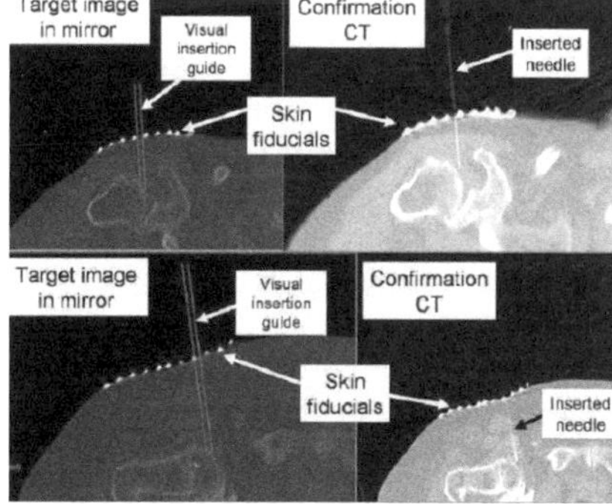

Figure 1. Functionally equivalent 2D image overlay device for CT scanners in a porcine trial (left) and preliminary joint arthrography results in human cadaver under CT Image Overlay guidance (right)

2. System Concept

The basic concept of the 2D image overlay is shown in Fig. 2 (left). The image overlay system shows axial MRI images on an LCD display, which are reflected back to the user from a semi-transparent mirror. Looking though the mirror, the anatomical image appears to be floating in the appropriate location in the body. Users from all viewpoints can share the same scene without any auxiliary tracking. The intersection of the mirror and display planes are marked with a laser plane parallel to the axial imaging plane. The laser is used for constraining the needle to the plane of the overlaid image while a virtual needle guide is displayed on the overlaid MR image controls in-plane rotation and depth.

The system creates the impression as if the image was inside the body in the correct pose and magnification, giving the physician a planar "tomographic vision." This technique can also be characterized as an in situ visualization tool, where the medical image is rendered right in the context of the procedure, spatially registered with the physical body. Perhaps the most promising aspect of image overlay is that the physician can execute the procedure without turning his/her attention away from the patient, and execute the same series of motions and actions as in conventional freehand procedures.

In most needle placement procedures, after the entry point is selected, three degrees-of-freedom (DOF) motion of the needle needs to be controlled. In this case, the physician uses the overlay image to control the in-plane insertion angle (first DOF), while holding the needle in the axial plane marked by the overlay device's laser light (second DOF). The insertion depth (third DOF) is controlled with a virtual depth gauge drawn on the overlay image. The advantages of 2D image overlay are numerous in comparison to other virtual reality or display augmentation methods reviewed earlier. Most significantly, 2D image overlay provides optically stable image without auxiliary tracking instrumentation and it requires only a simple alignment that does not need to be repeated for each patient. Although real-time imaging can not be used in the current design since the patient must be translated out of the bore for insertion, the overlay system assists the physician in detecting target motion and allows for gating the insertion with the use of skin fiducials.

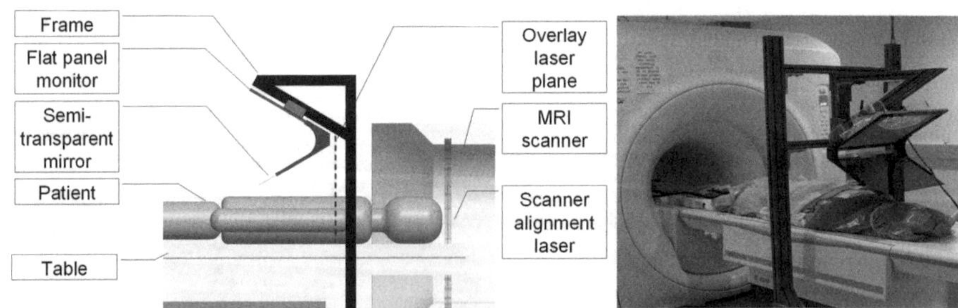

Figure 2. System concept of 2D image overlay device (left) and MRI image overlay device layout (right)

3. Materials and Methods

The MR overlay system is realized by mounting an MR-compatible LCD screen that is housed in an acrylic shell with an attached semi-transparent mirror to a modular extruded fiberglass frame as in Fig. 2 (right). The freestanding frame arches over the scanner bed and allows for images to be displayed on a patient when the encoded couch is translated out of the bore by a known amount. To maintain the goal of a very practical and low cost system, an off-the-shelf 19" LCD display was retrofitted to be MRI safe and RF shielded.

3.1. Calibration

Calibration is similar to that of the CT Image Overlay described in [6]. Calibration is accomplished in two steps: 1) make the overlay image coincide with the plane of the overlay's outer laser plane, and 2) determine the in-plane transformation between the overlaid MR image and the view of the physical object in the mirror. We fabricated a calibration phantom of perpendicular polycarbonate fiducial board with an embedded asymmetric set of 7mm diameter and 15mm long tubes of MR contrasts agent (Beekley MR-Spots, Beekley Corp., Bristol, CT). The calibration phantom also consists of a gel-filled box with targets embedded for validation as shown in Fig. 3(a).

The initial step of calibration is performed in the manufacture of the device to guarantee that the angle between the laser plane and the mirror and the mirror and the LCD are the same (60°). The laser is adjusted such that it passes though the intersection of the LCD and mirror planes while maintaining the correct angle. In the scanner room during an experiment, to ensure parallelism of the image plane, the calibration phantom is manually adjusted on the MR table until the scanner's axial laser plane sweeps the front face of the fiducial board and the overlay's laser does the same when the bed is translated out. The phantom is then translated into the scanner to take a single axial slice though the fiducial pattern; this image is then rendered on the overlay.

The first step of the in-plane registration process is image scaling. The overlay image must appear in correct size in the mirror, but there is variable linear scaling between the MR image and displayed image. The pixel size of the display is constant and it is either known from the manufacturer's specification or its measurement is trivial. The pixel size of the MR image is calculated as the ratio between the field of view (in millimeters) and image size (in pixel). The second step of in-plane registration is to determine a 3-DOF rigid body transformation. An MR image of the fiducial board and rendered on the overlay display, as seen in Fig. 3(a). The in-plane rotation and translation of the phantom's image is adjusted until each fiducial peg coincides with its mark in the image.

3.2. Workflow

Fiducials are first placed on the skin (Beekley MR-Spots) in the region of interest and are aligned with the axial direction. The subject is positioned and a small stack of MRI axial slices with a slice thickness appropriate for the given clinical application is acquired. A single MR slice is selected as the insertion plane, the patient is translated so that the appropriate slice lies in the scanner's alignment laser, and the appropriate entry point is marked on the skin with hollow IZI multi-modality markers (IZI Corp., Baltimore, MD). A single MRI image of this slice is then reacquired with the entry point fiducial in place. The image is transferred directly in DICOM format to the planning and control software implemented on a stand-alone PC. The computer is used to mark the target and entry points, draw a visual guide along the trajectory of insertion and mark the depth of insertion. This image is rendered on the Image Overlay device as shown in Fig. 3(b) and the patient is translated out so that the entry point fiducial lies in the laser plane of the overlay. The physician holds the needle at the entry point behind the mirror and adjusts the angle to the virtual needle guide while holding the needle in the plane of the laser (Fig. 3(c)). The Beekley MR-Spots and IZI fiducial are visible on both the patient and in the overlaid image; coincidence between the corresponding marks indicate correct calibration and entry point alignment respectively. This feature is particularly important for quality assurance, especially in applications when the target anatomy is prone to motion due to respiration or mechanical forces. The skin fiducials can be used to gate or synchronize the needle insertion to the respiratory cycle. After the needle is inserted, a confirmation image is acquired (Fig. 3(d)).

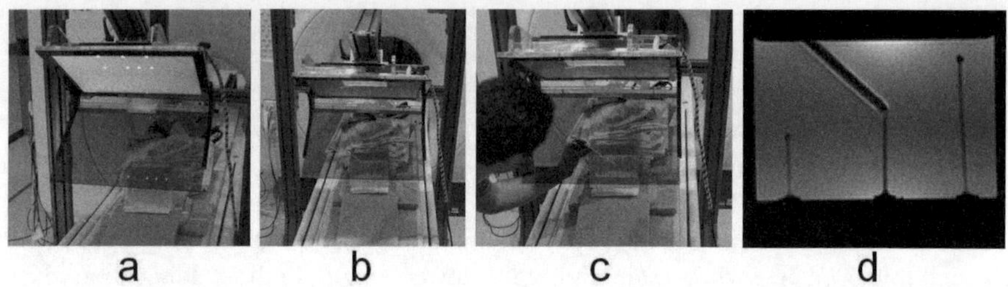

Figure 3. Workflow demonstrated in a phantom experiment: calibration(a), overlaid guide(b), needle insertion(c) and confirmation(d).

4. Results

The MR overlay system as shown in Fig. 2 (right) has been successfully tested in 1.5T and 3T scanners for compatibility. Experiments with a functionally equivalent CT guided version of the device as shown in Fig. 1 (left), a precursor to the current innovation [6,7], have very promising results. In the target application of joint arthrography, four trials were performed under CT overlay guidance. In all trials, the joint space was accessed successfully on the first insertion attempt as shown in Fig. 1 (right).

With the MRI Image Overlay, preliminary experiments in a 1.5T GE Signa Excite MRI scanner have so far been promising. The image overlay being applied to MRI-guided shoulder arthrography in a post-euthenasia porcine trial is shown in Fig. 4. In this experiment, an 18 gauge by 10cm MR-compatible diamond-tip needle (EZ-EM, Inc., Lake Success, NY) was successfully inserted into the joint space of the right shoulder. Contrast was injected, but distribution was not uniform due to the stiff tissue in the porcine cadaver. Statistical analysis of the insertion accuracy will be performed after more trials have been completed.

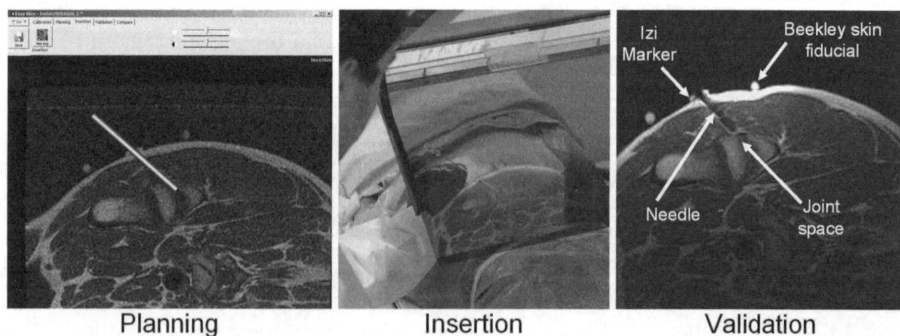

Figure 4. MRI Overlay guided direct MR arthrography in porcine trials. Targeting image with overlaid guide (left) insertion under overlay guidance (center) and confirmation image using an external imaging coil (right)

5. Conclusion

Experiments with the MRI Image Overlay device are underway and have so far shown great promise. Detailed, statistically significant accuracy trials have not yet been performed. However, since an equivalent test of the CT overlay has been successful in cadaver and ventilated porcine trials in [6] and [7], it is expected that similarly excellent results will be achieved in forthcoming MRA trials with the MRI overlay device. Animal and cadaver studies currently in progress are expected to prove the hypothesis that MR overlay will allow for accurate needle placement while significantly simplifying and speeding up the MRA procedure by eliminating the need for a separate, traditional radiographically (fluoroscopy or CT) guided contrast injection. The next generation of the device will be a smaller version that can be set up in a short bore magnet where the patient will not be shuttled in and out and we will enjoy near real-time imaging update.

Acknowledgements

The authors would like to acknowledge Iulian Iordachita for assistance in manufacturing the overlay and Csaba Csoma for help with development of the software. Partial funding for this project was provided by NSF Engineering Research Center Grant #EEC-97-31478, Siemens Corporate Research and Johns Hopkins Internal Funds.

References

[1] Jolesz FA. : Interventional and intraoperative MRI: A general overview of the field, *J Magn Reson Imaging* **8(1)** (1998), 3–7.

[2] Lenchik L, Dovgan DJ and Kier R : CT of the iliopsoas compartment: value in differentiating tumor, abscess, and hematoma, *Am J Roentgenol* **162** (1994) 83–86.

[3] Lewin JS, Nour SG and Duerk JL : Magnetic resonance image-guided biopsy and aspiration. *Top Magn Reson Imaging* **11(3)** (2000) 173–183.

[4] Krieger A, Susil RC, Menard C, Coleman JA, Fichtinger G, Atalar E and Whitcomb LL : Design of A Novel MRI Compatible Manipulator for Image Guided Prostate Intervention, *IEEE Trans. Biomed. Eng.* **52(2)** (2005) 306–313.

[5] DiMaio SP, Pieper S, Chinzei K, Fichtinger G and Kikinis R : Robot assisted percutaneous intervention in open-MRI, *5th Interventional MRI Symposium* (2004) 155.

[6] Fichtinger G, Deguet A, Masamune K, Fischer G, Balogh E, Mathieu H, Taylor RH, SJ Zinreich and Fayad LM : Image Overlay Guidance for Needle Insertions in CT Scanner, *IEEE Transactions on Biomedical Engineering* **52** (2005), 1415–1424.

[7] Fichtinger G, Deguet A, Fischer G, Balogh E, Masamune K, Taylor RH, Fayad LM and SJ Zinreich : CT Image Overlay for Percutaneous Needle Insertions, *Journal of Computer Assisted Surgery* **1(4)** (2005).

[8] Stetten GD, Chib VS.: Overlaying ultrasonographic images on direct vision, *J Ultrasound Med.* **20** (2001), 235–240.

[9] Schulte-Altedorneburg G, Gebhard M, Wohlgemuth WA, Fischer W, Zentner J, Wegener R, Balzer T, Bohndorf K. : MR arthrography: pharmacology, efficacy and safety in clinical trials, *Skeletal Radiology* **32** (2003), 1–12.

[10] Binkert CA, Verdun FR, Zanetti M, Pfirrmann CW and Hodler J. : CT arthrography of the glenohumeral joint: CT fluoroscopy versus conventional CT and fluoroscopy–comparison of image-guidance techniques, *Radiology* **229(1)** (2003) 153–158.

[11] Hilfiker PR, Weishaupt D, Schmid M, Dubno B, Hodler J and Debatin JF : Real-time MR-guided joint puncture and arthrography, *Eur Radiol.* **9(2)** (1999) 201–204.

Medicine Meets Virtual Reality 14
J.D. Westwood et al. (Eds.)
IOS Press, 2006

Control System Architecture for a Minimally Invasive Surgical Robot

Kenneth Fodero II+ BSEE, H. Hawkeye King+ BACS, Mitchell J.H. Lum+ MSEE,
Clint Bland+, Jacob Rosen+ Ph.D, Mika Sinanan++ M.D., Ph.D, Blake Hannaford+ Ph.D.

+ Department of Electrical Engineering, ++ Department of Surgery,
University of Washington, Seattle, WA, USA
E-mail:<kfodero, hawkeye1, mitchlum, cbland, rosen, mssurg,
blake>@u.washington.edu

Abstract. As the field of surgical robotics continues to evolve, it is important to keep patient safety in mind. This paper describes a safety control architecture aimed at moving an experimental system in the direction of intrinsically safe operation. The system includes safety features such as: a small number of states, Programmable Logic Controller (PLC) state transition control, active enable, brakes, E-STOP, and a surgeon foot pedal.

Keywords. Surgical Robot, Safety, Teleoperation, Telesurgery, PLC

1. Introduction

Surgical robotics is revolutionizing the way in which clinicians deliver health care. As the field of surgical robotics continues to evolve, it is important to keep patient safety in mind. In this paper we look at moving an experimental system in the direction of intrinsically safe operation. Although the resulting system is several steps short of a level of safety suitable for human surgery, we hope to evaluate concepts for a safety system which could facilitate a human rated design.

Safety has been considered by several other teams working on surgical robotics [1,2]. As early as 1991, a system with an emergency stop, foot pedal, and brakes was developed by Taylor, et al. [3]. Rovetta et al. looked at safety in terms of relevant industry standards [4]. Currently, the DaVinci, an FDA approved and human rated surgical robot system, includes such safety features as redundant sensors, hardware watchdog timers, and real-time error detection [5].

In this study, our main focus is on ways to increase our confidence that a highly complex system of software and hardware will always "do the right thing" or "fail safe." Our approach will rely on the following assumptions:

- A system with a small number of well defined states is inherently safer.
- Programmable Logic Controllers (PLCs) are a highly reliable off-the-shelf technology that can easily and reliably be programmed for small numbers of states.

- PLC implementation is more reliable than implementation of equivalent functions in a computer.
- Most of the complex real-time control functions will be managed by software.

This paper describes the design of a safety system for a surgical robot now under development in our laboratory.

2. Architecture

Based on an extensive database of dissection and suturing tasks performed by 30 surgeons, it was determined that 95% of the time surgical tools operated in a conical range of motion with a vertex angle 60 degrees [6]. We used these results to design the arms of our surgical manipulator with a numerical optimization process [7]. The safety system described in this paper is being developed for highly reliable operation of this manipulator in planned animal surgical experiments.

The basic hardware architecture of the system consists of a PC running a real-time version of the Linux operating system (RTAI). The PC communicates with a USB 2.0 interface card, designed in our lab. The interface card passes commands and information to and from the Linux host to the sensors, power amplifiers, and the PLC every 125us. The surgeon's foot pedal may be connected directly to the PLC for local operation or passed in through the network and I/O Board for remote operation. This allows remote or local operation of the pedal. Brakes on each motor engage if power fails or in the Pedal up or E-stop states under direct control of the PLC. The brake system is independent of possible bugs in the control software. The hardware architecture is shown in Figure 1.

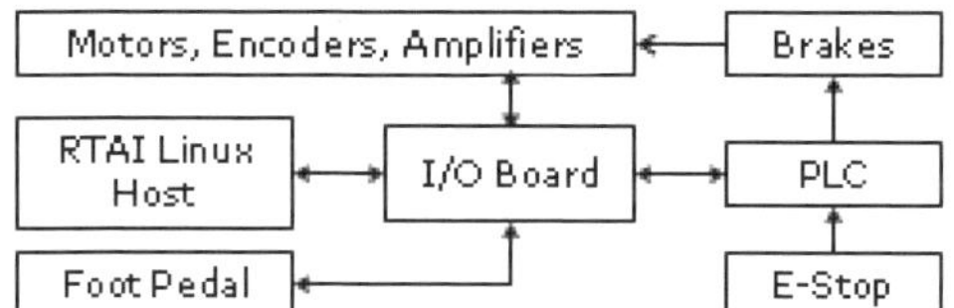

Figure 1. Hardware Architecture

The software for the system consists of a set of kernel modules under RTAI Linux. The Control Module contains the I/O, kinematics, control, and other functionality of the system. This module communicates with the system hardware through the USB 2.0 interface card. A function in the Control Module produces a 10Hz square wave for a watchdog timer function implemented in the PLC. User inputs are collected through engineer and surgeons interfaces. The networking module serves as an intermediary between these interfaces modules and the control module. The software architecture is shown in Figure 2. Allocation of software modules to computing hardware is flexible except for the I/O Board software and the PLC ladder logic.

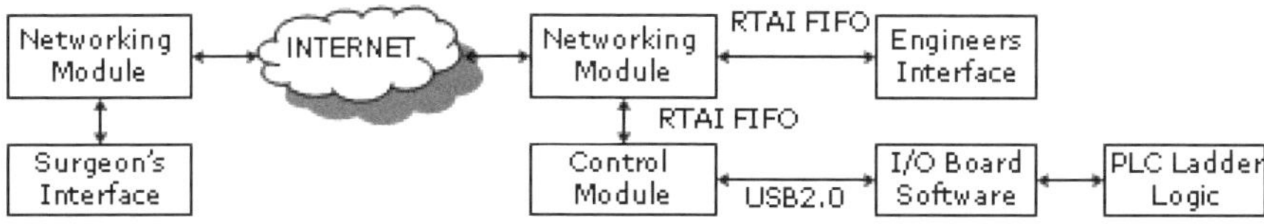

Figure 2. Software Architecture

The system operates in four states. These states are: Emergency Stop (E-Stop), Initialization, Pedal up, Pedal down. A Direct Logic 05 PLC (Figure 4) contains the state transition logic, and manages the transitions between the states. PLC state variables are connected to the USB I/O card and read by the Linux computer. The real-time Linux software (Control Module) will contain the same four states, but it transitions between states only in response to transitions of the PLC state machine. Transitions between pedal up and pedal down are controlled by surgeon inputs, either directly wired or relayed to the PLC. The state transition diagram for the system is shown in Figure 3.

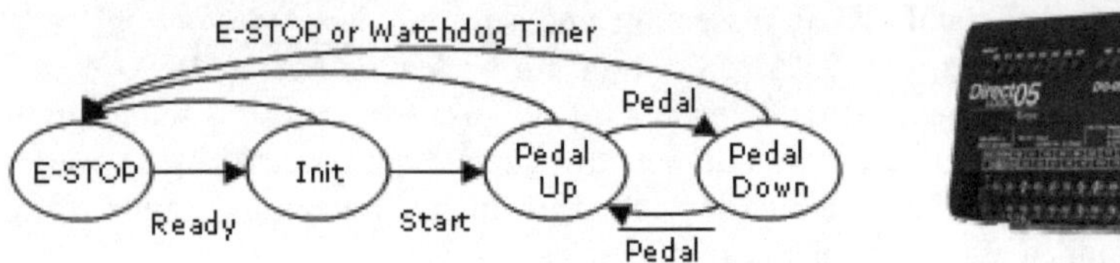

Figure 3. State Transition Diagram   **Figure 4.** Direct Logic 05

The PLC contains watchdog timer logic which detects loss of the 10Hz square wave (in either 1 or 0 position) indicating a crash of the controller software, and initiates a transition to the E-Stop state, within 100ms. A faster watchdog timer would be desirable for more rapid shutdown, but reliable detection of signals faster than 10Hz was not possible with the selected PLC.

3. Conclusions

The control system architecture described in this paper is a crucial element in the overall surgical robot system under development in the University of Washington BioRobotics Lab. We expect our system will provide a level of predictability, reliability, and robustness sufficient for animal surgery evaluation.

References

[1]   Davies B.L. "The safety of medical robots." In Proceedings of 29th ISR Conference on Advanced Robotics: Beyond 2000, Birmingham, April, 1998.
[2]   Varley, P. "Techniques for Development of Safety-Related Software for Surgical Robots." IEEE Transactions on Information Technology in Biomedicine, Vol. 3, No. 4, Dec 1999.
[3]   Taylor, R., et. al., "Taming the Bull: Safety in a Precise Surgical Robot" IEEE International Conference on Advanced Robotics. Pisa, Italy, June, 1991.
[4]   Rovetta, A, "Telerobotic Surgery Control and Safety," IEEE International Conference on Robotics and Automation, vol. 4, pp. 2895-2900, 2000.
[5]   Guthart, G. "The Intuitive™ Telesurgery System: Overview and Application," IEEE International Conference on Robotics and Automation pp. 618-621, San Francisco, USA, April 2000.
[6]   J.D. Brown, et. al., 'Design and Performance of a Surgical Tool Tracking System for Minimally Invasive Surgery,' Engineering Congress and Exposition: Advances in Bioengineering, BED, vol. 51, pp. 169-170, ASME, New York, Nov. 11-16, 2001.
[7]   Lum, M., et. al., "Kinematic Optimization of a Spherical Mechanism for a Minimally Invasive Surgical Robot" 2004 IEEE International Conference on Robotics and Automation pp. 829-834, New Orleans, USA, April, 2004.

Medicine Meets Virtual Reality 14
J.D. Westwood et al. (Eds.)
IOS Press, 2006

Metrics for an Interventional Radiology Curriculum: A Case for Standardisation?

Derek A GOULD[a], Andrew E HEALEY[a,b], Sheena Joanne JOHNSON[c], William Edward LEWANDOWSKI[d], David Oliver KESSEL[e]

[a]*Dept of Radiology, Royal Liverpool University Hospital, Prescot St, Liverpool, UK*
[b]*Dept of Medical Imaging, University of Liverpool, Brownlow Hill, Liverpool, UK*
[c]*School of Psychology, University of Liverpool, Liverpool, UK*
[d]*William E. Lewandowski Consulting, Shepherdstown, West Virginia, US*
[e]*Department of Radiology, St James' Hospital, Leeds.*

Abstract Interventional radiology training and assessment would benefit greatly from the introduction of simulation. Assessment methods should facilitate the highest standards of training and therefore must be chosen on the basis of evidence of impact on learning. A study of assessment in a training model shows the need for specialty specific metrics which were derived from a task analysis of interventional procedures.

Keywords Interventional radiology, metrics, validation, standards, simulation.

1. Background Problem

Interventional radiology (IR) is a generic term for imaging guidance of needles, guide wires and catheters to remote targets to treat patients. IR training programmes are patient centered, based on a defined curriculum and with certification incumbent on the satisfactory acquisition of the necessary knowledge, practical skills and attitudes to practice competently. Current training in interventional radiology relies on an apprenticeship where proficiency is attained by gaining experience on patients under the mentorship of an expert. Pressures to train more rapidly [1], and replacement of simple, invasive diagnostic training procedures by non-invasive imaging, are making it difficult to conduct training in an efficient and effective manner [2,3]. IR assessment follows content which is in keeping with a practice model for the speciality and this allows the results of assessment to provide legitimate evidence for award of a certification [4]. Objective assessment of skills is becoming important to certification in surgery, where observer-based checklists and global scoring systems have been studied for real world tasks [5-7] and virtual reality tools have been investigated [8,9]. While some work has been performed on objective assessment in IR using time path analysis [10], there is generally a lack of objectivity in the assessment of proficiency in IR, which currently uses log books and non-criterion based direct observation of procedures: this is subjective and lack reproducibility, reliability and proven validity. Models may train some skills, and in this study we have used a model, created by rapid prototyping, to assess skills proficiency. The use of virtual reality in simulation modelling is also being explored for training and assessment in interventional radiology, but its role has yet to be clearly defined. It is our position, that before being used in interventional radiology training, the clinical content of medical simulators needs to be validated. In addition, before being used to assess proficiency, the test content of the simulator must not only be clinically validated, it also must be reasonably proven to be able to discriminate between masters and non-masters, as part of an integrated testing regimen.

To be defensible, a strategy for developing a performance test should at the least be transparent and documented, including the methodologies used and outcomes obtained in defining metrics as well as performing validation. Assessment should apply to a range of test scenarios, and be objective, valid, reliable, blinded, fair, unbiased, accountable, cost effective and feasible [11], while providing opportunities for feedback to inform the trainee of their development, progress and learning needs [12]. The objective criteria used in testing, must be carefully chosen, so as to be truly indicative of the desired type of behavior and level of performance under real-world conditions. While there are no set rules in psychometric testing, high stakes examinations generally require a basis in an analysis of the job or task to be tested, performed by occupational psychologists and subject matter experts. Cognitive task analysis shows the key points at which decisions are made, and which information or cues are used by the expert to make those decisions. This includes the subconscious actions which are not immediately recalled by the subject experts. We have previously performed such an analysis, within an IR training curriculum [13] and are developing assessment metrics, as described in this paper.

Having developed an assessment methodology, its application, whether using real cases, models or a virtual reality simulator, requires great care to ensure legitimacy and accuracy of test scores, and the inferences drawn. Defensibility is founded in the thoroughness used to select test content, the expertise of the test item writers, rigorous standard setting, care of scoring and an appeal process for the examinee. In determining the validity (veracity of measurement) of the interpretation of, and inferences drawn from, test scores, a number of 'validation tests' can be used and have been well described previously [14]. Of the various studies described, face and content validity are regarded as of great importance; however, concurrent and predictive validity are also critical to evaluating the effectiveness of a given test. Concurrent validity is the ability of a test to discriminate between masters and non-masters, and predictive validity is the assessment of a test's ability to predict future competence over time [14]. The reason that face and content validity alone are insufficient when evaluating testing programs is that these measures do not indicate a test's ability to measure or classify performance [14]. Certainly, face and content validity are important in the overall scheme of evaluating the validity of a test, but they cannot stand alone. Notwithstanding this, and despite as yet, an apparent lack of either concurrent or predictive validity using endovascular simulators, there have been recommendations that training on VR simulators should be an essential prerequisite for carotid artery stenting [15,16].

2. Method

2.1 Cognitive Task Analysis (TA) and Metrics

Subject experts were approached to define the tasks in which candidates are expected to be competent and, although not exhaustive, six procedures (arterial, venous, kidney, liver needle puncture and generic ultrasound or computed tomography guided biopsy) within the UK, Royal College of Radiologists' Curriculum were selected for inclusion in the research. TA using observation (direct and video-record) and interview of experts was performed [13]. After production of an outline hierarchical and cognitive task analysis for each procedure, formal interviews with experienced operators enabled more detailed analysis of each procedure. The TA protocols were used in the identification of performance objectives by 3 subject experts, and will guide future simulator design. Three characteristics for each step within the TA were graded using a linear, visual analogue scale: skill threshold, range of skill, and level of criticality. Experts marked on the scale a cross where they felt the task would be best represented, the left extreme of the scale being minimum and the right maximum. Distance along the scale was measured to provide a quantitative value. The data for each subject expert, and each step in the task analysis, were recorded in a hierarchical format, allowing identification and comparison of the steps that require a similar amount of skill to complete.

2.2 Fixed Model Study

A transparent, silicon, fixed model of a human vascular tree (Elstrat, Switzerland) was set up with two surveillance video cameras recording simultaneously (using a video multiplex device), the activity of a manipulated catheter and the operators' hands. The model was mounted on a custom light box to allow through transmission illumination. A plain abdominal radiograph was placed between model and light box to simulate anatomical landmarks. The model was filled with a saline / low friction lubricant mix (Elstrat, Switzerland) to improve realism of catheter manipulations within the model, and to reduce optical refraction artefacts. Access to the model was via a 7 Fr (French) vascular access sheath (Terumo, UK). Full local research ethics committee approval was obtained prior to the study.

55 volunteer participants (36 expert, 19 novice) gave written consent to participate and, following the exercise, were interviewed to determine level of expertise and the realism of the test experience. Participants were permitted a single attempt on the model with no prior practice. Experts and novices were asked to sequentially cannulate first the right and then the left 'renal artery' using a standard 5 Fr Cobra 2 catheter (Cook, Letchworth, UK) with the aid of a .035" Glide wire (Terumo, UK). A time limit of 300 seconds was set. All procedures were video recorded (for hand motion and catheter positioning) enabling precise timings for task completion to be noted. The model was also used by a subject matter expert and an experienced trainee. Both were asked to repeatedly cannulate the right and then the left renal arteries. The video of both participants was then sent to two independent subject matter experts, who were blinded to the participants. Each assessing subject matter expert was asked to assess

overall skill level, catheter manipulation skill level, wire manipulation skill level, economy of movement. The assessors were asked to score on a visual analogue scale 0 being no skill/poor economy of movement, 10 being excellent skill/economy of movement. The individual scores were then totalled to give a total skill/economy of movement score.

3. Results.

3.1 Task Analysis and Metrics

Detailed task descriptions and decision protocols were produced for the six procedures. Common operator mistakes were established and pertinent cues and decision points identified and included in the task descriptions. Additionally, complexities deviating from the simplest method in each procedure were identified. Data to determine metrics were derived from subject matter experts (i.e. skill value, range of skills, criticality). Significant correlations ($p < 0.001$) between raters were found for these metrics indicating agreement between experts on the key points within procedures.

3.2 Validation of Catheterisation Model

Content validity (0.0 is not realistic and 1.0 totally realistic): In the model, experts determined content as having a realism rating of 0.6 (range .4 to .8). Amongst comments received were: "'feel' was realistic, despite the simple nature of the model" and "unconvinced of the long term effectiveness of training on such a model", and "a trainee would simply become skilled on the model but would not be able to transfer those skills to patients".

Construct validity: All 36 experts completed the test in an average of 96 seconds (range 225 - 33). 19 trainees with minimal angiographic experience were unable to complete the test within a 300 second time limit, only 2 completing the test in an unlimited period.

Concurrent validity: A subject matter expert and a trainee were asked to have repeated attempts at cannulation of the right and then left renal arteries. The expert demonstrates more consistent performance at a superior level of skill/economy of movement and with a reduced time to complete. The trainee has wide ranging performance and times. The data suggest that time to completion correlates to subject matter expert assessment of skill/economy of movement although both experts and trainees demonstrated improvement (in time taken) with repeated attempts.

4. Discussion

Simulations of all types (physical, electronic, and digital) have the potential to facilitate the learning of both cognitive and psychomotor skills. These various types of simulations have varying levels of fidelity based on their ability to replicate the sensory inputs of the real world. By senses, we don't just mean vision, audition, olfactory, taste and touch; we also mean cold, warmth, pain, kinaesthetic and vestibular [17]. Sensory inputs provide performance cues of varying levels of importance in the performance of a task, and we generally equate the "accuracy" or "realism" of a simulation with the presence (or lack of presence), and fidelity, of the sensory stimuli perceived by the learner. The more advanced simulation systems also have the ability to collect objective performance data and provide that information to the learner as either formative (during the performance) or summative (after the performance) feedback. The utility of a given simulation is directly related to its ability to replicate the nature and complexity of the sensory cues necessary to correctly perform a given task, and its ability to provide performance feedback to the learner. Less complex simulations can be used effectively to train either less complex tasks or specific subcomponents of more complex tasks. The key to effectively using a simulation in training is to understand the nature of the target task, to identify those sensory inputs which serve as key performance cues, and to identify the most effective type of performance feedback for the task.

Since tasks are always performed within some sort of context, to accurately describe behaviour, tasks must be converted into behavioural or performance objectives. The TA and assessment formulation outlined in this paper described a process of identification of key performance objectives in IR procedures. Performance objectives describe the conditions under which the task must be performed and the standards to which the task must be performed [18]. Once you have created the performance objectives, you can then identify the metrics required to determine relative accomplishment. The greater the ability of a given simulation to replicate a task, to replicate the conditions under which a task is performed, and to record the appropriate metrics, the more useful it is in testing. The study of the fixed vascular model suggested that time to completion, as a surrogate end point, may have limited value as an assessment tool (i.e. both experts and trainees reduced time to complete task after repeated attempts), and this may also apply to the subjective nature of operator skill based on catheter and hand motion. This helps to confirm the assertion, that in addition to conducting a traditional task analysis, one must attend to identifying critical performance cues, and then convert the tasks into performance objectives from which appropriate metrics can be derived. Additional rating of our performance objectives will therefore be performed by experts to determine the more critical metrics for use in checklists, global scoring systems or simulators. Such speciality specific metrics should allow reproducible, objective and fair assessments to be made, e.g. using blinded, video observation to distinguish between experts and novices.

Training curriculum should be based on validated performance objectives. The various instructional strategies and tools that make up a curriculum (lecture, simulation, structured experience, etc.) must all be designed and utilized in a systematic approach to allow learners to obtain mastery of these objectives. A training curriculum indicating the proficiencies required by the learner would normally be developed by the certifying organisation, which would also develop any test items for assessment, and determine the standards required. It follows that to be considered as part of a certifying organisation's curriculum, a simulation would need to be similarly aligned. While interventional radiology training in the UK is integral to the radiology curriculum of the Royal College of Radiologists [19], there appears to be few, or no, existing, specialist curricula for interventional radiology. A solution might exist in a uniform curriculum that is developed by the various recognised professional interventional radiology societies, working in concert, and using a documented, systematic approach starting with a task analysis, and ending with a validated, testing regimen. Once this has been accomplished, the interventional radiology societies will have then created the standards and criteria for the incorporation, with confidence, of new technology in instruction and testing such as virtual reality simulation.

References

[1]   Department Trade and Industry Working Time Regulations http://www.dti.gov.uk/er/work_time _regs/wtr2.htm#Special (accessed 28th July 2005)

[2]   Bridges M, Diamond DL. The financial impact of training surgical residents in the operating room. *Am J Surg* 1999;177:28-32

[3]   Crofts TJ, Griffiths JM, Sharma S J et al. Surgical training: an objective assessment of recent changes for a single health board. *BMJ* 1997;314: 814

[4]   Dauphinee WD. Licensure and certification. In: *International Handbook of Research in Medical Education, Part 2*. Norman GR, Van der Vleuten CPM, Newlble DI (Eds). Kluwer Academic Publishers 2002. p836

[5]   Martin J, Regehr G, Reznick R et al. Objective structured assessment of technical skill (OSATS) for surgical residents. *Br J Surg* 1997; *84*, 2, 273-278

[6]   Taffinder N, Smith S, Jansen J et al. Objective measurement of surgical dexterity -validation of Imperial College Surgical Assessment Device. *Minimally Invasive Ther and Allied Techniques 7(suppl 1)* 1998; 11: 2, 13

[7]   Moorthy K, Munz Y, Sarker SK et al. Objective assessment of technical skills in surgery. *BMJ* 2003; *327*, 1032-1037

[8]   Seymour NE. Gallagher AG. Roman SA et al. Virtual Reality training improves operating room performance: results of a randomised, double-blinded study. Yale University & Queen's University, Belfast. *Annals of Surgery*. 2002 Oct 236(4):458-63; discussion 463-4

[9]   Taffinder N, McManus I, Jansen J et al. An objective assessment of surgeons' psychomotor skills: validation of the MIST-VR laparoscopic simulator. *Br J Surg* 1998; 85(suppl 1): 75

[10] Bakker NH, Tanase D, Reekers JA et al. Evaluation of vascular and interventional procedures with time-action analysis: a pilot study. *J Vasc Interv Radiol*. 2002. 13:483-488

[11] Skills for the new millennium: report of societal needs working group. *CanMEDS 2000 Project* 1996.

[12] Southgate L, Grant J. *Principles for an assessment system for postgraduate medical training.* A working paper for the Postgraduate Medical Education Training Board. September 2004

[13] Johnson SJ, Healey AE, Evans JC, Murphy MG, Crawshaw M, Gould DA. Physical and cognitive task analysis in interventional radiology. *Journal of Clinical Radiology*: In Press

[14] Coscarelli W, Eyres P, Shrock S. *Criterion-Referenced Test Development (2nd ed.)*. Washington, DC: The International Society for Performance Improvement. 2000. p 140-147

[15] *Clinical Competence Statement on Carotid Stenting: Training and Credentialing for Carotid Stenting-Multispeciality Consensus Recommendations.* A report of SCAI/SVMB/SVS writing committee to develop clinical competence statement on carotid interventions. Catheterisation cardiovasc interventions 2005. 64:1-11

[16] Gallagher AG, Cates CU. Approval of Virtual Reality Training for Carotid Stenting; what this means for procedural-based medicine. *JAMA*, Dec 22/29, Vol. 292: 24. 3025-6

[17] Bailey, RW, *Human Performance Engineering: Using Human Factors / Ergonomics to Achieve Computer System Usability (2nd ed.)*. Englewood Cliffs, New Jersey: Prentice-Hall. 1989. p. 50

[18] Dick, WO, Carey L, Carey JO. *The Systematic Design of Instruction, (4th ed.)*. 1996. New York: Harper Collins. Chapters 3 and 6

[19] *Structured Training in Clinical Radiology*. 4th Ed. Editorial Board of the Faculty of Clinical Radiology, Royal College of Radiologists (2004)

Medicine Meets Virtual Reality 14
J.D. Westwood et al. (Eds.)
IOS Press, 2006

Surgical Multimedia Academic, Research and Training (S.M.A.R.T.) Tool:

A Comparative Analysis of Cognitive Efficiency for Two Multimedia Learning Interfaces that Teach the Pre-procedural Processes for Carpal Tunnel Release

Tiffany GRUNWALD, M.D.[a], Charisse CORSBIE-MASSAY, M.A.[b],

[a]*Plastic and Reconstructive Surgery, USC Keck School of Medicine*
grunwald@usc.edu
[b]*Critical Studies, USC School of Cinema Television*
charisse@alum.mit.edu

Abstract: This study proposes a series of guidelines for designing multimedia educational interfaces that combine educational strategies with cognitive load theory. There is a large body of research that confirms multimedia education is at least as effective as the traditional approach, but there is no discussion regarding the effectiveness of the interface design. This trial compares two interfaces to determine which design techniques are most cognitively efficient for the learner.

Keywords: Cognitive process, multimedia learning, interface design

1. Introduction

Multimedia instruction has provided a sophisticated method whereby traditional text and illustrations can be incorporated into interactive, multi-dimensional software. A presentation using text, illustrations, animations and video can assist the learner in building a mental model of the material. Students who receive well-constructed multimedia messages perform better on transfer tests designed to measure overall comprehension and problem solving ability, than do students who receive messages through traditional didactic method [1]. The authors assert that students learning through advanced multimedia interfaces that account for theories of cognitive load will achieve better comprehension of given lesson as compared to interfaces that do not.

As technologies become integrated at all educational levels, it is necessary to establish what design techniques are most successful in creating multimedia learning tools. Despite enthusiasm for incorporating multimedia, the assumption that interactive media alone will advance learning is simplistic. Merely translating a preexisting curriculum to a multimedia format is insufficient; rather, new curriculums and lesson plans must be designed for multimedia environments. This experiment serves to quantify the efficacy of trends in multimedia education and offers design guidelines that address the cognitive properties utilized in the learning process.

2.   Background

This experiment utilizes a literature review conducted by Grunwald and Corsbie-Massay entitled "Guidelines for Cognitively Efficient Multimedia Learning Tools: A review of literature relating to educational strategies, cognitive load and interface design"[2]. This review combines existing educational strategies and cognitive load theory to propose a series of guidelines for designing a cognitively efficient multimedia interface.

When developing a multimedia learning tool (MML), it is necessary to distinguish between media, which delivers the message, and the symbolic systems used to convey the message [3]. Many quantitative studies neglect to make this distinction thereby confusing the source of changes in learning. According to Mayer, "it is not possible to separate the effects of the medium from the effects of instructional method... learning outcomes depend on the quality of the instructional method rather than on the medium per se" [4]. In other words, learning is influenced by instructional methods, not the media by which it is delivered [2]. Therefore, a successful education strategy, one that assists students in retaining information in their long-term memory despite a limited working memory, must be developed *before* designing an MML. The following guidelines help create active learners and encourage long-term retention of newly acquired knowledge.

1. Create active, self-directed learners
2. Involve student in goal planning and agenda development
3. Maintain authentic context
4. Provide student sensitive instructional feedback
5. Provide student sensitive environment
6. Reflect on learning goals

Cognitive load theory is based on information processing assumptions, including Mayer's 'dual channel assumption,' which states that humans possess separate information processing channels for visual and auditory material (text information is interpreted through the auditory pathway), and the 'limited capacity assumption,' which limits the amount of information can that be consumed by either channel at one time (See Figure 1) [4]. Combined, the human working memory is capable of holding an average of seven items at once [5]. The number of elements that are consciously or unconsciously attended to by the learner is necessary in calculating the total cognitive load of an interface. The student must integrate the discreet bundles of information into a limitless long-term memory and the expanse of this long-term memory determines his or her proficiency with a given subject [2]. The following guidelines assist in creating an interface that reduces cognitive load.

1. Synchronize audio and visual information
2. Eliminate multi-tasking
3. Optimize representations/Approachable interface

4.   Maintain stable learning environment
5.   Eliminate redundant information
6.   Manage navigational control
7.   Maintain authentic context

The currently available research is lacking in studies specifically regarding the supplemental features of an MML such as a glossary and image control functions. Statistics regarding additional learning resources including the electronic notebook, lecture/surgery notes or Frequently Asked Questions (FAQs) are scarce. Baumlin et al. [6] conducted trials of EMCyberSchool that featured a supplementary online program with an extended resource of additional cases and images. The program proved successful without addressing the role of the additional resources in this success. Although additional materials are considered essential to learning, their usage rates are not addressed. Medical MML developers assume that more is better, but without strong evidence as to their utility and efficacy, money, time and effort may be wasted. Further research is necessary to discover what groups of learners benefit most from which resources.

The S.M.A.R.T. Tool seeks to discover the best synchronization of audio-visual information while documenting the learner's use of various learning resources to quantify when and how they are utilized. The experiment also tallies the student's interaction with the provided images.

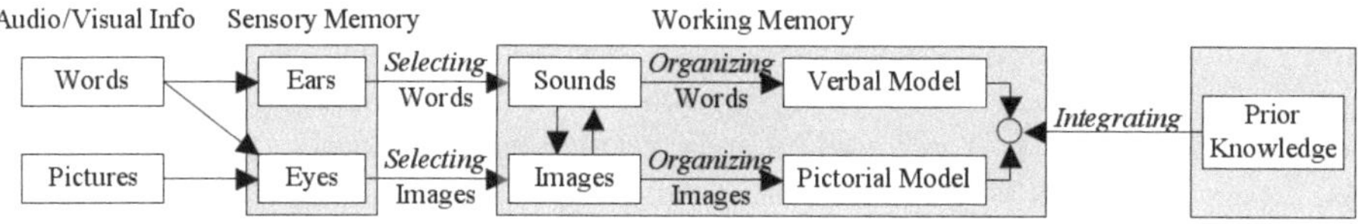

Figure 1. Dual Channel Assumption [4]

3.   Study Design

This study is a randomized controlled trial that quantitatively assesses the efficiency of different interface designs. Two dynamic interfaces were designed specifically for this study. Both teach the preliminary processes of carpal tunnel release, but vary in presentation to cater to the students' cognitive and educational needs.

3.1   Subjects

Our subjects include 80 medical students from the USC Keck Medical School. Subjects are randomly assigned to either interface A or interface B; each subject interacts with the program for a maximum of 15 minutes, followed by a cognitive assessment to determine the educational efficiency of each interface. Subjects were observed to discover *how* they interact with the interface and *what* learning resources they choose to utilize. By observing the student's interaction with the program, we hope to distinguish what resources are beneficial.

3.2   *Program Development*

This experiment utilizes a custom designed Flash MX program that teaches basic surgical and procedural concepts for carpal tunnel release. This dynamic program provides text images and audio to create an immersive media environment for the learner. The monitor is divided into two windows, a text window and an image window (see Figure 2). The text script was taken from an available teaching module for carpal tunnel syndrome. The image window plays a simple movie during the audio presentation after which the user is free to interact with highlighted text. These links control the image window and/or provide additional information. The program offers a variety of optional learning resources to assist the student including a hyperlinked glossary and expandable images.

The control interface (A) provides a simplistic multimedia interpretation of the material, similar to that of an existing multimedia textbook: the audio script is presented in the text window. The experimental interface (B) rephrases the visual delivery of the text; key terms and phrases are reorganized into an outline format that is revealed line by line in synch with the audio presentation.

The experimental interface is designed to test two design guidelines provided in the authors' aforementioned review: the appropriate presentation of audio and visual information and eliminating redundant material. The outline format visually reinforces the information provided in the audio channel and reduces redundant information, thereby utilizing the dual channel pathway to maximize the number of distinct items retained in the working memory. By revealing each line in conjunction with its audio reading, small chunks of information are presented simultaneously; each complement the others within the short-term working memory to better integrate into long-term memory.

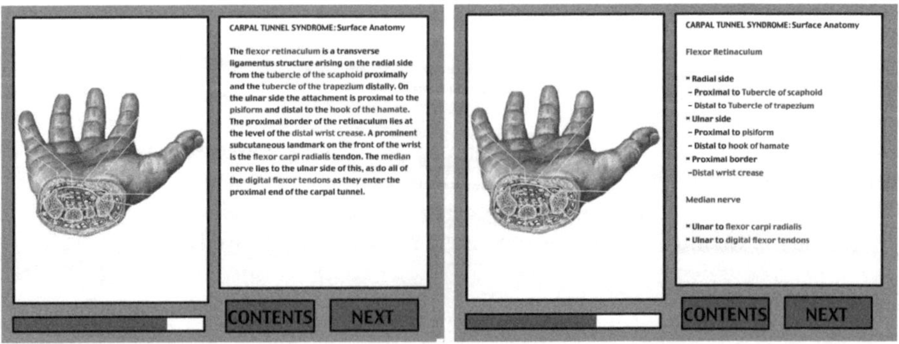

Figure 2. S.M.A.R.T. Tool, control and experimental interfaces

4.   Discussion

The ultimate goal of the S.M.A.R.T. Project is to design a fully comprehensive multimedia educational environment that can reduce the time necessary to acquire and perfect a skill as well as the monetary and temporal demands on the teaching hospital and its faculty. Our intention is not eliminate teaching in the operating room; rather, we are working specifically with fundamental surgical skills and decision making to allow for advanced teaching in the operating room.

This experiment will discover the best interface design for disseminating information regardless of the lesson or the field of inquiry. It will provide statistical data to confirm what presentation is most cognitively efficient for the user as well as an investigation into the learner's use of various learning resources. During testing, subjects were observed to discover the time spent with each module and how learning resources were utilized.

Although several MMLs provide supplemental glossaries and other learning resources, their efficacy is not quantified, rather the learning resources are assumed to enhance the MML without accounting for how they are used. By correlating performance on assessment tools with the time spent within each learning module and the student's interaction with the available supplemental image, the authors will present the best method of integrating various learning resources.

Existing multimedia learning tools fail to address cognitive load when anticipating the learner's interaction with the program. This study investigates MMLs that account for cognitive load and compares them with available learning tools. We will discuss a series of guidelines that can be employed by designers of medical education software as well as areas for future research.

References

[1] Grundman J, Wigton, R., Nickol, D. A Controlled Trial of an Interactive, Web-based Virtual Reality Program for Teaching Physical Diagnosis Skills to Medical Students. *Academic Medicine.* October Supplement 2000;75(10):S47-S49.

[2] Grunwald, T., Corsbie-Massay, C. Guidelines for Cognitively Efficient Multimedia Learning Tools: A review of literature relating to educational strategies, cognitive load theory, and interface design. *Academic Medicine.* March 2006 (in press)

[3] Clark R. Research on Web-Based Learning: A Half-full Glass. In: Bruning R, Horn, C. & PytlikZillig, ed. *Web-Based Learning: What do we know? Where do we go?* Greenwich: Information Age Publishing; 2003.

[4] Mayer R. *Multimedia Learning.* New York: Cambridge University Press; 2001.

[5] Miller GA. The Magical Number Seven, Plus or Minus Two: Some Limits on our Capacity for Processing Information. *Psychology Review.* 1956; 63: 81-97.

[6] Baumlin KM, Bessette MJ, Lewis C, Richardson LD. EMCyberSchool: an evaluation of computer-assisted instruction on the Internet.[see comment]. *Academic Emergency Medicine.* 2000;7(8):959-962.

Medicine Meets Virtual Reality 14
J.D. Westwood et al. (Eds.)
IOS Press, 2006

The Use of a GripForce System to Map Force Distribution Patterns of Laparoscopic Instruments

Neil GUPTA, Fernando BELLO[1], Herbert ARNARSSON, Philippe RIVIERE,
Suzannah HOULT and Ara DARZI
Department of Biosurgery and Surgical Technology,
Imperial College London.

Abstract. While it is acknowledged that the forces required to manipulate laparoscopic instruments can be significant and are important in terms of potential discomfort after prolonged use, no systematic study has been conducted. In this paper we present a GripForce system that allows for the mapping of force distribution patterns of laparoscopic instruments. Initial results showed significant differences in force distribution between various instrument handles, thus demonstrating the viability of the system and proposed methodology. Analysis of force distribution patterns of laparoscopic instruments can help towards improving instrument design, better understanding the relationship between force applied and performance, as well as provide useful feedback to trainees and surgeons.

Keywords. Force distribution, Force Patterns, Force Mapping, Laparoscopic Surgery

1. Introduction

Since the advent of laparoscopic surgery, surgeons have complained about uncomfortable instruments [1] and stressful working positions [2]. Laparoscopic instruments seem to have been developed with the purpose in mind but not the operator. Not only are the instruments uncomfortable, but it is well documented that many actually cause neuropraxia [3] and pain [4]. Relatively few researchers and doctors have published on the ergonomics of laparoscopic handle design but manufacturers are increasingly developing new handles with ergonomics in mind. It is acknowledged that the forces required to manipulate the instruments are important and that compressive forces can be concentrated at certain points on the hand in some instrument designs. This can cause blood flow reduction and may lead to tingling or numbness.

This paper introduces a GripForce system for the acquisition and analysis of force distribution patterns of laparoscopic instruments. Being able to study these patterns can

---

[1] Corresponding Author: Dr Fernando Bello, Dept. of Biosurgery and Surgical Technology, 10th Floor QEQM Building, St Mary's Hospital, Praed St, London W2 1NY, UK; E-mail: F.Bello@imperial.ac.uk

help towards improving instrument design as well as providing useful feedback to trainees and surgeons. We explore the use of the system in the context of ergonomic instrument design and study force distribution using different instrument handles to perform a simple cutting task.

2. Force studies in Laparoscopic Surgery

The force applied to tissues or perceived by a surgeon through a laparoscopic instrument has been studied by several authors with the purpose of characterizing tissue compliance [5], incorporating realistic force feedback into training systems [6,7] and assessing performance [8]. *In vivo* quantification of mechanical interactions between laparoscopic instruments and anatomical structures is of great interest for the modeling of the mechanical behaviour of living organs, the introduction of force feedback in surgical simulators and the design of new surgical instruments. Quantification of such manipulations is also relevant in the assessment of surgical practice.

On the other hand, little attention has been paid to estimating the forces applied by the surgeon to the instrument handles. Such forces may vary depending on the task being performed, dimensions of the hand, handle design and proficiency. Although ergonomics in surgery has been a driving force for some time, the ergonomics of laparoscopic instruments has only become increasingly relevant in recent years [9-14]. There are a few select research groups working on this topic and therefore the literature is relatively limited. These groups all identify similar ergonomic requirements for laparoscopic instruments [9,12,14]:

a) The **posture of the hand and arm** is important. Therefore the instruments should allow a relaxed working position in a neutral zone of hand movements.
b) The **forces required to manipulate** the instruments are important and so design must take into account the strengths of the different muscles in the hand and arm.
c) **Concentration of compressive forces** should be avoided by using the larger possible contact area.
d) It has been suggested that the **thumb should manipulate** any knobs on instruments, as it is the only finger which has strong abductors and adductors as well as flexors and extensors.
e) **Left-handed** users must be taken into account.
f) Consider the **hand dimensions** (anthropometry) of instrument users.

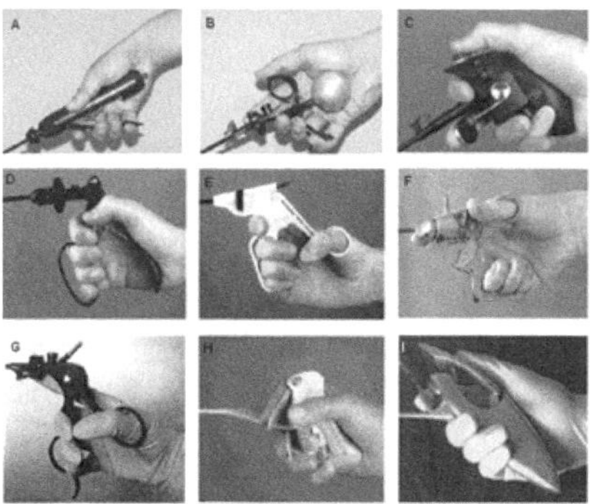

Fig. 1 Various handle designs: A. Aesculap inline axial handle PM 953 R; B. Experimental vario handle; Karl Storz Endoskope multifunctional handle CE 33124 M; D. Wilo 25.00 pistol grip shank handle; E. Autosuture endoshears 30531; F. Microsurge 01-1007; G. Pilling Weck access plus ring handle model 385202A; H. MFEHG Schafreuter multifunctional handle; I. Experimental handle design.

Following these criteria and comments from surgeons, manufacturers have altered the designs of laparoscopic handles over the years. Fig. 1 shows examples of various handle designs.

3. GripForce System

The GripForce system consists of a number of small force sensors, data acquisition hardware, a standard Webcam and bespoke software. A previous version of the system has already been used successfully to assess the force distribution patterns on the hands whilst driving a car and hitting a golf ball [15]. We now proceed to describe the various components of the system.

3.1. Force Sensors

We used the A201-25 FlexiForce® sensors supplied by Tekscan [16]. They are thin and unobtrusive piezoresistive force sensors with a force range covering the possible forces used in surgery and do not impede the movements of the hands whilst performing complex tasks. Fig. 2(a) illustrates the mounting of the sensors using Tegaderm transparent dressing.

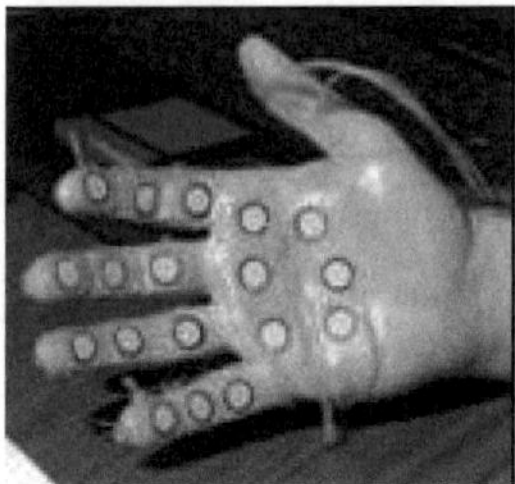 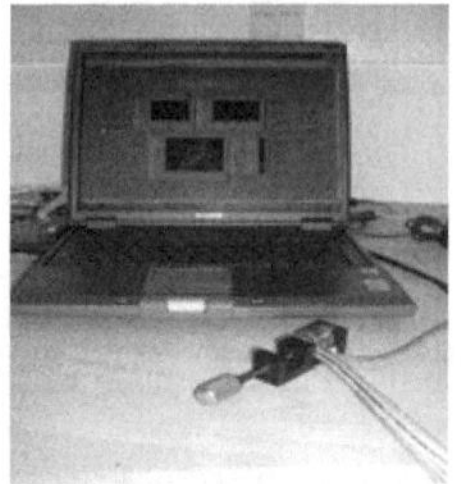

Fig. 2 (a) Mounting of the sensors. (b) Sensor calibration

3.2. Sensor Calibration

Calibration of the sensors involves the use of a force washer mechanism as described in [15] and shown in Fig. 2(b). Between 5-10 sensors can be placed in the mechanism and an increasing load exerted on the system by a vice. By tightening the clamp, the same force is exerted on the force sensors and the force washer. Repeating this process a number of times and plotting the readings of the sensors against the readings from the force washer it is possible to obtain the gain for each sensor.

3.3. Data Acquisition

The signal from each sensor is conditioned using a standard non-inverting amplifier and read through an AD132 Elan Data Acquisition Card [17]. For the purpose of this study only twelve out of the sixteen available channels were utilized as twelve sensors were considered sufficient.

3.4. Webcam

The quantitative force measurements generated by the sensors are complemented with simultaneous web camera footage providing qualitative information about the handling of the instrument. This information proved extremely valuable to understand and interpret the force measurements, as well as to validate the placement of the sensors.

3.5. Software

We chose as our development platform LabVIEW™, a graphical development environment for creating test, measurement and control applications [18]. The software has two separate components: Calibration and Acquisition / Analysis. The Calibration screen reads sensor data, calculates, displays and stores the gain for each sensor, while the Acquisition / Analysis screen contains the live video feed, a colour coded display of each sensor as placed on the hand, and a combined plot of force amplitude, with the possibility of storing both video and sensor data (see Fig. 3).

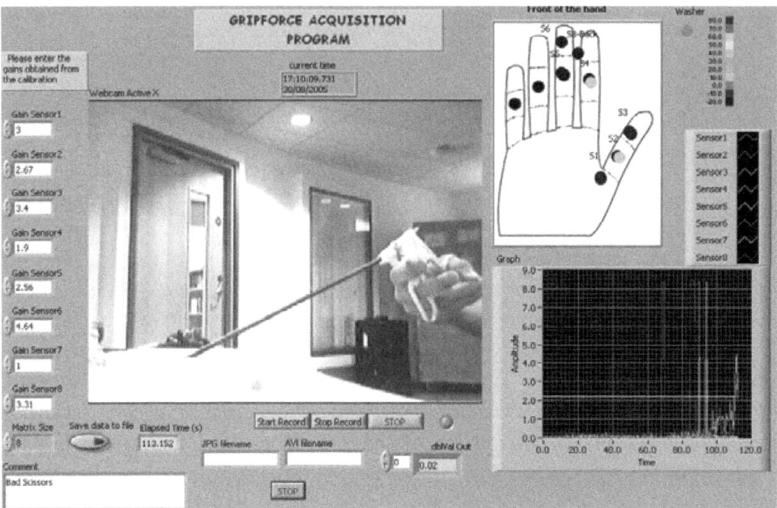

Fig. 3 GripForce Acquisition / Analysis software.

4. Experiments

We conducted a study with five subjects of varying laparoscopic experience: two Specialist Registrars with several years practice, two Senior House Officers with limited experience, and a medical student with basic knowledge of laparoscopic surgery and limited experience on laparoscopic simulators. They were instructed to perform a cutting task with four different instruments (see Fig. 4(a) – (d)) while force sensors on their hand measured the forces applied. A fifth handle (Fig. 4(e)) was also evaluated separately from the main study.

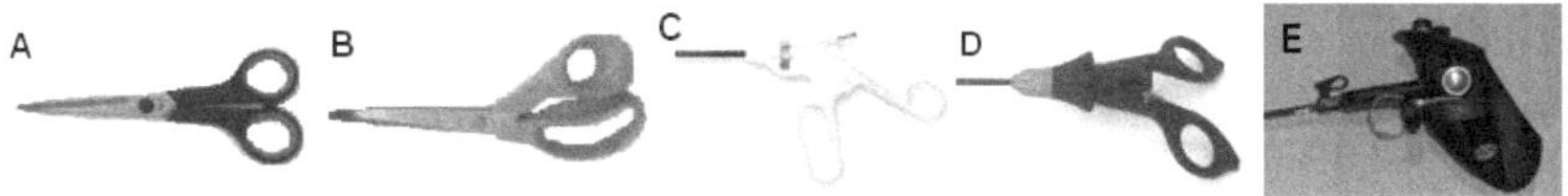

Fig. 4 A. Pair of household scissors; B. Pair of material shears; C. Autosuture EndoShears Pistol Grip Handle Laparoscopic Scissors; D. Karl Storz 33124 Inline Handle Laparoscopic Scissors; E. Karl Storz Endoskope multifunctional handle.

4.1. Sensor Placement

To gain a perspective on the ideal location of sensors on the hand, a method of inking and gloving was employed. This involved painting the instruments in ink and then using a gloved hand to perform a cutting task. This resulted on a contact map for each instrument. By assessing all the contact maps, twelve key areas were identified and sensors placed accordingly (Fig. 5).

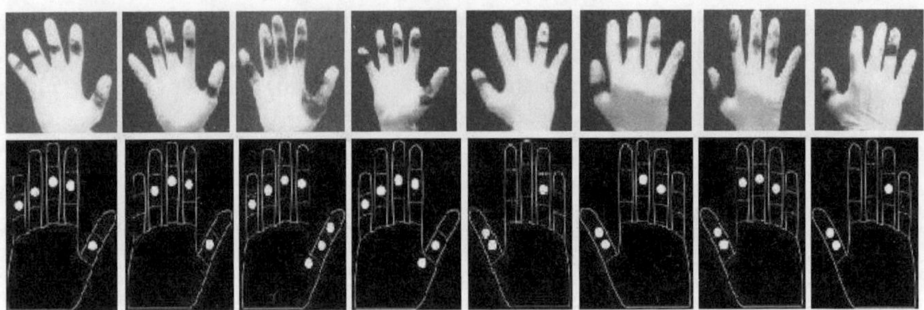

Fig. 5 Contact maps for the right hand.(front and back).

4.2. Task

All subjects were asked to cut a straight line through a piece of sponge using each of the four instruments in turn. The emphasis was not on the task performed, but on the actual forces applied by the hand. The order in which each subject used the instruments was randomised. Webcam and sensor data were stored and analysed for each subject. The sensors which recorded force whilst opening the instrument were plotted on the same graph and, similarly, the sensors which recorded force whilst closing the instrument were plotted onto a separate graph. This resulted in 2 graphs being produced for each of the subjects whilst using a particular instrument. As there were 5 subjects and 4 instruments, this resulted in a total of 40 graphs being plotted.

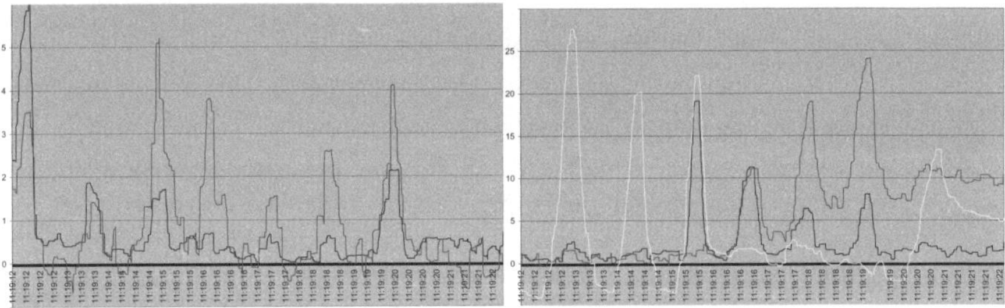

Fig. 6 Sample graphs for opening (L) and closing (R) of Karl Storz Inline Handle Scissors (N vs t).

After the task, the subjects were asked to rate the instruments for comfort and ease of use. For the laparoscopic instruments, all subjects said they preferred the Karl Storz Inline Handle to the Autosuture EndoShears. For the non-laparoscopic instruments all subjects preferred the material shears to the household scissors.

5. Results and Discussion

We studied the obtained graphs and charted the maximum and average values for each sensor during opening and closing. By comparing the maximum force detected by a particular sensor using different instruments we were able to observe the differing force distribution patterns of each tool. While it is difficult to compare the chosen non-surgical and laparoscopic equipment, the results showed that instruments acknowledged as more comfortable and having ergonomic designs had different force distribution patterns. Poor ergonomically designed instruments showed concentration of large forces on small areas of the hand whilst ergonomic instruments allowed for a greater spread of force (see Fig. 7). The recorded video footage illustrated the difference in handling techniques highlighting the importance of proper sensor placement and helping towards the interpretation of the sensor data.

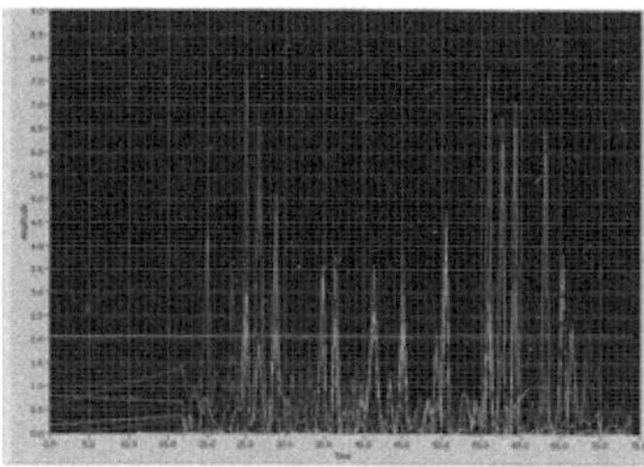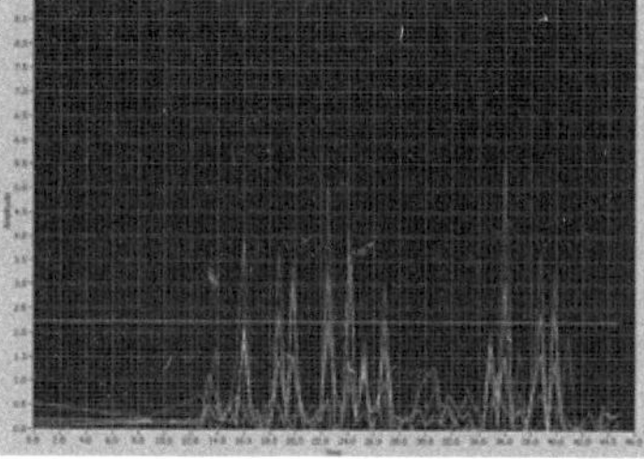

Fig. 7 Combined force distribution patterns for Autosuture Endoshears (L) and Karl Storz Endoskope (H).

6. Conclusions and Future Work

The results obtained from this study demonstrate that the GripForce system is able to record the force distribution patterns for different instruments and that these patterns can be related to accepted ergonomic design guidelines. Having proven the feasibility of the system, we will now conduct a larger study assessing laparoscopic instruments and handling expertise. We will also explore the potential use of force distribution patterns in the training and assessment of surgical trainees.

Acknowledgements

A Nikonovas for his help and advice with the original system and Dr. med. Ulrich Matern for his comments and arranging the loan of the Karl Storz Endoskope handle.

References

[1]   Matern U, Kuttler G, Giebmeyer C, Waller P, Faist M (2004) Ergonomic aspects of five different types of laparoscopic instrument handles under dynamic conditions with respect to specific laparoscopic tasks: An electromyographic-based study. Surg Endosc 18: 1231–1241.
[2]   Emam T, Frank T, Hanna G, Cuschieri A(2001) Influence of handle design on the surgeon's upper limb movements, muscle recruitment, and fatigue during endoscopic suturing. Surg Endosc 15: 667–672.
[3]   Horgan LF, O'Brian DC, Doctor N (1997) Neuropraxia following laparoscopic procedures: an occupational injury. Min Invas Ther Allied Technol 6: 33–35.
[4]   Majeed AW, Jacob G *et. a.l* (1993) Laparoscopist's thumb: an occupational hazard. Arch Surg 128: 357.
[5]   Carter FJ, Frank TG, Davies PJ, McLean D, Cuschieri A (2001) Measurements and modelling of the compliance of human and porcine organs. Med Image Anal 5: 231–236.
[6]   Ottensmeyer MP *et. al.* (2000) Input and output for surgical simulation: devices to measure tissue properties in vivo and a haptic interface for laparoscopy simulators. St Health Technol Inf 70: 236–242.
[7]   Brouwer I, Ustin J, Bentley L, Sherman A, Dhruv N, Tendick F (2001) Measuring in vivo animal soft tissue properties for haptic modeling in surgical simulation. Stud Health Technol Inform 81: 69–74.
[8]   Rosen J *et. al.* (2001) Markov modeling of minimally invasive surgery based on tool/tissue interaction and force/torque signatures for evaluating surgical skills. IEEE Trans Biomed Eng 48: 579–591.
[9]   Patkin M (1997) A check-list for handle design. Ergonomics Australia On-Line 11(2).
[10] Berguer R (1998) Surg. Tech. and the ergonomics of lapar. instruments. Surg Endosc 12: 458-462.
[11] Van Veelen MA, Meijer DW (1999) Ergonomics and design of laparoscopic instruments: results of a survey among laparoscopic surgeons. J Laparoendosc Adv Surg Techiques A 9: 481–489.
[12] Matern U, Waller P (1999) Instruments for minimally invasive surgery: principles of ergonomic handles. Surg Endosc 13: 174–182.
[13] Matern U (2001) Principles of ergonomic instrument handles. Min Inv Ther All Technol 10: 169–173.
[14] Van Veelen MA, Meijer DW, Goossens RHM, Snijers CJ (2001) New ergonomic criteria for handles of laparoscopic dissection forceps. J Laparoendosc Adv Surg Techniques 11: 17-26.
[15] Nikonovas A, Harrison AJL, Hoult S, Sammut D (2004) The application of force-sensing resistor sensors for measuring forces developed by the human hand. IMechE Vol. 218 Part H.
[16] www.tekscan.com
[17] www.elandigitalsystems.com
[18] www.ni.com/labview/

Medicine Meets Virtual Reality 14
J.D. Westwood et al. (Eds.)
IOS Press, 2006

Highly-Realistic, Immersive Training Environment for Hysteroscopy

Matthias Harders [a,1], Michael Bajka [b], Ulrich Spaelter [c], Stefan Tuchschmid [a],
Hannes Bleuler [c], Gabor Szekely [a]

[a] *Virtual Reality in Medicine Group, Computer Vision Lab, ETH Zurich, Switzerland*
[b] *Clinic of Gynecology, Dept OB/GYN, University Hospital Zurich, Switzerland*
[c] *Laboratoire de Systemes Robotiques, Institut de Production et Robotique, EPF Lausanne, Switzerland*

Abstract. The primary driving application of our current research is the development of a generic surgical training simulator for hysteroscopy. A key target is to go beyond rehearsal of basic manipulative skills, and enable training of procedural skills like decision making and problem solving. In this respect, the sense of presence plays an important role in the achievable training effect. To enable user immersion into the training environment, the surrounding and interaction metaphors should be the same as during the real intervention. To this end, we replicated an OR in our lab, provided standard hysteroscopic tools for interaction, and generate a new virtual scene for every session. In this setting, the training starts, as soon as the trainees enter the OR, and ends when they leave the room.

Keywords. surgical simulation, immersive environment

1. Background

Therapeutic hysteroscopy has become a common technique in gynecological practice [5]. Nevertheless, a number of potentially dangerous complications exist - the most common being uterine wall perforation, intra-uterine bleeding, and mismanagement of distension fluid. Therefore, specialized training is necessary to reduce the rate of complications. Virtual Reality based surgical simulation [6] is one option to provide a corresponding learning environment. In contrast to existing systems and products [7,8,9,10], our work aims at achieving the highest possible realism. A key target is to go beyond rehearsal of basic manipulative skills, and enable training of procedural skills like decision making and problem solving.

In this respect, the sense of presence [1] plays an important role in the training effect, which can be achieved. Therefore, a user should feel emotionally and cognitively present in the simulated environment [12]. In order to achieve suspen-

---

[1] Correspondence to: mharders@vision.ee.ethz.ch

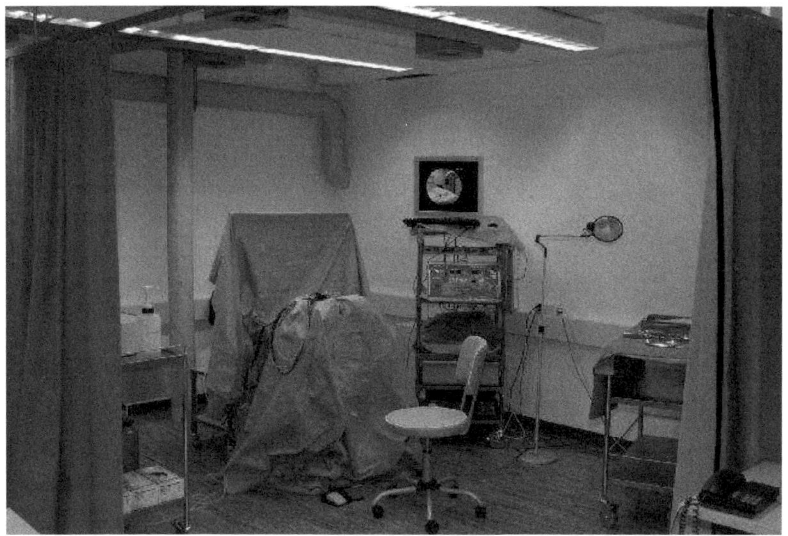

Figure 1. View of the complete OR.

sion of disbelief, a multi-sensory, first-person experience has to be provided [13]. Especially, if actions could lead to negative consequences in reality, it is vital, that the learning environment engages the trainee and seems real.

To enable user immersion into the training environment, the surrounding and interaction metaphors should be the same as during the real intervention. To this end, we replicated an OR in our lab, including standard hysteroscopic tools and surgical devices, and we provide multi-sensory feedback. Moreover, individualized problem cases are presented, by generating new virtual scenes for every session. In this setting, the training starts, when the trainee enters the OR, and it ends, when she leaves the room.

2. Tools and Methods

The first element of our immersive setup is the training environment. We outfitted our OR with real tools and equipment (Figure 1). These tools are actually needed to access the surgical site. For instance, the first step of an intervention is to enable access to the cervix with the specula, and then fixate it with surgical forceps.

The female pelvic region is represented by a Limbs&Things model [2]. It has been modified to our needs in order to be able to house the haptic device. It mainly provides the tissue models for vulva, vagina, and cervix. The latter are directly connected to the haptic device, thus hiding the mechanism from the user. Moreover, the model contains the bony structures of the pelvic region, as well as the abdominal wall. For further realism, two legs obtained from a patient model from Ruediger Anatomie [3] were added.

Since interaction should be carried out with real tools instead via a mouse, we use an original resectoscope, which has been equipped with sensors to interact with the simulation. Valves for controlling in- and outflow of the distension fluid

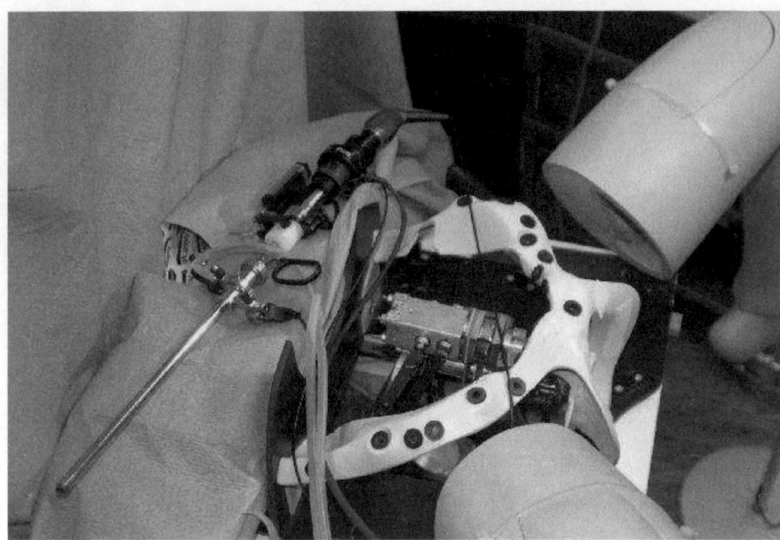

Figure 2. Haptic mechanism inside dummy.

are included. Displacement of the loop electrode is done with a standard handle, while current for tissue cutting or cauterization is controlled by foot pedals. The endoscopic camera is attached to the end of the tool and provides rotational Degrees-of-Freedom (DOF), as well as adjustment of focus. Thus, all typical manipulations of the original tool can be performed in the immersive setup and the simulation appropriately controlled. Moreover, the resectoscope itself can be completely dis- and reassembled from its individual components. All of the above allows the trainee to also get acquainted with the full complexity of tool handling.

The hardware allows insertion and complete removal of the surgical tool. After cervix fixation with the forceps, the hysteroscope is inserted into the uterine cavity, where it connects seamlessly with the haptic mechanism inside of the pelvic dummy, without any noticeable mechanical constraints. Triggered by the insertion of the tool, the visual display of the virtual scene starts automatically with a view obtained after passing the cervix. This permits a smooth transition into the fully immersive scenario instead of the well known simulation on/off experience.

The haptic device provides 4-DOFs for hysteroscopy [14]. Two DOFs for spherical displacement around a virtual pivot point are possible, as well as tracking and force-feedback for tool translation along and rotation around the tool axis. Friction and inertia from the haptic device are compensated by closed-loop control. During the simulation session, all gestures of the surgeon are tracked, permitting not only simple playback, but also making evaluation of the recorded session possible. The components inside of the mock-up (without the tissue elements) are depicted in Figure 2. During simulation the mechanical hardware remains completely hidden from eye-view.

A further element in the immersive environment is the auditory feedback. Characteristic sound sources are the electrocardiogram, hysteroscopy pump, artificial respiration, warning sounds for electrotomy and coagulation. These provide important cues to a gynecologist, and thus have to be integrated into a training

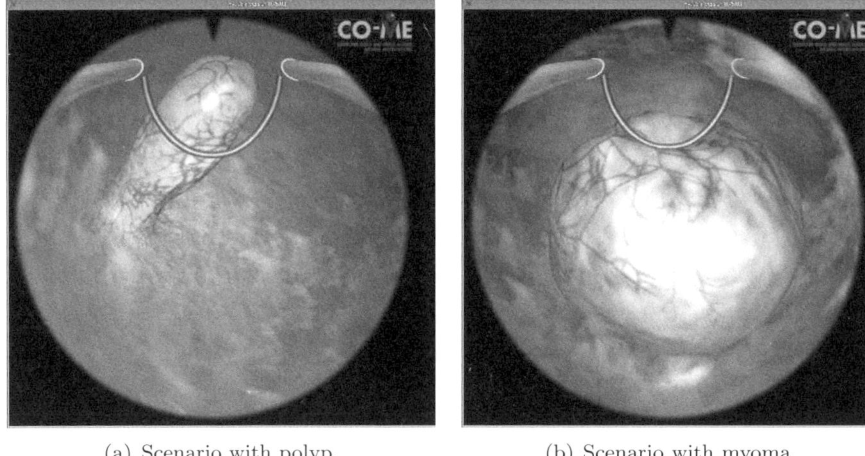

(a) Scenario with polyp.   (b) Scenario with myoma.

Figure 3. Individual training scenes with different pathologies.

system. To this end, a hysteroscopic intervention has been recorded with studio microphones and a highly sensitive sound level meter (room size 6 x 4 x 3 m). Measured sound pressure levels have been in general between 57 - 65 dB(A). The rhythmic beep of the ECG was by far the most audible source. Based on these data, sound samples were extracted, which are synthesized in real-time stereo during the simulation and adapted to the actual surgical action, e.g. regulating in-/outflow of the hysteroscopy pump.

The final element of the system is a complete process for creating individual training scenes [4]. Based on real data (i.e. 3D ultrasound and MRI datasets, intra-uterine videos acquired during interventions, and in-vivo tissue measurements), statistical models were generated, enabling the creation of new instances of surgical scenarios. This includes the variability of healthy anatomy, modeling of pathology growth, incorporation of vascular structures, attachment of textures, and specification of deformation parameters. Thus, just like in real life, no two (virtual) patients will be the same. In Figure 3 two training scenarios are depicted, showing a polyp and a myoma inside the uterine cavity.

Screenshots, movies of sample interventions and further descriptions of the simulator modules can be found one our project web (http://www.hystsim.ethz.ch).

3. Conclusions

In order to increase the sense of presence, and thus improve the training outcome, we created an immersive environment for hysteroscopy simulation. This includes the surroundings, surgical tools, haptic, visual, and auditory feedback, and a virtual training scene generation process. Further modules of the simulator include real-time collision detection and response, tissue deformation, and fluid models. The complete system is depicted in Figure 4.

In future work, we will focus on further enhancement of the surgical suite. In order to increase realism, real surgical devices, e.g. fluid pump, electrocardio-

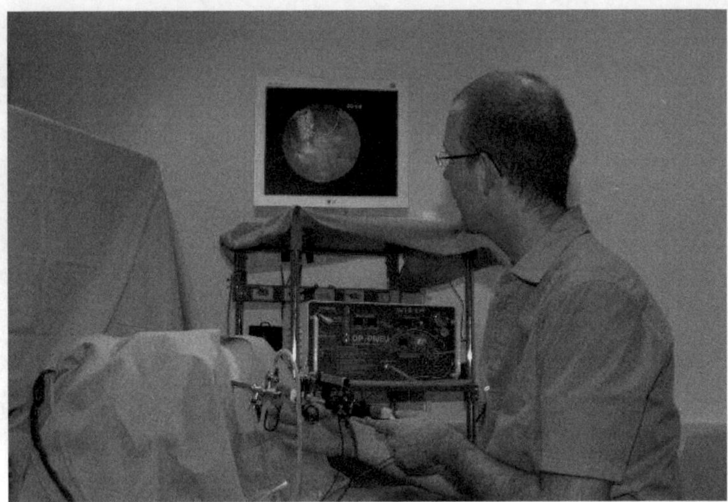

Figure 4. Close-up of the system.

gram, will be connected to and controlled by the simulation. Additionally, we will integrate real management of distension fluid with the simulation. Finally, an extension of the setup to team training possibilities will be examined.

Acknowledgment

This research has been supported by the NCCR Co-Me of the Swiss National Science Foundation. The authors would like to thank all developers of the hysteroscopy simulator project. We also are grateful to the support of the Ecole Cantonale d'Art de Lausanne and Mad Synthetics for creating the table for the simulator mock-up.

References

[1] M. Slater and A. Steed A Virtual Presence Counter. In *Presence: Teleoperators and Virtual Environments*, 9(5), 413-434, 2000.

[2] http://www.limbsandthings.com

[3] http://www.berlin-anatomie.de/

[4] R. Sierra, M. Bajka, C. Karadogan, G. Szekely and M. Harders Coherent Scene Generation for Surgical Simulators Medical Simulation Symposium ISMS, 221 - 229, 2004..

[5] ACOG Tech. Bulletin. Hysteroscopy. Int J Gyn. Obstet., May 1994. 45(2): 175-180.

[6] A. Liu, F. Tendick, K. Cleary and C.R. Kaufmann A survey of surgical simulation: Applications, technology, and education. *Presence: Teleoperators & Virtual Environments*, 12(6):599–614, 2003.

[7] J.S. Levy. Virtual reality hysteroscopy. *J Am Assoc Gyn. Laparosc.*, 3, 1996.

[8] Immersion Medical. AccuTouch system. Company webpage (visited Mar 2005).

[9] K. Montgomery, L. Heinrichs, C. Bruyns, S. Wildermuth , C. Hasser, S. Ozenne and D. Bailey Surgical simulator for hysteroscopy: A case study of visualization in surgical training. In *IEEE Visualization*, 449-452, 2001.

[10] W.K. Muller-Wittig, A. Bisler, U. Bockholt, J.L. Los Arcos, P. Oppelt and J. Stahler LAHYSTOTRAIN - development and evaluation of a complex training system for hysteroscopy. In *MMVR Proceedings*,81:336-340, 2001.

[11] M. Roussos, A. Johnson, T. Moher, J. Leigh, C. Vasilakis and C. Barnes Learning and building together in an immersive virtual world In *Presence: Teleoperators and Virtual Environments*, 8, 247-263, 1999.

[12] F. Mantovani and G. Castelnuovo Sense of Presence in Virtual Training: Enhancing Skills Acquisition and Transfer of Knowledge through Learning Experience in Virtual Environments In *Being There: Concepts, effects and measurement of user presence in synthetic environments*, G. Riva, F. Davide and W. IJsselsteijn (Eds.), 168-181, Ios Press, 2003.

[13] D. Romano and P. Brna Presence and reflection in training: support for learning to improve quality decision-making skills under time limitations In *Cyberpsychology and Behavior*, 4: 265-277, 2001.

[14] U. Spaelter, T. Moix, D. Ilic, M. Bajka and H. Bleuler A 4-dof Haptic Device for Hysteroscopy Simulation In *IROS 2004, IEEE/RSJ*, 4: p. 3257-3263, 2004.

Medicine Meets Virtual Reality 14
J.D. Westwood et al. (Eds.)
IOS Press, 2006

PelvicSim – A Computational-Experimental System for Biomechanical Evaluation of Female Pelvic Floor Organ Disorders and Associated Minimally Invasive Interventions

Balakrishna HARIDAS[a], Hyundae HONG[b], Ryo MINOGUCHI[b],
Steve OWENS[c], Thomas OSBORN[b]
[a]*University of Cincinnati, Cincinnati, OH;*
[b]*Procter & Gamble Company, Cincinnati, OH;*
[c]*SAEC/Kinetic Vision, Cincinnati, OH.*

Abstract. In this paper we describe the prototype of a new computational simulation system, PelvicSim. This system is being developed to simulate the in vivo biomechanics of the female pelvic floor organ system with the intent to provide clinical researchers, medical device designers with a virtual environment to understand the various biomechanical pathologies occurring in the pelvic floor. This information can then be used to develop new reconstructive surgical techniques, or design non surgical/surgical devices for the treatment of urinary incontinence and pelvic organ prolapse. In this paper, we provide the initial results from the development of the PelvicSim modules which combine in vivo sensing experiments, Ultrasound and MRI imaging datasets, and an inverse finite element modeling technology based on hyperviscoelastic constitutive modeling of the pelvic floor organs and tissues.

Keywords. Female pelvic organ disorders, Nonlinear hyperviscoelastic constitutive models, nonlinear finite element modeling, In Vivo Tissue Properties, Inverse finite element analysis, In Vivo Measurement, Tissue Deflection, Stress Relaxation, Balloon Loading and Pressure Sensing, MR Imaging and 3D reconstruction, Ultrasound B mode and M Mode Imaging.

1. Introduction

Pelvic Organ Prolapse (POP), Urinary Incontinence (UI), and Fecal Incontinence (FI) are a continuum of significant pathologies of the feminine pelvic floor organ system, rapidly becoming a significant health care problem in the United States [1,2]. Described as a "hidden-epidemic" [1], POP, UI, and FI occur due to damage to the pelvic floor support system consisting of the levator ani muscle, endopelvic fascia, and nerves organized as a complex load bearing apparatus in the pelvis. A significant percentage of women (11% - [2]) have to consider non-surgical treatment using transvaginal devices [3] to support/augment the pelvic floor, or reconstructive surgery with or without implantable devices. Over 400,000 pelvic floor surgeries are performed annually, with over 30% revision rates [1,2], representing a growing health care crisis in the aging female population. In a recent paper [1] an important goal of a 25% prevention and a 25% treatment improvement (a *"25/25"* strategy) was proposed for POP/UI. As a step towards the implementation of this strategy, we have initiated the development of PelvicSim, a computational modeling system based on a fusion of patient specific clinical imaging, in vivo sensing , and advanced nonlinear finite element based biomechanical modeling technologies. We envision this system to be released as a flexible architecture computational environment that will

a)　Serve as a research tool to enable studies on the natural history of POP as a function of parity, gravidity, age, menopause, neuropathy, pulmonary disease, ethnicity, obesity, smoking, and other risk factors

b)　Serve as a virtual biomechanical modeling environment to evaluate device-pelvic organ biomechanics and develop safe and effective innovations intended to detect, manage, and treat POP.

c)　Assist practicing clinicians to better quantify and potentially detect *a priori*, signs of pelvic floor dysfunction and POP. This will enable clinicians to take proactive actions to prevent progression to more severe states requiring surgical intervention.

2. Methods

The method underlying PelvicSim is the concept of inverse finite element modeling (FEM) and analysis of soft tissue mechanics [4-8]. In a typical FE simulation, the deformation of a structure in response to external loads is calculated. In the case of the pelvic floor organ system, FEM inputs would include the following

* *3D geometry of the uterus, cervix, bladder, vagina, levator ani muscle, endopelvic fascia, and distal rectum in a relatively stress free or reference state.*
* *Hyper-viscoelastic material properties of the various tissues*
* *External loading and boundary motions applied to the organs (elevated abdominal pressure, pelvic floor tightening, coughing, valsalva maneuvers)*

Assuming that the above three inputs are available, i.e., a well posed boundary value problem-BVP [9], an FE model can be solved to determine the outputs, i.e. tissue deformations and stresses. For pelvic organs and tissues, the inputs required for adequate definition of the BVP, are largely unknown.

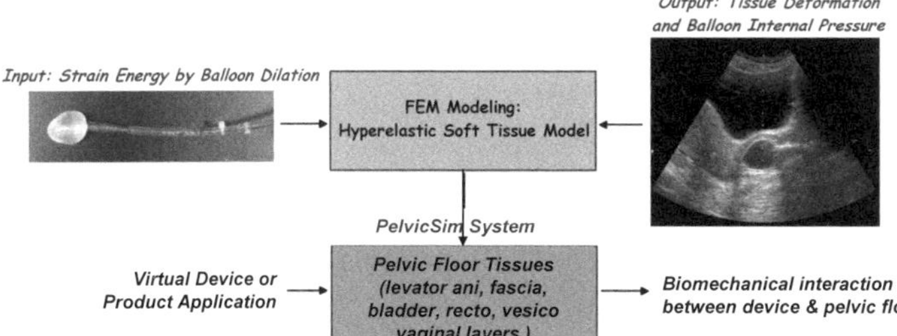

Figure 1. Schematic of inverse finite element modeling strategy in PelvicSim.

The goal of inverse FE analysis is to estimate hyperviscoelastic properties from *in vivo* experiments. Imaging is used to measure the geometry as well as the deformations of the pelvic organs and connective tissues in response to known in vivo loads. Loads are generated by minimally invasive, or non invasive devices (e.g. a transvaginal balloon). A finite element model is run iteratively to estimate the unknown hyperviscoelastic material properties of the soft tissues in the vicinity of the loading function. This process proceeds until predicted tissue deformations from the FE analysis match the measured (imaged) deformations. With the constitutive relationships determined and validated using this technique, the model can be used to *predict* the response of the pelvic floor organ system to other independent loading conditions.

2.1 Hyperelasticity theory for soft tissues

Over the past 25-30 years, there have been significant advances in the field of soft tissue constitutive modeling and finite element analysis [4-8]. Recent applications include the modeling nonlinear hyperviscoelasticity in anisotropic tissues with fiber reinforcements [5,7]. The framework of hyperelasticity theory requires stresses be derived from a stored elastic energy function [5,7]. For an isotropic material, the Cauchy stress σ, can be derived from a strain energy function $W(I_1, I_2, I_3)$, as

$$\sigma = \frac{2}{J} F \frac{\partial W}{\partial C} F^T \tag{1}$$

where $F = \dfrac{\partial x}{\partial X}$ is the material deformation gradient with x and X being current and

original positions of the material point respectively. I_1, I_2, and I_3 are the invariants of the right Cauchy Green deformation tensor C. $J = det(F)$ is the volume change.

Several forms of such functions have been identified [5,7]. A classical example of such a function is the generalized Mooney-Rivlin energy function,

$$W(I_1, I_2, I_3) = \sum_{l,m,n=0}^{\infty} A_{lmn} (I_1 - 3)^l (I_2 - 3)^m (I_3 - 1)^n \tag{2}$$

where A_{lmn} are material coefficients determined by fitting the above equation to experimental data. For soft tissues like tendons, ligaments, articular cartilage, and arteries, investigators have employed exponential forms of W,

$$W(I_1, I_2, I_3) = \alpha_0 \frac{e^{\alpha_1 (I_1 - 3) + \alpha_2 (I_2 - 3)}}{I_3^{\beta}} \tag{3}$$

where α_0, α_1, α_2 are positive constants, and $\beta = \alpha_1 + 2\alpha_2$. All these functions handle only isotropic classes of materials. A recently developed poro-hyperelastic constitutive model for tissues (tendons, ligaments, arteries) can simulate two independent fiber families oriented in various directions [5]. We have employed the most general form of finite strain viscoelasticity to represent nonlinearities in the constitutive relationship in addition to time dependence[8]. In this approach, the strain energy function/volume, W, is cast in a time dependent form using convolution integrals as

$$[\sigma(t)] = \int_{0+}^{t} \frac{\partial[\sigma]}{\partial[C]} \frac{\partial[C(\tau)]}{\partial\tau}\left(1 - \sum_{k=1}^{n} g'_k\left[1 - e^{-(t-\tau)/\tau_k}\right]\right)d\tau \qquad (4)$$

$g(\tau)$, is a normalized (reduced) stress relaxation function of the form,

$$g(t) = \left(1 - \sum_{i=1}^{n} g'_i\left[1 - e^{-t/\tau_i}\right]\right) \qquad (5)$$

In this paper we focus on the time independent, hyperelastic material constants required to model the tissues and organs in the female pelvic floor system.

2.2 MRI Imaging and Finite Element Model of Pelvic Organ System

MRI data from a single subject recruited IRB approved protocols was evaluated in Materialise Corporation's MIMICS software. Organ and tissue boundaries were identified and reconstructed in 3D (Fig 2)

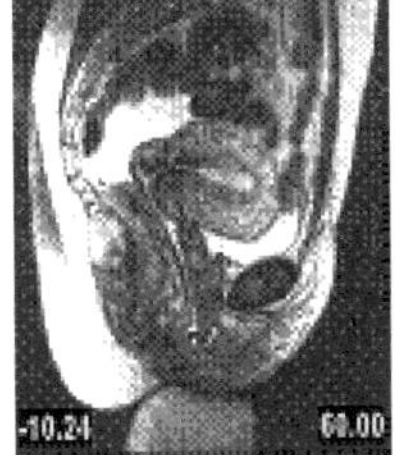
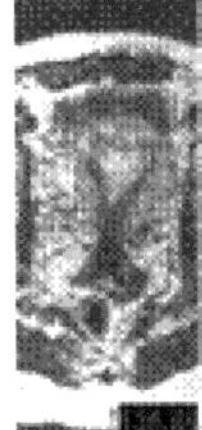
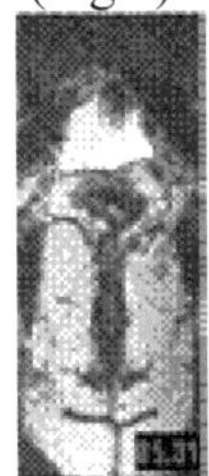
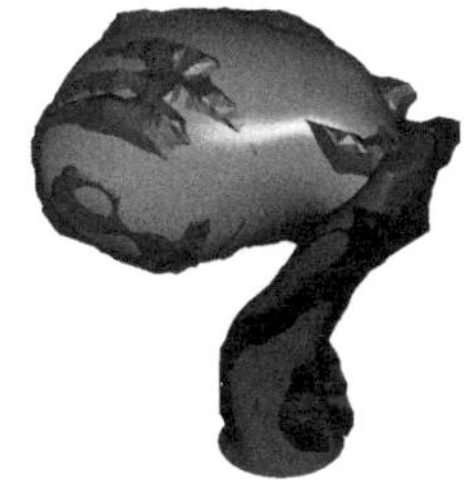

Figure 2. MRI Data (Subject #15)   **Figure 3. Raw MIMICS STL Data and "Smoothed" Geometry**

The geometry is exported from MIMICS in STL format and imported into a CAD package (I-DEAS from UGS Corp.) for finite element model creation. Due to the inherent irregularities in the data, representative "smoothed" Non-Uniform Rational B-Spline (NURBS) surfaces are created for each organ for finite element modeling. Figure 3 illustrates the raw MIMICS data and corresponding smoothed geometry of the vagina and uterus. The finite element model of the pelvic organ system is then created using this smoothed geometry. The model consists of shell and solid elements and is constructed to treat the anterior and posterior regions relative to the vagina lumen as homogenous hyperelastic solid regions (Fig 4) The mesh for the FE model was exported to the LS-DYNA code [10], which uses explicit time integration to solve the equations of motion and deformation.

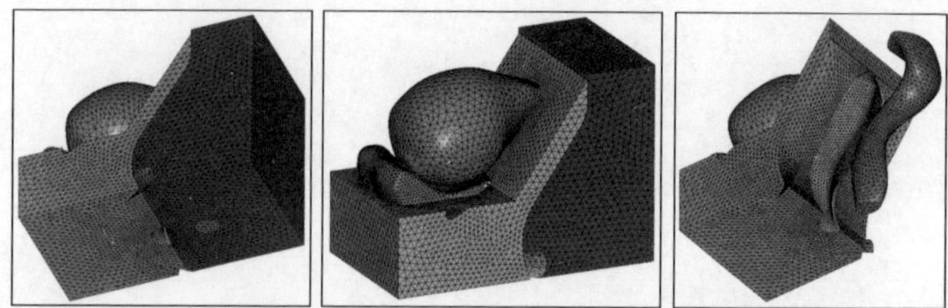

Figure 4. Pelvic Organ System - Finite Element Model

2.3 Inverse FEM identification of hyperelastic material constants of vaginal tissues

The MRI and Ultrasound imaging data was used to conduct a 3D nonlinear finite element simulation of the pelvic floor organs and support system. A bladder filling MRI study was first conducted to estimate the hyperelastic constitutive constants for the bladder wall. Bladder deformations in subject #15 were measured using MRI imaging and the FEM model was used to match these deformations based on input typical bladder pressures measured in vivo in recent studies [11]. Following this, an inverse analysis of the transvaginal balloon dilation was conducted to iteratively determine the local hyperelastic constitutive properties of the pelvic floor tissues.

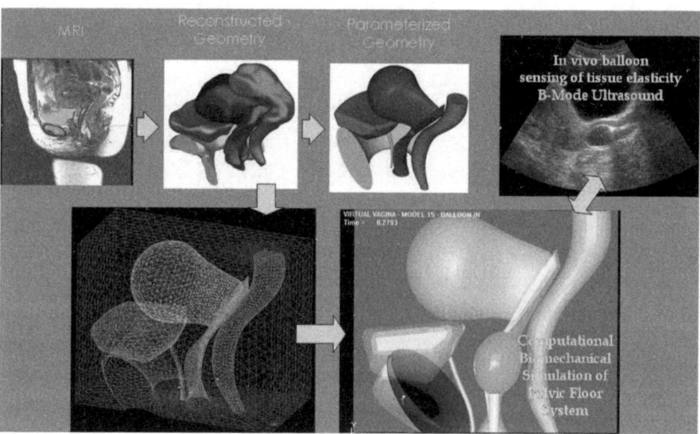

Figure 5. PelvicSim -Various Steps in Model Development

Three dimensional subject-specific finite element models of the pelvic floor organ system were constructed via segmentation of MRI images in the supine position. Results of simulation of the tissue loading by inflated balloon device show the deformations of the vesico-vaginal, and recto-vaginal tissues as well as the bladder wall. These models are validated against B and M-mode ultrasound images gathered during the experiments on the subject (Figure 5).

3.0 Results

Hyperelastic models (Table 1) in LS DYNA [10] were identified for the various tissue systems using the data from transvaginal balloon dilation. The inverse finite element model utilized a Blatz-Ko hyperelastic material formulation for the anterior and posterior homogeneous solid regions. The bladder wall was represented using a two-parameter Mooney-Rivlin hyperelastic material formation. Modeled using shell elements with a specified wall thickness of 1mm in the evacuated state, bladder material constants were adjusted to achieve a targeted bladder pressure between 1.5-2.0 kPa based on published data [11].

Table 1. Material Constants Calculated Using Inverse Modeling

Organ/Tissue	Strain Energy Function or Material Model Formulation	Property calculated using inverse FEM analysis
Vesico Vagina layers	Blatz-Ko	Shear Modulus: 2.5 kPa
Recto Vagina layers	Blatz-Ko	Shear Modulus: 1.25 kPa
Bladder Wall	Mooney-Rivlin	Constant A: 7.5 kPa Constant B: 2.5 kPa
Rectum	Elastic	Modulus of Elasticity: 900 kPa
Uterus	Elastic	Modulus of Elasticity: 50 kPa
Urethra	Blatz-Ko	Shear Modulus: 100 kPa

4.0 Conclusions

Good correlations are obtained between model predictions of tissue deformations and in vivo image data. This represents to our knowledge, one of the first attempts towards the development of a modeling environment and the estimation of in vivo hyperviscoelastic material constants for the pelvic floor organs. Future studies will expand this research to extract more biomechanical parameters, experimental, and computational model development across a range of subjects (preparous, post-parous, ethnicity), that will provide a virtual biomechanics modeling tool to OB/GYN surgeons, and medical device developers attempting to innovate new non-invasive and minimally invasive treatment for pelvic floor organ disorders.

References

[1]   DeLancey JO: The hidden epidemic of pelvic floor dysfunction: Achievable goals for improved prevention and treatment. *American Journal of Obstetrics and Gynecology* **192(5):** 1488-1495, 2005

[2]   Olsen AL, et al: Epidemiology of surgically managed pelvic organ prolapse and urinary incontinence. *Obstetrics and Gynecology* **89(4):** 501-506, 1997

[3]   Weber AM, et al: *Office Urogynecology.* McGraw-Hill, 2004.

[4]   Simon BR: Multiphase poroelastic finite element models for soft tissue structures. Applied Mechanics Reviews **(45):** 191-218, 1992

[5]   Haridas B, et al: Orthotropic hyperelasticity with two fiber families: A study of the effect of fiber organization on continuum mechanical properties in soft tissues. In *International Symposium on Ligaments and Tendons*, 2004

[6]   Lien, K. C., et al. 2004. Levator ani muscle stretch induced by simulated vaginal birth. *Obstetrics and Gynecology* 103, (1) (Jan): 31-40.

[7]   Weiss J.A., et al.: Finite element implementation of incompressible transversely isotropic hyperelasticity. *Computer Methods in Applied Mechanics and Engineering* **(135):** 107-128, 1996

[8]   Haridas B, Matice CJ: Performance evaluation of poly-ethylene terephthalate angioplasty balloons via blow molding simulation and structural analysis. *Journal of Applied Medical Polymers* **5(2):** 2001

[9]   Becker AA: *The Boundary Element Method in Engineering.* McGraw Hill Book Company, 1992.

[10]   Livermore Software Technology Corporation (LSTC): LS-DYNA theory manual. 2005.

[11]   Kim K, Ashton-Miller J: The vesico-urethral pressuregram analysis of urethral function under stress. Journal of Biomechanics **30(1):** 19-25, 1997

Medicine Meets Virtual Reality 14
J.D. Westwood et al. (Eds.)
IOS Press, 2006

Working Memory and Image Guided Surgical Simulation

Leif HEDMAN, *PhD*[a,c] , Torkel KLINGBERG *MD, PhD*[d], Ann KJELLIN, *MD, PhD*[b],
Torsten WREDMARK, *MD, PhD*[a], Lars ENOCHSSON, *MD, PhD*[b] , Li
FELLÄNDER-TSAI, *MD, PhD*[a,1]

[a] *Department for Clinical Science Intervention and Technology (CLINTEC), division of orthopaedics, Karolinska Institutet and Center for Advanced Medical Simulation at Karolinska University Hospital Huddinge, SE-141 86 Stockholm, Sweden, Phone +46 8 585 82102, Fax + 46 8 585 82224*
[b] *CLINTEC, division of surgery, and Center for Advanced Medical Simulation*
[c] *Department of Psychology, Umeå University, SE-901 87 Umeå, Sweden*
[d] *Department of Children and Womens Health, Karolinska Institutet*

Abstract. We report on a study that investigates the relationship between visual working memory and verbal working memory and a performance measure in endoscopic instrument navigation in MIST and GI Mentor II (a simulator for gastroendoscopy). Integrated cognitive neuroscience in state-of-the-art simulator training curriculum will take safety science in health care one step ahead. Current simulator validation focuses on <u>how</u> to train. In the light of recent research it is now prime time to ask <u>why</u> in search of mechanisms rather than to repeatedly show that training has effect. This will help tailor training to maximize individual output in procedures that require a high level of dexterity. WM training is a unique learning aid in simulator training and should be used alongside clinical practice in order to improve the quality of complex clinical intervention in the field of image guided surgical simulation.

Keywords. Image guided surgery, simulation, virtual reality and working memory

1. Introduction

Executive function of the human brain is a broad concept that includes, among other functions, the ability to inhibit a prepotent response, to plan, to reason, and also

---

[1] Corresponding author and reprint request: Li Felländer-Tsai at the above address and E-mail address: li.tsai@ki.se

working memory (WM). WM is the ability to retain information during a delay and then to make a response based on that internal representation. Furthermore, WM is often regarded as a more fundamental function, underlying other executive functions such as reasoning.

Extensive research on training in most other domains of knowledge has clearly shown that individual factors (that trainees bring to the training situation) can be more important than events occurring during as well as after training [1]. For example, little systematic attention has been paid to the cognitive processes involved in surgical proficiency, which also seems to be less understood by surgeons. One aspect of cognition that has received almost no consideration in the surgical research is surgeon's limited attentional capacity [2]. Most kinds of surgery contain multiplex tasks and requirements entailing a rigorous demand on attention level [3], and where a mental slip can result in fatal errors. Because there are clear limitations in the amount of information one can attend to or be conscious of, as well as in the amount of information that can be maintained in working memory, it is widely acknowledged that the constructs of working memory and attention are related to one another.

The WM system is thought to consist of verbal and spatial short-term stores and executive processes that operate on the contents of these stores. Executive WM is likely to be comprised of a number of distinct processes such as: multiple task coordination, set shifting, interference resolution, and memory updating, thought to be essential for high-level thought processes. Analysis of the controlling central executive has proved more challenging, leading to a proposed clarification in which the executive is assumed to be a limited capacity attention system. This sketchpad is assumed to be capable of temporarily maintaining and manipulating visuospatial as well as verbal information, accessed either through the senses or from LTM. Both neuropsychological evidence and functional imaging evidence support the view of the sketchpad as a multicomponent system, with occipital lobe activation presumably reflecting the visual pattern component, parietal regions representing spatial aspects, and frontal activation responsible for coordination and control [4].

Hence, WM, as a limited-capacity store for performing mental operations, might be very important to the surgeon for learning a new procedure or set of skills. Visual working memory and verbal working memory scores (three tasks were taken from the WAIS III test battery) [5] may correlate significantly with endoscopic simulator performance.

Even if many skills are needed to become a competent surgeon, a surgeon cannot be competent without a certain level of technical skills. Since the image guided surgical techniques are more difficult to learn, a focus on technical skills has become even more important. During the last decade there has been an increasing interest in Virtual Reality (VR) simulators for standardized training of technical surgical skills and for standardized and objective evaluation, assessment and certification of technical skills. In this environment it could also be possible to tailor critical, expensive and rare procedures.

Advanced simulators for intervention are increasingly used in training of physicians in order to improve patient safety [6,7,8]. Psychomotor skill acquisition is

     L. Hedman et al. / Working Memory and Image Guided Surgical Simulation

among other skills such as perceptual ability a prerequisite for safe image guided surgery. Several studies show correlation between innate visual spatial and surgical performamce in novices. Research in the field of cognition has indicated that Working Memory (WM) seems to be a limited capacity system that temporarily stores and processes information. It has been considered as a measure of information processing capacity that underlies cognitive skills [9,10]. WM can be viewed as a four-component model with a central executive coordinating attention activities and governing responses. Baddeley's three-component model of the working memory contains a central executive and two subsidiary slave systems – the phonological loop and the visuo-spatial sketchpad. Both the visual working memory, rehearsal processed based, and the verbal working memory falls within the phonological loop category – when using digit span tasks.

We hypothesize that the visual working memory test scores will correlate with the simulator performance measure. We also hypothesize that tasks involving a higher degree of central executive functions will be more discriminate in correlation with the performance measure. We have added the verbal working memory task to distinguish and rule out verbal working memory as a major factor for predicting endoscopic simulator performance – and thus define and elucidate the visual working memory phonological loop function for predicting endoscopic simulator performance.

2. Material and Methods

32 medical students participated in the study. None of the subjects had any previous experience from image-guided intervention. The study was approved by the local ethical committe. Performance data (Gastroscopy case 1 module 1) from the GI Mentor II (Simbionix, Cleveland, Ohio USA) (Figure 1) and MIST (MD level easy) (Mentice, Göteborg, Sweden) were compared with WM data from the WAIS test battery [5]. In another group of 13 students, the corresponding simulator data were compared with scores from a computer program (11) for training WM (RoboMemo ,CogMed, Sweden) (Figure 2).

The selected GI Mentor performance score measures the efficiency of screening (ES). The working memory (WM) tasks were taken from the WAIS III test battery [5]: Forward digit span task (FDS), backward digit span task (BDS) and an alphanumerical task (ANT) – with the forward digit span being the least demanding on the central executive function and with the alphanumerical task being the most demanding.

Pearson product moment correlation analysis was performed (level of significance set at $p<0.05$).

3. Results

There were significant Pearson's r correlations found between the visual working memory test scores and the simulator performance score and between the verbal visual working memory test score ANT and the simulator performance score (Table 1). Significant correlations were found between visual working memory scores and the simulator performance scores. Both efficiency of screening, total time, movement economy and total score were positively correlated to WM.

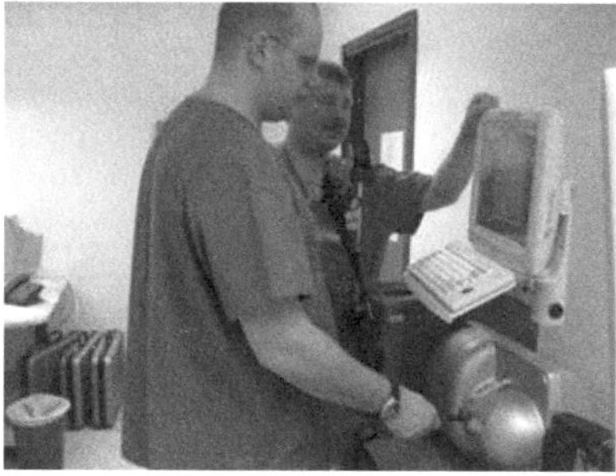

Figure 1. Virtual Gastroscopy on the GI Mentor II (Simbionix, Cleveland, Ohio USA).

Table 1. Pearson´s r correlations between performance score (ES) in the GI Mentor II simulator, Visual Working Memory and Verbal Working Memory Scores.

Visual WM task	Verbal WM task
Fds r=0.607, p=0.031	Fds r=0.306, p=0.166
Bds r=0.570, p=0.043	Bds r=0.324, p=0.152
Ant r=0.617, p=0.029	Ant r=0.639 p=0.013
ES	ES

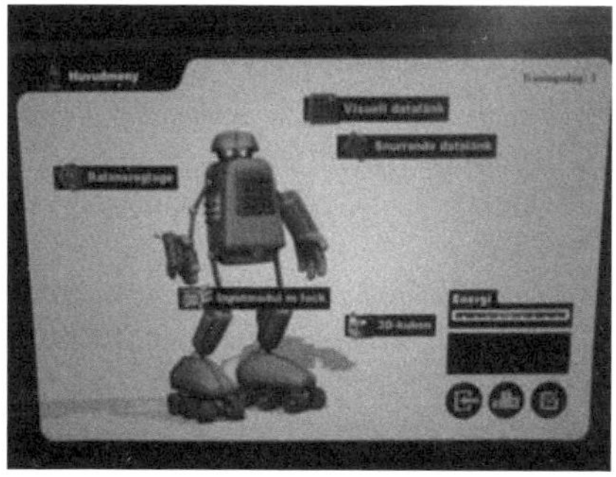

Figure 2. A computer program (Klingberg 2005) for training WM (RoboMemo,CogMed, Sweden).

4. Discussion

Our findings suggest that visual working memory significantly correlates with the simulation performance measure and that WM performance is a good predictor for image guided interventional simulator performance. The verbal working memory is dependent on more advanced central executive functions to discriminate significant differences for the performance tasks while the visual working memory tasks show a more uniform result regardless of central executive effort.

For many practitioners, it may be difficult to meet the professional guidelines for maintenance of competence established because they do not treat enough patients; thus training on a simulator may take the place of performance on patients to help prevent skills decay. The underlying assumption is that individuals who have performed the required number of procedures will be safe practitioners, but this ignores variability in individual learning rates. In fact "learning curves/performance curves" for the performance of medical procedures vary extensively between individuals. Individualized WM training could play a significant role in proficiency gains of surgical skills.

Recent studies presented by Klingberg and collaborators suggest that WM also can be improved by extensive training. It follows that the traditional view of WM capacity as a constant, innate ability had to be modified. In several studies [11] children with ADHD represented one group of subjects with a WM deficit, attributed to an impairment of the frontal lobe. The researchers used a new training paradigm with intensive and adaptive training of WM tasks and evaluated the effect of training with a double blind, placebo controlled design. Intensive and adaptive, computerized WM training gradually increased the amount of information that the subjects could keep in WM. Training has been shown to improve the WM performance of the subjects and result in increased brain activity in the dorsolateral prefrontal and parietal association cortices, indicating plasticity of the neural systems underlying WM [12]. With resource sharing the WM capacity can be stretched to increase cognitive load.

5. Conclusion

Working memory capacity relates to performance in advanced simulators for image-guided intervention, which in turn seems to be dependent on advanced central executive functions. The possibility to specific computerized WM training opens up new possibilities for adjuvant and individualized practice and optimizing of advanced image guided intervention setting high demands on central executive functions. Our findings further emphasise the importance of individualized practice of complex skills required in advanced image guided surgery in state-of-the art training in modern health care. More studies will be needed to confirm the training effects in other populations and to answer additional questions about the mechanisms underlying training-induced improvements of WM. An extension of this study is currently exploring these findings further.

6. Acknowledgments

This study was supported by research grants from Karolinska Institutet, Karolinska University Hospital AB and the European Commission Goal 1: North of Sweden.

References

1. Salas E and Cannon-Bowers J.A. The science of training: A decade of progress. *Annual Rev. Psychol* 2001: *52*, 471–99.
2. Gallagher, A.G,   Ritter, E.M, Champion, H, Higgins, G, Fried, M.P, Moses, G, Smith, D, and Satava, R.M. Virtual Reality Simulation for the Operating Room: Proficiency-Based Training as a Paradigm Shift in Surgical Skills Training. *Annals of Surgery,* 2005; 241(2): 364-372.
3. Malik, R, White, PS, & Macewen, CJ. Using human reliability analysis to detect surgical error in endoscopic DCR surgery. *Clinical Otolalaryngology & Allied Sciences*, 2003; 28: 456-60.
4. Smith E .E. and Jonides J. Working memory in humans: Neuropsychological evidence. *In M. Gazzaniga (Ed.) The cognitive neurosciences,* (1009–1020), 1996, Cambridge, MA: MIT Press.
5. Wechsler D. Wais III. Manual. San Antonio, TX, USA 2003. The Psychological Corporation.
6. Strom P, Kjellin A, Hedman L, Johnson E, Wredmark T, Fellander-Tsai L. Validation and learning in the Procedicus KSA virtual reality surgical simulator. *Surg Endosc* 2003;17(2):227-31.
7. Strom P, Kjellin A, Hedman L, Wredmark T, Fellander-Tsai L. Training in tasks with different visual-spatial components does not improve virtual arthroscopy performance. *Surg Endosc* 2004;18(1):115-20.
8. Felländer-Tsai L, Kjellin A, Wredmark T, et al. Basic Accreditation for Invasive Image-guided Intervention: A Shift of Paradigm in High Technology Education, Embedding Performance Criterion Levels in Advanced Medical Simulators in a Modern Educational Curriculum. *J Inform Technol Healthcare* 2004;3(2):165-73.
9. Baddeley A. Is working memory still working? *European Psychologist* 2002:7,2:85-97.
10. Cabeza R and Nyberg L. Neural bases of learning and memory: functional neuroimaging evidence. *Curr Opin Neurol.* 2000   Aug;13, 4:415-21.
11. Klingberg T, Fernell E, Olesen PJ, Johnsson M, Gustafsson M, Dahlström K, Gillberg CG, Forrsberg H, Westerberg H. Computerized training of working memory in children with ADHD--a randomized,controlled trial. *J Am Acad Child Adolesc Psychiatry.* 2005 Feb;44(2):177-86.
12. Olesen P, Westerberg H, Klingberg T. Increased prefrontal and parietal brain activity after training of working memory. *Nat Neurosci* 2004: 7:75-79.

Medicine Meets Virtual Reality 14
J.D. Westwood et al. (Eds.)
IOS Press, 2006

Virtual Acupuncture Human Based on Chinese Visible Human Dataset

Pheng-Ann Heng[1], Yongming Xie, Xinghe Wang, Yim-Pan Chui, Tien-Tsin Wong
Department of Computer Science and Engineering,
The Chinese University of Hong Kong, Hong Kong

Abstract. In this paper, we present our application of latest information technology in assisting the Chinese acupuncture research. Having integrated the Chinese Visible Human (CVH) data, virtual reality, visualization and imaging techniques, we have constructed a 3-dimensional digital human model for acupuncture. This model integrates the meridian positioning, acupoint positioning, arbitrary cutting-plane visualization, multi-layer dissection, needle puncturing simulation, as well as the common diseases-therapy information. Our work can be widely applied to Chinese acupuncture education, clinical usage and scientific research.

Keywords. Chinese Acupuncture, medical imaging, virtual reality, visualization, force feedback

Introduction

The outstanding therapeutic performance of Chinese Acupuncture has aroused the interest of many medical professionals worldwide. However, the high complexity of the acupuncture system has imposed great difficulties in the learning process for novice acupuncturists. In the light of this, we have developed advanced information technologies for the computer-assisted Chinese acupuncture training and research. By optimally integrating the virtual reality, visualization and imaging techniques, we have constructed a detailed virtual acupuncture digital human model based on the ultra-high resolution Chinese Visible Human dataset (CVH) [1].

1. Methods

Our virtual acupuncture system provides a multi-layer visualization capability, so we have to pre-process the CVH data and segment the original dataset into different parts (such as bone, muscle etc…). Our system can present six different models including the skin, the skeleton, the multi-dissected layers, the twelve skin-region, the flow of meridians, and the atlas of acupuncture points (See Fig 1). In particular, the multi-dissected layers model can be deployed for the haptic training of needle puncturing.

To deliver a high-quality and precise virtual acupuncture system, we have combined both the volume and surface representations in our rendering kernel. In order

---

[1] Corresponding Author: Pheng-Ann Heng, Department of Computer Science and Engineering, the Chinese University of Hong Kong, Hong Kong SAR, China; E-mail: pheng@cse.cuhk.edu.hk

to handle the huge CVH dataset in the rendering process, we have deployed the advanced GPU Shader Language programming techniques in order to generate a photorealistic effect.

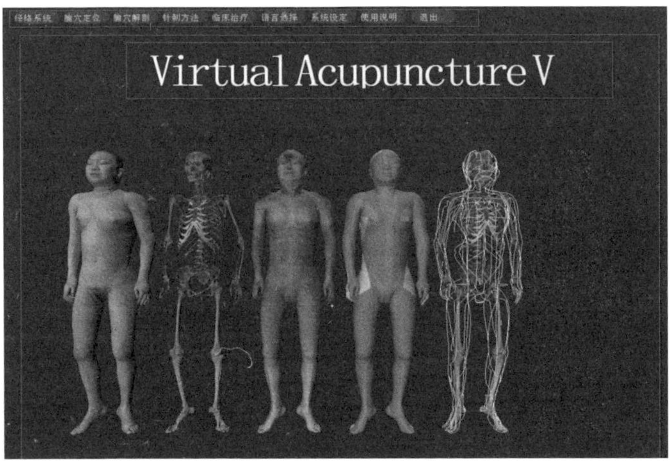

Figure 1. User Interface - the meridian system

2. User Interface

Having deployed the CVH data, advanced virtual reality and visualization technologies, we build a systematic virtual acupuncture human digital model which integrates the meridian system positioning (see Fig. 2), and 3-dimensional acupuncture point positioning. This can help acupuncture novices to acquire positioning concept in a much faster manner. Our system can serve as a very user-friendly acupuncture learning platform.

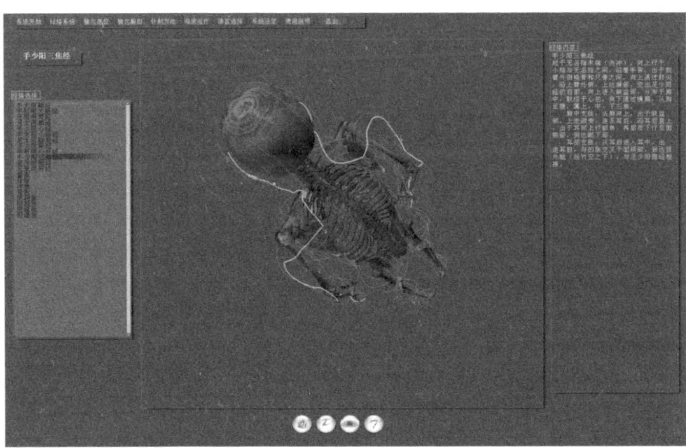

Figure 2. Interactive visualization of the meridian system.

In addition, arbitrary cutting-plane visualization (Fig. 3), multi-layer dissection (see Fig. 4) is also supported. User can interactively zoom in or zoom out in order to view highly detailed dissected information. With an integration of anatomical information, traditional surface location can be related to the underlying dissected structures. In this sense, scientific research on traditional Chinese acupuncture theory can be carried out in depth.

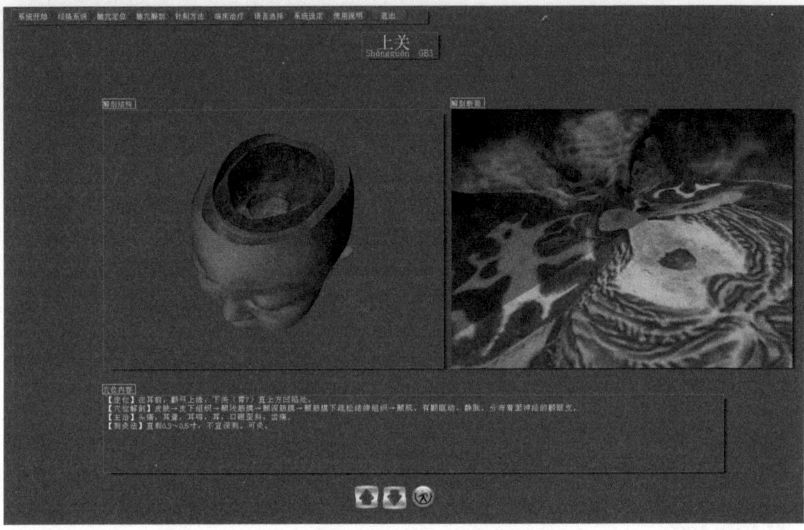

Figure 3. Multi-layer dissection visualization

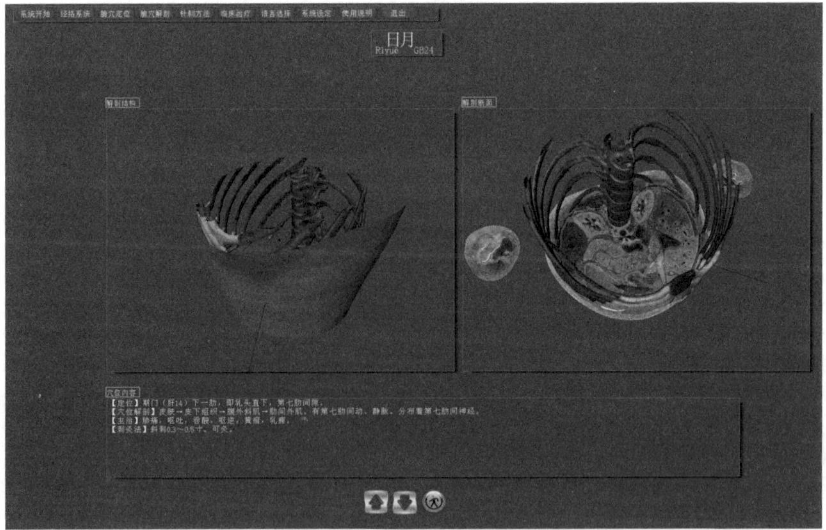

Figure 4. Anatomic view of the acupuncture point, Riyue, which is located at the abdomen.

In daily clinical practice of Chinese acupuncture, needle puncturing is crucial for its therapeutic effectiveness. Our system provides needle puncturing simulation and training (see Fig. 5), as well as the common diseases-therapy information. This training platform can also act as an objective evaluation system of puncturing techniques such as frequency and depth of needling. Such a digital platform can contribute to future Chinese acupuncture research as well.

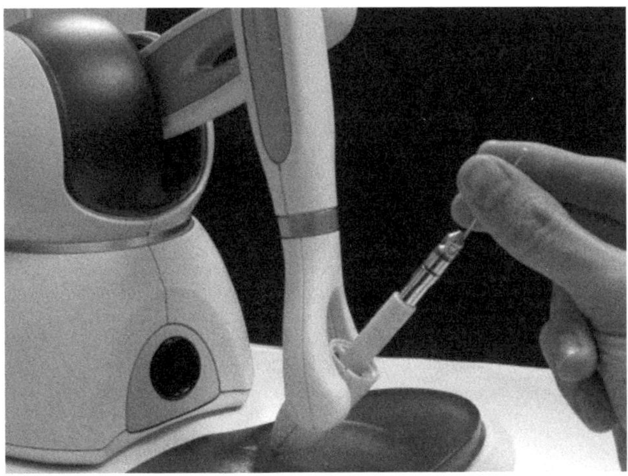

Figure 5. Haptic user interface.

3. Conclusion

In addition to the multi-modality and multi-lingual support, we are developing an open and comprehensive information-enhanced digital platform to support modern research in Chinese medicine. Our work can be widely applied to acupuncture education, clinical applications, as well as biomedical and digital human research.

Acknowledgment

This work described in this paper was supported by a grant from the Research Grants Council of the Hong Kong Special Administrative Region, China (Project No. CUHK4223/04E) and CUHK Shun Hing Institute of Advanced Engineering.

References

[1] S. X. Zhang, P. A. Heng et al., The Chinese Visible Human (CVH) Datasets Incorporate Technical and Imaging Advances on Earlier Digital Humans, Journal of Anatomy, Vol.204, 2004, pp.165-173.

Medicine Meets Virtual Reality 14
J.D. Westwood et al. (Eds.)
IOS Press, 2006

Visualization of a Stationary CPG-Revealing Spinal Wave

A. HIEBERT, E. JONCKHEERE[1], P. LOHSOONTHORN, V. MAHAJAN, S. MUSUVATHY, M. STEFANOVIC
University of Southern California, Los Angeles, CA

Abstract: Central Pattern Generator (CPG) is still an elusive concept that has a visual manifestation as a rhythmic oscillation commanded from the spine, but that also has another manifestation as a train of bursts in the surface electromyographic (sEMG) signals recorded on the para-spinal muscles. This leads to the challenging problem of correlating the visually observed spinal wave with the sEMG signals recorded during the session. This paper develops a mathematical model of the spinal wave phenomenon, which, when driven by the sEMG data, yields such visually observable features as wave nodes.

Keywords: Central Pattern Generator, surface electromyography.

1. Background/Problem:

Network Spinal Analysis (NSA) is a technique through which the practitioner sensitizes two specific points along the spine by applying light pressure: i) the cervical region where the dura is attached to the vertebra [1] and ii) the sacral area where the *filum terminale* attaches to the coccyx. These attachments indeed provide feedback mechanisms [6,7] which, when the areas are sensitized enough by the pressure contacts, create spontaneous oscillations. The early sequence of events is, first, an oscillation localized in the sacral area, then an upward propagation of the oscillation towards the cervical area, and finally a cervical oscillation elicited by the upward propagation phenomenon. During the initial phase, the oscillators are out of synchronization, traveling waves are moving in opposite directions, and the spine is in a non-periodic motion. However, after a few seconds, the sacral and cervical oscillators become synchronized, at which time the spine goes into a stationary wave pattern. Next to the above paradigm of two oscillators at the distal ends of a propagation medium, there are other more elusive wave patterns, like the wave pattern lumped in the sacro-lumbar area [3]. These wave patterns already point towards a CPG hypothesis [4] of these spinal oscillations.

The goals are i) to positively establish the wave phenomenon by correlation analysis of the sEMG signals recorded at various points along the para-spinal muscles and 2) to correlate the mathematically established wave phenomenon with the actual wave pattern as seen from a video clip.

---

[1] Corresponding author, Univ. of South. Calif., 3740 McClintock, Los Angeles, CA 90889-2563; e-mail: jonckhee@usc.edu.

2. Tools and Methods:

The data collection protocol is the same as that of [3]. All research subjects had signed the informed consent form approved by the Institutional Review Board of the University of Southern California (case USC UPIRB #01-01-009).

3. Results:

Let $x_i(t), i = 1,2,3,4$ be the signals recorded at the cervical, thoracic, lumbar, and sacral levels, resp. Let $y_i(t)$ be the D8 subband of the DB3 wavelet decomposition of the signal $x_i(t)$. The purpose of this filtering is to compensate for some analog problems and, more importantly, to capture a single fiber signal [9]. The canonical correlations $\sum_t y_i(t) y_j(t+s)/(\| y_i \| \cdot \| y_j \|)$ exhibit consistent zero crossings for some time shifts s as shown in Fig. 1. This is indicative of a stationary wave pattern [7]. Multimedia video footages integrated with sEMG display will be made available on http://eudoxus.usc.edu/CHAOS/nsa.html and will provide visual confirmation of the standing wave. A bank of Auto Regressive Integrated Moving Average (ARIMA) models were developed and the model best matching the data in a window around the specific time was found and plotted versus the time as shown in Fig. 2. This latter is a rather unique finding, as it shows a clear switching among ARIMA models, hence a bifurcation, occurring in the sacro-lumbar area.

4. Discussion/Conclusion:

The neurosurgical foundation of the sensitization of the cervical area is Breig's theory of dural vertebral attachments [1], which are conjectured to create sensory motor instabilities [7]. The neural pathways are hypothesized to be confined to the spine without higher cerebral function involvement, as demonstrated on a quadriplegic subject who was able to sustain the wave despite a C4-C5 injury [6,7]. This rhythmic motion sustained without external stimuli, with nervous pathways localized in the spine, and in a stationary wave pattern are indicative of a Central Pattern Generator (CPG) [2]. A recent paper [3] showed that patterned locomotor activity (stepping knee movement) of the lower limbs can be induced in paraplegic subjects by applying non-patterned epidural electrical stimulation on the sacro-lumbar area of the spine (in particular, L2). It provides another confirmation of the conjecture that the sacro-lumbar oscillator of the human gait can be elicited (see also [2]). Whether the sacro-lumbar phenomenon shown in Fig. 2 is related to the gait CPG is currently being investigated. Further investigation is underway aiming to understand the neuronal level organization of the human spine CPG oscillators (similar results have been reported on the mice population [8]).

References:

[1] A. Breig, *Adverse Mechanical Tension in the Central Nervous System*, John Wiley, New York, 1987.

[2] V. Dietz and S. J. Harkema, Locomotor activity in spinal cord-injured persons, *Journal of Applied Physiology* **96** (2004), 1954-1960.

[3] M.R. Dimitrijevic, Y. Gerasimenko, M.M.. Pinter, Evidence for a spinal central pattern generator in humans, *Annals of the New York Academy of Sciences* **860** (1998), 360-376.

[4] C. Eliasmith and C. H. Anderson. Rethinking central pattern generators: A general framework. *Neurocomputing.* **32-33(1-4)** (2000), 735-740.

[5] E. A. Jonckheere, P. Lohsoonthorn and V. Mahajan, ChiroSensor---An array of non-invasive sEMG electrodes, *The 13th Annual Medicine Meets Virtual Reality Conference (MMVR 13)*, Long Beach, CA, January 26-29, 2005. (available at http://eudoxus.usc.edu/CHAOS/nsa.html.)

[6] E. A. Jonckheere and P. Lohsoonthorn, Spatio-temporal analysis of an electrophysiological wave phenomenon, *International Symposium on the Mathematical Theory of Network and Systems (MTNS2004)*, Leuven, Belgium, July 5-9, 2004. (available at http://eudoxus.usc.edu/CHAOS/nsa.html.)

[7] E. A. Jonckheere, P. Lohsoonthorn, and V. Mahajan, Sensory motor instability and Central Pattern Generator in spinal oscillations," *Asian Journal on Control, Special Issue on Control Biology--Emerging Field of Life Science that Connects Biology and Control*, submitted, 2005. (available at http://eudoxus.usc.edu/CHAOS/nsa.html.)

[8] K. Kullander, S. Butt, J. M. Lebret, L. Lundfald, C.E. Restrepo, A. Rydstrom, R. Klein, O. Kiehn, Role of EphA4 and EphrinB3 in local neuronal circuits that control walking, *Science* **299** (2003), 1889-1891.

[9] W.M. Sloboda and V.M. Zatsiorsky, Wavelet Analysis of EMG Signals, *Twenty-First Annual Meeting of the American Society of Biomechanics*, Clemson University, South Carolina, September 24-27, 1997.

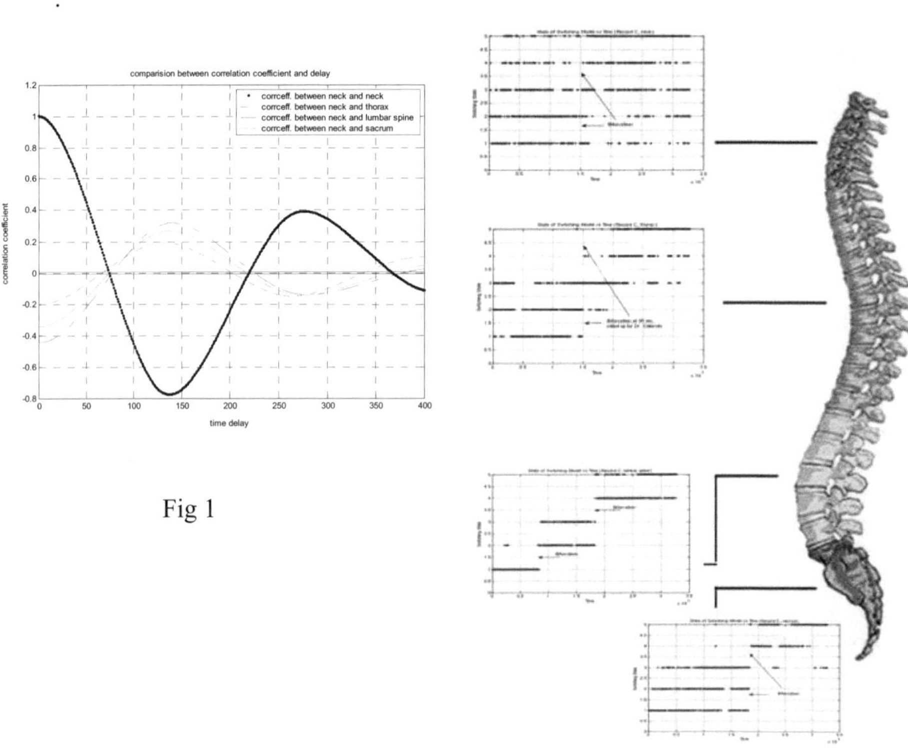

Fig 1

Fig 2

Medicine Meets Virtual Reality 14
J.D. Westwood et al. (Eds.)
IOS Press, 2006

Establishing Navigated Control in Head Surgery

Hofer, M.[a1]; Strauss, G.[a, d]; Koulechov, K.[b]; Strauß, M.[b]; Stopp, S.[b]; Pankau, A.[a]
Korb, W.[a]; Trantakis, Ch.[a, c]; Meixensberger, J.[a, c]; Dietz, A.[a, d]; Lüth, T.[b]

[a] *BMBF-Innovation Center Computer Assisted Surgery ICCAS, University of Leipzig*

[b] *Institute for Micromedicine-MiMed, Technical University of Munich*

[c] *University Hospital, Neurosurgery Department, University of Leipzig*

[d] *University Hospital, ENT Department / Plastic Surgery, University of Leipzig*

Abstract. Navigated Control (NC) describes an additional control for a tracked power driven instrument within a preoperatively segmented work space. In head surgery the authors first implemented NC in functional endoscopic sinus surgery (FESS). Recently the feasibility of NC for surgery on the petrosal bone is evaluated. NC in FESS and in petrosal bone surgery may reduce the risk of co-morbidity and the time effort compared to the conventional surgical interventions.

Keywords. Navigation, Navigated Control, FESS, Mastoid

Background

1. Navigated Control

Surgical instruments can be tracked by optical navigation systems [1]. **Navigated Control** (NC) describes a regular control for a power driven instrument by a surgeon and an **additional** control of the tracked instrument which is only powered within a preoperatively segmented work space. The guiding principle is to integrate the navigation data directly into a power driven instrument. In this way it is possible to fill the missing link between navigation used as a pure orientation device and manual preparation by the surgeon with the NC-Unit [2]. The goal is to reach a level of robustness of navigated control for the surgeon to rely on. Thus, a reduction in

---

[1] Mathias Hofer
Innovation Center Computer Assisted Surgery (ICCAS)
University of Leipzig
Philipp-Rosenthal-Strasse 55
04103 Leipzig, Germany
Tel: +49-341-9712005 Fax: +49-341-9712009
Mathias.Hofer@medizin.uni-leipzig.de

interruption regarding the hand-eye-coordination will be achieved. NC was first described for dental surgery [3] [4].

1.1. FESS-Control

The authors believe NC can reduce the risk of an injury in Functional Endoscopic Sinus Surgery (FESS) wherein the orbital cavity, the frontal scull base and the carotid artery are at risk. Orientation in the paranasal sinuses is very difficult for a surgeon. Usually the intervention site is observed with an endoscope. Atypical anatomy (low scull base, former operation, missing bone tissue) increase complexity and elevate the risk of an iatrogenic injury.

Taking the afore-mentioned risks into account the authors implemented NC in the year 2004 in a first study on a technical demonstrator where the system's feasibility for FESS was shown [2]. Due to unsatisfactory accuracy results, the authors proceeded with a second investigation with technical modifications.

An ethics committee approval for FESS-control was received in August 2005. Thus, the first clinical application of FESS-Control starts in October 2005 at the ENT department of the university clinic of Leipzig.

1.2. NC for Petrosal Bone Surgery

Recently a feasibility study of NC for a mastoidectomy (surgery on the petrosal bone) was conducted. The difficulty in this type of surgery is the identification and, therefore, the protection of risk structures such as the facial nerve, the sigmoid sinus, the inner ear, the organ of equilibrium and the lateral skull base with an immense time effort in order the trace them [5].

The material the surgeon drills on mainly is cortical bone and spongiosa. Reducing the time effort and, particularly, establishing reliable risk structure protections are the two main goals of future clinical application. Evaluation of the quality of the resection process is undertaken by the technical demonstrator.

2. Tools and Method

The system consists of an optical navigation system (LapDoc Accedo) and a shaver, respective a drill (Karl Storz GmbH&Co.KG, Tuttlingen, Germany) (figure 1 and 2).

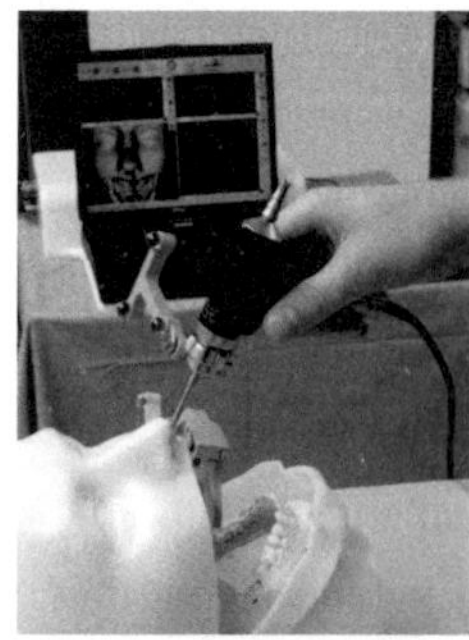

Figure 1. Technical setup for FESS-Control

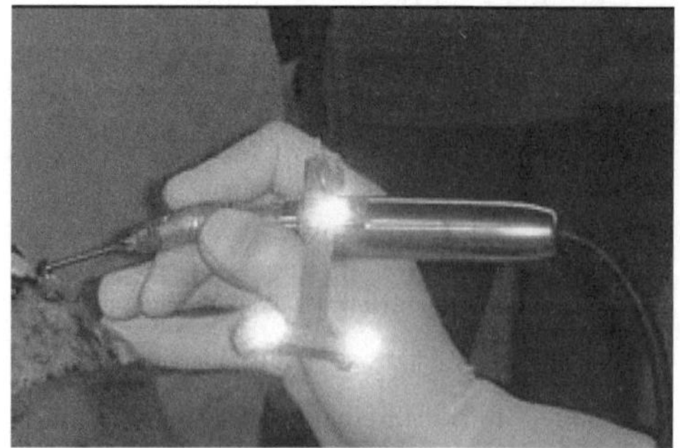

Figure 2. Drill used for mastoidectomy

For standardized and reproducible measurements, a demonstration model is required. A demonstrator consisting of a plastic human head with different receptacles and an upper jaw with teeth for a dental splint with an integrated navigation arc for registration was developed. Different soft tissue models (phenol foam "Steckfix-Dry-Phenolschaum", Smithers-Oasis GmbH u. Co. KG, Grünstadt, Germany) that represent the nasal cavity and rapid prototyping models of the petrosal bone (3di GmbH, Jena, Germany) [6] [7] can be reproducibly connected to the receptacles (figure 3 and 4).

The complete demonstrator with the replaceable models was CT scanned with clinical routine protocols (Volume Zoom plus 4, 120 kV, 90 mAs, 4 slice, collimation 0.5, increment 1, FOV 200x200mm2, Matrix 512x512, Siemens, Erlangen, Germany). Anatomic proportions were respected for the segmentation, the distance and angle between the model and the dental splint.

The demonstrator's position during the investigation was equivalent to a surgical intervention. Navigated-controlled resection of the segmented volume was then undertaken. This was compared with the conventionally navigated and freehand resection. Subsequently, all resected cavities are measured with high precision 3D-coordinates measurement systems (LH-65 (Wenzel GearTec GmbH, Karlsruhe, Germany), Faro-Titanium-Arm (Faro Technologies Inc.)).

For FESS-Control we segmented a volume to an average ethmoid cells' extent within the soft tissue model ($3 \times 2.4 \times 2.4$ cm^3) and defined it as the allowed working space. We investigated the surgical accuracy by touching fiducials in the sinus area of the anatomical models with the shaver tip in 417 measurements. The study also investigated the resection volume. 5 cavities were shaved with FESS-Control (Version 0.4), for each cavity 5 planes were evaluated by measuring them with a 3D-coordinates measurement system. The final cavities were compared to the planned ones. An evaluation of the time factor involved for a simulated surgical operation was undertaken for the navigated-controlled resection of the planned volume compared with the conventionally navigated (also 5 cavities) and freehand resection (5 cavities).

The first step for investigating on NC in mastoidectomies was finding suitable models (figure 4). Those models are petrosal bone models generated with the so-called rapid prototyping method based on original patient data. Initially, the risk structures within the petrosal bone model were enriched with contrast dye in order to guarantee their visibility in the CT scan. For the technical set up so far the focus lies on the facial nerve and the horizontal semicircular duct. In a second model set up, the facial nerve and semicircular duct were left as air filled channels. After the model's CT scan, these can then be determined and used for segmenting the workspace (figure 5) in demarcation to the risk structures. The cavities of the mastoidectomy in the

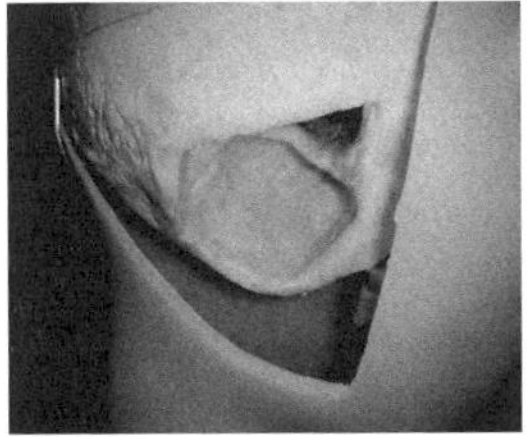

Figure 3: Demonstrator's receptable place (courtesy by MiMed)

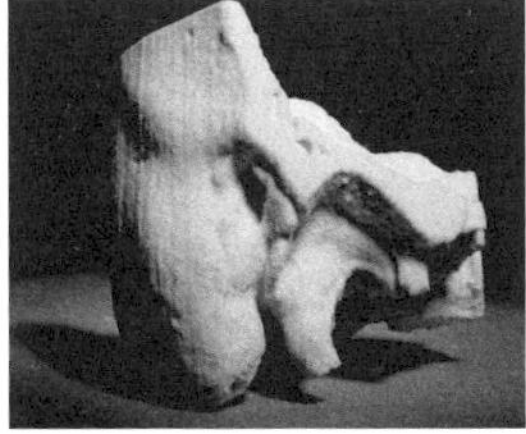

Figure 4: Rapid prototyping modell of the petrosal bone

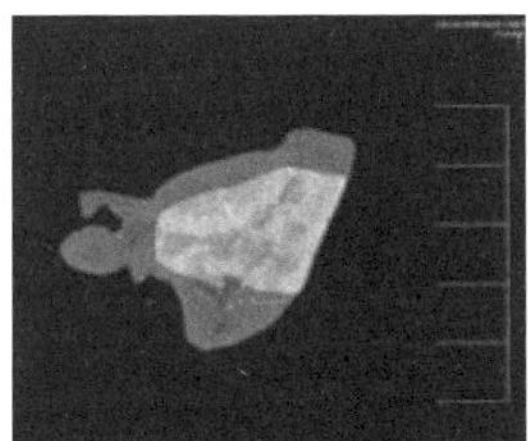

Figure 5: Segmenting the workspace in the CT scan

demonstrator are planned by an experienced surgeon, in order to work on a clinically realistic workspace. Afterwards, the navigated controlled resection is executed by inexperienced test persons for 5 cavities. With NC 5 additional mastoidectomies will be carried out by experienced surgeons. In the end, the experienced surgeon who planned the cavity resects it 5 times without any assistance. All cavities will be measured with the 3D coordinates measurement system.

3. Results

3.1. FESS-Control

For FESS-Control the current demonstrator overcame the deficits of previous works [2] (instability of the shaver blade, yielding foam) and led to better results for the surgical accuracy and the cavity resection. The <u>maximum</u> deviation value of the instrument's tip (surgical accuracy) proved to be 1.93 mm. Values between 0.95mm and 1.78mm for <u>maximum</u> deviation between the planned and the 5 cavities shaved with FESS-Control were ascertained. The lowest deviation was ascertained at the opposite wall (relative to the surgeon). The mean value for exceeding a cavity was 0.4mm for all cavities.

The <u>maximum</u> time for the navigated controlled resection amounted to 10 min. The conventionally navigated cavities consumed a <u>maximum</u> time effort of 20 min, whereas 12 min for freehand resection was the <u>maximum</u> value (table 1)

Table 1. Resection time for FESS surgery in different modalities

Cavity	Shaver	Time [min]
1	FESS-Control	8
2	FESS-Control	8
3	FESS-Control	9
4	FESS-Control	10
5	FESS-Control	10
6	navigated	16
7	navigated	15,5
8	navigated	18
9	navigated	18
10	navigated	20
11	free hand	12
12	free hand	10
13	free hand	10
14	free hand	10
15	Freehand	10

3.2. NC for Petrosal Bone Surgery

The described demonstrator proved to be suitable for the close-to-application tests for surgical accuracy. Adding the contrast dye to the 3D printer's ink led to clotting the printer jet, therefore this method had to be abandoned. With the air space filled in place, a suitable demonstrator could be corroborated. The material of the rapid prototyping model compared to human bone material is not identical, but close; it consists of a type of plaster (calcium sulphate).

4. Conclusion

4.1. FESS-Control

In contrast to the initial study [2], this study focuses on the presently existing clinical applicability of the navigated-controlled shaver in the paranasal sinus surgery.

Surgical accuracy of FESS-Control is satisfactory. A planned cavity can be realized with sufficient accuracy and high comfort. Because a deviation between the test result and the reference value (planned value) never can be equal to zero [8], it is necessary to have a correction factor included in the system. In the demonstrator, the lowest deviation was at the wall opposite the surgeon. This is, in our interpretation, due to the shaver design: The shaver knife is not opened directly at the tip of the instrument (figure 6), thus the 90° angle resection will result in exceeding the cavity only minimally, but the intra-operative condition for the structures at risk is an angle of 0-30° between shaver knife and resection surface.

The results from the time invested in FESS-Control can only mark a trend: It is possible to reduce operating time with the system and demand has been confirmed for the navigated-controlled resection of the planned volume, when compared with the conventionally navigated and freehand resection. Still, the actual intervention is too complex to be compared to the demonstrator setup in this study.

In October 2005, the clinical trial of FESS-Control on patients will provide better evidence for this frequent intervention in our clinic (200 per year). The particular aspects of the principle, such as cognitive relief of the surgeon and human-machine communication, will be investigated during the clinical trial.

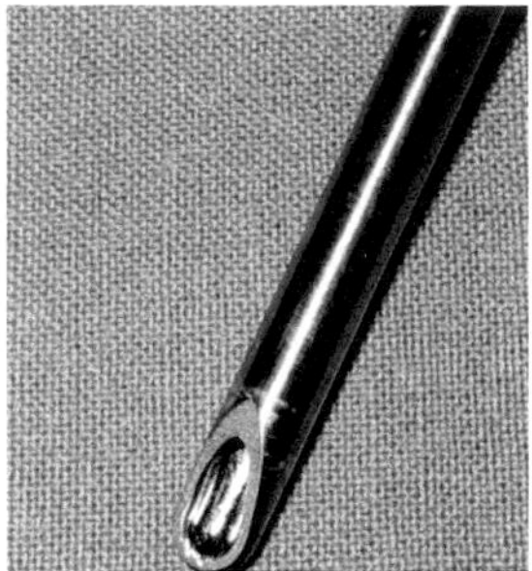

Figure 6. Shaver tip

4.2. NC for Petrosal Bone Surgery

For NC on the petrosal bone, a promising technical model was established in our test lab. With it we can resect closer-to-practice than with the technical model used for FESS-Control. If clinically satisfactory results occur, the authors will propose an ethics committee approval for clinical testing.

From our clinical perspective the maximum deviation for the resection must be below 2mm. The time-consuming mastoidectomy is conducted about 50 times per year in our clinic.

With NC the usability and comfort of a navigation system would be increased. The change in the technical setup for NC in the operating room is minimal, since the fundamental systems are already integrated. The actual surgery remains nearly unchanged in its procedure, both for FESS-Control and for NC in petrosal bone surgery. The instrument is controlled directly by the surgeon, which means that the surgeon can profit from the performance of up-to-date technology in an almost unnoticed manner

Promotion and Sponsors

This treatise is supported by means from the European Fund for Regional Evolution (EFFRE), the German Ministry of Education and Research (BMBF), the Alfried Krupp zu Bohlen und Halbach-Stiftung und the Deutsche Forschungsgemeinschaft (DFG). The Karl Storz GmbH & Co. KG, Tuttlingen, Germany kindly provided the surgical systems and technical support.

References

[1] M. Caversaccio, L. Nolte, R. Hausler,Present state and future perspectives of computer aided surgery in the field of ENT and skull base,Acta Otorhinolaryngol Belg, 56 (2002), 51-9

[2] G. Strauss, K. Koulechov, R. Richter, A. Dietz, J. Meixensberger, C. Trantakis, T. Luth,Navigated Control: Ein neues Konzept fur die Computer-Assistierte-HNO-Chirurgie,Laryngorhinootologie, 84 (2005), 567-76

[3] J. Glagau, O. Schermeier, A. Hein, T. Lüth, R. Kah, D. Hildebrandt, J. Bier 2002. Navigated Control in der Dentalen Implantologie. Leipzig

[4] K. Koulechov, T. Lueth 2004. A new metric for drill location for Navigated Control in navigated dental implantology. Elsevier

[5] A.R. Gunkel, M. Vogele, A. Martin, R.J. Bale, W.F. Thumfart, W. Freysinger,Computer-aided surgery in the petrous bone,Laryngoscope, 109 (1999), 1793-9

[6] K. Schwager, J.M. Gilyoma,Keramisches Arbeitsmodell fur Felsenbeinubungen— eine Alternative zum humanen Felsenbein? Laryngorhinootologie, 82 (2003), 683-6

[7] G. Schneider, A. Muller,Multicenterstudie zum Jenaer Felsenbeinmodell,Laryngorhinootologie, 83 (2004), 363-6

[8] G. Strauss, M. Hofer, W. Korb, C. Trantakis, D. Winkler, O. Burgert, T. Schulz, A. Dietz, J. Meixensberger, K. Koulechov, Genauigkeit und Prazision in der Bewertung von chirurgischen Navigations- und Assistenzsystemen Eine Begriffsbestimmung, HNO, (2005)

Medicine Meets Virtual Reality 14
J.D. Westwood et al. (Eds.)
IOS Press, 2006

Can Augmented Force Feedback Facilitate Virtual Target Acquisition Tasks?

Adrianus J.M. Houtsma [a,1] and Hilde Keuning [b]
[a] *U.S. Army Aeromedical Research Laboratory, Bldg 6901, Ft Rucker, AL 36362, USA*
[b] *Technology Management Dept., Technische Universiteit Eindhoven, The Netherlands*

Abstract. This study investigates facilitation of a manual target acquisition task by the application of appropriate force feedback through the control device (e.g., mouse, joystick, trackball). Typical manual movements with these devices were measured, and models of such movements were used to predict an intended target location from an initial portion of a trace. Preferred shapes and sizes for feedback force functions to be applied were empirically determined by collecting preference ratings and measuring task completion times. The general experimental task that is typical for an office situation, but findings appear generalizable to some medical and surgical situations (e.g. laparoscopy, catheterization) where a certain target has to be reached whose precise location may be known or unknown.

Keywords. Target acquisition, Force Feedback, Augmented Reality

Introduction

The purpose of this study is to investigate to what degree augmented force feedback facilitates a manual target acquisition task in terms of operation efficiency and user satisfaction. The experimental paradigm, moving a cursor from a central position on a flat screen to a suddenly appearing target elsewhere on the screen with a mouse or trackball-like device, may be more typical for an office than for a medical or surgical setting. Some of the control principles involved, however, may easily extrapolate to medical procedures such as laparoscopy or catheterization.

The general strategy of the study is first to investigate how consistent, and therefore, how predictable human hand and arm movements are, given a certain control device. An attempt is then made to predict, on the basis of an initial portion of an observed movement and the known variance of this type of movement, which target the subject has chosen to move to. For the sake of simplicity, alternative targets are always positioned at a constant radius from the starting position, and equidistant to one another. Hence, the difficult and challenging problem of detecting the choice of a target that is hidden behind another target is not addressed in this study.

Once the system knows, within a margin of certainty, where a selected target is located, it will apply a force to the control device that will help the user to reach that target. A first question addressed in the study is whether there is an ideal or preferred profile for such a feedback force. Given that the direction of the force will always be toward the selected target, its instantaneous magnitude can follow many different profiles. Since voluntary movements are generally not constant in velocity or acceleration [1] and muscle forces tend to vary during such movements, it is likely that an externally applied augmented force should have a particular matching profile to be effective and satisfying to the user.

The second question concerns the size or extent of the force field or, equivalently, the moment during the movement where it is turned on. This is by construction a trade-off between the degree of certainty the system will have about the selected target (it will grow with distance traveled), and the force field's effectiveness (the closer the cursor already is to the target, the less useful an augmented force will be).

1. Movement Kinematics

If a cursor is moved by means of a handheld control device (e.g., mouse, trackball, joystick), the actual path traveled greatly depends on the mechanics of the device and the hand/arm physiology of the user. Figure 1 shows results of repeated paths toward eight equidistant targets, obtained from a single user with a mechanical mouse (a), an optical (infra-red) mouse (b), and an optical trackball (c). For all three cases the average paths turn out to be rather straight. One can easily see, however, that the variance increases significantly for control devices (a) through (c), and also that variance depends somewhat on direction of movement. The former may, to some extent, be caused by the greater familiarity that most users have with mouse-like compared with trackball-like devices, which could imply that variance should become more similar with practice. The latter may be partially caused by limited coordination between arm, wrist, and finger movement, since the variance is clearly smallest for the horizontal (x) direction where only arm movement is used. Another potential contributor to variance could be the mechanical behavior of certain control devices that track more easily in the x- and y directions than in oblique directions.

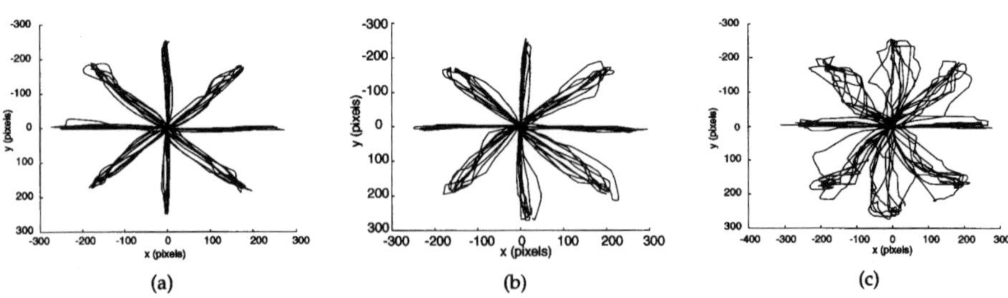

(a)   (b)   (c)

Figure 1. Cursor paths created by a single subject using (a) a mechanical mouse, (b) an optical mouse, and (c) an optical track ball. The eight targets were located in 45-degree angles at a radius of 250 pixels from the starting position at the center.

Trace statistics such as mean curvature and variability are useful for determining how far potential targets can be spaced apart, given a certain control device, to yield sufficiently reliable target location estimates, and also for the development of efficient target estimation algorithms.

2. Force Function Profile

Three general force function profiles, all circular in form and centered on the target, were comparatively investigated: (a) a constant force with a steep rise at the onset, and a steep fall when the target is reached; (b) a constant force with a slow rise, and an abrupt fall once the target is reached; (c) a constant force with an abrupt rise, and a slow fall when the target is approached. They are illustrated in Figure 2 in the form of half cross sections of a hole (top) and forward force of a ball rolling into such a hole (bottom), referred to as Shapes A, B and C.

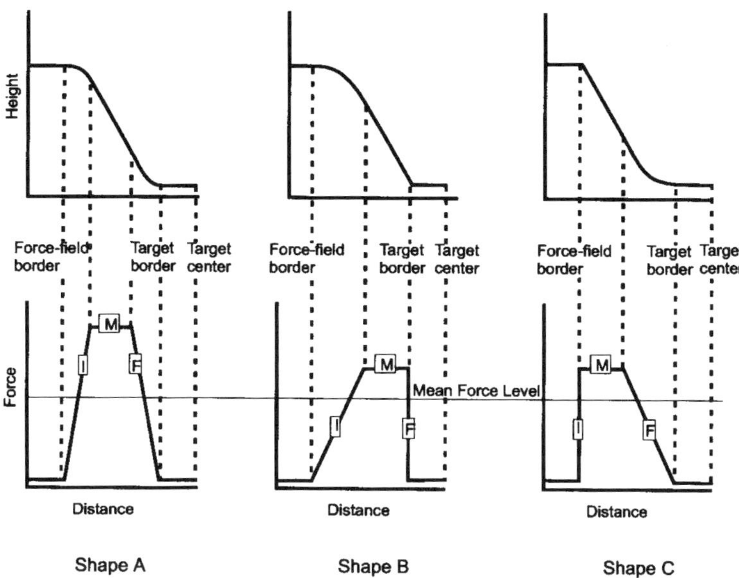

Figure 2. Three gravity-type force field profiles used in the experiment. The mean force level in the bottom graph designates the average force for the initial (I), middle (M) and final (F) phases of the movement.

The control device was an electro-mechanical trackball with force feedback [2]. Twelve participants were asked to move a cursor to one out of eight experimenter-selected targets, positioned as shown in Fig. 1. Participants were divided into two groups, because in an earlier pilot experiment seven had shown a preference for a relatively large mean force level (340 mN) and five had preferred a much smaller mean force level (140 mN). In separate experiments, satisfaction scores (ratings on a 7-point scale) and task completion times were measured for each group of participants, referred to as 'high' and 'low' respectively.

The results are illustrated in Figure 3. One can see that the group preferring the low mean force level does actually not care about the force field profile, as reflected by preference scores, but actually does benefit from profile B as reflected by task completion times. The group that prefers the high mean force level shows a definite satisfaction preference for profile B and also profits from this profile in task completion time [3].

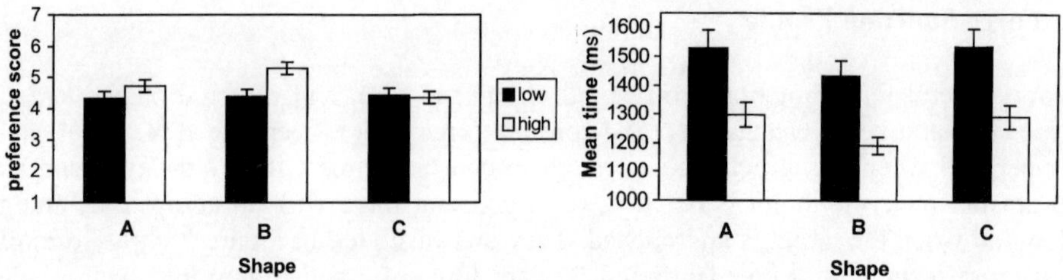

Figure 3. Average satisfaction scores (left) and task completion times (right) for 12 users, divided into two groups according to mean force preference level. Error bars designate data standard deviations.

There is a good intuitive reason for expecting a preference for, and improved performance with a force field profile of shape B. Its gradual start may allow the user to integrate the force that is externally applied to the track ball with the internally applied muscle forces, without having an annoying startling effect. The abrupt drop in force when the target area has been reached appears to have a functional effect, signaling the user to stop pushing. Profile C has neither of these properties, whereas profile A still may cause an initial startling effect. This general finding is likely not to be trackball specific, but may be generalizable to other types of manual operations and control tools.

3. Force Function Extent

If a target location is known in advance, as is often the case in medical applications, it is obvious that a facilitating force that guides the user toward the target should be turned on at the very beginning of the movement and thus extend over the entire work area. If, however, the target location is unknown and must be estimated from the user's initial movement, a force cannot be turned on until the target's location has been estimated with a sufficient amount of certainty. Turning a force on too early (large-size force field) causes frequent estimation errors, with the force pulling toward the wrong target. Turning the force on when a larger portion of the path has been completed yields better estimates of intended target, but leaves less space for the user to benefit from the augmented force.

An experiment was performed with eight closely spaced targets, positioned equidistant from a central starting point along a quarter-arc of a circle [4]. A single target estimate was made by the system after either 30% (large field), 60% (medium) or 80% (small) of the path toward the target had been completed. At this point a force field of profile B, centered on the target and with a mean force level of 340 mN, was turned on. The 'medium' force field approximately corresponds to the point along the path where the ballistic 'distance covering phase' ends and the fine-tuning 'homing in phase' begins ([1,5]. A no-force condition was used as a control.

Twelve participants were asked to move the cursor and click on a lit-up target with self-assigned speed-accuracy tradeoff, and provide a satisfaction rating in relation to the no-force control condition. The results are shown in Figure 4. On the left hand side one can see that the large force field, initiated halfway through the distance covering phase, scores very poorly in satisfaction compared with the no-force control condition (which is 0 on the scale by construction). The results also show that there is little or no change in participants' satisfaction scores in a repeat experiment after a break. The smallest field, initiated after 80% of the path to the target has been completed, scores mildly positive compared with the no-force condition.

On the right hand side, however, one can see that force fields of any size do not clearly improve efficiency. On the contrary, despite the large variance in the data the trend is for task completion time to be shortest without any force feedback, longest with the large force field, and to become shorter when the force field turn-on is delayed till the cursor is closer to the target. The principal reason for this behavior appears to be that with the large force field that is turned on early in the path to a selected target, the system makes too many estimation errors, sending the user to a wrong unintended target

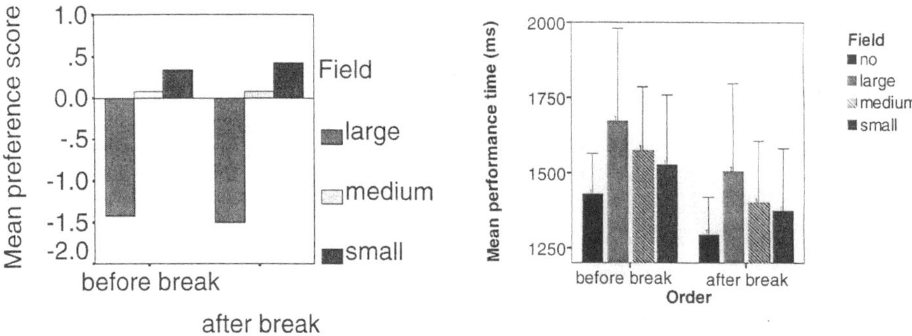

Figure 4. Preference scores (left) and task completion times (right) for 4 different force conditions. Error bars designate data standard deviations.

Further experiments investigated the effects of an iterative target estimation algorithm, where an intended target estimate is made at 30%, and again at 60% and 80% of the total path, and the direction of the applied force is corrected accordingly. This procedure has yielded satisfaction scores well above the 'no force' control condition, but task completion times that are still insignificantly different from no-force control condition [6].

It therefore seems that force feedback is generally effective in making a manual operation task 'feel' more pleasant, as is reflected by user satisfaction scores, but that, at least within the conditions investigated, it does not demonstrably improve task performance.

4. Conclusions

- When an augmented force is applied to aid manual movement of a virtual object to a target location, users prefer a smooth, gradual onset of the augmented force, and appreciate an abrupt offset as a signal that a target has been reached.

- Augmented force feedback generally enhances user satisfaction, but does not appear to add significantly to operation performance and efficiency
- User satisfaction and target acquisition performance are negatively affected by system errors in correctly estimating an intended target's location.

5. References

[1] Woodworth, R. The accuracy of voluntary movement. Psychological Review, 3, No. 13, 1899 (Special Issue).

[2] Engel, F., Goosens, P. & Haakma, R. Improved efficiency through I-and E-feedback: A trackball with contextual force feedback. Int. J. of Hum-Comp Stud., 41, 949–974, 1990.

[3] Keuning, H., Monné, Y, IJsselsteijn, W. & Houtsma, A. The form of augmented force-feedback fields and the efficiency and satisfaction in computer-aided pointing tasks. Human Factors 47, 418–429 2005.

[4] Keuning, H., van Galen, G. & Houtsma, A. The role of size of an augmented force field in computer-aided target acquisition tasks. Int. J. of Human-Comp. Interaction, 18, 219–232, 2005.

[5] VandeVen, J. Getting a grip on workload. PhD Thesis, Radbout University, Nijmegen, 2002.

[6] Keuning, H. Augmented force feedback to facilitate target acquisition in human-computer interaction. PhD thesis, Tech. Univ. Eindhoven, 2003, ISBN 90-386-1698-8.

1 Opinions, interpretations, and conclusions contained in this article are those of the authors and are not necessarily endorsed by the U.S. Army or the Department of Defense

Medicine Meets Virtual Reality 14
J.D. Westwood et al. (Eds.)
IOS Press, 2006

Effectiveness of Haptic Feedback in Open Surgery Simulation and Training Systems

John HU[a][1], Chu-Yin CHANG[a], Neil TARDELLA[a], Janey PRATT[b], James ENGLISH[b]
[a] *Energid Technologies Corporation*
[b] *Massachusetts General Hospital*

Abstract. This paper presents progress in the development of an untethered haptic feedback system for open surgery simulation and training being developed by Energid Technologies. A key innovation in our simulation is an untethered haptic feedback method. In this paper, we describe our approach to developing an effective untethered haptic feedback system, and our current progress. We also present the results of a haptic feedback effectiveness study which explores how haptic rendering accuracy behaves as a function of sampling rate for tool tracking.

Keywords. Open surgery, magnetic haptic feedback, surgery simulation [1,2,3], effectiveness, training, untethered

Introduction

Haptic feedback or touch sensation is important in surgical simulation. This may be more true in open surgery than in laparoscopic since the instruments in open surgery are not tethered to ports as in laparoscopic surgery. Very often haptics is used in open surgery where visualization is not possible. The surgeon depends on haptic feedback when identifying blood vessels under other tissues, differentiating between solid masses or fluid filled structures, gauging the amount of force being applied to an organ or tissue and in blunt and sharp dissection of tissues. Since open surgery depends on haptic feedback in an untethered instrument or directly to the surgeons hand, open surgical simulation would ideally provide the same sensations to the operator.

We have developed a method for accurately tracking surgical tools and generating appropriate haptic feedback as a function of modeled tool tissue interaction. A surgical tool can be tracked by means of a camera [4], magnetic sensors and optical sensors, and haptic force feedback can be created magnetically on the surgical tool with high fidelity [5]. This system will allow trainees to interface with a virtual surgical environment in the most natural and cognitively correct manner, namely with standard, untethered surgical tools.

This paper presents the development of an untethered magnetic haptic feedback system for an open surgery simulation and training system, a cooperative effort for the Army by personnel from Energid, MGH, and the MIT Touch Lab. In the paper, we introduce the magnetic haptic feedback system design and describe an analysis of the effectiveness of haptic feedback (tethered [6] vs. untethered) in open surgery simulation. We also explore system bandwidth requirements and report our findings.

---

[1] Corresponding Author: Principal Robotics Scientist, Energid Technologies Corporation, 124 Mount Auburn Street, Suite 200 North, Cambridge, MA 02138; E-mail: jju@energid.com.

1. Open Surgery Simulation System

Figure 1 shows the top-level framework for the open surgery simulation system. We capture information on tools using the tracker and use that information for visualization and performance assessment. There are seven modules in the system: visual tool tracking [4] (spatial processor & object tracker), tissue deformation [6] and bone dissection, visualization, haptics, audio feedback, metrics (used for real-time quality assessment through a database of "expert" values), and a database of surgery procedures. We are exploring hardware alternatives for the optical sensors, visualization devices, and the haptic feedback system [4,5].

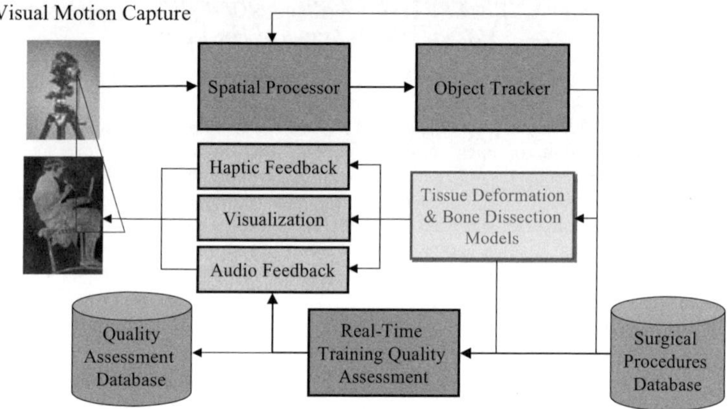

Figure 1: A Framework for the Surgical Trainer of Energid Technologies.

1. Effectiveness of Haptic Feedback

Effective haptic feedback is very important in open surgical simulation. Inaccurate haptic feedback may actually be harmful in the training process. In open surgical simulation, the haptic feedback system should use tools that are identical to those used in the operating room. These tools should not be tethered mechanically to an electronic tracing device or the platform, which would limit the natural tool-trainee interactions. Free-space, full-degree-of-freedom haptic feedback becomes impossible when using tethered devices. In addition, all surgical tools are typically simulated with a single stylus—detracting from the realism. Energid's magnetic haptic system overcomes the shortcomings of tethered devices, and, as such, is a natural choice for open surgery simulation. Figure 2 shows the complexity of open surgery procedures. Limiting the surgeon's hand motion in any way would prove to be unacceptable for the simulator.

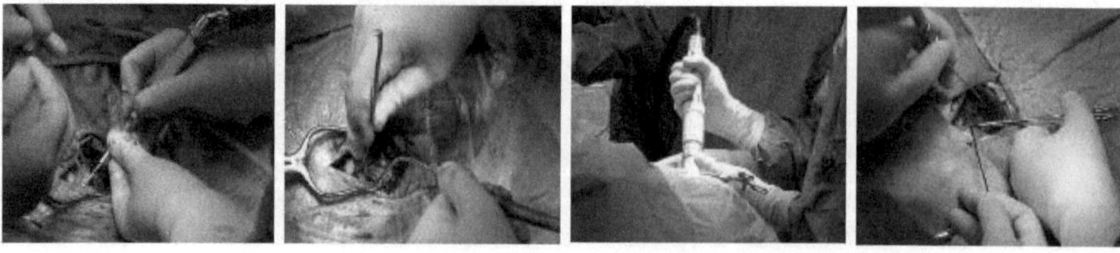

Figure 2: Scenarios of surgical tools applied in open surgeries.

To generate effective haptic feedback for open surgery, the following conditions need to be satisfied: (1) accurate tissue or bone model; (2) high-resolution tool tracking; (3) high-fidelity haptic feedback, and (4) a large unconstrained workspace for haptic rendering.

In past development of surgical simulation and training systems, much work has gone into tissues and bone modeling and high fidelity haptic devices. However, not enough emphasis has been placed on high resolution tool tracking and it's influence on haptic rendering. We have found some tool tracking done in laparoscopic surgical simulation, but open surgery tool tracking requires six degrees of freedom.

Figure 3 below shows how tool orientation affects haptic feedback in open surgery. Two scenarios are shown in this figure: one for tool-organ poking, another for tissue cutting. The reaction force depends on the organ tissue model, tool tip position relative to the organ, and cutting or poking direction. In this case if there is only three dimensional (X, Y, Z) position information available for the tool without tool orientation it is not possible to determine accurate haptic feedback

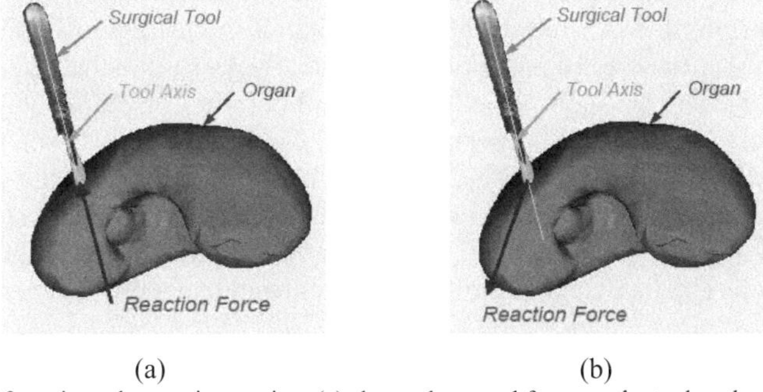

(a)   (b)

Figure 3: Reaction force in tool organ interaction. (a) shows the actual force on the tool as the organ is poked by a scalpel, and (b) shows the reaction force on the scalpel as the tissue is cut.

2. Untethered Haptic Feedback in Open Surgery Simulation

An untethered magnetic haptic feedback system is under development at Energid. It uses our vision-based surgical-tool tracking algorithm to determine the pose of the tool. For haptic feedback, each tool is magnetized with a strong permanent magnet. Force will be applied to the magnet using multiple electromagnets in a movable magnetic actuator. This approach is illustrated in the left part of Figure 4 below.

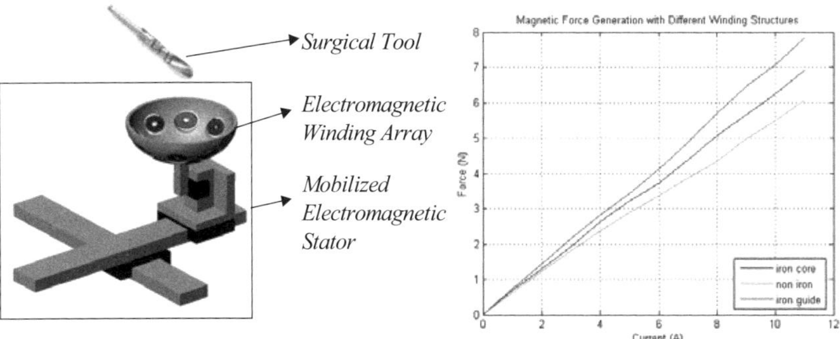

Figure 4: The untethered magnetic haptic feedback system (Left). On the right is the magnetic force data generated from a 1 D magnetic haptic test platform.

Force Feedback Loop: The force-feedback system includes two modules: mobile stage control and magnetic force generation. The desired position signal will be provided by means of a vision-based tool-tracking module in the surgery simulator, and the desired force resulting from tool-tissue interaction will be computed using the tissue models. The desired force vector is realized by adjusting the distribution of the spatial electromagnetic field and the excitation currents in the field winding array.

Sensory Measurement: Sufficient sensory information must be provided for the magnetic haptic control system. The sensory measurement should be accurate and fast. Live video cameras and magnetic sensors, such as Hall sensors are used to capture the surgical tool motion and posture variations. We use cameras to provide spatial information of tool-tissue interaction in a relatively low bandwidth, and the Hall sensors and optical sensors will be considered for high bandwidth in the local control loop of the haptic system.

Actuator Positioning Loop: The mobile stage expands the effective motion range for the magnetic haptic system. The typical motion range for an effective free space magnetic force interaction is limited. It is desirable to control the mobile stage so that the electromagnetic stator can always follow the magnetized tool and the surgery tool tip stays close to the central point of the electromagnetic field, and hence sufficient magnetic interaction force can be created.

Magnetic Force Control: The right figure of Figure 4 shows the force generation with a magnetic haptic device test platform in 1D. A maximum force of 8N was generated in our experiment. Higher force can be produced by means of adjusting the structural parameters in the haptic system and the control current values.

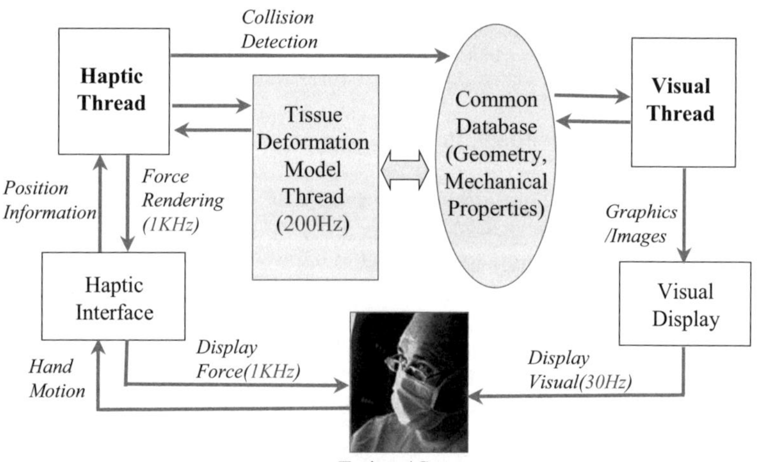

Figure 5: Diagram for haptic rendering.

Haptic Rendering: Figure 5 shows a diagram for our design implementing haptic rendering. There are four modules (haptic interface, tissue deformation model, patient organ information database and visualization) and two processes (haptic rendering and a related visual rendering). In our design, we will use the following bandwidths 1000Hz, 200Hz, and 30Hz for haptic rendering, tissue deformation computation, and visualization. Our minimum requirement for the haptic rendering is chosen as 300Hz preliminarily.

3. Bandwidth Requirement for Effective Haptic Feedback

There have been few systematic studies addressing bandwidth requirements for haptic fidelity. It is widely accepted that a sampling rate between 300Hz-1000Hz should be used for haptic feedback [7]. We were interested in understanding if it was possible to reduce the frequency without significant degradation of haptic rendering fidelity for our application. We specifically set out to understand the relationship between tracking error and sampling rate.

Position data was collected from a Sensible Technology Phantom^{TM} device. The data was generated by moving the stylus in a free hand motion that mimicked what would be expected from a surgeon performing a delicate surgery. A frequency analysis of the dimension containing the highest amplitude data can be seen in upper figures of Figure 6 below. Note that 95% of the energy is within the first 1.5 Hz. Even though the Nyquist sampling theorem suggests that a sampling rate of 3 Hz will capture 95% of the information, this is not necessarily sufficient for accurate estimation of future states.

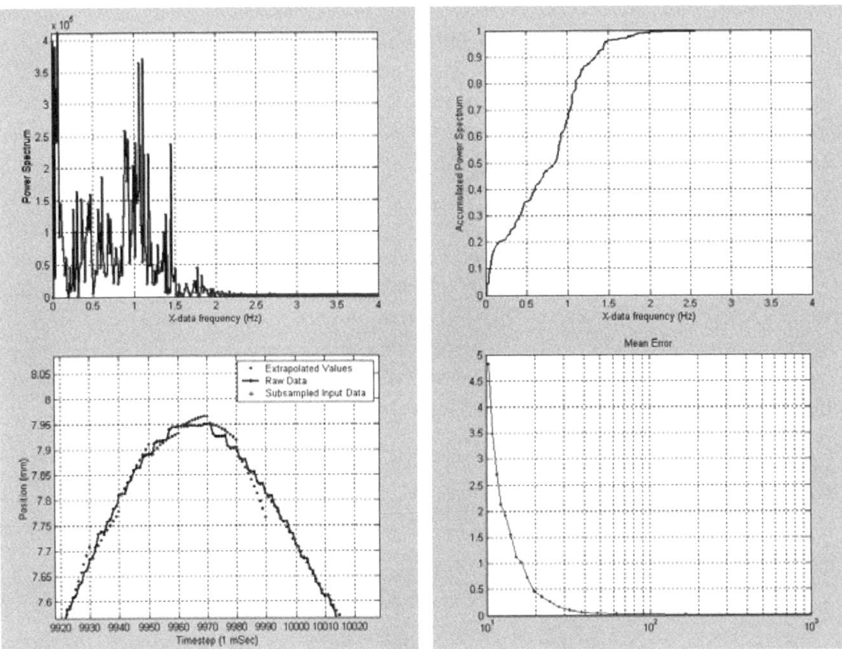

Figure 6: Tracking data bandwidth analysis. Upper left: The power spectrum of the position data. Upper right: The accumulated power, noticeable is 95% of the energy falls below 1.5 Hz. Lower left: a challenging portion of the collected position data with the extrapolated data points shown in between the subsampled data points. Lower right: mean tracking error as a function of sampling rate, which includes both extrapolation error and sensor error.

To assess the error as a function of sampling rate, 1000 Hz data was subsampled at various points and a Kalman filter was applied to the subsampled data. Between subsampled data points, the state was propagated forward assuming a constant acceleration. Figure 6 shows a portion of the position data. The subsampled data points in the lower left figure in Figure 6 are used by the Kalman filter. In the case shown, every tenth point was taken from the 1 KHz data resulting in an effective sampling rate of 100 Hz.   The extrapolated values in between the subsampled data points were computed from the last apriori state estimate returned by the filter. It is noticeable that the estimator does a fairly good job of tracking the data though there are cases of both overshoot and undershoot.

The average error was determined by comparison of the estimated measurement with the colleted data. To understand how the sampling rate impacted the error, trials were run over a span of 10Hz to 1000Hz, where 1000Hz corresponded to no subsampling of the input data. The resulting curve is shown below in lower right figure of Figure 6.

Our data analysis showed that a tool tracking bandwidth (sampling rate) of 300 Hz yields an error bound of less than 0.1mm, which is consistent with our expectations. For a sample rate of 100Hz the tracking error bound is about 0.16mm.

4. Conclusion and Future Work

In this paper, we have introduced our progress on an untethered magnetic haptic feedback system. The effectiveness of haptic feedback for open surgery simulation has been discussed, and a systematic data analysis on our experimental tracking data has been presented. In the future, we will further investigate the effectiveness of the untethered magnetic haptic feedback system for open surgery simulation, and we will quantify its performance through validation studies.

Acknowledgements

The authors gratefully acknowledge collaboration with Dr. Mandayam Srinivasan and Dr. James Biggs at MIT Touch Lab for their support in surgery modeling and haptic feedback. The contribution from Dr. Gill Pratt at Olin College Robotics Center was also highly appreciated. The work described above has been partially supported by the U.S. Army's Telemedicine and Advanced Technology Research Center, through the direction of Mr. Harvey Magee, Dr. Kenneth Curley, and Dr. Gerry Moses.

References

[1]   A. Liu, F. Tendick, K. Cleary, and C. Kaufmann, "A Survey of Surgical Simulation: Applications, Technology, and Education," *Presence,* vol. 12, issue 6, Dec. 2003.

[2]   S. Dawson, M. Ottensmeyer, "The VIRGIL Trauma Training System", *TATRC's 4th Annual Advanced Medical Technology Review*, Newport Beach, CA, Wednesday, January 14, 2004.

[3]   J, Kim, S. De, M. A. Srinivasan, "Computationally Efficient Techniques for Real Time Surgical Simulations with Force Feedback,*" IEEE Proc. 10th Symp. On Haptic Interfaces For Virt. Env. & Teleop. Systems,* 2002.

[4]   J. English, C. Chang, N. Tardella, and J. Hu, "A vision-based surgical tool tracking approach for untethered surgery simulations and training", *MMVR 13*, San Diego, IOS Press, 2005.

[5]   J. Hu, (Energid Technologies), US Patent Pending: Magnetic Haptic Feedback Systems and Methods for Virtual Reality Environments, filed at June 1, 2005.

[6]   H. Kim, D.W. Rattner and M.A. Srinivasan (2003). "The Role of Simulation Fidelity in Laparoscopic Surgical Training." *6th International Medical Image Computing & Computer Assisted Intervention (MICCAI) Conference*, Montreal, Canada, pp. 1-8, 2003.

[7]   G. Picinbono, J. Lombardo, H. Delingette and N. Ayache, "Improving Realism of a Surgery Simulator: Linear Anisotropic Elasticity, Complex Interactions and Force Extrapolation", Project Report, INRIA Sophia Antipolis, France, September, 2000.

Medicine Meets Virtual Reality 14
J.D. Westwood et al. (Eds.)
IOS Press, 2006

A Flexible Infrastructure for Delivering Augmented Reality Enabled Transcranial Magnetic Stimulation

Chris J Hughes [1] and Nigel W John
University of Wales, Bangor

Abstract. Transcranial Magnetic Stimulation (TMS) is the process in which electrical activity in the brain is influenced by a pulsed magnetic field. Common practice is to align an electromagnetic coil with points of interest identified on the surface of the brain, from an MRI scan of the subject. The coil can be tracked using optical sensors, enabling the targeting information to be calculated and displayed on a local workstation. In this paper we explore the hypothesis that using an Augmented Reality (AR) interface for TMS will improve the efficiency of carrying out the procedure. We also aim to provide a flexible infrastructure that if required, can seamlessly deploy processing power from a remote high performance computing resource.

Keywords. Augmented Reality (AR), Transcranial Magnetic Stimulation (TMS), Tracking, Visualization, High performance computing,

1. Introduction

Augmented Reality (AR) applications superimpose computer-generated artifacts onto an existing view of the real world. These artifacts must be correctly orientated with the viewing direction of the user who typically wears a suitable Head Mounted Display (HMD). AR is a technology growing in popularity in medicine, manufacturing, architectural visualization, remote human collaboration, and the military [1,2].

The use of AR in medicine has great potential and many clinical areas are currently being addressed [3], particularly for image guided surgery and similar applications. However, no previous work has been published on applying AR to Transcranial Magnetic Stimulation (TMS), a procedure in which electrical activity in the brain is influenced by a pulsed magnetic field [4]. TMS is extremely important for researchers as it allows them to accurately stimulate different points of the cortex and by recording the responses it is possible to validate the function of different areas of the brain. TMS has also been found to be useful in therapy and has had positive results when attempting to treat severe depression, auditory hallucinations and tinnitus as well as other drug resistant mental illnesses such as epilepsy. Common practice during the TMS procedure is to place an electromagnetic coil on the subject's head so that it is aligned with a region of interest

---

[1]Correspondence to: Chris J Hughes, School of Informatics, University of Wales - Bangor, Dean Street, Bangor, Gwynedd, LL57 1UT. Tel.: (0) +44 1248 382686; E-mail: chughes@informatics.bangor.ac.uk

on the cortex of their brain. The coil and subject's head can be tracked using optical sensors, and targeting information is calculated and displayed on a local workstation. This procedure allows analysis of the visual induced perceptions related to the cortical site stimulated. The Brainsight, frameless image-guided, TMS system (Magstim, UK) used during this project, incorporates a Polaris optical tracking system for tracking.

In this paper we explore the hypothesis that using an AR interface for TMS will improve the efficiency of carrying out the procedure. A complete implementation of this application requires more computational resource than is currently available on a local workstation. We therefore also aim to provide a flexible infrastructure that if required, can seamlessly deploy processing power from a remote high performance computing resource.

2. Implementation

We have written our own software for interfacing with the Brainsight tracking system that allows us to find the quaternion and translation position of each of the tools (coil or patient marker). We then use a custom written OpenGL application to render the subject's brain according to the operator's viewpoint, allowing for a calibration of the markers being tracked and movement of the patient. In order to accurately render the subject's brain from the view point of the operator, we need to know the orientation of both the subject's head and the view point of the operator. The Polaris Optical tracking system is supplied with several tools, which include a head position tracker and a probe that is used for the accurate pinpointing of positions in the trackers view. We use the head position marker to represent the subject and the probe to identify the position of the operators viewpoint through the HMD - see figure 1.

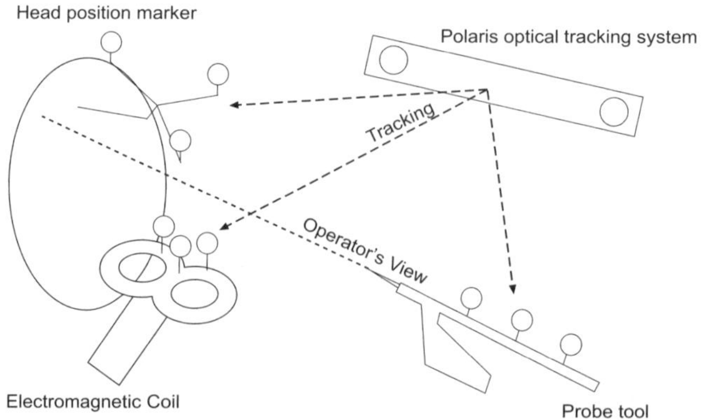

Figure 1. The tools being tracked

The operator's HMD utilizes a USB webcam to capture a video stream from their viewpoint. This video stream is then combined with the graphics rendered with our software to produce the final image that the operator will see during the procedure.

2.1. Polaris Interface

Communication between the operator's laptop and the Tracking System is achieved by sending ASCII text messages from the serial port of the laptop using the RS232 standard as shown in figure 2. All communications are initiated by the laptop which sends a message and will in response receive a reply either containing the requested information or a flag indicating whether or not the last command was successful. A 16-bit Cyclic Redundancy Check (CRC) is used to validate the integrity of each command using the polynomial $x^{16} + x^{15} + x^2 + 1$ [5].

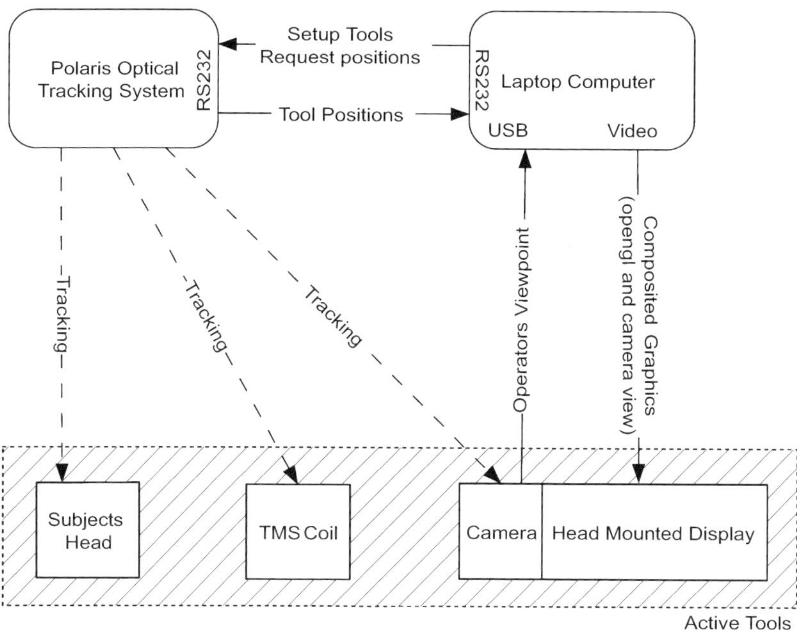

Figure 2. System Diagram showing the flow of data and the tools which are being tracked.

The description of the marker configuration for each tool is specified in a ROM file, which is provided by the manufacturer, and each tool is "plugged" into the tracker by passing the contents of these ROM files in messages. It is then possible to simply query the tracker as to the position of each tool, which it returns as a quaternion and translation pair.

2.2. Drawing the graphics

In order to correctly align the subject's brain the position of each tool is requested from the tracker and returned in quaternion and transformation form. $Q0, Qx, Qy, Qz$ represent the quaternion rotation of the tool and Tx, Ty, Tz represent the translational components of the transformation. To enable the rotation to be used in our OpenGL application, the quaternion representation is converted into a rotation matrix [6]:

$$RotationMatrix = \begin{bmatrix} a & b & c \\ d & e & f \\ g & h & i \end{bmatrix}$$

$$a = (Q0 \times Q0) + (Qx \times Qx) - (Qy \times Qy) - (Qz \times Qz)$$
$$b = 2 \times ((Qx \times Qy) - (Q0 \times Qz))$$
$$c = 2 \times ((Qx \times Qz) + (Q0 \times Qy))$$
$$d = 2 \times ((Qx \times Qy) + (Q0 \times Qz))$$
$$e = (Q0 \times Q0) - (Qx \times Qx) + (Qy \times Qy) - (Qz \times Qz)$$
$$f = 2 \times ((Qy \times Qz) - (Q0 \times Qx))$$
$$g = 2 \times ((Qx \times Qz) - (Q0 \times Qy))$$
$$h = 2 \times ((Qy \times Qz) + (Q0 \times Qx))$$
$$i = (Q0 \times Q0) - (Qx \times Qx) - (Qy \times Qy) + (Qz \times Qz)$$

Using OpenGL we can then simply transform to the position of the subject's head and draw the brain, then transform to the operator's viewpoint using an offset established during calibration to produce the final viewpoint. This view is then composited onto the video stream from the camera and presented back to the operator via the HMD.

3. Utilizing High Performance Computing Resources

The prototype developed is indicating that our initial hypothesis is correct. Although a full validation study is outside the scope of this project, favourable comments about the ease of use of the AR interface have been obtained from the Brainsight operator's in the School of Psychology. As shown in figure 3 the alignment is accurate, and the AR interface for positioning the coil is more natural than having to look between the subject and the results displayed on the workstation monitor (even if the workstation display is also projected onto the wall). However there are some limitations as to how well the software can perform. The laptop computer only has basic graphics capabilities and as such can only render the graphics at a low screen resolution, whilst maintaining real time performance.

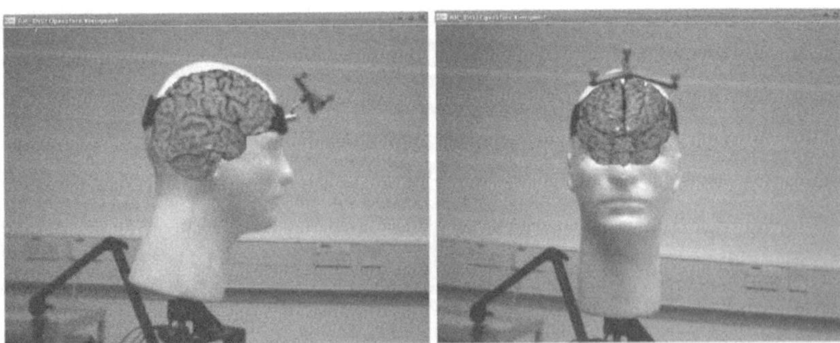

Figure 3. The operator's view showing accurate alignment of the real world and the computer graphics

One solution to this is to utilize high performance graphics resources on a remote server either across a local network or using the computational Grid [7]. This raises many issues such as providing redundancy in mission critical situations, avoiding latency problems, and maintaining real time performance. It is essential that the rendering is produced in real time to ensure that the illusion of AR is not lost and also inaccurate alignment can occur should the operator be working with graphics that are a few seconds late.

The e-Viz project [9] is currently under development and aims to provide a generic flexible infrastructure for remote visualization using the Grid [8]. e-Viz intends to address many of the issues using a combination of intelligent scheduling for new rendering pipelines and the monitoring and optimisation of running pipelines, all based on information held in a knowledge base. Our application has been developed specifically to allow easy integration with the e-Viz framework by implementing our software as an e-Viz client, as shown in figure 4. This means that once we receive the orientation of each tool we can render the desired representation of the subject's brain using any appropriate high performance visualization resources rather than drawing it locally using the often limited graphics resources available on the workstation. The operator, however, is unaware that the system is utilising remote resources.

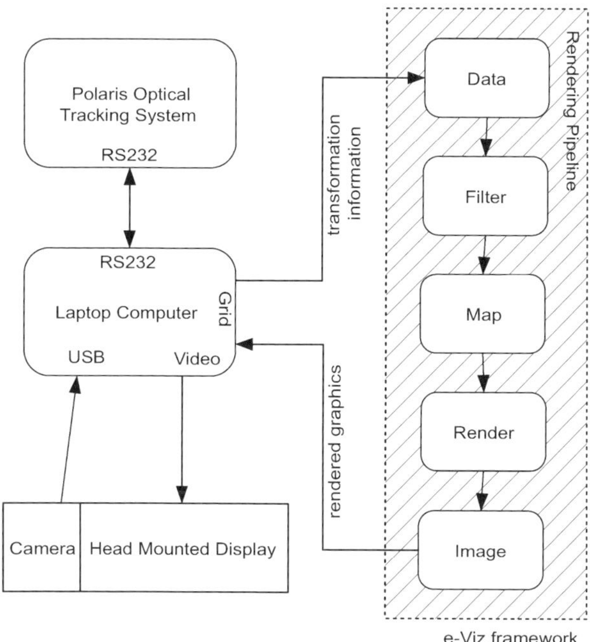

Figure 4. System Diagram extended to use e-Viz.

4. Discussion and Conclusions

We are working to improve the accuracy and quality of the computer generated results, whilst maintaining real time performance. We also need to extend the functionality of the system, for example, to allow the operator to look inside the brain during the targeting process. This involves using volume rendering as well as surface rendering, and using clip planes within the AR environment. A future aim is also to provide a version of the TMS procedure that is not reliant on optical tracking equipment. There has recently been new research into performing tracking by extracting feature points from the camera view generated using simple edge and corner detection ideas [10]. Over a series of frames these feature points can then be used to estimate the pose of an object in view and with basic calibration this can provide an effective tracking mechanism for our AR application. This novel method of tracking has to be integrated directly into the e-Viz framework as a user defined control, and would use the data gathered from the camera directly to steer the viewpoint rendering of the brain rather than just a set of transformations.

All of the above improvements to the system will mean that the processing requirement is too large for the local workstation alone to be able to achieve. Our solution is therefore to integrate our system with the e-Viz framework and so enable access to remote high performance computing resources.

Acknowledgements

We would like to thank Jason Lauder and Bob Rafal from the School of Psychology, University of Wales, Bangor, for allowing us access to their TMS laboratory and for supplying data from past experiments. This research is supported by the EPSRC within the scope of the project: "An Enhanced Environment for Enabling Visual Supercomputing" (GR/S46567/01). Many thanks to the e-Viz team at Manchester, Leeds and Swansea for their help and support.

References

[1] Azuma, R. T., "A survey of augmented reality. Presence: Teleoperators & Virtual Environments"', 1997 6(4): 355-385.

[2] Azuma, R. T., Baillot, Y., Behringer, R., Feiner, S., Julier, S., MacIntyre, B., "Recent Advances in Augmented Reality", IEEE Computer Graphics and Applications 21, 6 (Nov/Dec 2001), 34-47.

[3] Vidal, F. P., Bello, F., Brodlie, K., John, N.W., Gould, D., Phillips, R., Avis, N., "Medical Visualizaton and Virtual Environments", State-of-the-art Report, Eurographics 2004, Grenoble, September 2004.

[4] Paus, T., Jech, .R, Thompson, C. J., Comeau, R., Peters, T., Evans, A.C., "Transcranial magnetic stimulation during positron emission tomography: a new method for studying connectivity of the human cerebral cortex". J Neurosci. May 1 1997; 17(9):3178–3184.

[5] POLARIS Host Protocol Specification, Northern Digital Inc., November 2000

[6] Hart, J. C., Francis, G. K., Kauffman, L. H., "Visualizing Quaternion Rotation", ACM Transactions on Graphics, 1994, 13(3):256–276.

[7] Foster, I., Kesselman, C., "The Grid: Blueprint for a New Computing Infrastructure", Morgan Kaufmann, 1999.

[8] Riding, M., Wood, J., Brodlie, k., Brooke, J., Chen, M., Chisnall, D., Hughes, C., John, N. W., Jones, M. W., Roard, N., "e-Viz: Towards an Integrated Framework for High Performance Visualization", In Proc. UK e-Science All Hands Meeting 2005, Nottingham, 1026-1032.

[9] e-Viz project Web site, http://www.eviz.org/ Last accessed 22 October 2005.

[10] Fua, P., Lepetit, V., "Vision based 3D Tracking and pose Estimation for Mixed Reality", Eurographics 2005 Tutorial, Dublin.

Medicine Meets Virtual Reality 14
J.D. Westwood et al. (Eds.)
IOS Press, 2006

225

Fast Assessment of Acetabular Coverage Using Stereoscopic Volume Rendering

Jiro Inoue [a], Marta Kersten [a], Burton Ma [a], James Stewart [a], John Rudan [b],
Randy E. Ellis [a,b,c]

[a] *School of Computing, Queen's University, Canada*
[b] *Department of Surgery, Queen's University, Canada*
[c] *Corresponding author: ellis@bwh.harvard.edu*

Abstract. Previous CT-based methods of measuring acetabular coverage of the femoral head have either been labor-intensive or have required extensive pre-processing of the data prior to visualization. We propose a method of measuring acetabular coverage using stereoscopic digitally reconstructed radiographs that required very little labor or image preprocessing time. Taking a craniocaudal view of the pelvis, we measured both preoperative and postoperative CTs of 10 patients treated with transtrochanteric periacetabular osteotomy. Measurements were then made in both monocular and stereoscopic rendering modes. Our method is fast, easy, and provides an intuitive means of visualizing an orthopedic parameter that is important in the progression of early hip arthritis.

Keywords. volume rendering, stereo, acetabular coverage, digitally reconstructed radiograph

1. Introduction

Acetabular dysplasia is typically assessed by measuring the amount of acetabular coverage over the femoral head, but current 2D methods (such as center-edge (CE) angle of Wiberg [1]), used to assess acetabular coverage are inaccurate due to the 3D nature of the local anatomy [2,3,4,5]. Attempts at extrapolating 3D coverage from 2D images [4,6] have met with limited success due to the necessity of making assumptions about the joint geometry.

CT based approaches take advantage of the third dimension of the image to provide multidimensional acetabular coverage information. While the increased radiation exposure associated with acquiring a 3D image from CT is a concern, in cases treated by computer-assisted periactabular osteotomy [7,8], a CT scan is taken as a matter of course. The same data can be used to assess the acetabular coverage without additional imaging. Metrics such as the acetabular roof-anteversion angle [9], radially parameterized CE angle curves [2], and the surface area of acetabular overlap over the femoral head [3,5] can be used to characterize acetabular coverage with greater precision than X-ray based methods, but are time-intensive

The long term goal of our research is to develop a fast, accurate method of measuring acetabular coverage area. We hypothesize that, by using craniocaudal-view digitally

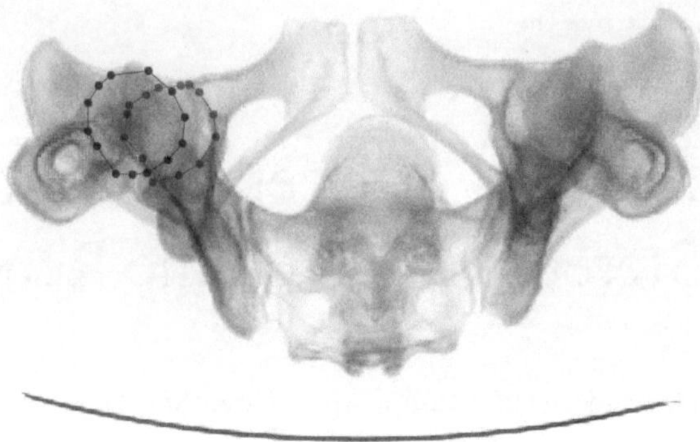

Figure 1. A craniocaudal DRR of the pelvis with outlined acetabulum and femoral head.

reconstructed radiographs (DRRs) and stereoscopic rendering, it will be possible for a physician to quickly and accurately measure acetabular coverage without making many separate measurements.

In this paper, we outline our experiences in using DRRs and stereoscopic rendering to measure the acetabular coverage area. We describe our method of visualizing the hip, and measuring the coverage area. We present some some preliminary results regarding the reliability of our methods.

2. Tools and Methods

DRRs were generated and displayed in real-time on a PC with a 2.8GHz Pentium 4 CPU, 1 GB of RAM, an nVidia Quadro FX1100 video card, and a ViewSonic Professional Series P95f+ CRT monitor. Wireless 3D glasses (eDimensional 3D Vision System) were used for stereoscopic visualization.

Our data consisted of pre-operative and post-operative CTs collected from ten volunteers previously treated with computer-assisted periacetabular osteotomy (20 total data sets). The CTs were taken for the purposes of treatment by image-guided surgery, prior to the conception of our research. The subject of the experiment was a graduate student with experience in processing CT data for computer-assisted orthopaedic surgeries.

The data were aligned in the CT coordinate frame and displayed as DRRs in a craniocaudal view. The subject picked the outlines of the acetabulum and femoral head in both monocular and stereoscopic rendering modes for each of the 20 data sets for a total of 40 tests. The order of the 40 tests was randomized. A DRR, with femoral and acetabular outlines, is shown in Figure 1.

3. Results and Discussions

The average time for outlining the overlapping areas was 39 seconds for the monocular renderings, and 42 seconds for the stereoscopic ones. Because there is no "gold standard" for area-based acetabular coverage assessment, it is difficult to validate our technique. We chose to compare to the method of Mechlenburg *et al.* [5] since the method is both straightforward and eminently reasonable. Two–way independent–sample t–tests showed that stereoscopic DRR based measurements correlated with the method of Mechlenburg($t = -0.825, p = 0.415$), while the monocular DRR based measurements did not($t = -2.148, p = 0.038$).

The positive correlation of the stereoscopic measurements with the method of Mechlenburg *et al.* suggests that there is a benefit to using stereoscopic visualization, and that our method is an accurate method of measuring acetabular coverage. Furthermore, our method is fast, taking under a minute to perform. We hypothesize that in the case of the monoscopic renderings, the visual cues present were insufficient to distinguish the articular surfaces from other artifacts in the image. This is consistent with the observations of Nakamura *et al.* [9] that in a full pelvic view from the top down, occluding features make measurements difficult even with translucency.

Our method is capable of coverage area measurements similar to Klaue *et al.*[3] but with far fewer measurements and on a single image as opposed to approximately 20 images. Compared to Nakamura *et al.*[9], our method requires much less pre-processing of CTs. The method of Mechlenburg *et al.* also measures the same coverage area, but from a sagittal view, and requires visualizing many slices individually.

The next phase of this research will involve refinement of our system to allow streamlined testing and the recruitment of radiologist subjects to validate the accuracy of our method, followed by pilot clinical testing of this method in the context of computer-aided surgery.

References

[1] G. Wiberg. Studies on dysplastic acetabula and congenital subluxation of the hip joint with special reference to the complication of osteoarthritis. *Acta Chir. Scand.*, 83(Suppl. 58), 1939.

[2] D.L. Janzen, S.E. Aippersbach, P.L. Munk, D.F. Sallomi, D. Garbuz, J. Werier, and C.P. Duncan. Three-dimensional CT measurement of adult acetabular dysplasia: technique, preliminary results in normal subjects, and potential applications. *Skeletal Radiol.*, 27:352–358, 1998.

[3] K. Klaue, A. Wallin, and R. Ganz. CT evaluation of coverage and congruency of the hip prior to osteotomy. *Clin. Orthop.*, 232:15–25, 1988.

[4] A. Kojima, T. Nakagawa, and A. Tohkura. Simulation of acetabular coverage of femoral head using aneteroposterior pelvic radiographs. *Arch. Orthop. Trauma Surg.*, 117:330–336, 1998.

[5] I. Mechlenburg, J. Nyengaard, L. Rømer, and K. Søballe. Changes in load-bearing area after Ganz periacetabular osteotomy evaluated by multislice CT scanning and stereology. *Acta Orthop. Scand.*, 75(2):147–153, 2004.

[6] N. Konishi and T. Mieno. Determination of acetabular coverage of the femoral head with use of a single anteroposterior radiograph. *J. Bone Joint Surg. [Am]*, 75-A(9):1318–1333, 1993.

[7] F. Langlotz, M. Stucki, R. Bächler, C. Scheer, R. Ganz, U. Berlemann, and L.-P. Nolte. The first twelve cases of computer assisted periacetabular osteotomy. *Comp. Aid. Surg.*, 2(6):317–326, 1997.

[8] D.J. Mayman, J. Rudan, J. Yach, R. Ellis. The Kingston periacetabular osteotomy utilizing computer enhancement: a new technique *Comp. Aid. Surg.*, 7(3):179–186, 2002.

[9] S. Nakamura, J. Yorikawa, K. Otsuka, K. Takeshita, A. Harasawa, and T. Matsushita. Evaluation of acetabular dysplasia using a top view of the hip on three-dimensional CT. *J. Orthop. Sci.*, 5:533–539, 2000.

Medicine Meets Virtual Reality 14
J.D. Westwood et al. (Eds.)
IOS Press, 2006

Ballistic Injury Simulation Using the Material Point Method

Irina IONESCU[a,b], Jeffrey A. WEISS[a,b], James GUILKEY[c],
Martin COLE[a], Robert M. KIRBY[a,d], Martin BERZINS[a,d1]
[a] Scientific Computing and Imaging Institute
[b] Department of Bioengineering
[c] Department of Mechanical Engineering
[d] School of Computing
University of Utah

Abstract: The Material Point Method is used in the computational simulation of ballistic projectile damage to the heart. A transversely isotropic hyperelastic material model is used to model the myocardium. Computed estimates of tissue damage are used to characterize damaged tissue. The method's potential to estimate the damaged tissue in the complete torso is considered.

Keywords: Material Point Method, soft tissue, failure, hyperelastic constitutive model.

Introduction

Penetrating trauma injuries are frequent, occurring in both civilian situations and in combat. They present a high socio-economic cost and represent a significant source of morbidity [1]. In the case of torso injury, regardless of the injury type and source (e.g., projectile, fragment, blunt trauma, and blast), structural damage to the hard and soft tissues determines subsequent changes in physiology and morbidity. Clinical and ballistics data associated with penetrating injuries are available in the literature [1,2], but the mechanisms of soft tissue failure are still poorly understood.

Modeling the mechanical failure of soft tissue can help calculate the type and extent of spatial damage, providing information necessary to predict physiology and outcome. Torso penetrating injuries are among the most dangerous and lethal, as the heart and lungs are at high risk. The objective of the present research was to use the Material Point Method (MPM) [3] and a previously developed hyperelastic soft tissue failure model [4,5] to study ballistic wounds to the heart. This method is used within a large-scale problem solving environment to model injuries to the heart and a simple torso model.

---

[1] Corresponding author: Martin Berzins, Scientific Computing and Imaging Institute and School of Computing, University of Utah, 50 S. Central Campus Dr. Rm. 3190, Salt Lake City, UT 84112, mb@sci.utah.edu

The conclusion from this work is that the MPM is a flexible computational technique that can robustly model soft tissue failure to the heart and may provide the basic framework for simulating complete torso injuries.

1. Materials and Methods

1.1. Constitutive framework

The majority of soft tissues can be represented as composite materials, comprised of a ground matrix reinforced by one or more fiber families. Such is the case of the myocardium, for which a single fiber family reinforces the ground matrix and dictates local material symmetry [6]. In the present research, a transversely isotropic hyperelastic constitutive model was used to represent the myocardium: an isotropic Mooney-Rivlin model was used for the ground matrix and an elastic model for the fiber family. A two surface strain based failure criteria, developed to incorporate the different failure mechanisms presented by the fibers and matrix substance [5], was used to quantify the damage. The material response was assumed to be the sum of the material responses of the constituents. Local failure of the matrix or fibers was dictated by critical values of the strains (Table 1). In case of failure the material response of fibers or matrix, respectively, was annulled.

Numerical modeling of tissue failure using Finite Elements (FE) would be a computationally expensive and cumbersome task, due to the need to re-mesh the models geometry as it changed due to excessive deformation, failure and/or contact. To this end, the equations of motion were discretized in space using the Material Point Method (MPM) [3,7], a quasi-meshless numerical method, suitable to model large deformations and fragmentations. The MPM algorithm was implemented in the Uintah Computational Framework (UCF) [8], an infrastructure for large scale parallel scientific computing on structured Cartesian grids.   The UCF used domain decomposition and the Message Passing Interface (MPI) [9] to achieve parallelism on distributed memory clusters. Previous experiments have shown that the MPM can scale up to nearly 1000 processors [8].

1.2. Model Geometry

A finite element model of a porcine heart using hexahedral elements (Figure 1a) [10] was used to obtain MPM geometry (Figure 1b). Each element of the volume was discretized further into particles by regular sampling relative to the element shape. Each particle was assigned volume relative to its portion in the sample. The local fiber directions were linearly interpolated within the element at each particle. The ventricle chambers were modeled using the internal surfaces of the of the ventricle walls, which were closed, by adding triangles across the top of the ventricles. Using libraries from Cubit [11], linked into SCIRun [12], the closed surface ventricles were transformed into a tetrahedral volume. Once more, particles were created within the tetrahedral elements using the method described above. These particles represented the blood volume and were assigned elastic (neo-Hookean) properties.

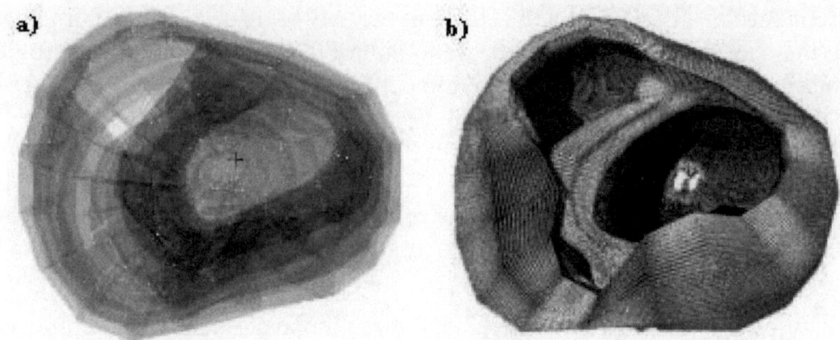

Figure 1. a) FE mesh of the myocardial wall; **b)** the resulting MPM particle distribution (top views).

A projectile measuring 9 mm in diameter and 14 mm in length, with a slanted end (Figure 2) was modeled with neo-hookean elastic material properties and assumed to have an initial velocity of 150 m/s. Simulations were performed for bullet initial velocities in the 'low-speed' range, i.e. less than 1000 ft/s as low speed projectiles have been shown to produce most of their damage by crushing the tissue, and almost no damage due to cavitation [2], as presently the model does not accommodate the capability of modeling cavitation effects, i.e. temporary cavity. Table 1 contains the list of material properties used for the myocardium.

Frictional contact was prescribed at the tissue-fragment interface. A coefficient of friction of 0.08 was considered between the bullet and the soft tissue, based on the value for metal in water [13]. The model consisted of 3×10^6 particles, 2.35×10^6 degrees of freedom, and required 32 1GHz Opteron processors.

Table 1. Material properties.

Myocardium – Transversely Isotropic Material Properties [14]						
C_1	C_2	C_3	C_4	C_5	Bulk modulus	λ^*
2.1 KPa	0	0.14 KPa	22	100 KPa	100 KPa	1.4
Critical fiber strain 40% (based on [6])			Critical ground matrix strain 50% (based on [14])			

Blood			**Projectile** [15]		
μ	Bulk modulus		μ	Bulk modulus	Yield stress
1.0 KPa	1 GPa		5.6 GPa	46 GPa	18 MPa

* stretch at which the collagen fibers straighten

2. Results

The projectile penetrated the myocardial wall and left ventricle. The type of failure and the distribution of failed particles, recorded in the results, assisted in interpretation of the damage sustained by the tissue. The wound profile (Figure 2) showed an approximate circular central area of complete tissue disruption in the bullet path, presenting a diameter increase from entrance to exit.

A layered distribution of failed particles was observed in the adjoining area of 'injured' soft tissue. The strain-based criterion assumed that a particle could undergo matrix failure, fiber failure and/or total failure. The material was reinforced by collagen fibers; therefore only a small ratio of particles experienced fiber or matrix only failure in comparison to the number of totally failed particles. . As the bullet penetrated the slab, it transferred its energy to the surrounding tissue producing damage. The damage dissipated with the distance from the bullet tract, as physically expected. Approximately 6% of the particles were damaged.

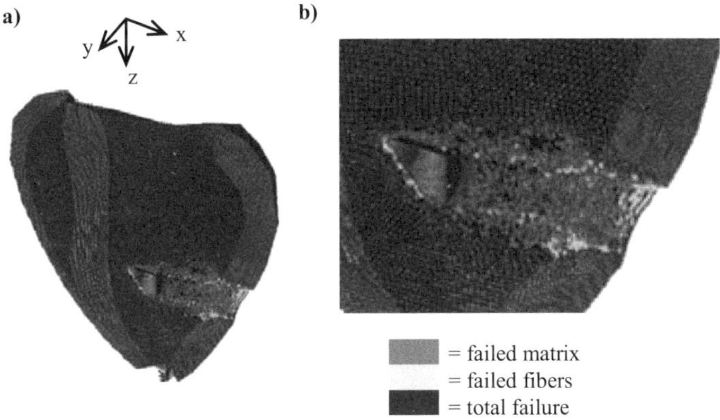

Figure 2. a) Heart wounding scenario; b) Detail of the injured area.

One of the important goals of this study was to predict physiological outcomes of trauma. The failure data recorded in the MPM simulation was exported to the initial FE mesh (Figure 3) and used to compute the response of the electromechanical heart model post-injury. At the wound location, the active mechanics of the myocardial model were disabled and the conduction in the electrophysiologic model features was reduced [10]. The distribution of myofiber strains and depolarization in the area around the wound was analyzed.

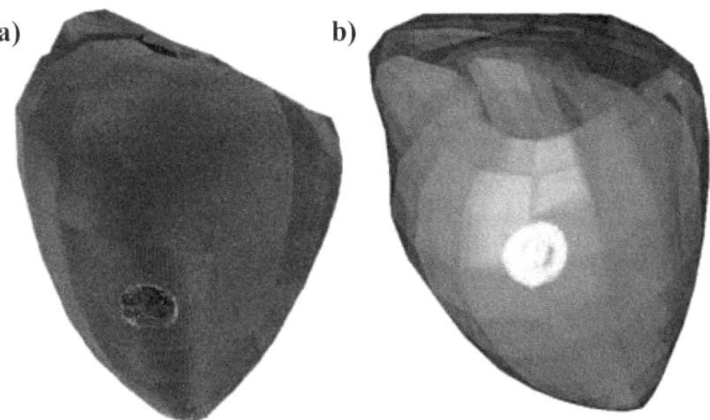

Figure 3. Injury data: a) MPM model; b) read into the FE electromechanical heart model.

A MPM model of the human torso containing detailed anatomical information (fat layer, internal organs, bone structure) (Figure 4) was used to simulate the path of the projectile through the external superficial tissues and into the left ventricle of the heart. The computational model is currently under refinement as different constitutive models with different embedded failure criteria are needed in order to accurately represent damage. Preliminary results have yielded information regarding the ballistic pathway and the resulting volume of damaged tissue for the entire torso (Figure 4).

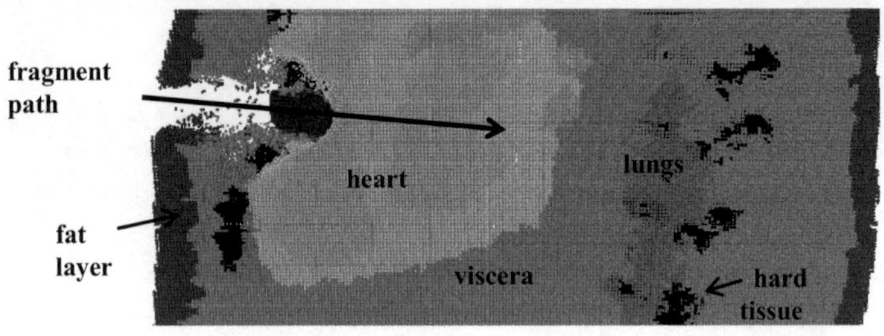

Figure 4. Torso injury scenario.

3. Discussion

A computational heart model, which included accurate anatomical details and realistic collagen fiber directions, was developed to model a ballistic injury scenario. A strain-based formulation was used to describe the failure of the material. This formulation incorporated two modes of failure: tensile failure for the collagen fibers and shear failure of the ground matrix. The results showed a realistic wound tract that reflects the geometry of wound tracts observed in experimental studies on cadaveric and animal tissue.

The main advantages of the present framework are the ease of discretizing complicated geometries, the ability to implement arbitrary constitutive models and to accommodate large computations with excellent parallel scaling. A similar FE model would have been cumbersome and computationally expensive to model using traditional finite element methods as re-meshing would have been necessary for every computational step to account for large changes in the contact surface between the bullet and tissue.

Failure predictions are specific to the criteria chosen. A more comprehensive failure criterion is needed to assess how damage propagates in the surrounding tissue as a result of trauma (e.g., adjacent blood vessels injury, swelling of tissue, etc.). The results obtained herein are both realistic and encouraging. The present framework allows for easy accommodation of alternative constitutive/failure formulations and could be extended to simulating the damage caused by a wide variety of penetrating wounds to the torso and heart.

Acknowledgement

This work was supported by a grant from the DARPA, executed by the U.S. Army Medical Research and Materiel Command/TATRC Cooperative Agreement, Contract # W81XWH-04-2-0012.

References

[1]　Gugala, Z. and Lindsey, R. W., 2003, "Classification of Gunshot Injuries in Civilians", Clin Orthop Relat Res, **1**, pp. 65-81.

[2]　Sellier, K. G. and Kneubuehl, B. P., 1994, *Wound Ballistics - and the Scientific Background.* Elsevier.

[3]　Sulsky, D. and Chen, Z., 1994, "A Particle Method for History Dependent Materials", Comp Meth Appl Mech Eng, **118**, pp. 179-196.

[4]　Ionescu, I., Guilkey, J., Berzins, M., Kirby, R. M., and Weiss, J. A., "Simulation of Soft Tissue Failure with the Material Point Method", presented at Summer Bioengineering Conference, Vail, Colorado, 2005.

[5]　Ionescu, I., Guilkey, J., Berzins, M., Kirby, R. M., and Weiss, J., 2005, "Computational Simulation of Penetrating Trauma in Biological Soft Tissues Using the Material Point Method", Stud Health Technol Inform, **111**, pp. 213-8.

[6]　Humphrey, J. D., 2002, *Cardiovascular Solid Mechanics. Cells, Tissues, and Organs.* Springer-Verlag.

[7]　Chen, Z. and Brannon, R., "An Evaluation of the Material Point Method", Sandia National Laboratories (SAND2002-0482) 2002.

[8]　Parker, S. G., 2002, "A Component-Based Architecture for Parallel Multi-Physics Pde Simulation", International Conference on Computational Science (ICCS2002) Workshop on PDE Software, Lecture Notes in Computer Science, eds. Sloot, P.M.A. et al., Springer Verlag, **2331**, pp. 719-734.

[9]　Gropp, W., et al., 1996, "A High-Performance, Portable Implementation of the Mpi Message Passing Interface Standard", Parallel Computing, **22**, pp. 789-828.

[10]　Usyk, T. and Kerckhoffs, R., 2005, "Three Dimensional Electromechanical Model of Porcine Heart with Penetrating Wound Injury", Stud Health Technol Inform, **111**, pp. 568-73.

[11]　Sandia_National_Laboratories, 2005, "Cubit Geometry and Mesh Generation Toolkit", http://cubit.sandia.gov.

[12]　Parker, S. G., Weinstein, D. M., and Johnson, C. R., 1997, "The Scirun Computational Steering Software System", in *Modern Software Tools in Scientific Computing*, E. Arge, A. M. Bruaset, and H. P. Langtangen, Eds. Birkh\auser Press, Boston, pp. 1-40.

[13]　Engineers Edge, 2000-2005, "Engineering, Manufacturing, Design Database and Tools", http://engineersedge.com.

[14]　Hunter, P. J., McCulloch, A. D., and ter Keurs, H. E., 1998, "Modelling the Mechanical Properties of Cardiac Muscle", Prog Biophys Mol Biol, **69**, pp. 289-331.

[15]　Automation Creations, 2004, "Material Property Data", http://www.matweb.com.

Medicine Meets Virtual Reality 14
J.D. Westwood et al. (Eds.)
IOS Press, 2006

Use of Surgical Videos for Realistic Simulation of Surgical Procedures

[1]Wei JIN, [1]Yi-Je LIM, [2]Tejinder P. SINGH and [1]Suvranu DE
[1]Department of Mechanical, Aerospace, and Nuclear Engineering
Rensselaer Polytechnic Institute, Troy, NY 12180
[2]Department of Surgery
Albany Medical College, Albany, NY 12208

Abstract. One of the major challenges in the development of virtual environments for medical simulations is photorealistic rendering, permitting high fidelity visual effects and user interaction. Digitized videos recorded from the laparoscopic camera are a rich source of information about surgical scenarios. How to fully utilize the information is important for improving the realism of the simulated scenarios. In reality, the camera viewpoint changes frequently and even for the same viewpoint, the scene is dynamic due to rhythmic heartbeat. Hence, the results of classical texture mapping are usually visually unappealing as they fail to capture the pulsatile effect, as well as other global illumination properties of the scene. In this paper we present a hybrid technique to improve the photorealistic rendering of the virtual surgery scenarios by spatio-temporally utilizing videos recorded during actual surgical procedures.

1. Introduction

One of the major challenges in the development of virtual environments for medical simulations is photorealistic rendering, permitting high fidelity visual effects and user interactions. In our previous work [1] we presented a synthetic solution by using various image-based rendering (IBR) methods [2] for realistic rendering of virtual surgery scenes. Digitized videos recorded from the laparoscopic camera are a rich source of information about surgical scenarios. How to fully utilize the information is important for improving the realism of the simulated scenarios.

Classical texture mapping, the method of choice for most realistic simulators developed to date, suffers from some major drawbacks which delimit its use in a fully realistic simulation. In reality, the camera viewpoint changes frequently and even for the same viewpoint, the scene is dynamic due to rhythmic heartbeat. Hence, the results of classical texture mapping are usually visually unappealing as they fail to capture the pulsatile effect, as well as the global illumination properties of the scene: radiosity, glistening and varying amounts of illumination from one part of the scene to the other. In this paper we present a hybrid technique to improve the photorealistic rendering of virtual surgery scenarios by spatio-temporally utilizing videos recorded during actual surgical procedures.

2. Methods and Tools

Each second of the digitized video usually contains 15-30 frames, which is a large amount of information (the "average" video bit rate is around 4 Mbps) [3], and how to utilize this information in IBR is an issue. To simulate the throbbing effect of the heartbeat, we searched and filtered the frames corresponding to relatively stable camera positions where the effect is prominent. These frames were then used dynamically as texture maps.

When the camera angle and position yawed and pitched in the surgical video, we extracted these frames and used them spatially with the IBR techniques: image mosaicing [4] and view dependent texture mapping (VDTM) [5]. Image mosaicing is used to expand the narrow view angle of the camera and VDTM is used to generate glistening effects of the tissue while the view angle changes. Physics-based computations are performed using a meshfree technique [6].

The background of a laparoscopic scene is usually complex due to

1) the presence of various types of organs and soft tissues, veins and the peritoneum,

2) a variety of colors and textures, and

3) dynamic glistening of the mucous membrane under the illumination of the head light attached to the laparoscopic camera.

At the same time, the background is more or less invariant compared to the foreground (except when the laparoscope is panned). It is, therefore, computationally effective not to generate separate 3D geometric models for the objects in the background. While static texture mapping is ineffective, a collection of images, obtained from videos of actual laparoscopic surgeries, with very few geometric primitives may be used to render novel views using the principles of IBR.

2.1. Spatial Utilization of Videos

Image mosaicing and view dependent texture mapping (VDTM) are two IBR technologies we have been using to enhance the realism of virtual surgery scenes. We summarized them as methods that are utilized to spatially augment the scenarios, in contrast to dynamic techniques described in section 2.2.

2.1.1. Generation of Background-specific Texture Using Image Mosaicing

The view-port of the laparoscopic camera is very narrow and each frame of the video captures only a small part of the surgical scene. Image mosaicing, an IBR technique, is well adapted to create the background texture from the segmented video frames. The main steps of image mosaicing include

1) Collecting images.
2) Image registration.
3) Eliminating seams by blending.

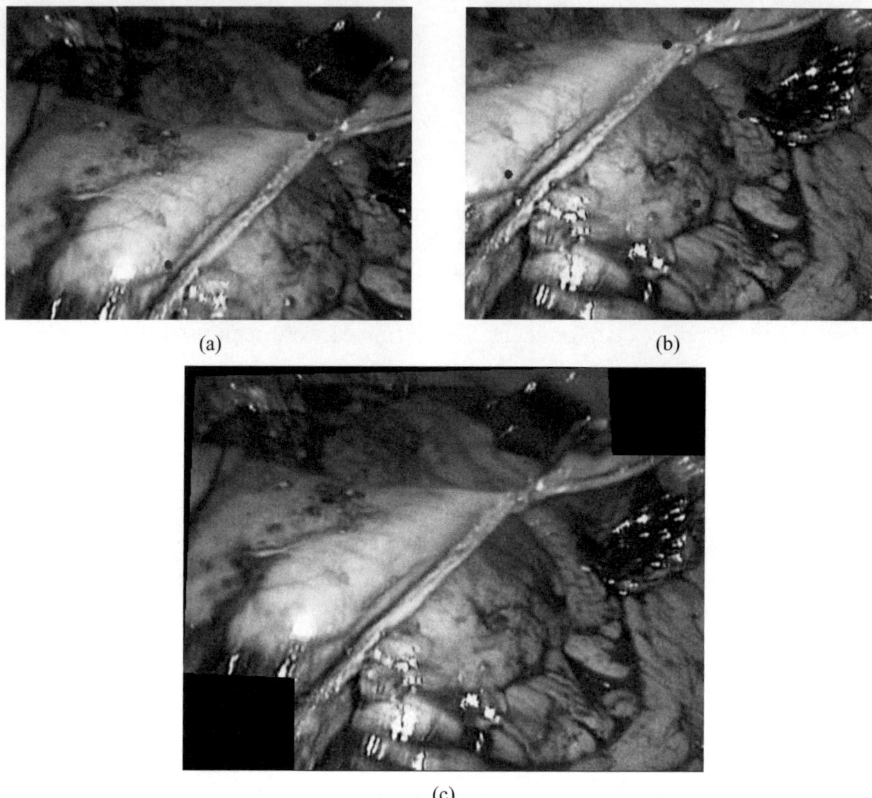

Figure 1. Generating background-specific texture using image mosaicing. (a) and (b) show two images extracted from laparoscopic surgical video. To find a projective transformation, or image registration, we choose four corresponding feature points in the image frames. The composite background images are shown in (c) using two images from (a) and (b).

In contrast to the creation of image mosaicing from indoor/outdoor scenes, the image registration using features of intra-abdominal tissue surfaces is difficult due to the variety of colors and textures of the skin and mucous membrane. Manual registration does not guarantee precision matching of features in two image frames. Error minimization algorithms are therefore necessary. To find a projective transformation, or image registration, we choose four corresponding feature points in the image frames. We minimize the sum of the squared intensity errors

$$E = \sum \left[I'(x_i', y_i') - I(x_i, y_i) \right]^2 \qquad (1)$$

over all corresponding pairs of pixels i in both images $I(x_i, y_i)$ and $I'(x_i', y_i')$ using the Levenberg-Marquardt minimization algorithm [7].

The next step is the elimination of seams by blending of the two images. In order for the edges not to be visible, the intensities of the images are weighted less for pixel locations closer to the edges. If the pixel location is closer to the center of one image but is near the edge of the other, then the pixel whose location is near the center of its image gets a greater weight in the blended image. An example of how the background can be created using image mosaicing is presented in Figure 1. The implementations were done using the image processing toolbox of MATLAB® (Mathworks, Inc.). An example of how the background may be created using image mosaicing is presented in Figure 1.

2.1.2. Generation of Glistening Effects Using VDTM

It is difficult to capture visual effects such as highlights, reflections, and transparency using a single texture-mapped model. We propose to use view dependent texture mapping (VDTM) [5], another IBR method, to generate the glistening background seen in surgical videos.

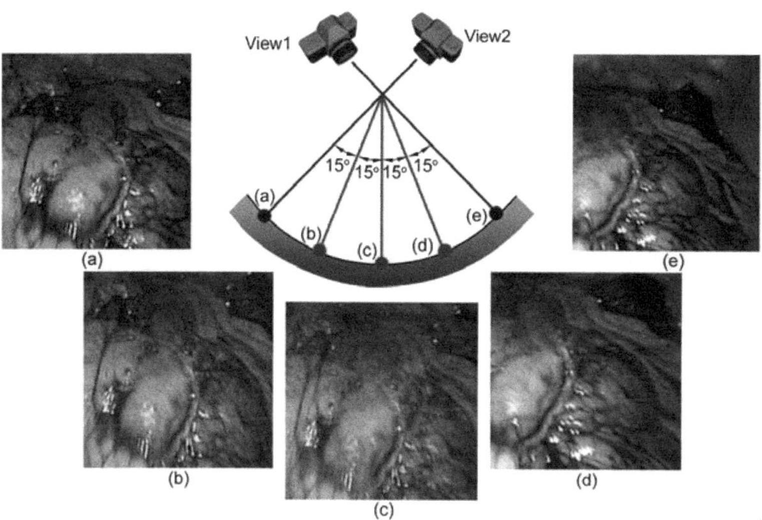

Figure 2. Background rendered using VDTM. Two images, (a) and (e), taken 60° apart are placed on a parabolic background. Intermediate views (b)-(d), 15° apart, are inferred by view interpolation using weights.

Developed for rendering architectural models [5], in the VDTM method, actual video images can be draped on an underlying geometry. In principle this technique is quite close to the texture mapping idea. However, rather than using one single texture map per polygon, several view-dependent images, originally captured from different angles, are smoothly warped and blended (using weights) to provide a new view.

The motivation of using VDTM to provide the glistening effect of the background is from the observation of the surgery scene. Tissues appear to glisten when the relative position of the laparoscopic camera changes. Since the real light source is attached to the camera, the displacement of the light source is identical to the change in viewpoint. Thus we sample a few images with different glistening effects from video sequences of actual surgical procedures, and selectively blend between the original images. As a result, the view-dependent texture mapping approach allows the renderings to be considerably more realistic than static texture-mapping. The rendering of the background in Figure 2 was created in real time using this technique.

2.2. Temporal Utilization of Videos

Due to the rhythmic heartbeat of the patient in surgery, the laparoscopic surgery scene is always dynamic. We extracted a series of continuous frames from the surgical video and texture mapped these images in the same order and generated a loop in the rendering to simulate rhythmic heartbeat (Figure 3).

2.2.1. Extracting a Continuous Sequence of Frames of Surgical Video

First, we went over the lengthy surgical videos to find a suitable clip (2-3 seconds) which included several complete loops of the throbbing scene. Then we cut this clip out using a movie editing software (Windows Movie Maker V2.1), and used an AVI to BMP convert tool (AVI2BMP V1.50) to get a series of images from the clip.

2.2.2. Using SubImage for Video Texture Mapping

Creating a texture may be more computationally expensive than modifying an existing one. In OpenGL Release 1.1, there are new routines to replace all or part of a texture image with new information. We used glTexSubImage2D() to repeatedly replace the texture data with new video images. Also, there are no size restrictions for glTexSubImage2D() that force the height or width to be a power of two. This is helpful for processing video images [8].

3. Results

In our preliminary results, we use a human kidney model, obtained from the segmented Visible Human data set [9] as the foreground. Using actual surgical videos, we have improved the virtual surgery scene with expected realistic features (Figure 3). The model is fully interactive through a haptic interface device (Phantom).

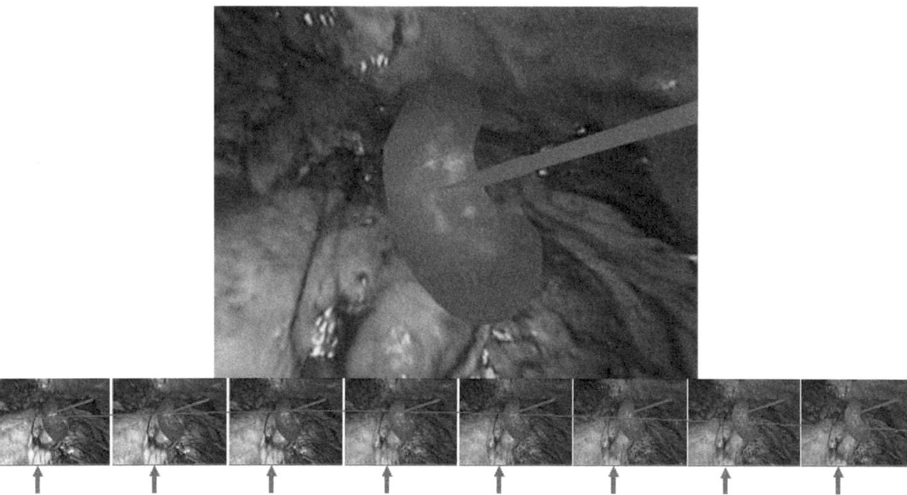

Figure 3. Sequence of snapshots showing the dynamic throbbing effect

4. Discussion

In this work we have developed a methodology for generating realistic virtual surgery scenes with glistening effect using a combination of various image-based rendering methods, including image mosaicing and VDTM coupled with a dynamic technique to represent dynamic throbbing of organs due to heartbeat. The visually realistic models are coupled to a physically-based computational scheme. This computational scheme has been presented in [6]. Realistic examples are presented to showcase the results.

Acknowledgements: This work was supported by grant R21 EB003547-01 from NIH/NIBIB.

References

[1]   W. Jin, Y.-J. Lim, X. G. Xu, T. P. Singh, S. De, "Improving the Visual Realism of Virtual Surgery", Proceeding of MMVR Conference, pp.227-233, 2005.
[2]   H.-Y. Shum, S. B. Kang, "A review of image-based rendering techniques", IEEE/SPIE Visual Communications and Image Processing, pp.2-13, 2000.
[3]   J. Taylor, "DVD Demystified, 2nd edition", McGraw-Hill Professional, 2000
[4]   R. Szeliski, "Image mosaicing for tele-reality applications", Proceeding of IEEE Workshop on Applications of Computer Vision, pp.44-53, 1994.
[5]   P. E. Debevec, Y. Yu, G. D. Borshukov, "Efficient view-dependent image-based rendering with projective texture-mapping", Eurographics Rendering Workshop, pp.105-116, 1998.
[6]   S. De, J. Kim, and M. A. Srinivasan, "A meshless numerical technique for physically based real time medical simulations", Proceeding of MMVR Conference, pp.113-118, 2001.
[7]   W.H. Press, S.A. Teukolsky, W.T. Vetterling, B.P. Flannery, "Numerical Recipes in C: The Art of Scientific Computing", 2nd edition, Cambridge Univ. Press, 1992.
[8]   OpenGL Architechture Review Board, D. Shreiner, J. Neider, M. Woo, T. Davis, "OpenGL programming guide: the official guide to learning OpenGL, Version 1.4", Addison-Wesley, 2003.
[9]   M. J. Ackerman, "The Visible Human project", Proceeding of MMVR Conference, pp.5-7, 1994.

Medicine Meets Virtual Reality 14
J.D. Westwood et al. (Eds.)
IOS Press, 2006

Pulse!! - A Virtual Learning Space Project

Claudia L. JOHNSTON, PhD[a], Doug WHATLEY[b]
[a]*Associate Vice President for Special Projects, Texas A&M University-Corpus Christi*
[b]*CEO – BreakAway, LTD*

Abstract. Game-based technology structured within an epistemic framework is revolutionizing learning. Intersecting military simulation technologies with modern pedagogical education practices, *Pulse!!* offers an epistemic framework for optimizing cognitive and psychomotor skills in clinical practices. Its intelligent authoring system is an integrated, fully immersive, interactive virtual learning simulation for civilian and military health care practitioners, providing opportunities to make mistakes and repeat actions.

Keywords. Virtual learning simulation, objective assessment, intelligent authoring system, high-fidelity complex modeling, internet-based simulation

Introduction

The health care delivery system, both military and civilian, is impacted by stressors threatening the system's viability. The Institute of Medicine reports that errors are responsible for 44,000 to 98,000 deaths annually [1] and the Agency for Healthcare Research and Quality estimates that related costs are between $17 billion and $29 billion annually [2]. Compounding the issue, patient length of stay is dramatically shortened – giving students significantly fewer opportunities for clinical expansion. Contributing to the safety issue is the growing shortage of nurses, as cited by the U. S. Department of Health and Human Services. The Department warns that, despite increases in nursing programs, projected demand for nurses substantially exceeds projected supply [3]. Capacity in nursing education programs is at a maximum, faculty are retiring in unprecedented numbers, care patterns are changing, and according to a 2005 report released by the National League for Nursing, 125,000 *qualified* nursing students, at all levels, were denied admission in 2004 [4]. To date, neither the military nor the civilian health care establishments have the education or training environment that provides the level of experiential training and education to prepare caregivers for responding to catastrophic health insults from terrorism and bioterrorism.

Textbooks and lectures, even when computer assisted, focus primarily on the creation of didactic content rather than real-time clinical experiences needed for the health professions' education and mission-critical training. While there are efficient authoring methodologies for network operations, those systems do not produce high-fidelity, persistent, first-person, educational content mirroring the real world. First-responders, military and civilian, require sharply coordinated skill sets that enable swift and precise responses to rapid change. Otolaryngologist-in-chief at Boston, Massachusetts's Children Hospital, Dr. Gerald B. Healy, relays the need for new training technologies for increasing patient safety. He states that medical simulation may reduce surgical error by screening potential surgeons for demonstrable aptitude, providing initial surgical training, promoting on-going education through a reproducible process, enabling periodic assessment of acquired surgical skills, and maintaining proficiency through rehearsal of complex, patient-specific procedures [5]. *Pulse!!* – a learning platform within the *Virtual Leaning Space Project*, is a complex, high-fidelity virtual clinical lab currently being designed to meet these cognitive, psychomotor, and real-time clinical learning needs.

Virtual Clinical Learning Methodologies

To date, despite the increasing sophistication traditionally structured e-learning environments have created for didactic instruction, nothing has yet been built that links and also bridges the asynchronous educational processes to immersive, first-person, real-time path planning experiences. According to Shaffer, Squire, Halverson, and Gee, game play, when situated within an epistemic framework, is a powerful learning tool, connecting with modern education pedagogies' recognized need for students to connect knowledge in social and experiential ways [6]. *Pulse!!* situates learning within a virtual epistemic framework, connecting learning to experience and replacing rote memorization of facts and information. It presents facts, but inter-contextually adds values, skills, and practices. *Pulse!!* motivates learners by actual "doing," and by increased performance incentive through game-level advancement. To succeed and "win" a medical scenario, the student must learn to think and act as an expert medical professional. Not only does the program analyze student performance, it also simulates numerous clinical emergencies. Achieving optimal outcomes in discrete tasks will also hone communication, organization, discipline, and empathy competencies. To deepen this learning immersion, *Pulse!!* realistically details patient and equipment visuals and sounds.

By associating a virtual medical clinic to an extensive patient simulation modeling system, *Pulse!!* creates a virtual clinical learning lab. It has an array of interactive tools for learning immersion and upgrade capability for reflecting new knowledge. This project constructs a life-like virtual world, using game-based technologies and development techniques, which serve as the organizing framework of a platform for post/co-didactic learning and training. First-responders, students, and practitioners in the healthcare disciplines will be able to acquire and practice critical experiential skills. This internet-based simulation platform is being built as a dynamic, multi-user, immersive environment with pedagogical linkages for situated learning.

In a life-like, interactive space, students master particular skills, performances, and procedures by taking on the role of either physician or nurse within a virtual medical health care delivery system. Clinical simulations may include complex combat injuries stemming from bomb blasts, gunshots, shrapnel, RPG, mortar burns, and MVA injuries.

Mark W. Scerbo, in analyzing the future of medical training, emphasizes the importance of virtual simulators. He points to a research report by Seymour et al., published in 2002, showing that medical residents trained on simulators needed 30%

less time to perform a genuine procedure than those trained according to the traditional method [7].

Pulse!! promotes critical skill set training anytime, anywhere, facilitating accelerated diagnosis and treatment of wounds, diseases, and other conditions as a result of rapidly changing weapons and agents intended to create harm. The intelligent authoring system will rapidly provide military health care practitioners with training scenarios for basic competency and critical military readiness skills for almost any battlefield environment. The project's iterative, play-based design employs or modifies cutting edge game-based technologies with continual prototyping and developing through performance feedback and on-line guidance. In a personal interview, Mark W. Bowyer indicated that simulation and virtual reality offers the opportunity to "see one, *practice many*, do one, teach one." [8] Training of military and civilian medical providers in the *Pulse!!* virtual learning platform will reduce the intensity of injuries, save lives and limbs, and provide a substantial reduction in errors and other risk inducing events.

Conclusion

The future landscape of education is rapidly evolving through the intersection of flight and military simulations with game-based technologies, for training and learning. *Pulse!!* intersects these sophisticated technologies with traditional medical education into an epistemic framework, optimizing cognitive and psychomotor skills. Game-based modeling will enable the student and practitioner to achieve never-before-possible proficiency and expertise in relevant skill sets. The programming interface is a self-contained component driving a complex, high-fidelity, first-person perspective, dynamically responding to real-world contextual inputs. *Pulse!!* creates an alternative pathway in a virtual clinical world for experiential learning independent from time and distance.

The virtual clinical learning lab - *Pulse!!* is a learning platform in the beginning stages of production. Funding for the project is provided to Texas A&M University–Corpus Christi, Office of Special Projects, through the Office of Naval Research.

References

[1]	Institute of Medicine. *To err is human: Building a safer health system.* Washington: National Academy Press; 1999 Nov.

[2]	Agency for Healthcare Research and Quality. *Injuries in hospitals pose a significant threat to patients and a substantial increase in health care costs.* Press Release: 2003 Oct 7.

[3]	U.S. Department of Health and Human Services. *National Center for Health Workforce Analysis*: 2002 July. < http://bhpr.hrsa.gov/healthworkforce/reports/rnproject/default.htm> Accessed 2005 Oct 24.

[4]	National League for Nursing. NLN Update Index 2005 May; VIII (10).

[5]	Healy, G. B. MD, FACS. *The college should be instrumental in adapting simulators to education. Bulletin of the American College of Surgeons* 2001 Nov; 87 (11): 10-11.

[6]	Shaffer, D. W., Squire K. R., Halverson, R., and Gee, J. P. 2004. *Video Games and the Future of Learning.* <http://www.academiccolab.org/gappspaer1.pdf> Accessed 2005 Oct 24.

[7]	Scerbo, M. W. *The Future of Medical Training and the Need for Human Factors.* Paper presented at the 49th Annual Meeting of the Human Factors and Ergonomics Society, FL: 2005 Sept.

[8]	Bowyer, M. W. Simulation and virtual reality training. 2004.

Medicine Meets Virtual Reality 14
J.D. Westwood et al. (Eds.)
IOS Press, 2006

243

Real-Time Augmented Feedback Benefits Robotic Laparoscopic Training

Timothy N. JUDKINS[a], Dmitry OLEYNIKOV MD[b], and Nick STERGIOU[a,1]
[a]HPER Biomechanics Lab, University of Nebraska at Omaha, Omaha, NE
[b]Dept of Surgery, University of Nebraska Medical Center, Omaha, NE

Abstract. Robotic laparoscopic surgery has revolutionized minimally invasive surgery for treatment of abdominal pathologies. However, current training techniques rely on subjective evaluation. There is a lack of research on the type of tasks that should be used for training. Robotic surgical systems also do not currently have the ability to provide feedback to the surgeon regarding success of performing tasks. We trained medical students on three laparoscopic tasks and provided real-time feedback of performance during training. We found that real-time feedback can benefit training if the feedback provides information that is not available through other means (grip force). Subjects that received grip force feedback applied less force when the feedback was removed. Other forms of feedback (speed and relative phase) did not aid or impede training. Secondly, a relatively short training period (10 trials for each task) significantly improved most objective measures of performance. We also showed that robotic surgical performance can be quantitatively measured and evaluated. Providing grip force feedback can make the surgeon more aware of the forces being applied to delicate tissue during surgery.

Keywords: robotic surgery, da Vinci, training, real-time feedback, haptic

Introduction

The advent of robotic surgical systems, such as the da Vinci Surgical System (dVSS, Intuitive Surgical, Inc., Mountain View, CA), have overcome some of the limitations of manual laparoscopy. The addition of three-dimensional visualization has provided depth perception [1], while wrist-like articulations of the instruments have also been shown to improve surgeons' dexterity [2, 3]. Tremor abolition and motion scaling have been shown to enhance dexterity when using robotic systems [3]. Regarding training, the coordinated hand and instrument movements have improved the training time of residents [4-6], with fewer errors committed and less time taken for surgical task completion [3, 7-10].

However, there is a lack of research on what type of tasks should be used to properly train surgeons. A universal training protocol is absent and proficiency in using robotic systems is judged subjectively. Furthermore, current robotic systems do not have the ability to provide any feedback to the surgeon regarding the success of

---

[1] Corresponding Author: HPER Biomechanics Lab, University of Nebraska at Omaha, 6001 Dodge St., Omaha, NE 68182; Webpage: http://www.unocoe.unomaha.edu/hper/bio/home.htm; E-mail: nstergiou@mail.unomaha.edu.

performing the task. Such feedback mechanisms could be especially beneficial for training with robotic systems. In the Motor Learning discipline, it has been repeatedly shown that external or augmented feedback is essential for skill acquisition [11-14]. Our goal was to investigate the use of real-time augmented visual feedback to improve training and performance while performing three different surgical tasks with the dVSS.

1. METHODS AND MATERIALS

1.1. Subjects

Twelve right-handed novice users of the dVSS, which were medical students (23.2±0.6 yrs) of the University of Nebraska Medical Center, gave consent to participate in accordance with university guidelines.

1.2. Tasks

Subjects performed three tasks (Figure 1): bimanual carrying (BC), needle passing (NP), and suture tying (ST). In the BC task, subjects simultaneously picked up two 15 x 2 mm rubber pieces (one each with left and right graspers) from 30 mm (diameter) metal caps and placed them in two other metal caps 50 mm away. The subjects repeated the movement 6 times in succession. In the NP task, they passed a 26 mm surgical needle through 6 holes in a latex tube. In the ST task, they tied two knots with a 100 mm x 0.5 mm suture around one of the holes in the latex using the intracorporeal knot. All tasks were cyclic and designed to mimic actual laparoscopic surgical tasks that require significant bimanual coordination.

1.3. Experimental protocol

The subjects were randomly assigned to one of four feedback groups: speed (SP), grip force (GRIP), relative phase between left and right grasper movement (RP), and control (CTRL). Speed feedback was presented as two green vertical bars (left and right arm). When the speed increased, the bar enlarged vertically. Similarly, grip force feedback (or haptic feedback) was presented as two red vertical bars. Relative phase was presented as a red circular dial with a moving needle. The needle pointed to the right for an in-phase (0°) relationship and to the left for an out-of-phase (180°). When the right and left grasper moved in the same direction and with the same speed, then we had an in-phase relationship between the two sides. The opposite is an out-of-phase relationship. Part of the dial was shaded green indicating the desired relative phase for the task as calculated from expert data from a previous experiment.

All subjects performed the 3 tasks for 3 pre-training trials (PRE), 10 training trials with feedback, and 3 post-training trials (POST). Prior to PRE trials, subjects were given verbal instruction on how to complete the task. Subjects were not allowed to practice before the experiment. Speed, grip force, and relative phase feedback were displayed visually in real-time during the training trials using a custom program written in Labview (National Instruments, Inc., Austin, TX). The feedback was overlaid on the visual display of the dVSS surgeon's console so subjects were able to see the feedback while performing the tasks. The control group received no real-time feedback during the training trials.

1.4. Data Collection and Analysis

Position and velocity of dVSS instruments were collected at 75 Hz. Eight dependent variables were analyzed for differences in performance with training: time to task completion (**TTC** in sec), distance traveled (**D** in mm), mean speed (**S** in mm/sec), grip force (**F**), median curvature (κ_{med} in mm^{-1}), 95% confidence intervals of curvature (κ_{CI} in mm^{-1}), mean relative phase (Φ_{mean} in deg), and standard deviation of relative phase (Φ_{SD}). **D**, **S**, **F**, κ_{med}, and κ_{CI} were measured for right and left grasper. **F** was provided by the dVSS Application Programmer's Interface and is a unitless measure related to force applied by the graspers of the robot. Relative phase measured the coordination between the right and left grasper (0° = in phase, 180° = out of phase). Group means were compared using two-way mixed ANOVAs, with condition (PRE, POST) as the within factor and feedback (SP, GRIP, RP, CTRL) as the between factor. Post-hoc pairwise comparisons with Bonferroni corrections were performed when factors were significant. All values reported are mean ± std. error. The statistical analysis was performed for each task and dependent variable.

2. RESULTS

2.1. Bimanual Carrying

Condition (PRE vs POST): TTC was significantly shorter POST training (p<0.0005; Table 1). Right and left **S** were both significantly faster POST training (p<0.0005). Right and left **F** were both significantly lower POST training (R: p<0.0005, L: p=0.016). Right and left κ_{med} were significantly smaller POST training indicating straighter movements (R: p=0.004, L: p=0.004). Right and left κ_{CI} were significantly smaller POST training indicating less varying curvature (R: p<0.0005, L: p=0.001). **D**, Φ_{mean} and Φ_{SD} were not significantly different.

   Feedback (SP vs GRIP vs RP vs CTRL): Right **F** was significantly different between groups (p=0.003), and specifically significant smaller (0.193 units) for GRIP as compared to SP. Right and left κ_{CI} were significantly different between groups (R: p=0.021, L: p=0.009), with right κ_{CI} significantly greater (0.125 mm^{-1}) for GRIP as compared to RP, and with left κ_{CI} significantly greater (0.070 mm^{-1}) for GRIP as compared to CTRL. All other measures were not significantly different.

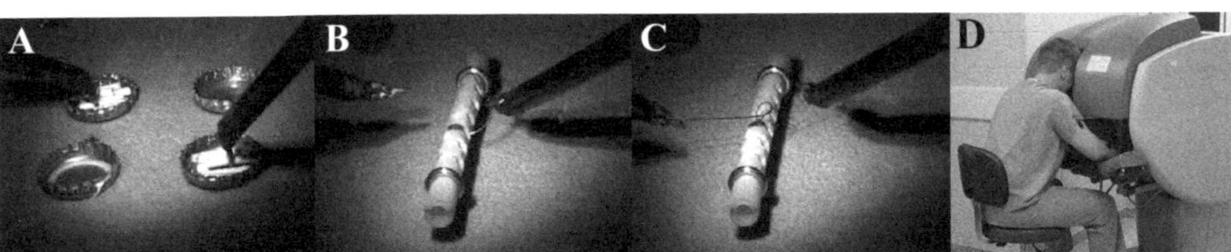

Figure 1: Experiment Setup. A) Bimanual Carrying. B) Needle Passing. C) Suture Tying. D) Subject seated at surgeon's console of dVSS.

Task	Mean Difference (PRE-POST)						
	TTC	Right D	Left D	Right S	Left S	Right F	Left F
BC	19.4 *	-42.5	-21.6	-11.52 *	-11.93 *	0.059 *	0.033 *
NP	42.4 *	296.3 *	154.6 *	-2.39 *	-3.93 *	0.066 *	-0.005
ST	60.5 *	532.7 *	531.5 *	-6.55 *	-5.31 *	0.086 *	0.07 *
	R. κ_{med}	L. κ_{med}	R. κ_{CI}	L. κ_{CI}	Φ_{mean}	Φ_{SD}	
BC	0.40 *	0.28 *	0.093 *	0.048 *	1.90	-0.036	
NP	0.24 *	0.99 *	0.008	0.164 *	-14.49	0.099	
ST	0.53 *	0.49 *	0.058 *	0.018	-9.18	-0.158 *	

Table 1: Within subject pairwise comparisons between conditions for all tasks and dependent variables. Mean differences are shown as PRE – POST. * indicates significance at the p=0.05 level.

Interaction effects: Interaction effects show if types of feedback affected condition performance in a different manner. Right and left **D** had significant interaction effects (R: p=0.02, L: p=0.05). For both, the SP group traveled farther POST training as compared to other feedback groups. Left **S** also had a significant interaction effect (p=0.042). The SP group moved faster POST training as compared to other feedback groups. Right and left **F** had significant interaction effects (R: p=0.003, L: p==0.004). In both cases, **F** was significantly smaller POST training for the GRIP group as compared to other feedback groups (Figure 2). No other interactions were found.

2.2. Needle Passing

Condition (PRE vs POST): TTC was significantly shorter POST training (p<0.0005; Table 1). Right and left **D** were significantly smaller POST training (R: p<0.0005, L: p=0.001). Right and left **S** were both significantly faster POST training (p<0.0005). Right **F** was significantly lower POST training (p<0.0005). Right and left κ_{med} were significantly smaller POST training indicating straighter movements (R: p=0.001, L: p<0.0005). Left κ_{CI} was significantly smaller POST training indicating less varying curvature (p<0.0005). Left **F**, right κ_{CI}, Φ_{mean} and Φ_{SD} were not significantly different.

Feedback (SP vs GRIP vs RP vs CTRL): TTC was significantly different between groups (p=0.037). RP took significantly more than CTRL. Right **D** was significantly different between groups (p=0.011), with being significantly smaller for GRIP and SPEED as compared to RP. Right and left **S** were significantly different between groups (R: p=0.017, L: p=0.024). Right **S** was significantly faster for CTRL as compared to GRIP. Left **S** was also significantly faster for CTRL as compared to GRIP. Right **F** was significantly different between groups (p=0.017). Right **F** was significant smaller for GRIP as compared to SP. Right and left κ_{med} were significantly different between groups (R: p=0.041, L: p=0.041). Right κ_{med} was significantly greater for GRIP as compared to CTRL. Left κ_{med} was significantly greater for GRIP as compared to CTRL. Right and left κ_{CI} were significantly different between groups (R: p=0.003, L: p=0.001). Right κ_{CI} was significantly smaller for CTRL and RP as compared to GRIP. Left κ_{CI} was significantly smaller for CTRL and RP as compared to GRIP. All other measures were not significantly different between groups.

Interaction effects: Right and left **F** had significant interaction effects (R: p=0.006, L: p=0.027). In both cases, **F** was significantly smaller POST training for the GRIP group as compared to other feedback groups (Figure 2). Right κ_{CI} had a significant

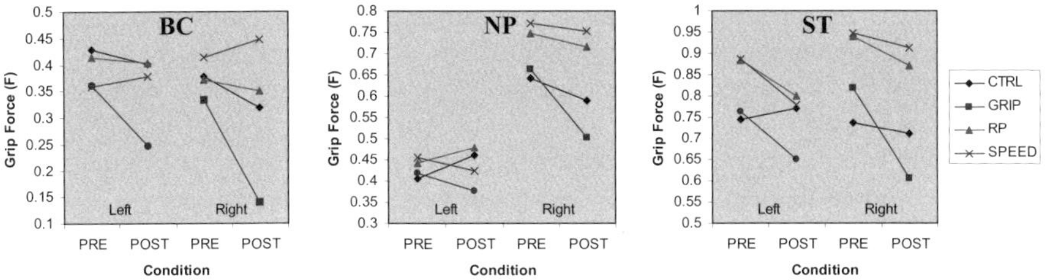

Figure 2: Interaction effect of Right and Left F during the BC, NP, and ST tasks. F is significantly smaller POST training for the GRIP feedback group compared to all other feedback groups.

interaction effect (p=0.041). GRIP made more varied movements POST training than other groups. No other measures had interaction effects.

2.3. Suture Tying

Condition (PRE vs POST): TTC was significantly shorter POST training (p<0.0005; Table 1). Right and left **D** were significantly smaller POST training (R: p=0.001, L: p<0.0005). Right and left **S** were both significantly faster POST training (p<0.0005). Right and left **F** were significantly lower POST training (R: p=0.001, L: p=0.001). Right and left κ_{med} were significantly smaller POST training indicating straighter movements (p<0.0005). Right κ_{CI} was significantly smaller POST training indicating less varying curvature (p=0.003). Φ_{SD} was significant larger POST training indicating more varied coordination patterns. Left κ_{CI} and Φ_{mean} were not significantly different.

Feedback (SP vs GRIP vs RP vs CTRL): Right **F** was significantly different between groups (p=0.001). Right **F** was significant smaller for CTRL and GRIP as compared to RP, and also for CTRL and GRIP as compared to SP. Right and left κ_{CI} were significantly different between groups (R: p=0.002, L: p=0.029). Right κ_{CI} was significantly larger for GRIP and SP as compared to RP. Left κ_{CI} was significantly larger for CTRL as compared to RP. No other significant differences were found.

Interaction effects: Right **F** had significant interaction effects (p=0.026). Right **F** was significantly smaller POST training for the GRIP group as compared to other groups (Figure 2). No other measures had interaction effects.

3. CONCLUSIONS

This study has shown that real-time augmented feedback during training can impact surgical performance based on the type of feedback given. It has been found previously that augmented feedback aids performance when task-intrinsic feedback (naturally-occurring sensory feedback) is not available [12, 14]. Particularly, grip force feedback, which is not directly available to the subject, reduces the forces applied while performing each task even after feedback is removed. All tasks showed a significant decrease in grip force after training for subjects that received grip force feedback while other feedback groups did not significantly decrease grip force after training. Thus, it is important for surgeons to be aware of the amount of force being applied to tissue so as not to damage the tissue during surgery. Grip force feedback during training may be an effective means to train the surgeon to use sufficient force. Furthermore, feedback seems to be parameter specific, as grip feedback revealed better results for grip force. It is possible that there is a need for variable feedback mechanisms based on the surgical task being performed.

Nearly all performance measures significantly improved post-training. Other studies have shown that residents can be trained faster on robotic surgery as compared to manual laparoscopy [4-6]. These studies attribute the faster learning to the intuitive movements of the dVSS; that is, the grasper movements match the hand movements. In addition, our study demonstrated that these performance improvements can be the result of relatively little training (10 trials per task).

We found that real-time feedback for robotic laparoscopic training can benefit robotic surgical training. Real-time haptic (force) feedback proved most beneficial and may reduce tissue injury. A relatively short training period is required to gain this added benefit. Future work will confirm that these subjects retain the skills learned after several weeks of no training. Furthermore, the quantitative improvements that we observed will be correlated with subjective evaluation by an expert robotic surgeon.

REFERENCES

[1]   D'Annibale, A.M.D., V.M.D. Fiscon, P.M.D. Trevisan, M.M.D. Pozzobon, V.M.D. Gianfreda, G.M.D. Sovernigo, E.M.D. Morpurgo, C.M.D. Orsini, and D.M.D. Del Monte, *The da Vinci Robot in Right Adrenalectomy: Considerations on Technique.* Surgical Laparoscopy, Endoscopy & Percutaneous Techniques, 2004. **14**(1): p. 38-41.

[2]   Munz, Y., K. Moorthy, A. Dosis, J. Hernandez, S.D. Bann, F. Bello, S. Martin, A. Darzi, and T. Rockall, *The benefits of stereoscopic vision in robotic-assisted performance on bench models.* Surg Endosc, 2004. **18**(4): p. 611-616.

[3]   Moorthy, K., Y. Munz, A. Dosis, J. Hernandez, S. Martin, F. Bello, T. Rockall, and A. Darzi, *Dexterity enhancement with robotic surgery.* Surgical Endoscopy, 2004. **18**(5): p. 790-795.

[4]   De Ugarte, D.A., D.A. Etzioni, C. Gracia, and J.B. Atkinson, *Robotic surgery and resident training.* Surg Endosc, 2003. **17**(6): p. 960-963.

[5]   Chang, L., R.M. Satava, C.A. Pellegrini, and M.N. Sinanan, *Robotic surgery: identifying the learning curve through objective measurement of skill.* Surg Endosc, 2003. **17**(11): p. 1744-1748.

[6]   Hernandez, J.D., S.D. Bann, Y. Munz, K. Moorthy, V. Datta, S. Martin, A. Dosis, F. Bello, A. Darzi, and T. Rockall, *Qualitative and quantitative analysis of the learning curve of a simulated surgical task on the da Vinci system.* J Gastrointest Surg, 2004. **18**(3): p. 372-378.

[7]   Hashizume, M., M. Shimada, M. Tomikawa, Y. Ikeda, I. Takahashi, R. Abe, F. Koga, N. Gotoh, K. Konish, S. Maehara, and K. Sugimachi, *Early experiences of endoscopic procedures in general surgery assisted by a computer-enhanced surgical system.* Surg Endosc, 2002. **16**: p. 1187-1191.

[8]   Hubens, G., H. Coveliers, L. Balliu, M. Ruppert, and W. Vaneerdeweg, *A performance study comparing manual and robotic assisted laparoscopic surgery using the da Vinci system.* Surgical Endoscopy, 2003. **17**(10): p. 1595-9.

[9]   Prasad, S.M., H.S. Maniar, N.J. Soper, R.J. Damiano, and M.E. Klingensmith, *The effect of robotic assistance on learning curves for basic laparoscopic skills.* Am J Surg, 2002. **183**(6): p. 702-707.

[10] Sarle, R., A. Tewari, A. Shrivastava, J. Peabody, and M. Menon, *Surgical Robotics and Laparoscopic Training Drills.* J Endourol, 2004. **18**(1): p. 63-67.

[11] Rose, D.J., *A multilevel approach to the study of motor control and learning.* 1997, Needham Heights, MA: Allyn & Bacon.

[12] Hadden, C.M., R.A. Magill, and B. Sidaway, Concurrent vs. terminal augmented feedback in the acquisition and retention of a discrete bimanual motor task. Journal of Sport & Exercise Psychology, 1995. **17**: p. S54.

[13] Kelso, J.A., *Phase transitions and critical behavior in human bimanual cooridination.* Am J Physiol Regul Integr Comp Physiol, 1984. **246**: p. 1000-1004.

[14] Magill, R.A., *Motor Learning: Concepts and applications.* 5th ed. 1998, Boston, MA: McGraw-Hill.

Medicine Meets Virtual Reality 14
J.D. Westwood et al. (Eds.)
IOS Press, 2006

Computer-Aided Forensics: Metal Object Detection

Timothy Kelliher[a], Bill Leue[a], Bill Lorensen[a], Alexandra Lauric[b]
[a]Imaging Technologies, GE Global Research, Niskayuna NY
[b]Tufts University

Abstract. Recently, forensic investigators1 have started using diagnostic radiology devices (MRI, CT) to acquire image data from cadavers. This new technology, called the virtual autopsy, has the potential to provide a low cost, non-invasive alternative or supplement to conventional autopsies. New image processing techniques are being developed to highlight forensically relevant information in the images. One such   technique is the detection and characterization of metal objects embedded in the cadaver. Analysis of this information across a population with similar causes of death can lead to developing improved safety and protection devices with a corresponding reduction in deaths

1. Problem

Modern X-RAY Computed Tomography (CT) and Magnetic Resonance Imaging (MRI) scanners are capable of providing high-resolution cross-sectional images of the interior of human bodies. Recently, forensic investigators have started using these diagnostic radiology devices to acquire image data from cadavers.[1] This new technology, called the virtual autopsy, has the potential to provide a low cost, non-invasive alternative or supplement to conventional autopsies. The whole body CT exams required for a virtual autopsy generate large datasets. Typically, cross-sectional images are 512x512 each with sub millimeter pixel spacing. A typical whole body CT scan can consist of 3000 of these images. Interactive examination of these large datasets by radiologists is time-consuming and expensive. We describe one technique in the emerging field of Computer-Aided Forensics (CAF) that uses image analysis techniques to locate and analyze foreign objects within virtual autopsies.

2. Method

The virtual autopsy begins with a whole body CT study (GE Lightspeed 16, GE Healthcare Technologies). The exams are constructed with .625 mm pixels and slices spaced 1.25 mm. The data is transferred to a radiology workstation (GE Advantage Windows) for review by radiologists. Currently, the radiologist uses a four-window display showing axial, coronal and sagittal cross-sections as well as a 3D volume rendering used for navigation. For CAF processing, we transfer the studies to Linux and Windows workstations using DICOM protocols.

The initial application of CAF is the analysis of metal fragment location, size and distribution. The first step to any CT-CAF process is to loate the body within the images. We generate a mask of the body using thresholding, masking, and connected component labeling[2]. In the protocol employed here, the body is scanned while it is still in the body bag to ensure as little pre-scan disruption as is possible. The threshold excludes the majority of clutter around the body, such as the bag and clothes. The masking is done to remove both the table and any reconstruction artifacts created where areas of the body fell outside the scanner's field of view. After masking and thresholding, connected components are used to find the remaining objects. The image statistics of these objects are then compared to decide if they represent parts of the body or foreign objects that were contained in the bag. They must be above a minimum size and have a mean intensity that falls within the range for bone and tissue. To accommodate the large volume, we generate the mask one slice at a time.

We create a digitally reconstructed radiograph, DRR in both lateral and AP views. The DRRs are used later in the process both as a quality control check to ensure proper mask generation and as a visualization aid in displaying the extracted metal.

We apply the body mask to the original gray-scale CT data and identify all voxels that exceed 1900 Hounsfield units. This value is sufficiently above any densities that exist naturally in the human body to distinguish the metal form the body. A connected component algorithm aggregates each group of voxels. Then a number of statistics are computed for each group including location, size, mass and orientation. We have created an atlas of the human body, dividing the body into head, neck, thorax, abdomen and upper/lower extremities. We adapt the atlas to each individual using deformable registration. Each metal object is associated with these regions. The quantitative results are exported in a form suitable for database insertion. We also produce a rendering of the body combined with surface models of the extracted metal [3].

3. Results

We have run the metal fragment extraction on hundreds of virtual autopsies containing anywhere from zero fragments to more than 2000 metal fragments. Figures 1,2 & 3 show results for one case. In this case the individual had a gunshot wound to the right shoulder as well as abdominal wounding. This example had 78 metal objects. The size of the metal objects varied from 1 mm to 14 mm. A distinct clustering of fragments is seen in the shoulder where the projectile hit the bone and fragmented into many pieces.

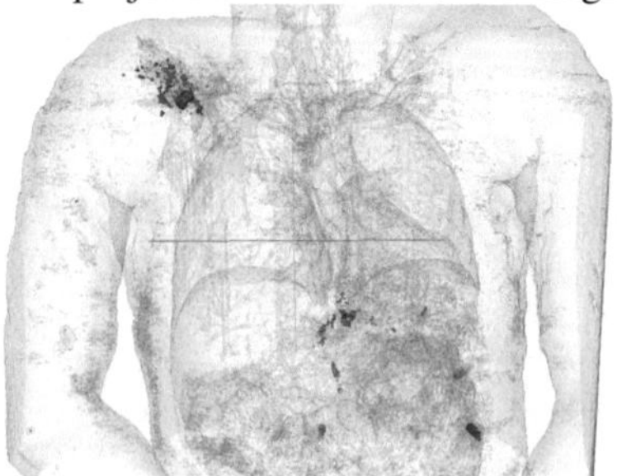

Figure 1: Metal fragments in the context of the body model. Fragments in the shoulder are from a gunshot.

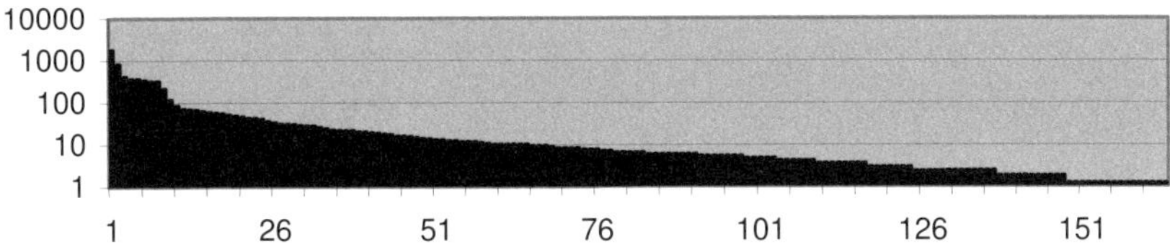

Figure 2: Histogram of fragment sizes (mm^3) found in the example case. (logarithmic scale)

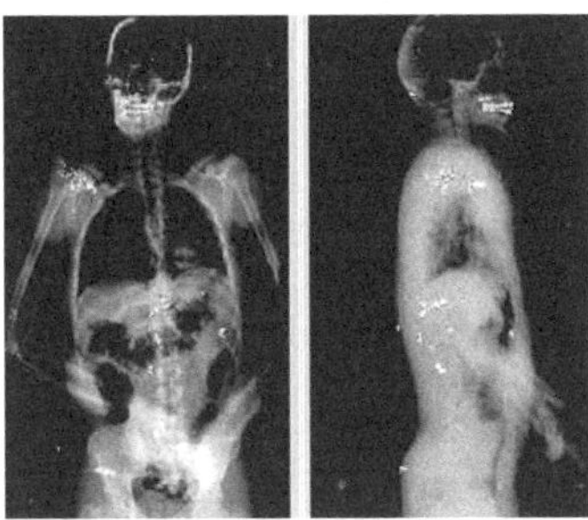

Figure 3: Digitally Reconstructed Radiographs, lateral and AP views with segmented metal highlighted.

4. Discussion

This work is the first in a series of investigations into the usefulness of automatic, objective analysis of virtual autopsy data. Radiologists are continually learning more about the reading and interpretation of post-mortem CT images. Our objective is to quickly develop automated techniques to translate this knowledge into an effective virtual autopsy that is reproducible from site to site. We plan to refine the regional atlas into further levels of detail, eventually down to the organ level. Additional information from the extracted metal objects may also be possible. For instance, various metal has differing X-RAY attenuation and it may be possible to characterize the extracted metal objects. Depth of penetration of the metal objects is also of forensic interest. Determination of the nature of the metal distribution is possible and may help find ballistic trajectories. These trajectories may facilitate automated wound path extraction.

This work was supported by a grant from DARPA, executed by the U.S. Army Medical Research and Materiel Command/TATRC Assistance Agreement, Contract # W81XWH-05-2-0059 "A" (Approved for Public Release, Distribution Unlimited).

References

[1]   Thali MJ, et.al., Virtopsy, a New Imaging Horizon in Forensic Pathology: Virtual Autopsy by Postmortem Multislice Computed Tomography (MSCT) and Magnetic Resonance Imaging (MRI) - a Feasibility Study. J Forensic Sci 2003 Mar; 48 (2): 386-403.
[2]   http://www.itk.org.
[3]   http://www.vtk.org.

Medicine Meets Virtual Reality 14
J.D. Westwood et al. (Eds.)
IOS Press, 2006

Parametric Modeling and Simulation of Trocar Insertion

T. Kesavadas, Govindarajan Srimathveeravalli, Velupillai Arulesan ({kesh, gks2, arulesan}@eng.buffalo.edu)
Virtual Reality Lab, Dept. of Mechanical and Aerospace Engineering
State University of New York at Buffalo, Buffalo, NY 14260

Abstract: Trocar insertion, the first step to most micro surgery procedures is a difficult procedure to learn and practice because procedure is carried out almost entirely without any visual feedback of the organs underlying the tissue being punctured. A majority of injuries is attributed to the excessive use of force by the surgeon. This paper looks at developing a haptic based trocar insertion simulator which will assist in training and skill advancement in carrying out this procedure. Different issues regarding development of force model and and trocar-tissue interaction is studied.

1. Introduction

Trocars play an important role in laparoscopy and thoracoscopy where they are used to puncture an opening before laparoscopic devices are inserted. According to a study by FDA (Food and Drug Administration) laparoscopic trocar insertion procedures are the most commonly named procedure in malpractice claims among laparoscopic surgery [1]. Interestingly, the analyses of the reports indicate that the trocar design identified in all fatality reports was either a "shielded" trocar or an "optical" trocar. This alludes to a fact that visual feedback alone is not sufficient to prevent injuries during trocar insertion. A majority of injuries are attributed to use of excessive force by the surgeon due to various factors [2]. Therefore, it is evident that new training methodlgies are required to improve the skill of the surgeon to reduce trocar related injuries. We intend to develop a trocar simulator that will assist in pre-operative training with the help of haptic feedback. The simulator will be built by collecting force displacement data from actual insertions, identifying parametric values of the tissues depending on insertion point and finally building the simulator capable of providing realistic position-force feedback. Early experiments suggests that tissue modeling is perhaps one of the most challenging problem due to difficulties in measuring physiological data and the nonlinear – anisotropic behavior of the tissue.

2. Force Modeling

The first step in modeling the tissue is to obtain relevant force and displacement data for known loading conditions and identifying a suitable dynamic model that will capture the information from the experiments. Different models for tissue modeling have been discussed in literature ranging from mass spring models based on Voigt and Maxwell elements which are simple and best equipped for real time applications to complex Finite Element Method (FEM) models. We use the discrete element combination method to model the viscoelasticity properties of tissues. The force is modeled along the lines of soft tissue needle insertion system described by Okamura et al. [3]

$$Force = F_{stiffness} + F_{friction} + F_{cutting}$$

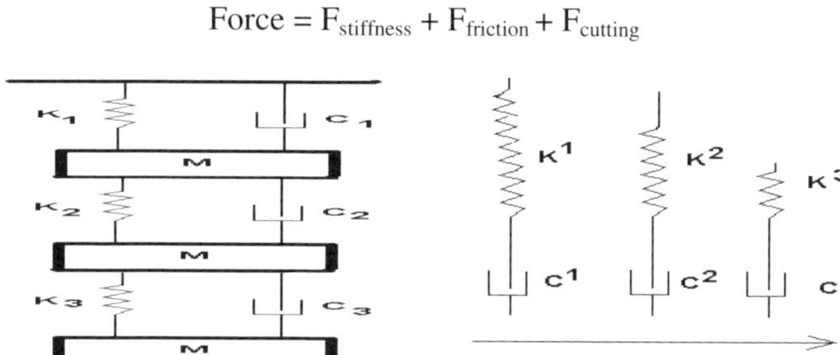

Figure 1: Spring Mass Damper setup for a three layered skin model

Figure 2: Gain Scheduling Setup for different force values

In our case we ignore the cutting force from our model and concentrate on the friction and stiffness forces. The simple spring damper mass model for the three layers of the abdominal wall that include Skin, fat and muscle is shown in Figure 1. The system is modeled using the Maxwell model using only stiffness and damping elements. We further assume the frictional force to be a constant throughout the procedure.

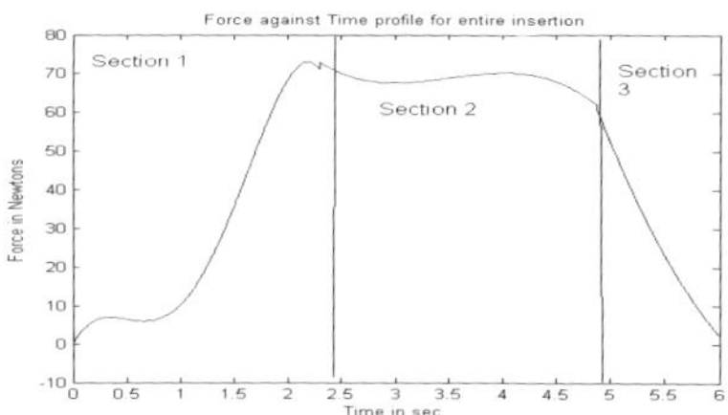

Figure 3: Force against Time profile

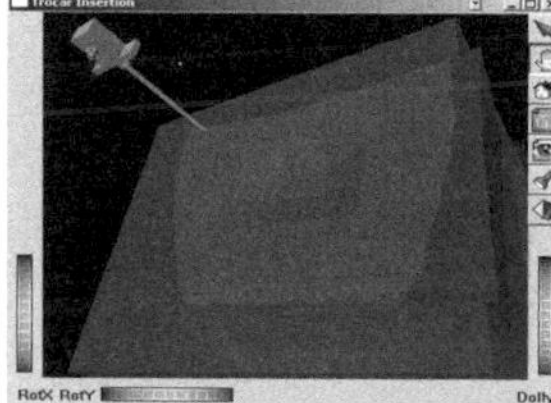

Figure 4: Screenshot of Simulator

The force pattern for the insertions of a 12mm bladeless trocar on a porcine model are non linear in nature as can be seen from Figure 3. The curve for the force profile is similar for a 5mm bladeless trocar as well, except that the peak force value was lower (about 35.84N). To try and model this force pattern we used a method known as gain scheduling wherein we use multiple linear systems to model sections of the non-linear pattern which is linear within a certain timeframe. We divide the force curve into three sections using a different parametric equation to model each section as in Figure 2. The three parametric equations used to model the three different regions are as follows:

$$F^1 = k_1x^4 + k_2x^3 + k_3x^2 + k_4x + d$$

$$F^2 = k_5x^3 + k_6x^2 + k_7x + d$$

$$F^3 = k_8x^2 + k_9x + d$$

The first section is modeled using a fourth order linear fit while the second is modeled using a cubic fit and the third section is modeled using a quadratic fit. The abdominal wall thickness is approximated to be between 10 to 30 mm for skin/fat layer and between 10 and 15 mm for muscle thickness of a male. The entire wall thickness is assumed to be about 35-45 mm in thickness.

3. Simulator

We have created a virtual simulator that simulates the deformation of the skin tissue as the trocar is inserted which is the first step towards creating a pre-operative training module. The simulator is a visualization tool which presents the deformation of the tissue as the trocar insertion takes place as can be seen in Figure 4. In the next version we intend to integrate the simulator with a PHANToM™ Desktop device to provide haptic feedback.

4. Future Work

After the completion of the haptic set up it will be evaluated using human subject trials. The input model for a range of patient data such as age, BMI, fat content etc will be used to determine the constants for the parametric equation determined by the data fitting procedure.

Acknowledgement
We thank Dr Celeste Hollands, MD, and Dr Stan Lau, MD of Women and Children's Hospital of Buffalo for their advice and guidance in this research.

References

[1]   Fuller, J., B.S. Ashar, and J. Carey-Corrado, Trocar-associated injuries and fatalities: An analysis of 1399 reports to the FDA. Journal of Minimally Invasive Gynecology, 2005. 12(4): p. 302.
[2]   Bhoyrul, S., et al., Trocar injuries in laparoscopic surgery. Journal of the American College of Surgeons, 2001. 192(6): p. 677.
[3]   Okamura, A.M., C. Simone, and M.D. O'Leary, Force modeling for needle insertion into soft tissue. Biomedical Engineering, IEEE Transactions on, 2004. 51(10): p. 1707.

Medicine Meets Virtual Reality 14
J.D. Westwood et al. (Eds.)
IOS Press, 2006

255

Exploiting Graphics Hardware
for Haptic Authoring

Minho Kim [a,1], Sukitti Punak [a], Juan Cendan [b], Sergei Kurenov [b], and Jörg Peters [a]

[a] *Dept. CISE, University of Florida*
[b] *Dept. Surgery, University of Florida*

Abstract. Real-time, plausible visual and haptic feedback of deformable objects without shape artifacts is important in surgical simulation environments to avoid distracting the user. We propose to leverage highly parallel stream processing, available on the newest generation graphics cards, to increase the level of both visual and haptic fidelity. We implemented this as part of the University of Florida's haptic surgical authoring kit.

Keywords. virtual surgery training, haptic rendering, GPU shader, subdivision surface, etc.

1. Introduction

Shape artifacts, such as the transition between facets of an insufficiently refined model, can distract both a user's visual and haptic senses from a given task. However, modeling a large scenario to a level of refinement that hides such representation artifacts, requires considerable computational resources. Fortunately, recently, the graphics processing units (GPU) of graphics cards have become more powerful, offering highly parallel stream processing with access via *graphics shader programming*; moreover, novel data structures have been developed to shift the work of finely evaluating high quality surface representations, so-called subdivision surfaces, from the central processing unit (CPU) to the GPU, freeing the CPU for higher-level and user-input tasks. While the state-of-the art research addresses the need for real-time visual animation of high-quality representations, the higher frequency of haptic update has not, at this point, been satisfactorily addressed in the literature.

We propose to leverage highly parallel stream processing, available on the newest generation graphics cards, to increase the level of both visual and haptic fidelity by taking advantage of (i) the locality of haptic probing (Figure 4) and (ii) an improved communication channel (bus) between the GPU and CPU.

As a proof of concept, we implemented the visual and haptic improvement in the University of Florida's haptic surgical authoring kit. This haptic authoring kit is a low cost environment that allows the specialist surgeon to author haptic and multimedia training exercises. A key issue in such a haptic simulation is to determine the minimal level

---

[1] Correspondence to: SurfLab, Dept. CISE, CSE Bldg E325, University of Florida, Gainesville, FL 32611. Tel.: +1 352 392 1255; Fax: +1 352 392 1220; E-mail: {mhkim,jorg}@cise.ufl.edu.

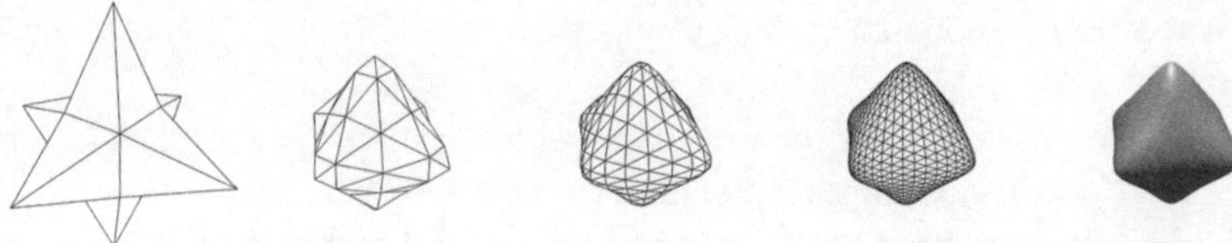

Figure 1. Surface mesh refinement (depth 0,1,2,3) and rendering of using Loop's Subdivision.

of visual and haptic fidelity required to make the exercise effective. We had found earlier that the consistent interplay between visual and haptic feedback is important to avoid distracting the author form the task. However, modelling the surfaces of organs, vessels and tissues as visually and haptically smooth surfaces results in an equally undesirable time-lag, especially when surfaces are allowed to deform.

Recently, many applications have been developed that leverage the parallel processing power of the modern GPUs. One of these applications is the run-time evaluation of subdivision surfaces (1) using programmable graphics hardwares, called *GPU shaders*. Since most of the human organs can be modeled compactly using subdivision surfaces, we adapt this approach using GPU shaders not only for visual rendering but also for haptic rendering for our authoring environment. By tracking the current position of the haptic device, we can localize the evaluation thus reducing rendering overhead for high-frequency rendering of deforming objects.

2. Background: Subdivision Algorithms, Spatial Data Structures and Shaders

Subdivision algorithms create smooth surface approximations by recursively refining the connectivity and smoothing the geometry of a polyhedral input mesh, known as the *control mesh* (see e.g. [1,2], 1). In all popular algorithms the position of a new mesh node is obtained as the weighted average of old nodes of a small submesh, whose graph is called *stencil*. One such refinement pattern splits each triangle into four and is called Loop subdivision (Figure 1).

Modern GPUs provide programmable parallel stream processing in the form of *vertex shaders* and *fragment shaders* [3]. Vertex shaders process attributes, such as positions, normals, and texture coordinates, of a single vertex without connectivity. The downstream fragment shaders process the rasterized data (i.e. attributes per pixel) and assign the resulting pixels. Fragment shaders are the key computation units for most GPU algorithms (as well as ours) because of their computation power and ability to read and write data by rendering to the framebuffer and copying to readable texture images.

Strategies and techniques for computation on GPUs are collected in [4]. A number of important algorithms have been modified to rebalance the workload between CPU and GPU and take advantage of parallel execution streams in programmable graphics hardwares: particle systems [5], collision detection [6], cellular automata [7], global illumination [8] and other numerical computations [9,10]. The algorithmic component on the GPU, called *shader*s, rely essentially on accessing regularly laid out data, typified by the 2D array, to minimize workflow branching and maximize parallelism. Irregular access typically requires interaction with the CPU.

3. Real-time subdivision surface reevaluation on the GPU

Most recently, researchers succeeded in mapping the irregular access structure characterizing general subdivision surface evaluation, to a representation on the GPU [11].
A locality-preserving data access keeps all irregularities strictly inside overlapping, independently refinable pieces of the mesh, called *fragment meshes* (Figure 2), allowing
for parallel streams of work per fragment mesh and also per mesh node. The fragment
meshes are encoded into one-dimensional array as a texture, called *patch texture*, fed
into GPU pipeline in a parallel fashion, and subdivided *recursively* by fragment (pixel)
shaders in an off-screen framebuffer. Since all topology (connectivity) information is
lost in the one-dimensional array, a smart, pre-computed *stencil lookup table* is also sent
to GPU as a texture. The GPU then re-evaluates a freely deforming surface at interactive frame-rates (20-30 frames-per second) for moderately-sized control meshes (ca
100 nodes); see also Table 2. Thanks to recursive subdivision, it can model *semi-smooth
creases* (features that are sharp in the large scale, but rounded at the small scale) and
global boundaries i.e. surface pieces.

There are several implementation challenges for this approach. One is to guarantee
water-tight boundaries, i.e. no pixel-dropout artifacts between fragment meshes. Another
is to avoid the *redundant data round-trip* of the final subdivision data that current generation graphics cards enforce: the evaluated values are stored in pixel formats in an off-
screen framebuffer, the *pbuffer*, that cannot directly be rendered. In currently available
standard GPU interfaces, it needs to be copied back to system memory and then returned
to GPU pipeline again. This 'round-trip' of the refined data when it is the largest in size,
slows the rendering considerably. The feature that enables us to use the data in pixel formats (stored in a texture of framebuffer) as vertex array is called *render-to-vertex-array*
and there are several extensions for this purpose in OpenGL®, including the *PBO/VBO
extension* and the *überbuffer (supperbuffer) extension*; the upcoming OpenGL® *FBO
(framebuffer object) extension* is expected to replace and improve on both which should
help our implementation.

3.1. GPU implementation of Loop subdivision

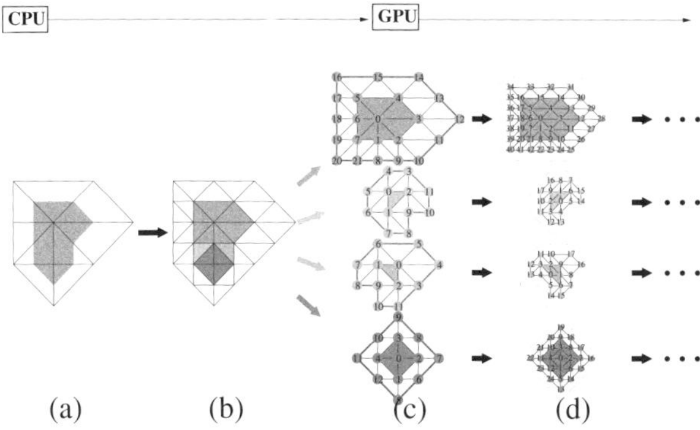

Figure 2. Workflow of GPU Loop subdivision kernel: (a) input control mesh (b) initial subdivision (c) fragment meshes and (d) fragment meshes subdivided in the GPU.

Most available mesh models consist of triangles and the natural subdivision scheme for triangulated data sets. Following the general approach of [11] we implemented Loop subdivision on the GPU solving two challenges specific to Loop subdivision. First, as Figure 2 shows, after one refinement on the CPU, we obtain *vertex fragment meshes* composed of two layers of triangles around each of the input control vertices. However, for each of the input facet, there is an additional center triangle that needs to separately treated as a *facet fragment mesh*. Its implementation, although the same over all facet fragment meshes, is nontrivial. Secondly, guaranteeing water-tight boundaries, especially where two facet and two vertex fragment meshes meet, despite rounding of intermediate results, requires a smart symmetric refinement.

4. Surgical Haptic Authoring

To address the constant need for practicing surgeons to quickly and conveniently refresh their knowledge of surgical procedures that they are not performing on a regular basis, the University of Florida surgical authoring kit provides a media rich and 'hands-on' channel for publishing procedures by a specialist surgeon (see Figure 3). A key point of this approach is that the specialist surgeon rather than a computer programmer will author the material to make the approach flexible and remove a level of indirection that slows publication and easily leads to wrong emphasis. Currently the kit's haptic component is based on the affordable Phantom® Omni™Haptic Device.

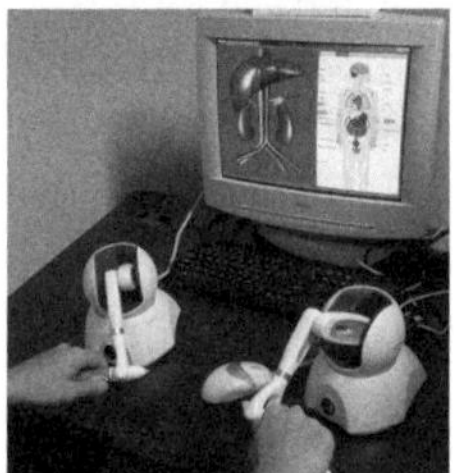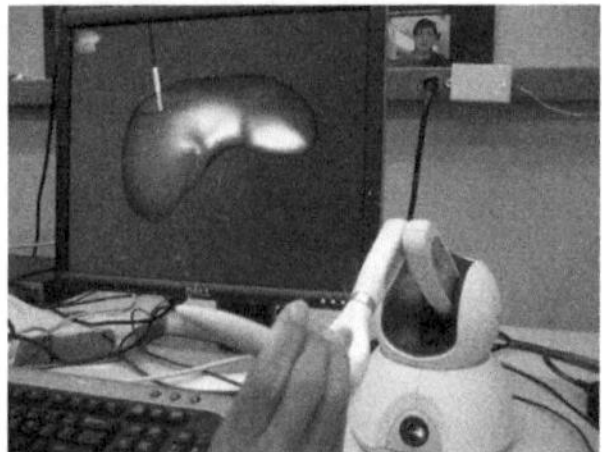

Figure 3. Screen shots from the University of Florida surgical authoring kit.

5. Haptic rendering exploiting the GPU subdivision kernel

The OpenHaptics™Toolkit is a popular SDK that enables developers to control several widespread haptic device lineups from SensAble Technologies, Inc.. One of its merits is that we can use the same OpenGL® geometry rendering modules for the haptic rendering. Since we already have the *finely subdivided* subdivision mesh calculated by GPU shaders for visual display, we should obviously use them again for haptic rendering.

We dramatically improve the haptic rendering performance, by bounding each fragment mesh to localize the haptic rendering of a deformable object. Since the geometry of the fragment meshes change as they are subdivided, such bounding boxes must enclose all the intermediate subdivided ones. Fortunately, in Loop subdivision, positions of all the vertices in the intermediate subdivided fragment meshes are convex combinations of

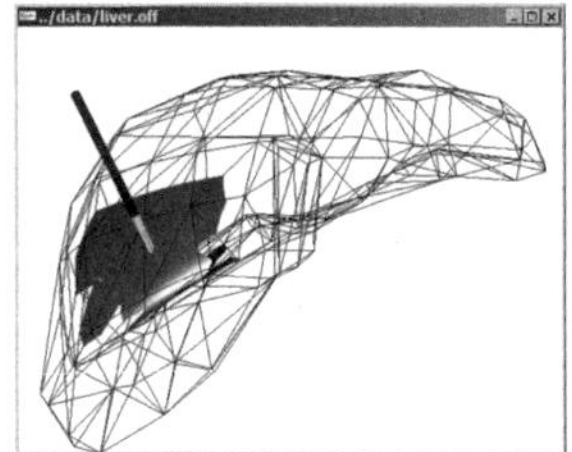
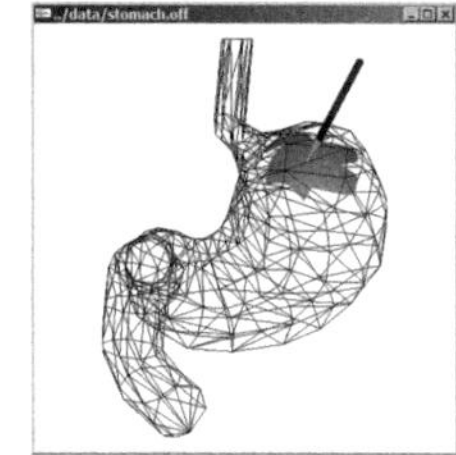

Figure 4. Visual display of the localized fragment meshes used for haptic rendering.

	CPU	GPU	system memory	video memory	shaders per patch	double buffer ing	buffer size	data round-trip removal
1	Pentium 4 (2.40GHz)	ATI Radeon 9700 Pro (Omega driver 2.5.97a)	1GB	128MB (AGP 4×)	2	no	2048×1024	none
2	Pentium 4 (3.00GHz)	nVidia GeForce 6800GT (driver 71.84)	1GB	256MB (AGP 8×)	1	yes	2048×256	PBO/VBO
3	Pentium M (1.60GHz)	nVidia GeForce 6200 (driver 70.87)	512MB	128MB (PCI Express 16×)	1	yes	2048×256	PBO/VBO
4	Pentium 4 (2.80GHz)	ATI Radeon X800 (Omega driver 2.5.97a)	1GB	256MB (AGP 8×)	1	no	2048×256	PBO/VBO

Table 1. Four hardware/shader configurations used for timings in Tables 2 and 3. All configurations use the pbuffer mechanism as off-screen framebuffer.

the initial ones and therefore stay inside of the convex hull of the initial fragment mesh. We enclose the convex hull by a bounding sphere to increase performance.

One of the bottlenecks when working with deformable objects are bounding box updates. However, the range of movement of the control vertices of deformable organs is limited, so that we can make the bounding spheres partially static, fixing its center position and adjusting only the radius. The radius depends on the deformation and the *speed of the haptic device*: if the device moves too quickly for the size of the bounding sphere, we may not detect the intersection of the device with the surface of the object but penetrate it to the interior, resulting in a well-known *falling-off* artifact. By calibrating the radius according to the speed of the haptic device, we can avoid this artifact.

Once the fragment meshes close to the haptic device are determined, only their GPU-subdivided meshes need to be handed to the haptic engine. Figure 4 visually illustrates the fragment meshes rendered for haptic feedback.

Results: Table 1 summarizes the four hardware/shader configurations tested for the visual feedback. Table 2 shows the resulting timings for purely visual feedback and Table 3 the frames per second for combined visual and local haptic rendering of real-time deforming of high-quality surfaces. The drop in performance with our current implementation can be as bad as 50% for small models on the older ATi9700, but is just 10-20% on the newer ATiX800. Considering that complete recomputation to depth 5 for each frame is beyond the need perceived by users, the numbers indicate that high-quality visual and local haptic rendering is now within reach of commodity PCs with high-end commodity graphics cards.

Acknowledgements This research was made possible in part by NSF Grants DMI-0400214 and CCF-0430891.

fps	liver		stomach		mechpart		venus	
	4	5	4	5	4	5	4	5
1	9.70	6.27	8.53	4.41	7.62	4.60	4.27	1.88
2	22.83	15.63	19.42	11.43	18.28	13.07	9.70	5.24
3	18.32	9.15	12.08	4.85	13.62	6.81	5.04	1.90
4	13.91	8.42	11.43	5.71	10.33	6.04	5.42	2.40

Table 2. Frames per second (fps) for visual rendering of the four configurations in Table 1; four data sets are refined to depth 4, respectively 5 (ca. 300K triangles for liver, 550K for stomach).

fps	liver		stomach	
	4	5	4	5
1	5.20	3.62	4.54	3.32
4	10.86	6.40	10.00	5.08

Table 3. Frames per second (fps) for visual rendering and haptic feedback on the two platforms/configurations 1 and 4 supporting the Omni and two surfaces relevant to our surgical authoring.

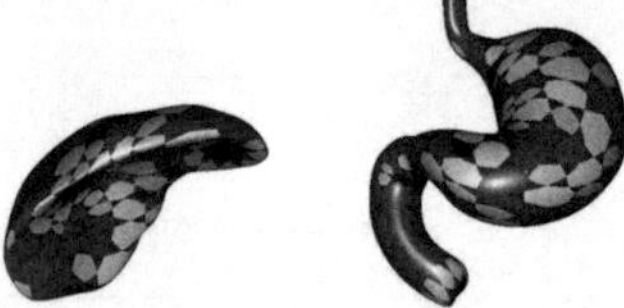

Figure 5.: Models liver and stomach shaded according to split into fragment meshes.

References

[1] Tony DeRose and Michael Kass and Tien Truong. Subdivision surfaces in character animation. In *SIGGRAPH '98 Conference Proceedings*, pages 85–94, 1998.

[2] Joe Warren and Henrik Weimer. *Subdivision Methods for Geometric Design*. Morgan Kaufmann Publishers, 2002.

[3] Erik Lindholm and Mark J. Kligard and Henry Moreton. A user-programmable vertex engine. In *SIGGRAPH '01 Conference Proceedings*, pages 149–158, 2001.

[4] Mark Harris and David Luebke and Ian Buck and Naga Govindaraju and Jens Krüger and Aaron E. Lefohn and Timothy J. Purcell and Cliff Woolley. GPGPU: General-purpose computation on graphics hardware. *Course notes 32 of SIGGRAPH 2004*, 2004.

[5] A. Kolb and L. Latta and C. Rezk-Salama. Hardware-based simulation and collision detection for large particle systems. In *Eurographics Symp Proc Gr Hardware*, 2004.

[6] Naga K. Govindaraju and Stephane Redon and Ming C. Lin and Dinesh Manocha. Cullide: interactive collision detection between complex models in large environments using graphics hardware. In *Proceedings of the Conference on Graphics Hardware*, pages 25–32. Eurographics Association, 2003.

[7] Mark J. Harris and William V. Baxter and Thorsten Scheuermann and Anselmo Lastra. Simulation of cloud dynamics on graphics hardware. In *Proceedings of the Conference on Graphics Hardware*, pages 92–101. Eurographics Association, 2003.

[8] Timothy J. Purcell and Craig Donner and Mike Cammarano and Henrik Wann Jensen and Pat Hanrahan. Photon mapping on programmable graphics hardware. In *Proceedings of the Symposium on Graphics Hardware*, pages 41–50. Eurographics Association, 2003.

[9] Jens Krüger and Rüdiger Westermann. Linear algebra operators for gpu implementation of numerical algorithms. In *SIGGRAPH '03 Conference Proceedings*, pages 908–916, 2003.

[10] Jeff Bolz and Ian Farmer and Eitan Grinspun and Peter Schröder. Sparse matrix solvers on the gpu: conjugate gradients and multigrid. In *SIGGRAPH '03 Conference Proceedings*, pages 917–924, 2003.

[11] Le-Jeng Shiue and Ian Jones and J. Peters. A realtime gpu subdivision kernel. In Marcus Gross, editor, *Siggraph 2005, Computer Graphics Proceedings*, Annual Conf Series, pages 1010–1015. ACM Press, 2005.

Medicine Meets Virtual Reality 14
J.D. Westwood et al. (Eds.)
IOS Press, 2006

An Interactive Stereoscopic Display for Cooperative Work – Volume Visualization and Manipulation with Multiple Users

Yoshifumi KITAMURA

Human Interface Engineering Lab., Osaka University, Japan

Abstract. A stereoscopic display table for cooperative work with a volume data is described. Adequate stereoscopic image generated from the volume data is displayed and shared by multiple users. All the users can observe and interact with the volume data displayed on the IllusionHole in a face-to-face environment. It displays each pair of stereoscopic images such that all users observe the 3D image at exactly the same position. An outline of the system is described in this paper.

Keywords. Virtual Reality, Computer Human Interaction, CSCW, 3D User Interfaces, medical diagnosis, surgery planning, IllusionHole

1. Introduction

Stereoscopic displays have been increasingly used in many applications to observe complicated 3D information intelligibly. Therefore, in some application areas, there is great demand for incorporating stereoscopic displays for sharing 3D images by multiple users. For example, in medical diagnosis, training and surgery planning it is common for several people to exchange their ideas in front of a computer display monitor. These situations require the use of an interactive stereoscopic display that allows multiple users to simultaneously observe a stereoscopic image adequately and correctly. However, such a display has not been developed yet.

IllusionHole is a unique interactive stereoscopic display that allows three or more observers to simultaneously observe a stereoscopic image from their individual viewpoints [1]. With a simple configuration, it provides intelligible 3D stereoscopic images free of flicker and distortion. Moreover, all users observe the 3D image at exactly the same position. Therefore, IllusionHole is useful for applications in which several people work together to perform tasks with a multiplier effect.

In this paper, an interactive volume data visualization and manipulation system based on the idea of IllusionHole is described. A volume data displayed on the IllusionHole is shared by multiple users, and is interactively manipulated through discussions in a face-to-face environment.

2. System Configuration

The IllusionHole display system consists of a normal display and a display mask with a hole in the center. In order to display delicate tones of images of volume data, a DLP projector (Barco, Galaxy, 5,000 ANSI lumens) is used, and parameters of the hardware are designed as follows; a 1,388-mm-wide and 1,140-mm-deep display surface, with 1,140 mm height from the floor. The display mask is placed over the display surface at a suitable distance. Here, the hole radius of the display mask is determined to be 200 mm. The head position of each user is tracked by a 3D positional tracker (Intersense IS-600 Mark 2 SoniDisc), which is attached to LCD shutter glasses (Stereographics, CrystalEyes3) used for field-sequential stereo viewing.

The stereoscopic image of volume data for each user is generated by using a volume rendering software (AZE Ltd. VirtualPlace) according to the measured head position. Here, two different types of user interfaces are developed for manipulation of volume data. The one is a graphical user interface on PC for the purpose of selection of volume data and general adjustment of parameters of images. The other is a 3D user interface on IllusionHole that allows users to directly manipulate volume data intuitively.

3. Application Examples

Figure 1 shows an example of a volume data of a human body displayed on IllusionHole. Figure 1(a) shows a snapshot of IllusionHole shared by four users as observed from the fourth user's viewpoint. Figures (b), (c), and (d) show images observed by individual users standing to the left, center, and right of IllusionHole in Fig. 1(a), respectively. All users observe the same object but from different directions according to their viewpoints. Examples of volume data manipulation interface on IllusionHole using a stylus device are shown in Fig. 2.

IllusionHole displays each pair of stereoscopic images so that all users observe the 3D image at exactly the same position. This is done by making sure that the two images for each user have adequate disparity according to the measured viewpoint. By utilizing this feature, IllusionHole can be applied to cooperative works in which all users share a 3D image as if a real object is placed instead of the virtual one. For example, several medical doctors can simultaneously observe the patient's symptoms from their own viewpoints and exchange their opinions. Consequently, IllusionHole can be a powerful tool for making quick and accurate diagnoses, surgery simulation and training, and other medically related tasks.

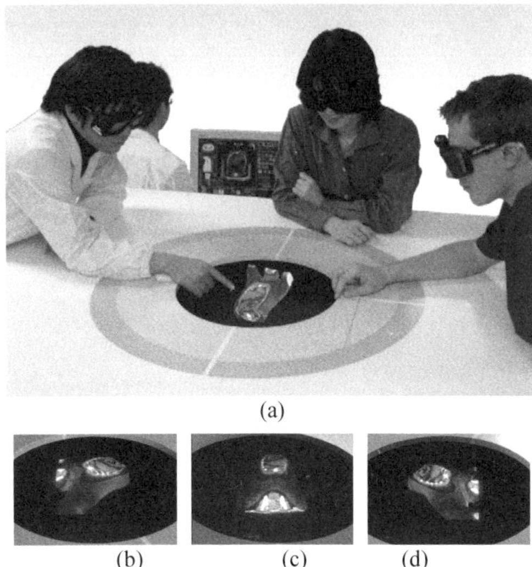

(a)

(b)　　　　(c)　　　　(d)

Figure 1. Volume data of a human body displayed on IllusionHole.

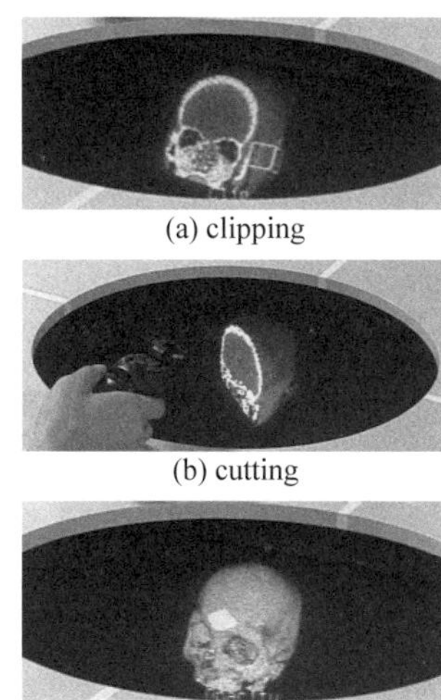

(a) clipping

(b) cutting

(c) adjusting of transparency

Figure 2. Examples of volume data manipulation interface on IllusionHole.

Acknowledgement

This research was supported in part by "Strategic Information and Communications R&D Promotion Programme (SCOPE)" of the Ministry of Internal Affairs and Communications, Japan.

References

[1]　Y. Kitamura, et al.: Interactive stereoscopic display for three or more users, *Computer Graphics Annual Conference Series (Proceedings of SIGGRAPH 2001)*, pp. 231–239 (2001).

Medicine Meets Virtual Reality 14
J.D. Westwood et al. (Eds.)
IOS Press, 2006

3D Live-Wires on Mosaic Volumes

Sebastian KÖNIG[1], Jürgen HESSER
Institute for Computational Medicine
Universities of Mannheim and Heidelberg
Germany

Abstract. The paper discusses the first evaluation of a 3D Live-Wire technique
that operates on over-segmented 3D mosaic volumes. Pre-processing normalizes
data by histogram spreading followed by over-segmentation with region growing.
This leads to a robust and intuitive parameter selection for various tissues and
image modalities without requiring problem specific knowledge.
During interactive segmentation from a set of user-defined seed points a triangle
mesh using Delaunay triangulation is generated. For each triangle, defined by three
seed points, a closed surface patch is generated by the 3D Live-Wire method.
For evaluation purpose white cerebral matter from MRI images is to be segmented.
A mean deviation from the correct object boundary extracted from available model
data of about 0.60 pixels (± 0.23) is observed while the required time was about
229.5 seconds (± 173.2).

Keywords. Segmentation, 3D Live-Wires, Volume Data.

Introduction

Segmentation decomposes an image into its constituent parts, i.e. the location and
outline of objects of interest in an image, whereby semiautomatic methods combine the
automatic processing with dedicated application specific knowledge of the user. By
identifying interesting image components the user can restrict the segmentation process
to relevant areas.

Live-Wires [1, 2] are an interactive, edge-based image segmentation method and
use gradient magnitude for the separation of the object from the background. Compared
to automatic segmentation methods like e.g. snakes or min-cuts, Live-Wires allow a
higher quality of segmentation and local optimization at the cost of a higher amount of
user interaction.

The original image data is transformed into a weighted graph [1, 7, 8] where
weights are derived from the image gradient. Next, the desired object boundary is
calculated piecewise as cost minimal paths between user selected seed points. Various
improvements were proposed, especially with focus on performance issues and the
extension of the original two-dimensional approach to volume data [3 – 8].

---

[1] Corresponding author: Sebastian König, University of Mannheim, Institute for Computational Medicine,
B6 23-29, 68131 Mannheim, Germany; E-mail: skoenig@rumms.uni-mannheim.de

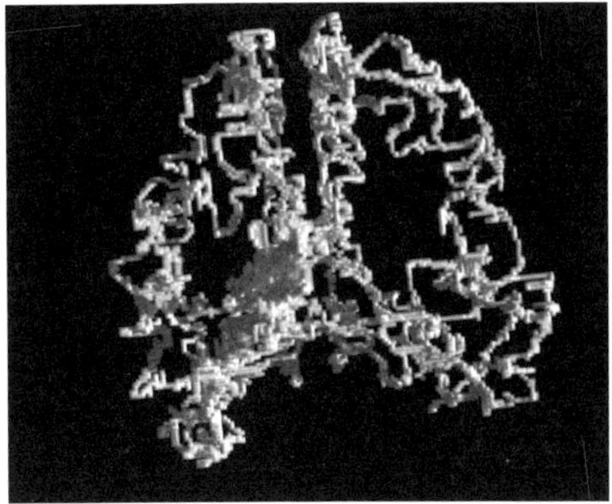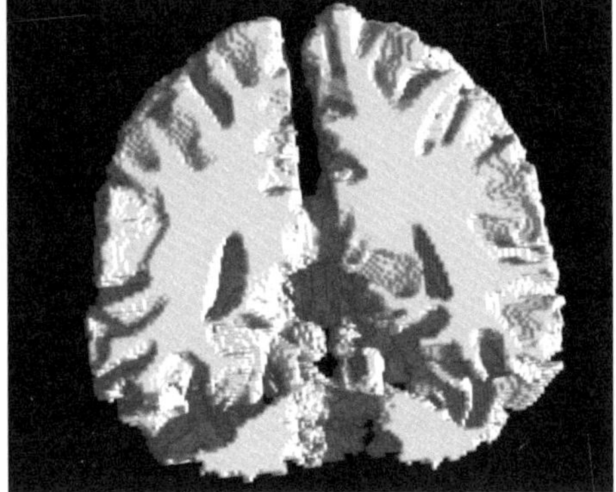

Figure 1. Left: Initial surface framework connecting the seeds. Right: Segmented white matter volume.

1. Methods

1.1. Automatic Pre-Segmentation and Graph Generation

The image volume is over-segmented into a mosaic volume using region growing in a first step, but selecting an optimal region growing threshold by hand is a non-trivial and error-prone task [7, 8].

To simplify this step and to improve the quality of the pre-segmentation histogram spreading is applied allowing for contrast independent pre-processing. Instead of tuning the region growing threshold the user's task is reduced to select typical gray values for object and background. Histogram spreading emphasizes regions of interest by normalizing the higher typical value to the maximum and the lower typical value to zero, thus suppressing gray values and structures below or above the typical interval. The region growing step is performed on this spread data allowing a fixed region growing threshold for all kind of tissues and modalities of MRI.

The graph for Live-Wires is constructed from the resulting mosaic volume by assigning surfaces between two homogeneous mosaic regions ("facets") as graph nodes and topological connecting lines as edges [8].

1.2. Surface Patch Segmentation from Three Seed Points

A surface patch defined by a triple of seed facets is calculated in three steps as described in detail in [8]. First, cost optimal paths between all seed pairs are computed leading to an initial frame (cf. figure 1). Cost terms used consist of a sophisticated dynamic term taking into account the typical user-defined gray values for object and background from the pre-processing. Additional spokes divide the initial frame into sub-frames. These spokes consist of paths calculated between one of the seeds and the opposite path. After a final gap filling step a closed object boundary patch is achieved.

1.3. Forming Larger Surfaces from a Set of Seeds

Surface patches sharing two seeds share the connecting path between them as well. Therefore, bigger surface areas can be composed by connected patches. A set of user selected seed facets on the desired surface or object boundary is transformed into a set of seed triples using Delaunay triangulation. These triples define the framework for the surface and lead to surface patches as described in subsection 1.2.

2. Results

In order to achieve an objective evaluation we use a synthetic MRI volume and model data taken from the BrainWeb database[2] (181×217×181 voxel, 8 bit, modality T1, slice thickness 1 mm, noise 3%, intensity non-uniformity 20%).

The region growing threshold was set to 0.2 for all segmentations. The segmentations were performed on a Pentium IV 3 GHz PC, 1 GByte RAM.

We analyzed 20 segmentations of the boundary between gray and white matter and achieved a mean deviation between the segmented surface patches and the model data of 0.596 pixels (± 0.225), 8.521% (± 9.628) false positives and 8.561% (± 4.334) false negatives. The mean computation time per surface was 229.5 seconds (± 173.2). On average 20.2 (± 5.0) user selected seed points were set per surface.

3. Conclusion

The histogram spreading allows a higher and more selective data reduction, a better segmentation quality and further simplifies the user interaction (cf. [8]). While the time for segmentation is still high, optimizations currently implemented could cut this cost by up to one order of magnitude, thus rendering this method to interactive.

References

[1]   E.N. Mortensen, B.S. Morse, W.A. Barrett, J.K. Udupa: *Adaptive Boundary Detection Using Live-Wire Two-Dimensional Dynamic Programming*. IEEE Proc. of Computers in Cardiology (CIC'92), pp. 635-638, 1992.

[2]   E.N. Mortensen, W.A. Barrett: *Intelligent Scissors for Image Composition*. Computer Graphics (SIGGRAPH `95), pp. 191-198, 1995.

[3]   E.N. Mortensen, W.A. Barrett: *Toboggan-Based Intelligent Scissors with a Four Parameter Edge Model*. IEEE: Computer Vision and Pattern Recognition, 2, pp. 452-458, IEEE Computer Society, 1999.

[4]   A.X. Falcao, J. Udupa, S. Samarasekera, S. Sharma: *User-Steered Image Segmentation Paradigms: Live Wire and Live Lane*. Graphical Models and Image Processing, 60(4), pp. 233-260, 1998.

[5]   A.X. Falcao, J. Udupa, F.K. Miyazawa: *An Ultra-Fast User-Steered Image Segmentation Paradigm: Live Wire on the Fly*. IEEE: Transactions on Medical Imaging, 19(1), pp. 55-61, 2000.

[6]   S. König, J. Hesser: *Live-Wires on Edges of Presegmented 2D-Data*. Bildverarbeitung für die Medizin 2003, T. Wittenberg et al., pp. 156-160, Springer, Erlangen (Germany), 2003.

[7]   S. König, J. Hesser: *Live-Wires Using Path Graphs*. Methods of Information in Medicine, 43, pp. 371-375, 2004.

[8]   S. König, J. Hesser: *3D Live-Wires on Pre-Segmented Volume Data*. Proc. of SPIE Medical Imaging 2005: Image Processing, pp. 1674-1679, 2005.

---

[2] BrainWeb: Simulated Brain Database. http://www.bic.mni.mcgill.ca/brainweb

Medicine Meets Virtual Reality 14
J.D. Westwood et al. (Eds.)
IOS Press, 2006

Surgical PACS
for the Digital Operating Room

Systems Engineering and Specification of User Requirements

Werner Korb [a,1], Stefan Bohn [a], Oliver Burgert [a], Andreas Dietz [a,b], Stephan Jacobs [a,c],
Volkmar Falk [a,c], Jürgen Meixensberger [a,d], Gero Strauß [a,b], Christos Trantakis [a,d] and
Heinz U. Lemke [a]

[a] *Innovation Center Computer Assisted Surgery, Leipzig, Germany.*
[b] *University Hospital Leipzig, Department of ENT Surgery, Leipzig Germany.*
[c] *Herzzentrum Leipzig, Department of Heartsurgery, University Leipzig, Germany.*
[d] *University Hospital Leipzig, Department of Neurosurgery, Leipzig Germany.*

Abstract. For better integration of surgical assist systems into the operating room,
a common communication and processing plattform that is based on the users
needs is needed. The development of such a system, a Surgical Picture Aquisition
and Communication System (S-PACS), according the systems engineering cycle is
oulined in this paper. The first two steps (concept and specification) for the engineering of the S-PACS are discussed.

A method for the systematic integration of the users needs', the Quality Function Deployment (QFD), is presented. The properties of QFD for the underlying
problem and first results are discussed. Finally, this leads to a first definition of an
S-PACS system.

Keywords. image-guided surgery, digital operating room, Surgical PACS, systems
engineering cycle, user requirements, surgical assist systems

1. Introduction

Unlike in the business and automation industry, there exists no communication platform
within the operating theatre that allows unified data exchange between imaging systems and other surgical assist systems (SAS) such as navigation or mechatronic devices
[1,2,3]. Many SASs have good functionality as stand-alone facilities, however they lack
plug-and-play features. SASs are required for surgical interventions and should be well
integrated into the surgical procedures to allow interoperability, e.g. smooth communication of data such as images and signals as well as the visualization of data.

The lack of proper human-machine interfaces in the digital operating room can be
considered as a main problem. As of today, surgeons and clinical personel need to be
specially motivated and require some technical ability as well as an interest in research

---

[1]Correspondence to: Werner Korb, Innovation Center Computer Assisted Surgery (ICCAS), Faculty of
Medicine, University of Leipzig, Philipp-Rosenthal Strasse 55, D-04103 Leipzig, Germany. Tel.: +49 341 97
12000; Fax: +49 341 97 12009; E-mail: werner.korb@iccas.de.

when they use SASs. Image aquisition, image selection, image processing and image visualization are often not possible according to the users' needs. The users are forced to be satisfied with limited technical features of current systems. Interconnection may improve the range of technical possiblities and allow more flexible user interaction.

One of the research focuses of the *Innovation Center Computer Assisted Surgery* (ICCAS) in Leipzig, Germany, addresses the above problems with the development of a *Surgical Picture Acquisition and Communication System (S-PACS)*. Other research topics of ICCAS include surgical workflow [4], information and communication technology (ICT) in surgery and systematic clinical evaluation of SASs.

2. Materials and Methods

2.1. Systems engineering cycle

For the prototype development of an S-PACS at ICCAS, the steps generally prescribed in the systems engineering cycle (SEC) will be followed: (a) concept, (b) specification, (c) modular and detail design, (d) implementation, (e) tests, (f) applications, (g) maintenance. Particular care should be given to the right organizational embedding of the SEC into the S-PACS project. In this context it is advisable to take account of an observation by the Standish Group [5,6], which surveyed IT executive managers for their opinions about why projects do or do not succeed. The three major reasons for success are user involvement (15.9% of responses), executive management support (13.9%), and a clear statement of requirements (13%). There are other success criteria, but with these three elements in place, the chances of success are higher. Without them, the chance of failure increases dramatically.

This survey shows the high importance of the integration of users and executive managers (in the case of ICCAS, the scientific/medical board) into the SEC. In ICCAS this involvement started from the first S-PACS concept, continued in the specification phase and also in subsequent steps, which are, however, not discussed in this paper. The scientific/medical board of 9 members includes 2/3 surgeons from three different disciplines (neuro-, ENT and cardiovascular surgery) and 1/3 engineers. The board members were all involved in working out the proposal for the project, which is currently funded by the federal government of Germany (**Concept Phase**). The user requirements and their importance ratings were elaborated in different workshops of the board (**Specification Phase**).

2.2. Risk factors

Some classical examples of risk factors for software engineering are outlined in [5]. The most important factors are collocated in Tab. 1 and completed with the relevance in the S-PACS project within ICCAS. The risk factors can be categorized into 4 main groups according the relative importance (cf. survey of the Standish Group) and the perceived level of control (see [5] and Fig. 1).

The items of category 1 (C1) are therefore most relevant for the development in software engineering projects and are the basis for the choice of the QFD method [7] that is described in the following section.

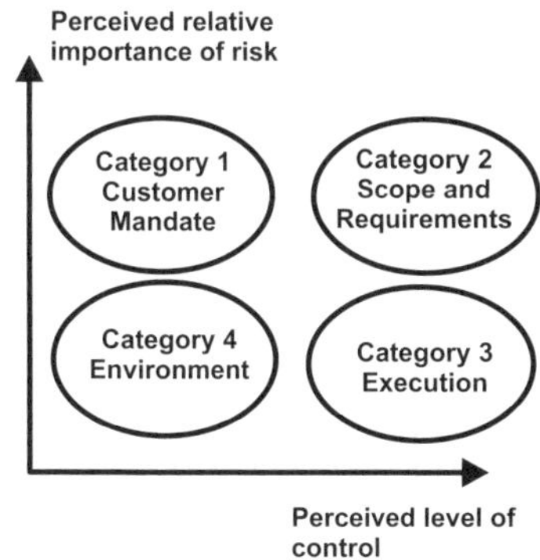

Figure 1. A risk categorization framework (developed by [5])

C	Risk Factor Description (cf. [5])	Relevance/Strategy in S-PACS Development (ICCAS)
1	Lack of user participation	At ICCAS, users from three surgical dispciplines are involved (^{1})
1	Conflict between users	Everyone involved understands challenge (^{2})
1	Users resistant to change or with negative attitudes towards the project	Generally surgeons may be sceptical to change; at ICCAS change is initiated by surgeons
1	Lack of cooperation from users	Record problems on-site in the operating room
1	Lack of top management support	Clinic directors have to be involved (^{3})
1	Lack/loss of organizational commitment	–
2	Undefined project-success criteria	Use of *Success Resource Deployment (SRD)*
2	Conflicting, unclear or incorrect system requirements	Use of *Quality Function Deployment (QFD)* simulation, test beds
2	Ill-defined project goals	Use of QFD and feedback from users
3	Social problems and team conflicts	–
3	New technology with high level of technical complexity	Potential risk for S-PACS development; therefore abstraction to formal level
3	Highly complex task being automated	Use of workflow analysis
3	Project affects a large number of user departments or units	Potential risk because different surgical disciplines are involved; early interaction is needed
3	One of the largest projects attempted by the organization	Potential risk for S-PACS development in ICCAS; definition of smaller sub-projects
3	Ineffective communication	Regular meetings/discussions with all involved parties.
4	Dependency on outside suppliers and other environmental risks	The standardisation working group *DICOM in surgery* is important and supported by ICCAS

Table 1. The project risk factors for the development of a Surgical PACS system within ICCAS only those risk factors from [5] are selected that are relevant for the S-PACS development; they are explained in the right column; (^{1}) - (^{3}) refer to section 2.3.

2.3. User involvement and user requirements

Quality function deployment (QFD) is a structured and quantitative method to identify customer needs under the umbrella of *constancy of purpose*. It can play an important role in systems engineering for implementations that are cross-functional and complex.

QFD begins with *brainstorming* any benefits the customer may require within the scope of the problem. The user requirements are then structured in a tree. Each node in the tree is assigned with an *importance rating (IR)* as agreed by the group of users. Based on the IRs, a rating (*impact factors IF*) of the entries in the tree is possible. The user requirements (quality) are combined with engineering attributes (function) in a matrix. The matrix allows an efficient implementation (prototyping) to be performed according to the user's needs, because the engineering attributes are mapped to the user requirements. In particular, the application of QFD within the S-PACS project allows (cf. category 1 in Tab. 1)

(^{1}) the surgeons to be involved in structured group discussions (this is carried out within a given limited time period, in order not to overload the tight working schedule of surgeons)

(^{2}) easy understanding of the challenge (based on a clear structure of discussion)

(^{3}) the ICCAS board (management) and the clinical directors to be involved

(^{4}) the requirements to be rated (based on the IRs of a reasonable number of surgeons, at the specification state also a quantitative expression of the requirements is possible)

3. Results

At ICCAS, three surgical disciplines (neuro-, ENT and cardiovascular surgery) and different engineering disciplines (computer science, medical informatics, applied mathematics, biomedical engineering) were involved in working out the QFD tree, which includes all the necessary components and systems characteristics as well as the project-management steps, to develop an S-PACS. On a first level, the tree consists of the branches:

1. systems components
2. systems characteristics
3. standards and interfaces
4. project management
5. validation and evaluation
6. collaborations

These branches will be further detailed according to a given relationship between the node descriptions. For example, it is only reasonable to finalize the systems characteristics as well as the standards and interfaces, after the systems components branch is established, etc. The user requirements mainly influence the first subtree *systems components*. In Fig. 2 the first two levels of this subtree are shown. A more detailed QFD tree of a Surgical PACS as specified by the ICCAS interdisciplinary workgroup is provided in www.surgical-pacs.org .

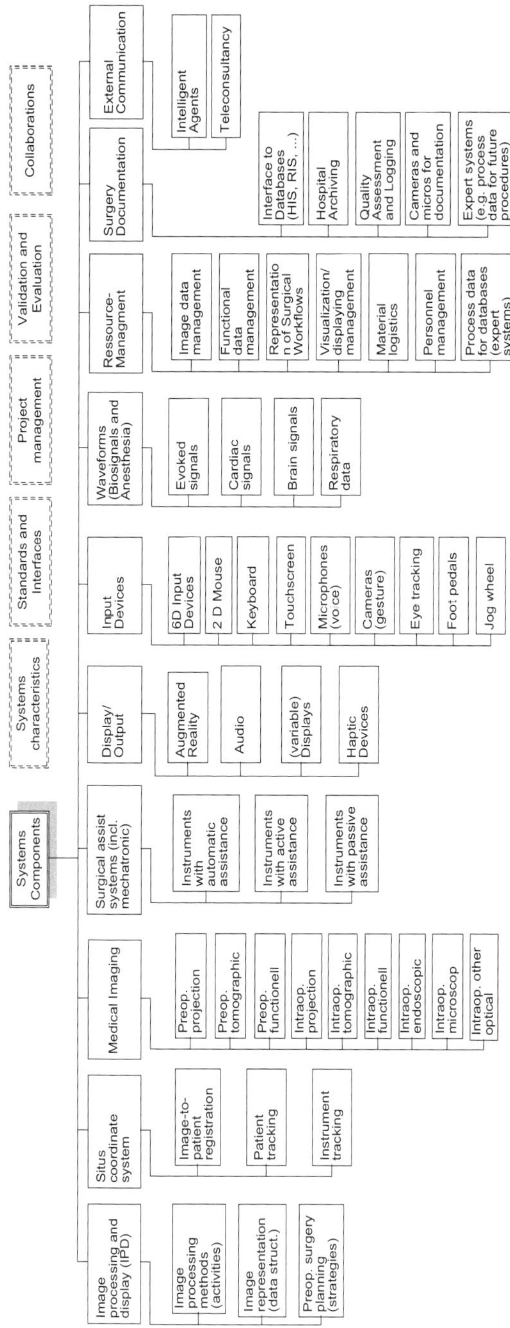

Figure 2. The *Systems Components* subtree of the S-PACS QFD tree (up to the third level).

4. Conclusion

From the preceding paragraphs we conclude with the following **definition of an S-PACS system**: The *Surgical Picture Aquisition and Communciation System* (in short: S-PACS) is a system for enabling management of images and associated information for image-guided surgery. It is a set of ICT devices, including software, that integrate surgical assist systems (SAS), as well as clinical-information systems. An S-PACS (optionally augmented with a workflow/ressource-management system) provides the IT infrastructure in the operating theatre. (cf. Fig. 2)

Development of an S-PACS should only be based on surgical workflow analysis and QFD specifications.

Possible prototype realizations of an S-PACS system are currently in development in ICCAS, such as a system for image-guided navigated neurosurgery including the usage of intraopative 3D sonography [8].

Acknowledgment

The presented work is supported by the Federal Ministry of Education and Research (BMBF) in Germany (Grant No. 03 ZIK 031 and 03 ZIK 032, *Centres for Innovation Competence: Create Excellence - Foster Talent*). ICCAS is also supported by the Saxon Ministry of Science and the Fine Arts (SMWK).

References

[1] Lemke HU, Osman MR, Horii SC: Workflow in the Operating Room: Review of Arrowhead 2004 Seminar on Imaging and Informatics, SPIE Conference on PACS and Imaging Informatics, Vol. 5748, 2005.

[2] Cleary K, Kinsella A, Mun SK: OR 2020 workshop report: operating room of the future. In: Lemke HU, Inamura K et al., eds. Computer Assisted Radiology and Surgery 2005, Berlin, Germany. Amsterdam: Elsevier, pp. 832-838, 2005.

[3] Schorr O, Pernozzoli A, Haag C, Brief J, Raczkowsky J, Hassfeld S, Woern H: Ein Prozess- und Architekturmodell für die Computer assistierte Chirurgie. In: Boenick U, Bolz A, eds. Beiträge zur 36. Jahrestagung der Deutschen Gesellschaft für Biomedizinische Technik (DGBMT) im VDE, pp. 86-89, 2002.

[4] Neumuth T, Durstewitz N, Fischer M, Strauss G, Dietz A, Jannin P, Cleary K, Lemke HU, Burgert O: Structured Recording of Intraoperative Surgical Workflows. In: Proceedings of the SPIE Conference on Medical Imaging, 11 - 16 February 2006, San Diego, California USA, 2006 (accepted for publication).

[5] Wallace L, Keil M: Software Project Risks and their Effect on Outcomes. Communications of the ACM 47(4), pp 68-73, 2004.

[6] www.standishgroup.com, CHAOS Report, 1994.

[7] Lemke HU, Heuser H, Pollack T, Niederlag W: Request for Proposal for PACS Planning and Evaluation. In: Lemke HU, Vannier MW et al., eds. Computer Assisted Radiology and Surgery. Amsterdam: Elsevier, pp. 871-6, 2000.

[8] Lindner D, Trantakis C, Arnold S, Schmitgen A, Schneider JP, Meixensberger J. Neuronavigation based on intraoperative 3D-Ultrasound during tumor resection. In: Lemke HU, Inamura K et al., eds. Computer Assisted Radiology and Surgery 2005, Berlin, Germany. Amsterdam: Elsevier, pp. 815-820, 2005.

Medicine Meets Virtual Reality 14
J.D. Westwood et al. (Eds.)
IOS Press, 2006

Smooth Vasculature Reconstruction with Circular and Elliptic Cross Sections

Karl Krissian[1], Xunlei Wu[2], and Vincent Luboz[2]

[1]*SPL, Brigham and Women's Hospital, http://splweb.bwh.harvard.edu,*
[2]*The SIM Group – CIMIT/MGH, http://www.medicalsim.org,*
karl@bwh.harvard.edu and {xwu4, vluboz}@partners.org

Abstract: This paper presents a method to segment and reconstruct vascular structure from patient volumetric scan. First, a semi-automatic segmentation phase leads to the vessels centerlines and the estimated circular or elliptic cross section description. Then, the skeleton data are used by the reconstruction phase to generate the three dimensional vascular surface. This structured surface is able to handle interactive visualization, real-time and robust physics-based modeling. The accuracy and consistency of our technique are evaluated on a vascular phantom as well as two clinical data sets. Experiments show that the proposed technique reaches a good balance in terms of mesh smoothness, compactness, and accuracy, where elliptic cross section estimation induces lower error.

1. Introduction

In the context of assisted vascular surgery, starting with a complete, accurate and robust vascular network is the key. Indeed, such a network could lead to real-time interventional radiology simulation system where physicians would be able to learn and practice without putting patients at risk. To fulfill these goals, this vasculature must be *smooth* for visualization, *structured* for blood flow computation, and *efficient* for real time collision detection/collision response. This paper presents a method to generate this complete vascular surface, as a part of the simulator developed at the SIM Group [1].

Most of the techniques generating vascular networks are based on two steps: segmentation followed by reconstruction. The segmentation uses either contour enhancement methods (including statistical approaches: Expectation Maximization [2], random Markov fields), or geometrical methods (region growing, adaptive thresholding, explicit or implicit active contours). The most famous technique, the level sets [3, 4], belongs to the implicit active contour family. It is usually preceded by a noise reduction step.

The reconstruction technique relies on the segmentation result. If the segmentation result is ridges then a "marching cube-like" algorithm [5] is applied to get the vascular surface. If it is a skeleton, then a meshing technique is used [6]. An up-to-date survey on surface reconstruction techniques is presented in [7].

2. Methodology

Our method, presented in details in [8, 9], follows the two main steps presented above: segmentation and reconstruction. It performs a streamlined process composed of: noise reduction, active contour segmentation, skeletonization, radius estimation, and surface reconstruction. The goal of this approach is to preserve the topology of the vasculature and generate a smooth and compact surface in order to suit the needs of the simulator [1].

2.1. Segmentation

Anisotropic diffusion precedes the segmentation to reduce the noise while enhancing small vascular structures. This filter, based on [10], enables better segmentation. Then, a set of morphological operations are applied to remove the bones and the skin. Their intensity values are similar to those of vessels. This might disturb the segmentation process.

A level set algorithm [3] is then used to segment the main vessels' contours. The equation is based on advection, smoothing and expansion terms. A skeletonization is then applied to the data set resulting from the level sets. It gives a simple representation of the network as a centerline set. The skeleton is obtained through homotopic thinning [11].

Pruning, connection and smoothing are then applied to the skeleton. The first one aims at small branches of the skeleton due to noise. The remaining lines are then connected to avoid centerline discontinuity and to get closer to a unique tree. This step is necessary to connect disconnected line sections, which go in the same direction, and are separated due to the medical data set resolution. To obtain a unique tree, manual line connection is often needed since it is not easy to determine if lines should be connected or not automatically. The resulting skeleton is then smoothed.

Finally, starting from the centerlines, the vasculature geometry is computed. In [8, 9], we estimate it through a circle fitting. A circle is grown in the plane of each cross-section and stopped when there is a relevant maximum of the intensity gradient of the data set.

Fitting an ellipse instead of a circle estimates the cross sections (CS) in a better way. This matches real vasculature geometry better without sacrificing the smoothness and the low complexity of the mesh. Based on initial estimated centerlines and a segmentation of the vascular network, ellipses are fitted in the planes of the vessel CS's. Each plane is orthogonal to the centerlines locally. The ellipses are fitted at points regularly distributed along each centerline. The fitting procedure uses a mean least square error described in [12] based on the points extracted from an iso-contour of the current cross-section. An iterative scheme improves both the fitted ellipses and the sub-voxel locations of the ellipse centers. This is done by updating the position of the centerline sampling points based on the center of the fitted ellipses and then using the updated centerline to estimate new ellipses. Two iterations are experimentally sufficient to reach almost convergence (displacements of the centerlines is less than *0.1mm*).

2.2. Surface Reconstruction

The proposed method reconstructs topologically preserving quadrilateral surface patches of branching tubular structure given the vascular centerlines and the description of either circular or elliptic cross section (CS) at each sampling point. The motivation of introducing elliptic CS estimation is that ellipse provides higher degree of freedom (DOF) than circles. The additional flexibility will improve the reconstruction accuracy at vessel joints, stenosis, aneurysm, and places whose CS shape is far from circles. And yet the abstract closed curve description retains the compactness and smoothness as in the case of circular CS.

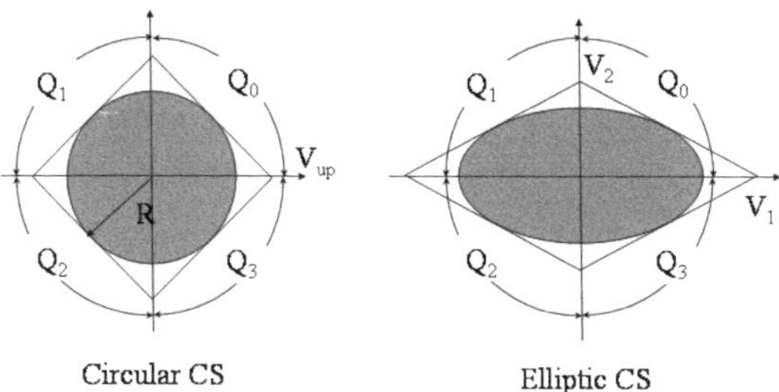

Figure 1: Illustration of the 4 quadrants placement under circular (*Left*) and elliptic (*Right*) CS.

The description of elliptic CS from skeletonization is more complex than circular CS. Only one scalar value is needed for the radius of each circle, whereas two ordered vectors, $\vec{v}_1$ and $\vec{v}_2$, the magnitude of which r_1 and r_2 reflects the main axes radii, are used for each ellipse. The order of such vectors is consistent with that of adjacent CS such that adjacent CS normal vectors, i.e. $\vec{n} = \vec{v}_1 \times \vec{v}_2 / |\vec{v}_1 \times \vec{v}_2|$, form an acute angle. $\vec{v}_1, \vec{v}_2, \vec{n}$ provide the local frame of each CS who is perpendicular to the tangent of local centerline.

Table 1: The differences of circular and elliptic CS estimation schemes.

	Circular CS	Elliptic CS
Data Representation	1 scalar	2 ordered vectors
Circumscribed Polygon	Square	Rhombus
V_{up} Propagation	Yes	No
CS Distribution	Radius+Curvature	Area+Curvature
Trunk Branch Selection	Radius+Angle	Area+Angle
Advantages	Minimize surface twist due vector propagation; Compact skeleton representation.	Improve the accuracy of reconstructed surface; Easier to implement.
Shortcomings	Deficient to represent non-circular sections.	Rely highly on segmentation quality.

There is no need to propagate the *"up"* vector as in circular CS case since the four quadrants $Q_{0...3}$ are determined by $\vec{v_1}$ and $\vec{v_2}$ naturally demonstrated in Fig. 1. Also, the adaptive CS distribution and the trunk branch selection are slightly modified to rely on ellipse's area rather than circle's radius in [9]. Tab. 1 summarizes the differences of circular and elliptic CS estimation approaches.

3. Tests and evaluation

3.1. Circular CS Results

These results are detailed in [8, 9]. Against a vascular phantom, our analysis shows that length variation stays within *1.0mm*, while $2\sigma_{length}=3.5mm$. The radius variation is always under *0.2mm*, with *0.6mm* inter pixel space. We also test our surface to an iso-surface by Marching-Cube [5], which is treated as the reference. From our reconstructed surface to the reference surface, *Hausdorff* distance error is computed using *MESH[1]*. The root mean square (RMS) error is always sub-voxel (*<0.6mm*). The error monotonically decays as the surface is refined. The surface smoothness, measured by the RMS of the minimal surface curvature, is *0.03* uniformly on our reconstructed surfaces with *5%* iso-surface triangles, which is 10 times smoother than any decimated surfaces (between *0.3* and *0.7*).

3.2. Elliptic CS Results

In the circular CS based test, the maximum *Hausdorff* distance error is *<3.5mm*, which is still quite large comparing to the sub-voxel RMS error. We observe the maximum error happens around vessel joints whose CS's are far from circles. When evaluating elliptic CS estimation against circular approach, *Hausdorff* distance analysis is used on the basilar artery session as shown in Fig 2.

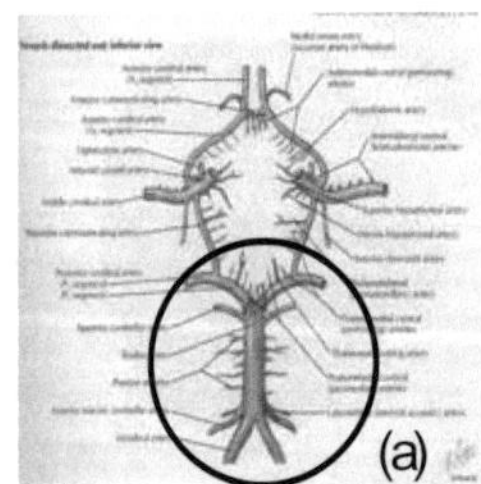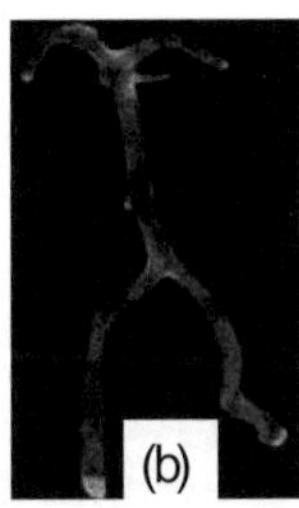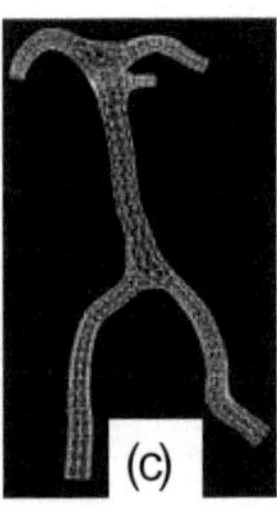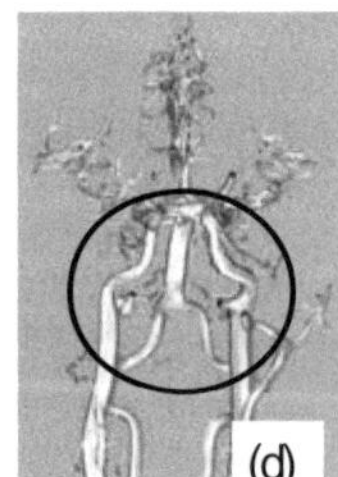

Figure 2: (a) Anatomy of the circle of Willis; (b) segmented iso-surface; error color code ranges from blue (0.0mm) to red (3.0mm), (c) reconstructed arterial surface. (d) zoom-out view of (c).

Fig. 3 shows the RMS and the maximum errors between the reconstructed surface and the iso-surface. By using elliptic CS estimation, the RMS error is consistently smaller than the circular CS counterpart as depicted in the upper half of Fig.3. The lower half of Fig. 3 is more encouraging since the maximum error decreases more than *40%* from *2.3mm* to *1.4mm* under no subdivision. Elliptic CS estimation based surface

---

[1] http://mesh.berlioz.de

patching achieves better accuracy and is more versatile in representing vessel joints and vessel malformation, e.g. stenosis and aneurysm whose shapes are far from a circle.

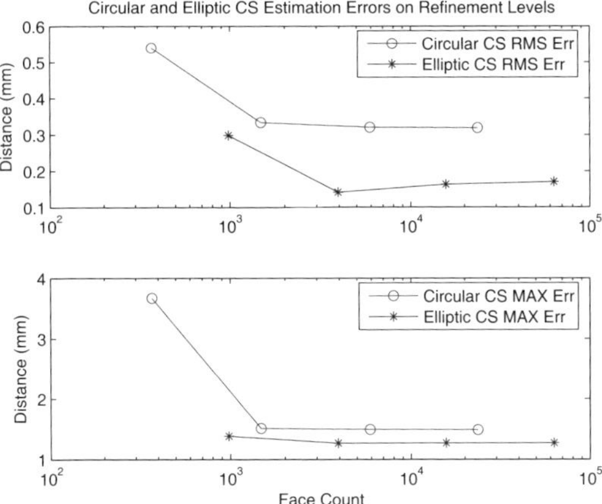

Figure 3: Elliptic CS based vascular surface patching consistently improves the surface accuracy over circular CS based technique in both RMS and maximum error tests.

4. Conclusion

A new method for segmenting and reconstructing a structured, smooth, and efficient vasculature is presented in this article. It consists in a streamlined process from a patient CTA scan to a 3D surface. The evaluation of our method on a phantom showed that it is producing homogeneous and accurate skeletons. The introduction of elliptic CS based surface patching has improved this accuracy, especially around non-circular areas, without losing the advantages of surface smoothness and compactness as in the circular CS case. Tested against both a vascular phantom and real clinical data sets, the reconstructed surfaces are at least *10* times smoother and yet uses *20* times less triangles than the decimated iso-surfaces. These results demonstrate the accuracy and robustness of our method.

The main drawback of our method is that it is not fully automatic and manual labor is often required to recover tiny vessels, whose diameters are of the same order as scan resolution. The skeleton of these tiny vessels appears as disconnected line segments after pruning. Also vessels located in proximity with others needs manual intervention. The amount of manual interaction would be greatly reduced by introducing a vascular atlas or template. Hence, tiny vessels and tangent vessels should be easier to identify. An automatic correction of centerline orientation is also under investigation based on graph theory. Finally, testing on more patient scans would help to validate the whole streamlined method proposed before integrating the process into the vascular interventional simulation system mentioned above.

5. Ongoing work

Our method is currently extended to a new application: the segmentation and the reconstruction of heart coronaries shown in Fig. 4 (a). The reconstructed coronaries are showed in Fig. 4 (b).

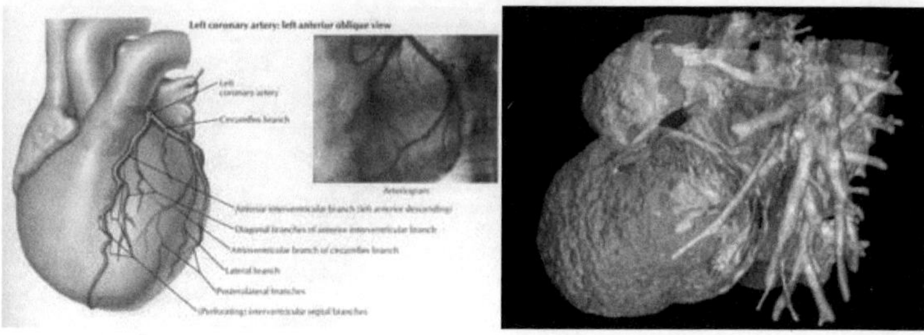

Figure 4: (a) Anatomy and angiography of the left coronary. (b) Reconstruction of the left coronary vessels in red overlaid over the heart iso-surface.

Under angiography, the heart scan does not have the artifacts presented in neuro-vascular regions. This primitive result is encouraging since the vascular surface is generated automatically from our proposed process without any manual interaction. Consequently, it seems possible to apply our technique to reconstruct the whole coronary vascular network with great detail with minimal manual intervention.

References:

[1] Duriez C., Lenoir J., Neumann P., Cotin S.: New approaches to catheter navigation for interventional radiology simulation. Proceedings of Medical Image Computing and Computer Assisted Intervention, MICCAI 2005.

[2] Wells, W. M. and Grimson, W. E. L. and Kikinis, Ron and Jolesz, Ferenc A. Adaptive Segmentation of MRI Data Springer-Verlag, 1995 , 905 , 59-69.

[3] Sethian, J.A. Level Set Methods and Fast Marching Methods: Evolving Interfaces in Comp. Geom., Fluid Mech., Comp. Vision and Materials Sci. Cambridge Univ. Press, 1999.

[4] Suri, J.S., Liu, K., Singh, S., Laxminarayan, S.N., Zeng, X., Reden, L.: Shape recovery algorithms using level sets in 2D/3D medical imagery: state-of-the-art review IEEE Transactions on Information Technology in Biomedicine, 2002 , vol. 6 , pp. 8-28.

[5] Lorensen W., Cline H.: Marching cubes: A high resolution 3d surface construction algorithm. In Computer Graphics Proceedings (1987), vol. 21, SIGGRAPH, pp. 163–169.

[6] Felkel, P., Wegenkittl, R., Bühler, K.: Surface Models of Tube Trees. Proceeding of CGI, 2004, pp. 70-77.

[7] Bühler, K., Felkel, P., La Cruz, A.: Geometric Methods for Vessel Visualization and Quantification - A Survey. VRVis Research Center, Austria, 2002, Technical Report, pp. 24-48.

[8] Luboz V., Wu X., Krissian K., Westin C.F., Kikinis R., Cotin S., & Dawson S. A segmentation and reconstruction technique for 3D vascular structures. P Proceedings of Medical Image Computing and Computer Assisted Intervention, MICCAI 2005, pp. 43-50.

[9] Wu X., Luboz V., and Krissian K. Smooth Vasculature Reconstruction from Patient Scan. Workshop On Virtual Reality Interaction and Physical Simulation (VRIPHYS), Pisa, Italy, November 2005.

[10] Krissian, Karl Flux-based anisotropic diffusion applied to enhancement of 3-D angiogram. IEEE Trans Med Imaging, 2002, 21, 1440-2.

[11] Malandain G., Bertrand G., Ayache N. Topological Segmentation of Discrete Surfaces International Journal of Computer Vision, vol.10, pp. 183-197, 1993.

[12] Fitzgibbon A., Pilu M. and Fisher R.B., 1999. Direct Least Square Fitting of Ellipses. IEEE Transactions on Pattern Analysis and Machine Intelligence (PAMI), vol. 21, no. 5.

Medicine Meets Virtual Reality 14
J.D. Westwood et al. (Eds.)
IOS Press, 2006

Towards a VR Trainer for EVAR Treatment

E. KUNST[a,1], S. RÖDEL[b], F. MOLL[c,d], C. VAN DEN BERG[d], J. TEIJINK[e], J. VAN HERWAARDEN[c,d], J. VAN DER PALEN[f], R. GEELKERKEN[b]
[a] Kunst & van Leerdam Medical Technology bv, Enschede, the Netherlands; ekunst@kvlmt.nl; [b] Department of Vascular Surgery, Medical Spectrum Twente, Enschede, NL; [c] Department of Vascular Surgery, University Medical Centre, Utrecht, NL; [d] Department of Surgery, Saint Antonius Hospital, Nieuwegein,NL; [e] Deparment of Surgery, Atrium Medical Centre, Heerlen, NL; [f] Department of Epidemiology, Medical Spectrum Twente, NL.

Abstract Endovascular repair of aortic abdominal aneurysms (AAA) is more and more becoming part of clinical practice. Up to approximately 30 clinical procedures however are necessary to obtain the surgical skills to make the procedure reliable and safe. The current study aims to generate a VR trainer to speed up the training process of experienced vascular surgeons to become experienced EVAR (endovascular AAA repair) surgeons by introducing a VR environment. This manuscript describes the contents and validation of the first step in the VREST – EVAR trainer, i.e. the proper definition of the knowledge and skills that need to be transferred.

1. Background / Problem

Endovascular repair of aortic abdominal aneurysms (AAA) is more and more becoming part of clinical practice[1,2,3,4]. Literature indicates that the reliability of the performance of such a highly specialized procedure requires a learning curve of approximately 30 cases[5].

The current study aims to generate a VR trainer to speed up the training process of experienced vascular surgeons to become experienced EVAR (endovascular AAA repair) surgeons by introducing a VR environment and to improve the reliability and safety of the clinical procedure. The VR trainer is being build on the VREST Platform for Virtual Medical Training[6].

The VREST – EVAR trainer involves three steps. The first focuses on the proper definition of the knowledge and skills that need to be transferred. The second stage offers an interactive simulation environment to become acquainted with the knowledge and EVAR protocol. The third step includes real-time 3D visual and haptic feedback.

---

[1] Corresponding Author: E.E. Kunst, MSc, PhD, Kunst & van Leerdam Medical Technology bv, P.O. Box 3536, NL – 7500 DM Enschede, The Netherlands; e-mail: ekunst@kvlmt.nl.

This manuscript describes the contents and validation of the first step in the VREST – EVAR trainer, also referred to as EAG tool (effective AAA graftmanship).

2. Tools and Methods

Proper patient – device selection is very important in the clinical procedure and thus in the training setting. This includes the determination whether a patient is suitable for a AAA endograft and the subsequent selection of the best device available for this patient. This may mean weighing up to 78 variables[7].

Each AAA is divided into 7 areas[7] that run from the suprarenal area (area 1) down to the common femoral artery (area 7, left and right), see Figure 1. The areas relevant for endograft sealing are denoted as possible landing zones for a AAA endograft. Each of the possible landing areas is judged on its complication rating for sealing and fixation, and for passage. A complication rating (on a scale from 0 to 100%) is a measure for the level of complications an experienced physician expects from a certain combination of physical parameters. The parameters that determine complication ratings include diameter, length, amount of thrombus, amount of calcification, angulation and shape.

Three vascular surgeons and two interventional radiologists each assessed 202 cases with three types of commercially available endografts, adding up to 3.030 assessments in total.

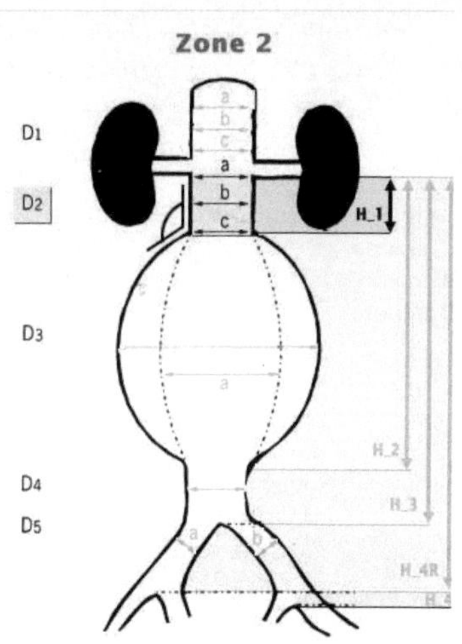

Figure 1. AAA, 7 area's

3. Results

The results of the assessments of each individual physician are compared to the outcome of the EAG tool. In 71.6% the EAG-tool fully agrees with the group of physicians. In 3.7% the EAG-tool produces a false negative outcome: the programme does not feel that a certain patient is fit for an endograft, whereas the group of physicians does find it possible. In 24.6% of the cases the EAG-tool promotes further discussion of the patient, and in only 0.2% the EAG-tool gives a false positive advise.

4. Conclusions / Discussion

Medical simulators will enhance there effectiveness if they contribute to the visual skills of the trainee, to the haptic skills of the trainee and to the decision-making skills of the trainee.

The current study shows that even in complicated surgical procedures, the knowledge and skills that need to be transferred to unexperienced surgeons can be made explicit. This opens the way to build medical simulators and VR trainers to transfer both knowledge and skills associated with the procedure, the 3D visuals, the 3D haptics and instrument choice. In this way medical simulators will truly become part of the medical training environment.

The current research is being pursued by enveloping the knowledge database that was developed with a VR training shell. This will be build within the VREST Platform for Virtual Medical Education, a combined effort of the VREST Consortium, a cooperation of University Medical Centres, large Teaching Hospitals, Technical Universities and SME's.

References

[1]　Armon MP, Yusuf SW et al. Anatomical suitability of abdominal aortic aneurysms for endovascular repair. Br J Surg 1997; 84: 178-180.

[2]　Albertini JN, Kalliafas S et al. Anatomical risk factors for proximal perigraft endoleak and graft migration following endovascular repair of abdominal aortic aneurysms. Eur J Vasc Endo Surg 2000; 19: 308-312.

[3]　Carpenter JP, Baum RA et al. Impact of exclusion criteria on patient selection for endovascular abdominal aortic aneurysm repair. J Vasc Surg 2001; 34: 1050-1054.

[4]　SternberghIII WC, Carter G et al. Aortic neck angulation predicts adverse outcome with endovascular abdominal aortic aneurysm repair. J Vasc Surg 2002; 35: 482-485.

[5]　Forbes TL, DeRose G et al. Cumulative sum failure analysis of the learning curve with endovascular abdominal aortic aneurysm repair, J Vasc Surg, 2004; 39: 102-108.

[6]　Kunst EE, Geelkerken RH, Sanders AJB. The VREST learning environment, MMVR13 Proceedings, 2005; 270-272.

[7]　Kunst EE, Geelkerken RH, Rödel SR. The EAG tool: a decision support system for selection of abdominal aorta aneurysm endografts, ICMCC 2004 Proceedings.

Medicine Meets Virtual Reality 14
J.D. Westwood et al. (Eds.)
IOS Press, 2006

Gestalt Operating Room Display Design for Perioperative Team Situation Awareness

Fuji LAI and Gabriel SPITZ, *Aptima, Inc., Woburn, MA*
Email: fujilai@aptima.com
Philip BRZEZINSKI, *LiveData, Inc., Cambridge, MA*

Abstract. The perioperative environment is a complex, high risk environment that requires real-time coordination by all perioperative team members and accurate, up-to-date information for situation assessment and decision-making. There is the need for a "Gestalt" holistic awareness of the perioperative environment to enable synthesis and contextualization of the salient information such as: patient information, case and procedure information, staff information, operative site view, physiological data, resource availability. One potential approach is to augment the medical toolkit with a large screen wall display that integrates and makes accessible information that currently resides in different data systems and care providers. The objectives are to promote safe workflows, team coordination and communication, and to enable diagnosis, anticipation of events, and information flow from upstream to downstream care providers. We used the human factors engineering design process to design and develop a display that provides a common operational picture for shared virtual perioperative team situation awareness to enhance patient safety.

Keywords. Perioperative, team, display, situation awareness, human factors, data integration, patient safety

1. Background

In the complex, high risk perioperative environment there is the need for real-time coordination by all perioperative team members and the need for accurate, up-to-date information for situation assessment and decision-making. Information needs to be shared not only between the immediate team in the Operating Room (OR), but also needs to flow seamlessly from upstream to downstream care providers as well. Dierks et al. [1] identified the areas of vulnerability: (1) intra-OR team communication; (2) communication with central core; (3) intraoperative consultation (e.g. radiology); (4) handoffs, in particular from the OR to the Post-Anesthesia Care Unit (PACU).

2. Methods

Human factors approaches were used to enhance information transfer in the identified areas of vulnerability. Human factors is the application of the understanding of human behaviors and abilities to identify human performance and work environment issues and then to design interventions such as tools, systems and environments that address the identified issues. The design process is iterative in nature: contextualizing the problem by understanding the work environment, conceptualizing a solution, and then designing a prototype that is put in front of representative users and stakeholders for feedback, which is folded back in to inform a revised design.

In the perioperative environment there is the need for a "Gestalt" holistic awareness to enable synthesis and contextualization of: patient information, case and procedure information, staff information, operative site view, physiological data, diagnostics such as pathology or radiology, resource availability, upstream and downstream components, OR schedule information. To design an information display that would meet these needs, we went through the participatory design process with clinical end users and stakeholders including surgeons, anesthesiologists, and nurses to identify the data needed on limited display real estate. Much time was spent in identifying: (1) the key pieces of information; (2) information priorities; (3) how to display the information in an intelligent way to enhance understanding of the salient information.

Objectives identified included the need: to promote safety protocols and workflow, information consistency and quality, collaboration and team orientation, communication, backup and monitoring, and information visualization; to enable trending and diagnosis, anticipation of events, teleconsultation, information flow; to provide immediate update and historical account to enhance efficiency.

3. Results

To address the identified needs we developed a large screen wall display that integrates and makes accessible information that currently resides in different data systems and care providers. This display provides a common operational picture for shared virtual OR team situation awareness and promotes: (1) information flow across geographical space—access by all parties; (2) information flow across time—upstream to downstream.

The display extracts information from data systems in the OR and bubbles up the most important information. Important patient identifying information and critical information such as allergies are featured prominently. Staffing information is clearly visible, which resonated with users. A progress log enables anyone walking in to come up to speed immediately on events thus far as well as current status of the case. Given that different pieces of information are important at different phases, center tabs were designed to be triggered by phase-specific events.

There is first a pre-incision screen to promote timeout brief and team huddle before starting. When the checklist has been completed, the display progresses to the intraoperative screen, which may have a heavier focus on information such as physiological trends. When the procedure is coming to a close the display proceeds to a closing screen that prompts the team to check counts and specify PACU orders. This display can be accessed via the web from the PACU so that PACU staff can see what is going on in the OR and can anticipate and prepare for patient arrival in the PACU accordingly. Finally there is a handoff screen to facilitate the handoff to PACU staff.

To minimize workload and enhance usability, effort was made to limit the amount of interaction and separate data entry required for this system.

4. Discussion

This product has been deployed in a working OR and is scheduled to be deployed in other ORs in early 2006. This will present the opportunity to assess the impact of such an information aid on performance as well as healthcare quality. The design and implementation of this display serves as an illustration of how human factors engineering approaches can be used to understand core issues and design and assess solutions that will form part of the future medical toolkit to enhance patient safety in the perioperative environment.

Acknowledgements

This work was conducted in collaboration with Massachusetts General Hospital (Boston, MA) and Memorial Sloan-Kettering Cancer Center (New York, NY). This work is supported by TATRC, U.S. Army Medical Research and Materiel Command under Contract No. W81XWH-04-C-0015 awarded to Live Data, Inc.

References

[1] Dierks, M., Roth, E., Lai, F., Entin, E.B., Sato, L., Surgical risk hot spots: Mapping adverse events and activity nodes to transitions using a high fidelity surgical process model, *Proceedings of the HFES 48th Annual Meeting* (2004).

Medicine Meets Virtual Reality 14
J.D. Westwood et al. (Eds.)
IOS Press, 2006

285

Integrating Surgical Robots into the Next Medical Toolkit

Fuji LAI and Eileen ENTIN, *Aptima, Inc., Woburn, MA*
Email: fujilai@aptima.com

Abstract. Surgical robots hold much promise for revolutionizing the field of surgery and improving surgical care. However, despite the potential advantages they offer, there are multiple barriers to adoption and integration into practice that may prevent these systems from realizing their full potential benefit. This study elucidated some of the most salient considerations that need to be addressed for integration of new technologies such as robotic systems into the operating room of the future as it evolves into a complex system of systems. We conducted in-depth interviews with operating room team members and other stakeholders to identify potential barriers in areas of workflow, teamwork, training, clinical acceptance, and human-system interaction. The findings of this study will inform an approach for the design and integration of robotics and related computer-assisted technologies into the next medical toolkit for "computer-enhanced surgery" to improve patient safety and healthcare quality.

Keywords. Surgical robotics, integration, barriers, computer-enhanced surgery, patient safety

1. Background

Surgical robotics and other innovative technologies for the operating room hold much promise for revolutionizing the field of surgery and improving patient safety. However, despite the potential advantages they offer, surgical robots have yet to realize the full potential impact to enhance surgical care. In many cases, for a variety of reasons, systems are relegated to sitting in the corner unused. The major causes of the current technology adoption "choke point" need to be identified and addressed. In tandem with technology considerations, social and cultural considerations need to be taken into account. What is needed now is to cross the chasm from the early adopters to the early majority and to demonstrate that surgical robots add real value and to make robotics an integral accepted part of the next medical toolkit. This call was made at a recent Telemedicine and Advanced Technologies Research Center (TATRC) sponsored Integrated Research Team meeting that brought together clinicians, researchers, developers, and other stakeholders to address these issues.

2. Methods

In support of the TATRC call, we conducted a study to identify the potential barriers to adoption and integration of robotic and other computer-assisted technologies into the operating room (OR) of the future. This was done through in-depth interviews with a variety of stakeholders identified as key individuals who would be able to offer insight. To understand various perspectives, our sample of 24 participants included 13 end users, seven academic researchers, and four developers. We were interested in uncovering specific experiences and in discovering new insights that might inform and help the integration of surgical robotic systems into the OR.

3. Results

Our analysis of the interview data revealed many common themes recurring throughout the interviews. The issues and barriers to acceptance that our interviewees perceived included the following.

3.1. System Size

Many robotic systems have large footprints and are difficult to fit into already overcrowded operating rooms. These systems can be difficult to move and set up. Once the robot is in the room it can limit access to the patient and become an obstacle that the surgical team must maneuver around. Systems need to be lightweight, have a small profile, and be modular, adaptable, and flexible.

3.2. Setup, Case Progression, and OR Throughput

Another major barrier is that many systems take too much time to set up and tear down. Furthermore, the use of a robot for procedures may result in increased overall procedure times which has the drawbacks of reducing the surgeon's case volume and reducing the OR throughput. Systems also need to allow ease of setup for multiple procedures.

3.3. Workflow Issues

The introduction of a robotic system into the OR undoubtedly disrupts the existing workflow. Interviewees indicated that in addition to the changes to each individual's tasks and cognitive and physical workload, there needs to be accommodation and adaptation imposed due to the fact that the robot is now a new surgical team member. New team coordination and communication strategies are needed as well. Furthermore, additional personnel support, such as an on-site technician, may be needed.

3.4. New Proficiencies and Training Needs

Many interviewees emphasized that robotic surgery requires a radical culture shift from traditional methods and also noted the steep learning curve involved in some instances. Robotic surgery changes the surgeon's role and tasks, and for robotic surgery new surgeon essential competencies may emerge. Training and the assessment of aptitudes and skills through appropriate metrics is an important issue that was raised.

Appropriate human-machine interface design is also an important factor in easing training demands.

3.5. Validation

A major stumbling block for integration has been the difficulty in demonstrating the actual benefits of robotic surgery to stakeholders. The basic questions are: 1) what are the surgical benefits for the patient, and 2) does robotic surgery enhance performance and patient safety. A number of interviewees felt that at this time there is little advantage in robotic surgery. The key is to demonstrate that surgical robots make difficult procedures simpler and make new procedures possible by affording computer-enhanced capability to allow: increased dexterity; precision; information augmentation for surgical planning, simulation, and rehearsal; integration of safety features; extension of the reach of surgical care and training through telesurgery.

3.6. Cost

Given the expense of these systems, it is critical to specify the business case for surgical robotics: will they result in overall hospital cost savings. The financial cost-benefit analysis needs to consider the larger context of the perioperative process and environment.

4. Discussion

The vision of the medical toolkit of the future is that of compatibility, interoperability, and modularity with the ability to leverage digital data for "computer-enhanced surgery." The findings of this study will inform an approach for the design and integration of robotics and other computer-assisted technologies into the OR of the future to enhance surgical care.

Acknowledgements

This work was supported by TATRC, U.S. Army Medical Research and Materiel Command under Contract No. W81XWH-04-P-1073. The views, opinions and/or findings contained in this report are those of the authors and should not be construed as an official Department of the Army position.

Medicine Meets Virtual Reality 14
J.D. Westwood et al. (Eds.)
IOS Press, 2006

Study of Laparoscopic Forces Perception for Defining Simulation Fidelity

Pablo LAMATA[1], Enrique J. GÓMEZ[1], Francisco M. SÁNCHEZ-MARGALLO[2],
Félix LAMATA[1,3], María ANTOLÍN[1], Samuel RODRÍGUEZ[1], Alfonso OLTRA[4],
Jesús USÓN[2]

[1] *Grupo de Bioingeniería y Telemedicina, Universidad Politécnica de Madrid, Spain,
{lamata, mantolin, srodrigu, egomez @gbt.tfo.upm.es}*
[2] *Minimally Invasive Surgery Centre, Cáceres, Spain, {msanchez, juson @ccmi.es}*
[3] *Dept. of Surgery, Hospital Clínico Universitario, Zaragoza, Spain,
{cgbh-fmata@hcu-lblesa.es}*
[4] *Biomechanical Institute of Valencia, Valencia, Spain {alfonso.oltra@ibv.upv.es}*

Abstract: One of the most controversial dilemmas in virtual reality laparoscopic simulators design is the incorporation of force feedback (FF). This issue is approached with an experimental design in which surgeons assess the resistance against pulling of four different tissues, which are characterized with the acquisition of interaction forces. Comparing subjective assessments with objective force parameters we aim to determine the fidelity boundary beyond which no more realism is necessary in simulation. Interaction pulling forces of four tissues have been characterized, which can constitute a basis for requirements of a FF algorithm. Results have also led to the hypothesis that surgeons are able to differentiate tissues and perceive somesthesic information although resulting interaction forces are of the same magnitude than interferences like trocar friction.

Keywords: laparoscopy, virtual reality, simulation requirements, force feedback

1. Introduction

Laparoscopic surgery is becoming a preferable alternative to open surgery in many procedures. However it requires a long and cost training process, in which virtual reality (VR) simulation can play an important role [1].

One of the most controversial dilemmas in VR simulation design is the incorporation of force feedback (FF). It has been studied how trocar friction could hide tactile information [2], but perception is enhanced with FF both in grasping [3] and pulling [4] maneuvers. One interesting methodological approach to assess the importance of FF is to compare user performance with and without FF, which has found results that supports the convenience of FF [5]. Following this line, degradation of haptic hardware has been modeled to explore the impact of its quality [6].

The approach taken in this study is to design a psychophysical experiment to understand how surgeons perceive pulling and pushing forces in the laparoscopic theatre. This is an extension of our former work studying consistency perception [4]. Therefore surgeons assess the resistance against pulling of four different tissues, which are characterized with the acquisition of interaction forces. Comparing subjective valorizations with objective force parameters we aim to assess the fidelity boundary beyond which no more realism is necessary in simulation.

This study aims to contribute to the definition of actual requirements of simulators in order to be an effective training tool. The design and validation of VR simulators is the main objective of the SINERGIA Spanish Research Collaborative Network (G03/135).

2. Tools and Methods

Subjective consistency perception is studied together with the acquisition of the interaction forces that deliver the consistency information. Four tissues of the pig abdominal cavity are selected and studied: diaphragmatic crus (t1), esophagus (t2), gastric fundus (t3) and greater omentum (t4). Description of both studies is made in following sections.

2.1. Consistency Perception Study

Tissue consistency is here understood as the resistance felt against the penetration (pushing) and withdrawal (pulling) of a grasper holding the tissue. It is measured by a scale from 0 to 10: value 0 corresponds to movements with an empty grasper, and value 10 corresponds to a grasper holding a rigid structure as a ligament in its bone junction. A total of 29 different surgeons were enrolled in the study.

The experiment has different stages in which surgeons assess tissue consistency with different sources of information: a written description of tissues being grasped in a questionnaire (Q), visual information of tissues being pulled and pushed from a video (VI), tactile information making maneuvers in the porcine model (TI) or visual and tactile information simultaneously (VTI). Details about this experiment can be found in [4].

2.2. In-vivo Interaction Forces Measurement

A laparoscopic grasper (Click Line, Storz medical, Germany) is equipped with a Force/Torque sensor (Mini40 F/T, ATI, USA) as shown in Figure 1. This device is similar to that described in [2;7]. It can be introduced through a trocar and acquire forces of all degrees of freedom of the laparoscopic tool but grasping. Nevertheless an indirect measure of grasping forces can be taken due to the mechanical transmission of grasping from the handle to the tip of the tool. The transmission is done through the inner metal axis, which is coupled to the outer black tube in which the sensor is attached (see Figure 1). This is more a limitation than an advantage, because when a grasp is closed it is acquired as a pushing force, i.e., there is a coupling between these two degrees of freedom. Another feature is the total weight of the device, 215g, which is more than double of the grasper alone (85g).

The device is therefore used in a controlled way, fixing grasping before making pulling and pushing maneuvers. An experienced surgeon is instructed in this way and performs three repetitions of five consecutive insertion and extraction maneuvers holding each of the four tissues of the pig model (t1-t4). In each repetition the tissue is grasped in a different place trying to bite the maximum amount of tissue. Measurements are made on the same pig model that is used for the perceptual experiment. Two parameters are obtained from each force profile: peak to peak value (N) and maximum temporal slope (N/s).

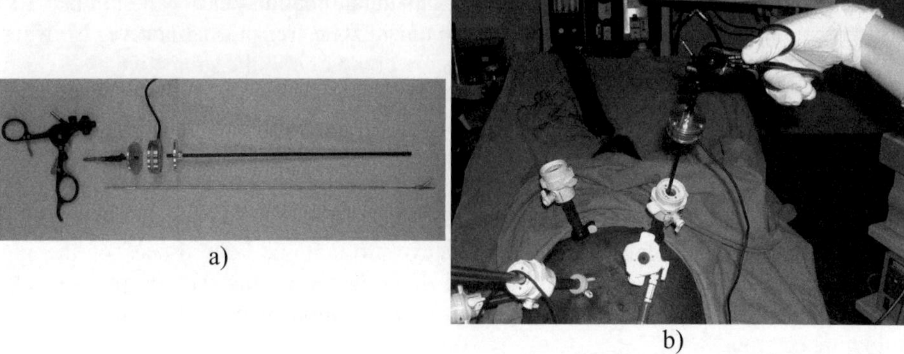

Figure 1: Device designed to acquire laparoscopic interaction forces. a) Device dismounted in its different components: the black tube has been cut and two metal plates have been designed to fix the F/T sensor. The metal axis is introduced in the black tube and is responsible for the transmission of the grasping movements. b) Device being used in the pig model through a trocar in the forces measurement study.

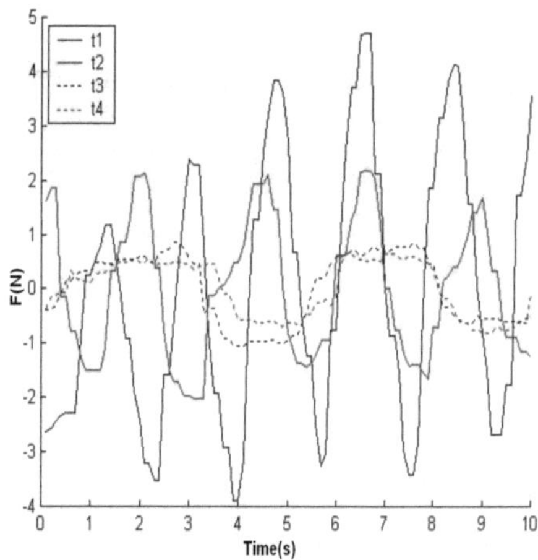

Figure 2: Interaction force profiles studied for different tissues. Profiles of t3 and t4 are complete, whereas those of t1 and t2 only show the first two pulling and pushing maneuvers.

Table 1. Results of the subjective perception of tissue consistency and the objective parameters obtained from the interaction forces profiles. Values shows mean ± standard deviation.

	t1	t2	t3	t4
Subjective perception of tissue consistency:				
TI (0 to 10)	8.8 ± 1.0	7.4 ± 1.1	2.8 ± 1.5	0.8 ± 0.8
VTI (0 to 10)	8.3 ± 0.9	6.7 ± 0.9	3.1 ± 1.2	0.9 ± 0.8
In-vivo interaction forces measurement:				
Vpp (N)	5.8 ± 1.2	3.3 ± 0.6	1.5 ± 0.2	1.6 ± 0.1
m (N/s)	7.4 ± 1.9	3.3 ± 1.1	0.9 ± 0.3	1.0 ± 0.2

3. Results

Interaction forces of four different tissues (t1-t4) are acquired. Examples of the force profiles are shown in Figure 2. Two parameters, peak-to-peak value (Vpp) and maximum slope (m) are used to characterize each of the five pulling-pushing cycles of each of the three repetitions. Average values are compared to the subjective assessment of tissue consistency by surgeons in a 0 to 10 scale [4] as shown in Table 1.

4. Discussion

The objective of present study is to understand how forces are perceived through laparoscopic tools. The complexity of a systematic study would be too high, as there are many variables influencing how forces are produced: attached organs, point of grasping, factors that change the biomechanical tissue properties (irrigation, disease conditions, age…), amount of tissue bitten… Our simplistic approach has been to compare the subjective perception of four "pulling scenarios" (section 2.1) with objective parameters obtained from force profiles of these scenarios (section 2.2).

The scope of the study is limited to one surgical maneuver, pulling. This is one of the most frequent maneuvers, but not the only one in which force information could be important. Nevertheless pulling enables a straightforward force acquisition and characterization with the device developed. Moreover, it originates force values that are higher than other delicate maneuvers, what makes it more robust to noise sources.

The force acquisition device built allows characterizing the pulling interaction forces in a controlled way. Acquisition of forces simultaneously with the perceptual analysis would be desirable, but the coupling of grasping with pushing information is not the only difficulty: the weight introduced with the F/T sensor would distort perception.

Results have shown how surgeons are able to distinguish between four different tissue consistencies with only force information. Interaction forces are perceived despite friction, and these forces deliver information about tissue consistency. On the other hand interaction pulling forces of four different tissues have been characterized with their peak to peak value and its maximum temporal slope, which can be used as a basis for requirements of a FF algorithm. Force measurements agree with ranges described in the literature [2;7].

What is interesting of present study is to compare results of both experiments (2.1 and 2.2). Surgeons performed free pulling of tissues to rank their consistency in 2.1, whereas force profiles of 2.2 belong to a controlled "standardized" pulling. This difference could lead to some discrepancies between parameters from forces obtained in 2.2 and forces perceived in 2.1, as there are different styles of pulling between surgeons. We think that this could affect to the maximum slope, but not much to the peak to peak value as all surgeons reached roughly the same maximum pulling. The other difference between 2.1 and 2.2 is the point of grasping the tissue, but results varying this point in 2.2 haven't shown differences in acquired forces. Both experiments are made with the same pig model and trocars.

Average perception values and force parameters are much correlated, as shown in Table 1. Nevertheless perception differences between t3 and t4 have not been explained with force parameters, probably hidden by friction forces which can be up to 3N [2]. In our experiment trocar friction forces had a maximum value around 0.7 N, which means a peak to peak value of 1.4N. This is a value similar to what was obtained in t3 and t4 (1.46N and 1.6N respectively). Nevertheless trocar friction didn't hinder surgeons to distinguish between t3 and t4.

These results lead to the next hypothesis: "surgeons are able to differentiate tissues and perceive somesthesic information although resulting interaction forces are of the same magnitude than interfering forces like trocar friction". It seems that surgeons learn to distinguish between friction forces, which are similar in every pulling and pushing maneuver, and resulting forces from the interaction with organs. This is opposed to the idea that "it is unlikely that the operator will be able to discriminate between somesthesic information generated by the organ and that generated by the resistance of the wall" [2].

5. Conclusion

Simulators require FF capability if tissue consistency information has to be delivered. Interaction pulling forces of four tissues have been characterized, which can constitute a basis for requirements of a FF algorithm. Results have lead to the hypothesis that surgeons are able to differentiate tissues and perceive somesthesic information although resulting interaction forces are of the same magnitude than interfering forces like trocar friction

Acknowledgements

This research has been partially funded by the SINERGIA Thematic Research Collaborative Network (G03/135) of the Spanish Ministry of Health & Education. Authors would like to express their gratitude to all members of the SINERGIA consortium. Our special thanks to S.Pascual and M.C.Tejonero (Sta. María del Puerto Hospital, Cádiz) and to J.B.Pagador and all the staff of the Minimally Invasive Surgery Centre of Cáceres.

References

[1] R. Aggarwal, K. Moorthy, and A. Darzi, "Laparoscopic skills training and assessment," Br J Surg, vol. 91, no. 12, pp. 1549-1558, Dec.2004.

[2] G. Picod, A. C. Jambon, D. Vinatier, and P. Dubois, "What can the operator actually feel when performing a laparoscopy?," Surg Endosc, vol. 19, no. 1, pp. 95-100, Oct.2005.

[3] G. Tholey, J. P. Desai, and A. E. Castellanos, "Force feedback plays a significant role in minimally invasive surgery - Results and analysis," Annals of Surgery, vol. 241, no. 1, pp. 102-109, 2005.

[4] P. Lamata, E. J. Gómez, F. M. Sánchez-Margallo, F. Lamata Hernández, F. del Pozo, and J. Usón Gargallo, "Study of consistency perception in laparoscopy for defining the level of fidelity in virtual reality simulation," Surgical Endoscopy, vol. (in press) 2005.

[5] H. K. Kim, D. W. Rattner, and M. A. Srinivasan, "The role of simulation fidelity in laparoscopic surgical training,", Lect Notes Comput Sc 2878 ed 2003, pp. 1-8.

[6] I. Brouwer, K. E. MacLean, and A. J. Hodgson, "Simulating cheap hardware: a platform for evaluating cost-performance trade-offs in haptic hardware design,", 1 ed 2004, pp. 770-775.

[7] C. Richards, J. Rosen, B. Hannaford, C. Pellegrini, and M. Sinanan, "Skills evaluation in minimally invasive surgery using force/torque signatures," Surg. Endosc., vol. 14, no. 9, pp. 791-798, Sept.2000.

Medicine Meets Virtual Reality 14
J.D. Westwood et al. (Eds.)
IOS Press, 2006

Computer Prediction of Balloon Angioplasty from Artery Imaging

Denis LAROCHE [a,1], Sebastien DELORME [a], Todd ANDERSON [b],
Jean BUITHIEU [c], and Robert DIRADDO [d]
[a] *Industrial Materials Institute, Boucherville, QC, Canada*
[b] *University of Calgary, AB, Canada*
[c] *McGill University Health Center, Montreal, QC, Canada*

Abstract. The success of angioplasty depends on a balance between two conflicting objectives: maximization of artery lumen patency and minimization of mechanical damage. A finite element model for the patient-specific prediction of angioplasty is proposed as a potential tool to assist clinicians. This paper describes the general methodology and the algorithm that computes device/artery friction work during balloon insertion and deployment. The potential of the model is demonstrated with examples that include artery model reconstruction and prediction of friction on the arterial wall during balloon insertion and deployment.

Keywords. Finite elements, model, angioplasty, multi-body contact, friction.

Introduction

Cardiovascular diseases are the first cause of death in the western world. Balloon angioplasty, the most practiced medical intervention worldwide, consists of dilating a stenosed artery with a polymeric balloon in order to restore blood flow to an acceptable level. Often, a metallic slotted tube called *stent* is deployed and permanently implanted inside the artery to prevent elastic recoil of the artery. The most frequent complication of angioplasty, restenosis, is an excessive repair reaction of the arterial wall, related to its mechanical damage during the intervention. Restenosis has been shown to be related to two types of mechanical damage: 1) overstretch injury of the arterial wall and 2) denudation of the endothelium (the cell monolayer that lines the interior part of the arterial wall) due to friction with the balloon. The specific contribution of both types of injury to restenosis is still debated [1,2]. Whether because of patients comeback after 6 months for target vessel revascularization or because of the use of expensive drug-eluting stents, it is generally recognized that restenosis increases by 25 to 30% the total cost of this intervention, which in Canada results in a 50M$ increase on the annual healthcare burden.

The success of angioplasty depends on a balance between two conflicting objectives: 1) maximizing the final deformation of the artery and 2) minimizing the mechanical damage to the arterial wall. Few research groups have attempted to simulate angioplasty with numerical or analytical models and predict its outcome.

---

[1] Corresponding Author : Denis Laroche, Industrial Materials Institute, 75 de Mortagne, Boucherville, QC, Canada, J4B 6Y4; E-mail : denis.laroche@cnrc-nrc.gc.ca

Angioplasty simulation, combined with current artery imaging technique such as intravascular ultrasound (IVUS), has the potential to become a clinical tool to assist in the selection of an appropriate intervention strategy for a specific patient. This could be done by virtually testing various strategies. However to render the tool clinically useful, two often competing requirements must be met: high accuracy of the predicted behavior and high computational speed.

This work presents improvements to a finite element model for predicting the device/artery behavior during angioplasty [3-5]. They consist of the integration of artery model reconstruction and the development of a new multi-body contact algorithm to reduce computational time and increase its robustness. Calculation of friction work is also proposed as an hypothesized predictor of endothelium denudation. To our knowledge, friction damage to the endothelium has never been considered in angioplasty simulations, possibly because of the difficulty of implementing a robust contact/slip algorithm for deforming bodies. An example of balloon angioplasty simulation on a coronary artery obtained from intravascular ultrasound imaging is presented to demonstrate the potential of the proposed model.

1. Methodology

A finite element modeling software developed for the analysis of large deformations of soft materials is used to solve angioplasty mechanics [3-5]. The model computes the device/artery interaction and large deformations that occur during device insertion and deployment into the diseased artery. It predicts the resulting artery lumen patency, including stress and strain distribution in the arterial wall, for a specific device and inflation pressure. The software uses conjugate gradient methods with various pre-conditioners to iteratively solve the system of equations.

1.1. Angioplasty Procedure Model

As described in a previous report [3], the angioplasty device model consists of a balloon being wrapped onto a rigid catheter. The balloon is modeled with membrane elements and the Ogden hyperelastic constitutive equation. The artery is modeled with incompressible solid elements and the Mooney-Rivlin hyperelastic constitutive model. Tetrahedral elements rather than hexahedral elements are proposed for the artery, thus allowing the use of automatic mesh generation from medical images, and reducing the time required for pre-processing the data. The simulation steps include the balloon pre-folding onto the rigid catheter, the insertion into the artery, and its complete deployment to dilate the target lesion. During balloon insertion, the friction exerted on the arterial wall significantly deforms it and depends upon the boundary conditions on the artery.

1.2. Implicit Multi-body Contact Algorithm

Contact algorithms are usually time consuming and limiting factors in complex finite element applications. They have been traditionally used in explicit software and include collision detection [6,7], non-penetration constraint and friction/slip capabilities [8,9]. Collision detection algorithms can be explicit (position based) or implicit (trajectory based). However, very few papers discuss the robustness of each approach and their application to implicit finite element computation, particularly the problems associated with the "dead-zone" or with the thin membrane collision detection.

An important contribution of this work is the development of a multi-body contact algorithm that is rapid and robust enough to handle complex contact and friction behaviors between the balloon and the artery. Collisions between virtual nodes and surfaces moving with large displacement steps are detected with an implicit iterative approach that fully respects the non-penetration constraint. At every displacement increment, the positions of the virtual nodes are computed as a minimization problem with the objective function F being their distance to the finite element mesh, subject to a non-penetration constraint g. The problem is given by Eqs. (1) and (2), with X_{Vi} and X_{FEi} being the positions of the virtual nodes and those of the finite element mesh, respectively.

$$F(X_{Vi}) = \sum_{i=1}^{N} |X_{Vi} - X_{FEi}| \tag{1}$$

$$g(X_{Vj}, X_{Vk}) = N_{Vk} \cdot (X_{Vk} - X_{Vj}) \leq 0 \tag{2}$$

Indices i represent all the surface nodes while j and k are for contacted nodes and surfaces, respectively. N_{Vk} and X_{Vj} are the virtual surface normal vector and the position of one of its connected nodes, respectively. This technique is stable for large displacement increments and is therefore directly applicable to implicit finite elements. Once contact is detected, it is handled with an augmented Lagrange algorithm that computes slip and friction forces.

2. Simulation Examples

The example includes two simulations of balloon angioplasty on the mid-LAD coronary artery of a patient. The various steps involved in the construction of the models for the artery and the angioplasty device, as well as the intervention simulation are presented. The contact algorithm used approximately 18% of the total computational time for each simulation.

2.1. Artery Model Reconstruction

The artery model was reconstructed from intravascular ultrasound (IVUS) images of a percutaneous coronary intervention (PCI). The intervention included several balloon deployments and the implantation of three stents. Three IVUS pullbacks were performed during the procedure at a pull-back speed of 0.5 mm/sec. The first IVUS sequence was used in this example to build the finite element mesh of a 66-mm long artery segment. Equally spaced images (one per cardiac cycle) were selected and imported into the Amira software (Mercury Computer Systems, Chelmsford, MA) as a 120x120x136 voxel field. The average cardiac cycle rate over the whole sequence was measured from observation of the images. The lumen and media-adventitia borders were identified through manual segmentation. Interpolation between image frames was used to compensate for shadow artifacts. An initial surface mesh was created using the marching cube algorithm. From this surface mesh, a tetrahedral mesh was then produced using the advancing front method. The 11553-node mesh was edited to avoid tetrahedrons with a large aspect ratio, in order to prevent ill-conditioning of the finite element problem.

2.2. Angioplasty Using a Short Balloon

In this example a 12-mm long angioplasty balloon having a deflated diameter of 3.2 mm (nominal diameter of 3.5 mm at 8 atm) was used. Previously mounted onto a rigid catheter and folded with the use of four folding blades, the balloon was gradually inserted into the artery up to the most stenosed segment. Then an internal pressure of 12 atm was gradually applied to fully deploy the balloon and dilate the artery lumen.

Figure 2 shows predicted deformations during the procedure. Figure 3 shows the balloon deployment mechanics and the balloon-artery interactions in a cross-section view. The distribution of stretch on the artery is represented in grey tones. As expected, the maximum stretch is located on the thinnest part of the arterial wall.

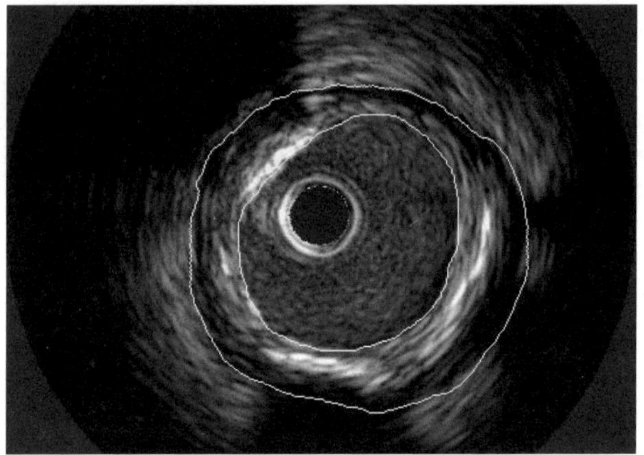

Figure 1: Example of segmented IVUS image showing lumen and media-adventitia borders.

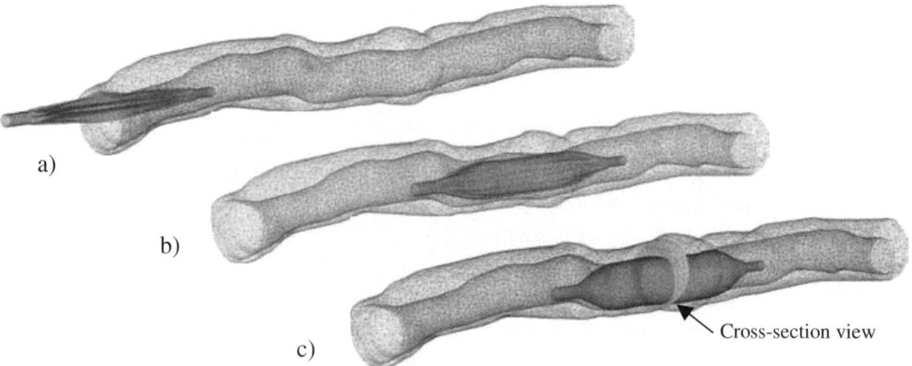

Figure 2: Simulation results for the 12mm long balloon. a) insertion; b) deployment; c) end of deployment.

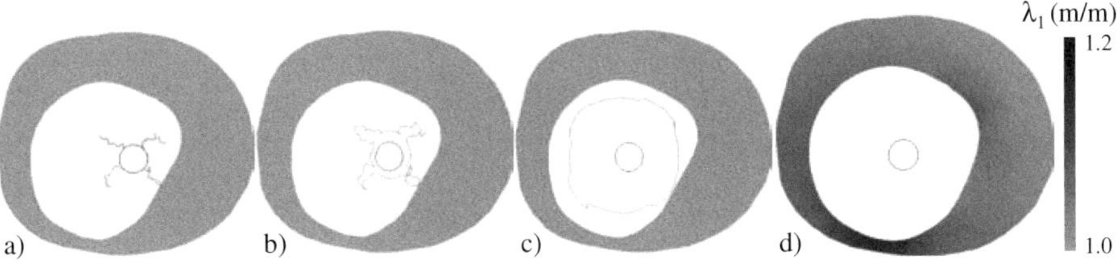

Figure 3: Cross-section view (Fig 1) of balloon deployment for the 12mm balloon. a) end of balloon insertion; b) and c) steps of deployment; d) end of deployment (12 atm).

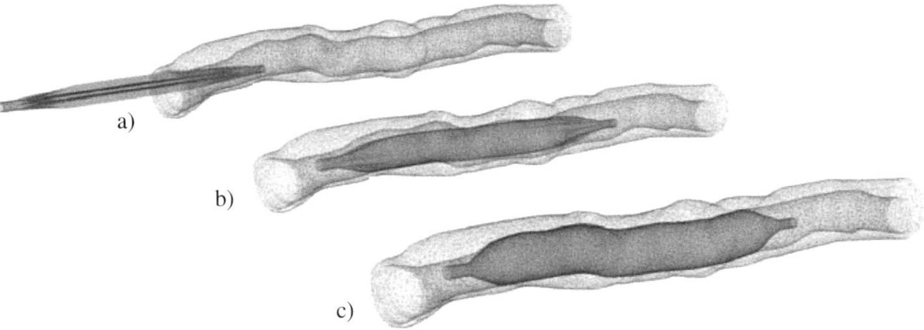

Figure 4: Simulation results for the 28mm long balloon. a) insertion; b) deployment; c) end of deployment (12 atm).

2.3. Angioplasty Using a Long Balloon

In this second example a 28-mm long balloon was used on the same artery segment. Similar simulation steps as for the short balloon were used to inflate at 12 atm. Figure 4 shows predicted deformations during the procedure. When compared to the short balloon example, the long balloon seems to deform and conform to the artery shape.

2.4. Prediction of Friction Work

In each simulation the cumulative friction work per unit area was computed. This is expected to give an indication of the amount of damage to the endothelial cells. Figure 5 shows predicted friction work density after balloon deployment for the two examples. It can be seen that for both short and long balloons, an average friction work density of 10 μJ/mm^2 was predicted on the artery where the deployment took place. Smaller yet unexpectedly high friction work due to the balloon insertion was also observed for both examples. These values can be explained by the use of a rigid catheter and by the high structural stiffness of balloon flaps. Friction work predicted on both insertion and deployment areas is high enough to potentially damage the endothelium.

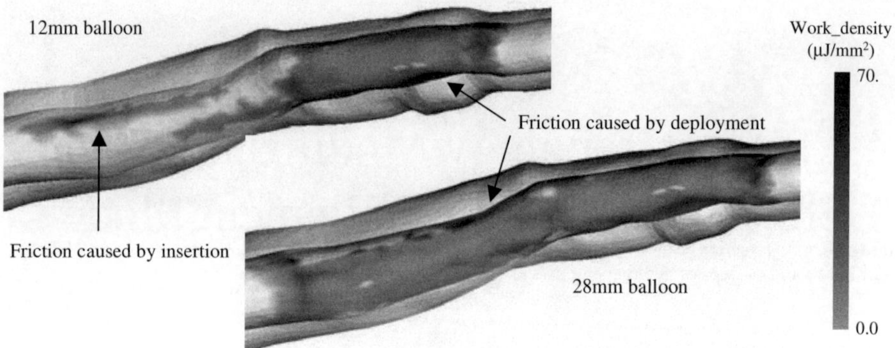

Figure 5: Predicted friction work density on the arterial wall for the 12 mm and the 28 mm balloons.

3. Conclusion

In this paper a finite element model for predicting balloon angioplasty from artery imaging was presented, with emphasis on new developments such as reconstruction of artery model from medical images and calculation of friction work from a new multi-body contact algorithm.   A numerical example on a human coronary artery demonstrated the potential of the model to predict the mechanical interaction between the balloon and the arterial wall.   In an effort to render the simulation clinically useful, the friction work exerted by the balloon was computed and presented as a potential indicator of endothelium damage.   Future work will focus on constitutive models for the artery and the use of deformable catheters to further improve the accuracy of the simulation.   Experimental work is underway to verify the relationship between friction work and endothelial denudation.

References

[1]   Clowes AW, Clowes MM, Fingerle J, Reidy MA.   Kinetics of cellular proliferation after arterial injury. V. Role of acute distension in the induction of smooth muscle proliferation. *Lab Invest* 1989; **60**:360-364.

[2]   Fingerle J, Au YP, Clowes AW, Reidy MA. Intimal lesion formation in rat carotid arteries after endothelial denudation in absence of medial injury. *Arteriosclerosis* 1990 **10**:1082-1087.

[3]   Delorme S, Laroche D, DiRaddo R, Buithieu J.   Modeling polymer balloons for angioplasty: from fabrication to deployment. *Proc Annual Technical Conference (ANTEC), SPE*, Chicago, IL, 2004.

[4]   Laroche D, Delorme S, DiRaddo R.   Computer simulation of balloon angioplasty: effect of balloon deployment on contact mechanics. *ASM Materials & Processes for Medical Devices Conference*, Anaheim, CA, 2003.

[5]   Laroche D, Delorme S, Buithieu J, DiRaddo R. A three-dimentional finite element model of balloon angioplasty and stent implantation. *Proc Comp Meth Biomech Biomed Eng* **5**, Madrid, 2004.

[6]   Hallquist JO, Goudreau GL, Benson DJ. Sliding interfaces with contact-impact in large-scale lagrangian computations. *Comp Meth App Mech Eng* 1985; **51**:107-137.

[7]   Zhong ZH. *Finite element procedures for contact-impact problems.* Oxford University Press, 1993.

[8]   Laursen TA, Simo JC. A continuum-based finite element formulation for the implicit solution of multibody, large deformation frictional contact problems. *Int J Num Meth Eng* 1993; **36**:3451-3485.

[9]   Puso MA, Laursen TA. A mortar segment-to-segment contact method for large deformation solid mechanics. *Comp Meth Appl Mech Eng* 2004; **193**:601-629.

Medicine Meets Virtual Reality 14
J.D. Westwood et al. (Eds.)
IOS Press, 2006

Efficient Topology Modification and Deformation for Finite Element Models Using Condensation

Bryan Lee [a,b,1], Dan C. Popescu [a] Bhautik Joshi [a,c] and Sébastien Ourselin [a]

[a] *BioMedIA Lab, Autonomous System Laboratory, CSIRO ICT Centre, Australia*
[b] *School of Electrical and Information Engineering, University of Sydney, Australia*
[c] *Graduate School of Biomedical Enginering, University of New South Wales, Australia*

Abstract. Cuts on deformable organs are a central task in the set of physical operations needed in many surgical simulation environments. Our BioMedIA surgical simulator structures are Finite Element Models, driven by displacements on the touched nodes as opposed to forces. This approach allows for realistic simulation of both deformation and haptic response at real-time rates. The integration of condensation into our system increases its efficiency, and allows for complex interaction on larger meshes than would normally be permitted with available memory. We present an extension of our novel algorithm for cuts in deformable organs, in the context of condensed matrices. We show results from our surgical simulation system with real-time haptic feedback.

Keywords. Surgical Simulation, FEM, Condensation, Cutting, Haptics, Real-time

1. Introduction

Recent developments in hardware and computer technologies have allowed for the design of simulation systems of increased complexity. Medicine is a beneficiary of these advances, with surgical simulation one of the real-time application areas that is most demanding in terms of computational power. The use of surgical simulators can have significant advantages over traditional methods of teaching and assessing surgical skills. They can replace the need for practising on cadavers or animal organs and provide a stable, reproducible and risk free training environment.

Haptic simulation systems enhance the virtual experience by adding a feeling of touch to the visual interaction. The addition of a tactile component comes with computational challenges of its own: typically, haptic devices need to be updated at rates in the range of 300 to over 1000 Hz, otherwise they might provide degraded mechanical experience, such as bumpy motion or unpleasant vibrations.

The current state-of-the-art in surgery simulations comprises a wealth of heterogeneous techniques, many of which still do not meet the accuracy requirements for widespread acceptance by medical practitioners. This is, however, a very active research area and the goal of building high fidelity complex simulators is continuously brought nearer.

---

[1]Correspondence to: Bryan C. Lee, CSIRO ICT Centre, Macquaire University, Locked Bag 17, North Ryde, NSW, 1670, Australia. Tel.: +612 9325 3267; Fax: +612 9325 3101; E-mail: BryanC.Lee@csiro.au.

Nealen *et al.* [4] provides a recent review on the various Physically Based Modelling (PBM) techniques for deformable models. The techniques covered include the Finite Element Method (FEM), mass-spring systems, particle systems, and mesh-free methods such as particles systems. The requirements of real-time haptic response is usually a trade-off with accuracy. The various techniques developed are designed to address these issues

Our BioMedIA surgical simulator structures are Finite Element Models. A key part of the algorithmic framework is that the interaction is driven by displacements on the touched nodes rather than forces from the interacting device. The integration of condensation of matrices into our system increases its efficiency, and allows for complex interaction on larger meshes than would normally be permitted with available memory. We have extended our work on topological modification (i.e. cuts) in our Physically Based Modelling (PBM) system, by allowing it to operate in the context of operating on condensed matrices.

2. Method

The cutting algorithm involves the integration of several components. In section 2.1 we describe our PBM procedure, which forms the backbone of the calculations to make real-time FEM for physical deformations a feasible proposition. By considering only nodes that are on the surface of deformable objects, section 2.2 describes how matrix condensation can be combined with PBM to permit the manipulation of large meshes. In section 2.3 we briefly summarise previous work [6] on support for toplogy modification within our PBM framework. In section 2.4, we describe our novel algorithm for adding support for condensed matrices for topology modification.

2.1. Physically Based Modelling

The realism of the interaction with virtual objects depends heavily on the type of model used to describe them. Non-physical models are simpler representations and therefore easier to update in real-time, but provide less realistic simulations. Physically based models are more complex representations, allowing for simulations of increased realism, but involve more sophisticated computation. They are generally derived directly from the physical equations governing the evolution of the modelled system. Finite Element (FE) models are frequently used because they are well known for producing accurate results when interacting with deformable soft-tissue models. The FE solver can be modified to allow for real-time interaction, and we have previously implemented such a technique, as described in [5], as part of our surgical simulation system.

Typically, an FE deformable model is described by a stiffness matrix, which encompasses the geometrical and physical properties of the object. A typical linear system would be a modelled using the Hookean spring equation, such that:

$$F = Kx \tag{1}$$

where F represents the forces at nodes, x represents the displacements of the nodes, and K is the stiffness matrix. FEMs commonly require at least the precomputation of the stiffness matrix. For increased efficiency, when a realistic interaction with haptic feedback needs to be modelled, the precomputation of the inverse of the stiffness matrix is also necessary [6,8]. Calculations of the stiffness and inverse stiffness matrices are computationally demanding and are only precomputed once before the simulation begins.

This inverse stiffness matrix can then be subsequently used to calculate the deformations due to interaction during simulations.

2.2. Condensation

As computational efficiency is a primary goal in surgical simulation systems, modifications to known algorithms are developed to achieve this. One such modification to the commonly used FEM is condensation, as detailed in [1,2]. Whilst the deformable organs are modeled as volumetric objects, interaction involves contact only with the surface of the model. Haptic feedback is received from the contact made with the surface nodes, and visual feedback only requires the surface of the model to be recalculated, as the position of the nodes within the model cannot be seen.

Once the inverse stiffness matrix has been calculated, only a small proportion of this matrix is required for further calculations. The submatrix required consists of only the rows and columns corresponding to surface nodes. This reduction in the size of the inverse stiffness matrix required, referred to as condensation, increases computational efficiency and reduces memory requirements, allowing larger models that would normally not be possible to simulate due to memory size.

2.3. Topology modification

Complex interactions with the organs, such as cutting, alter the structure of the model. Once the structure is modified, the precomputed, large size matrices associated with the model are no longer valid, and have to be recalculated. These calculations are too computationally demanding to be performed during the simulation. A solution to the cutting problem is to incrementally update the inverse stiffness matrix rather than recalculate it [2,6]. As this inverse matrix is, in general, not sparse, updating it under real-time haptic rate constraints becomes a considerable computational challenge.

Our work on topology modification for virtual organs [6] is based upon a particular form of the Sherman-Morrison-Woodbury formula for updating the inverse of a matrix. [7,9] have proposed similar cumulative topology updates, however their methods require the external forces as primary input for updating the deformation and cannot be used in the context of haptic feedback. In contrast to these other topology modification methods, our method allows for realistic simulation of both deformation and haptic response.

2.4. Modified Matrix Update Procedure

We use an extension of our work on topology modification [6] by integrating condensation to allow real-time interaction with larger models. Once calculated, the precomputed inverse stiffness matrix, referred to in the following text as the inverse matrix, is stored on disk such that it can be re-used in the future. The condensed inverse stiffness matrix, referred to in the following text as the condensed matrix, is extracted from the inverse stiffness matrix and stored in memory.

When the interaction with the model involves only deformation of the model, the condensed matrix allows for efficient calculations. When the interaction involves a modification to the topology, it is incrementally updated to reflect modifications in the structure of the model. Our update algorithm described in [6] can be summarised as follows:

We consider the case of a 3D tetrahedral mesh of n nodes, made up of tetrahedra indexed by an index spanning the set $\mathcal{I}$. The local stiffness matrix corresponding to tetrahedron i is:

$$K_i = v_i B_i^T C_i B_i \tag{2}$$

where v_i is the volume of the tetrahedron i, B_i is a 6×12 matrix depending only on the geometry of the tetrahedron, and C_i is a 6×6 matrix describing the physical attributes of the tetrahedron.

A global $3n \times 3n$ stiffness matrix K' for an object is obtained by adding the globalised versions of the local stiffness matrices:

$$K' = \sum_{i \in \mathcal{I}} G_i^T K_i G_i = \sum_{i \in \mathcal{I}} \bar{K}_i. \tag{3}$$

where G_i is a 0's and 1's "globalisation" matrix, and multiplications with this matrix only require the extraction of the corresponding rows and columns.

To remove one of the constituent tetrahedra, we use a particular form of the Sherman-Morrison-Woodbury formula for updating the inverse of a matrix, for the case when the subtracted low-rank matrix is positive semidefinite, i.e. can be written in the form $V^T V$:

$$(K - V^T V)^{-1} = K^{-1} + K^{-1} V^T (I - V K^{-1} V^T)^{-1} V K^{-1} \tag{4}$$

The second term from the right side of Eq. (4) is the "update" that needs to be performed on the inverse matrix. The final equation of the update matrix M becomes:

$$M = K^{-1} G_i^T U_i^T R^T \Lambda^{-1} R U_i G_i K^{-1} = W^T \Lambda^{-1} W. \tag{5}$$

where $W = R U_i G_i K^{-1}$. U_i is a precomputed 6×12 matrix, and only the 6×6 rotation matrix R and the 6×6 diagonal matrix Λ need to be computed in real-time. See [6] for a detailed explanation.

W is calculated by extracting the required rows, corresponding to the deleted tetrahedron, from the inverse matrix stored on disk and multiplication with RU_i. The update matrix M is then calculated by multiplication in blocks and written to disk such that the full $3n \times 3n$ matrix does not have to be stored in memory.

2.5. Simulator Architecture

The BioMedIA surgical simulator serves as a prototyping environment for physically based modelling algorithms. The deformable models are represented as tetrahedral meshes, and are automatically generated from patient-specific models. We have built upon our existing system to add cutting functionality [3]. The simulator primarily runs in two interactive and asynchronous loops: a graphics loop for rendering the deformed virtual organ to screen at 30 Hz, and a haptics loop, at 1 kHz, for rendering force feedback.

The stiffness matrices are double-buffered. When a cut event occurs, the stiffness matrix that is buffered is updated in the background while the interactive loops are running. When the buffered matrix update is complete, it is swapped with the active matrix along whilst simultaneously updating the deformed model to reflect the cut. This permits a much smoother interactive experience as neither the graphics or haptics appear to stall whilst the relatively expensive cut operation is executed.

3. Results

The integration of condensation into our scheme increases its efficiency, and allows for complex interaction on larger models, whilst maintaining accuracy of the model. Fig. 1

illustrates the deformations of a cube while cutting is performed. After each modification to the structure, the precomputed matrix is updated, and a change in deformation response can be seen.

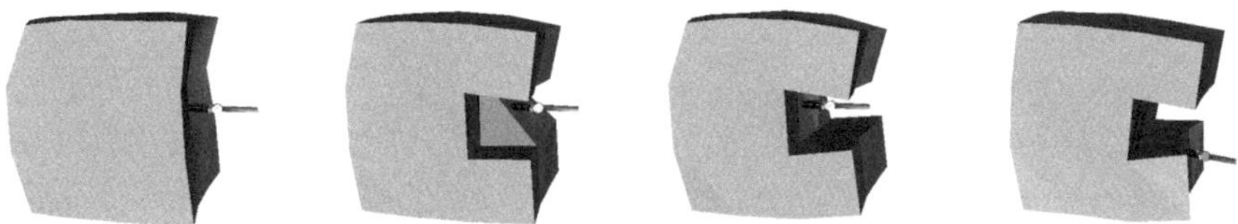

Figure 1. *Illustration of interaction between a surgical tool and deformable model of a cube while real-time cutting is performed. Far left: Original model before cutting. Middle left: Cut partially completed. Far and middle right: Cut completed, representing a modified structure. Note the difference in deformation responses after the cut has been performed.*

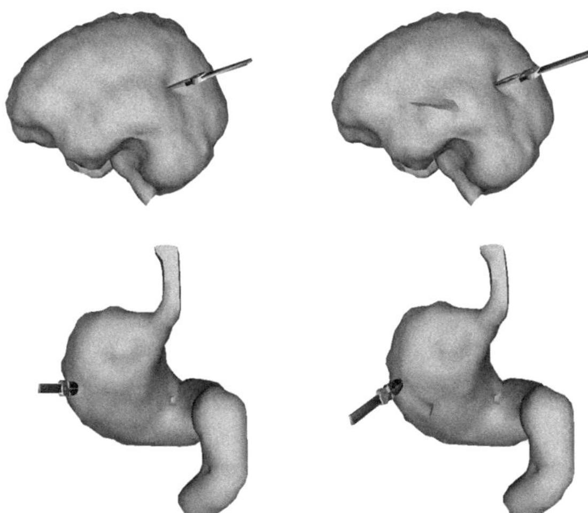

Figure 2. *Illustration of interaction between a surgical tool and deformable models while cutting is performed. Top: Model of a brain consisting of 7480 nodes and 39323 tetrahedra. Bottom: Model of a stomach consisting of 2736 nodes and 11954 tetrahedra.*

The performance of our topology modification algorithm has been measured on a 2.4 GHz Pentium 4. The results are shown in Fig. 3. The dotted line represents the timings without condensation and the solid line represents the timings with the condensation extension. By reducing memory requirements, condensation permits topology modification to be carried out on meshes that would not otherwise fit into conventional memory.

Condensation does however come with a cost. Manipulating matrices in memory is much quicker then file I/O. Furthermore, there exists extra overhead in managing a condensed matrix. The times required to delete a tetrahedron while integrating condensation are therefore greater than a deletion without condensation.

It is interesting to note that the timings for up to 500 nodes are almost identical regardless of the number of nodes. This can be attributed to the overhead required to access a file no matter how small the file is. Also, possible performance improvements could be made by experimenting with the size of the blocks used when accessing the data in the files.

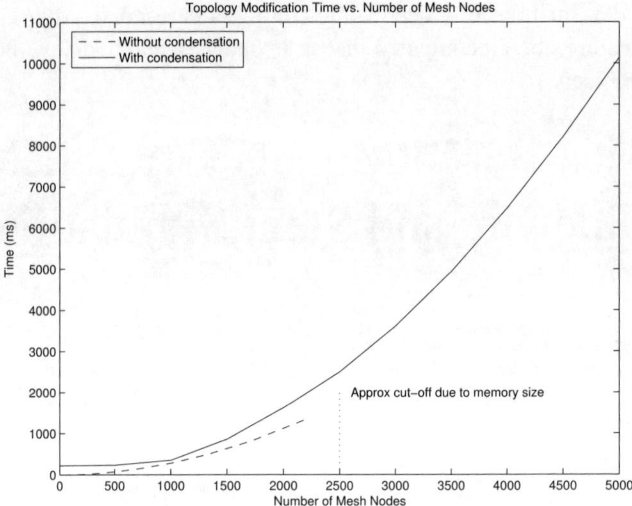

Figure 3. *Time necessary to delete a tetrahedron from a mesh, on a 2.4 GHz Pentium 4.*

4. Conclusion

We have presented the combination of cutting FE models and condensation, fully integrated into our surgical simulation system. The use of condensation has allowed complex interaction, including deformation and cutting, with larger models. It increases computational efficiency and decreases memory requirements to facilitate real-time visual and haptic interaction, in our surgical simulation environment.

References

[1] M. Bro-Nielsen and S. Cotin; *Real-time Volumetric Deformable Models for Surgery Simulation using Finite Elements and Condensation*, In Proceedings of Eurographics 1996.

[2] M. Bro-Nielsen; *Finite Element Modeling in Surgery Simulation*, In Proceedings of the IEEE, vol.86, no.3, 1998.

[3] B. Joshi and B. Lee and D. C. Popescu and S. Ourselin; *Multiple Contact Approach to Collision Modelling in Surgical Simulation*, Medicine Meets Virtual Reality 13 (MMVR2005), vol.111, pp.237-242, 2005.

[4] A. Nealen, M Muller, R. Keiser, E. Boxerman and M. Carlson; *Physically Based Deformable Models in Computer Graphics* , In Proceedings of Eurographics 2005.

[5] D. Popescu and M. Compton; *A Method for Efficient and Accurate Interaction with Elastic Objects in Haptic Virtual Environments*, In Proceedings of Graphite 2003, pp.245-249, 2003.

[6] D. C. Popescu, B. Joshi and S. Ourselin; *Real-time topology modification for Finite Element models with haptic feedback*, In Proceedings of The 11th International Conference on Computer Analysis of Images and Patterns, Springer, LNCS vol.3691, pp.846-853, 2005.

[7] W. Wu, J. Sun and P. A. Heng; *A Hybrid Condensed Finite Element Model for Interactive 3D Soft Tissue Cutting*, Medicine Meets Virtual Reality (MMVR 2003), vol.94, pp.401-403, 2003.

[8] H. Zhong, M. P. Wachowiak, T. M. Peters; *Enhanced Pre-computed Finite Element Models for Surgical Simulation*, Medicine Meets Virtual Reality 13 (MMVR 2005), vol.111, pp.622-628, 2005.

[9] H. Zhong, M. P. Wachowiak and T. M. Peters; *Adaptive Finite Element Technique for Cutting in Surgical Simulation*, In Proceedings of SPIE 2005, 2005.

Medicine Meets Virtual Reality 14
J.D. Westwood et al. (Eds.)
IOS Press, 2006

305

Physics-Based Models for Catheter, Guidewire and Stent Simulation

Julien Lenoir [a], Stephane Cotin [a,b], Christian Duriez [a] and Paul Neumann [a,b]

[a] *The Sim Group, CIMIT/MGH*   [b] *Harvard Medical School*

Abstract. For over 20 years, interventional methods have improved the outcomes of patients with cardiovascular disease or stroke. However, these procedures require an intricate combination of visual and tactile feedback and extensive training periods. An essential part of this training relates to the manipulation of diagnostic and therapeutic devices such as catheters, guidewires, or stents. In this paper, we propose a physics-based model of wire-like structures that can be used as a core representation for the real-time simulation of various devices. Our approach is computationally efficient, and physically realistic. A catheter/guidewire is simulated using a composite model, which can dynamically adapt its material properties to locally describe a combination of both devices. We also show that other devices, such as stents, can be modeled from the same core representation.

Keywords. Simulation, Interventional Radiology, Real-Time, Physics-based

1. Introduction

Over the last twenty years, interventional methods such as angioplasty, stenting, and catheter-based drug delivery have substantially improved the outcomes for patients with cardiovascular or neurovascular disease. However, these techniques require an intricate combination of tactile and visual feedback, and extensive training periods to attain competency. Traditionally, the best training environments on which to learn the anatomic-pathologic and therapeutic techniques have been animals or actual patients. Yet, the development of computer-based simulation can provide an excellent alternative to traditional training. To reach this goal, aspects of the real procedure need to be simulated, including catheter[1] and guidewire[2] manipulation is the most important, but also therapeutical devices usage, like stents. In a real procedure, after puncturing the femoral artery, a guidewire-catheter combination is advanced under fluoroscopic guidance through the arterial network to the target location (brain, heart, abdomen). There, various therapeutic devices (stent, balloon,...) can be deployed and treatment can be delivered. A few computer-based training systems focusing on interventional radiology have been developed or commercialized as of today [12,7,4]. These systems include interactive models of catheters but do not deal with the complex interactions between a device and the vessels or between catheter and guidewire. We propose a composite model of catheter/guidewire that handles these two problems. A physics-based device model is used to create a realistic and accurate behavior, while a specific visualization technique is proposed to render

---

[1] A hollow, flexible tube inserted into a vessel to allow the passage of fluids or other devices
[2] A flexible wire positioned in a vessel for the purpose of directing the passage of a catheter.

both objects from one unified model. Also, an update of the model's material properties is performed dynamically to describe a combination of both devices using a unique model. In addition, the core representation is derived to model stent devices.

This paper is organized as follows: previous work is discussed in section 2, then the physical core model is outlined in section 3, the composite model of catheter/guidewire is exposed in section 4, a stent model example is described in section 5 and preliminary results are presented in section 6.

2. Previous work

Previous work in the field of interventional radiology simulation has focused on the development of complete systems [4,12], visualization [11] and anatomical modeling [10]. In [12] the authors simulate the catheter using a linear elasticity FEM-based representation. In [4] the catheter simulation is based on a multi-body system composed of a set of rigid bodies and joints. This discrete model permits a good approximation of a catheter but requires many small links to represent a high degree of flexibility, thus leading to increased computation cost. Other work outside of the area of interventional radiology has focused on one-dimensional deformable models. For instance, Lenoir *et al* [9] proposed to simulate a surgical thread in real-time using a dynamic spline. Another way to model one-dimensional deformable objects is to use the Cosserat theory, as proposed by Pai [13]. This model is static and takes into account all possible deformations of a one-dimensional object. But contact handling with such a model is difficult and for catheter navigation, where collisions occur continuously along the length of the device, this remains an issue, and computation times for a large number of points can lead to non-interactive simulation times.

Finally, some recent work directly related to the simulation of a catheter or guidewire has been proposed by Cotin *et al* [3]. This physics-based model consists of a set of connected beam elements that can model bending, twist and other deformations in real-time. The simulation is based on a static finite element representation. Different aspects of this model are presented in section 3 while our contribution begins in section 4 by presenting its application on simulating a catheter/guidewire and a stent in section 5.

3. The core model

As previously mentioned, our approach is based on a physics-based model (described in details in [3]). The physical model is defined as a set of beam elements. Each element has 6 degrees of freedom, 3 in translation and 3 in rotation. The model is continuous and the equations are solved using a finite element approach. Since each element can bend, a lower number of elements is required to represent the catheter than with a rigid body approach [4]. The choice of a static over a dynamic model was made since the catheter or guidewire navigate inside blood vessels where the blood induces a damping factor. Under this assumption, the equations of the mechanical system can be written as: $[K]U = F$, where U represents the degrees of freedom, F the forces and torques applied on each nodes and $[K]$ the stiffness matrix of the system. Yet, the significant flexibility of a catheter or guidewire can generate geometric non-linearities when navigating inside twisted parts of the vascular system. Since this cannot be handled by a linear model, we overcome this problem by defining $[K]$ as a function of the degrees of freedom U: $[K(U)]U = F$.

The system is then solved using an incremental approach [3] which permits faster computation times compared to other techniques. Additionally, the system of equations can be re-written by decomposing the model as a set of substructures [3], which improves even further the computation times. To control the deformation and navigation of the device, we use a combination of external forces and boundary conditions. Since the device (catheter, guidewire or stent) is manipulated by the interventional radiologist using only a combination of translations and rotations about the main axis of the device, this is taken into account in the model via a set of boundary conditions. Those constraints are transmitted along the all entire model via its deformations, according to the material properties.

This physics-based representation will serve as the core of the two models we will introduce in the following sections.

4. Composite catheter-guidewire representation

In this section we describe how catheter/guidewire combination (i.e. a configuration where the guidewire is partially or totally inserted inside a catheter) can be modeled as a composite model, involving the physics-based component introduced above and an animation component. By simulating only one model, we avoid the problems of handling numerous contact between the catheter and the guidewire, since both devices are co-axial. This proposition is detailed in [8] and is exposed briefly in this section as one example of a model that can be based on this generic core representation.

4.1. Animation component

The animation part is based on the visual appearance of the catheter and the guidewire, which is needed to distinguish between them. A parameter *limit* represents the curvilinear position of the guidewire tip relatively to the catheter tip. Typically, the value of this parameter is zero when both device tips are at the same location, negative when the guidewire tip is inside the catheter and positive when it is outside. A change in the value of *limit* happens only when either the catheter or the guidewire is pushed or pulled. This modification is shown during the rendering of the model, by using the *limit* value to define two different objects. Both objects are rendered as generalized cylinders [1,2]

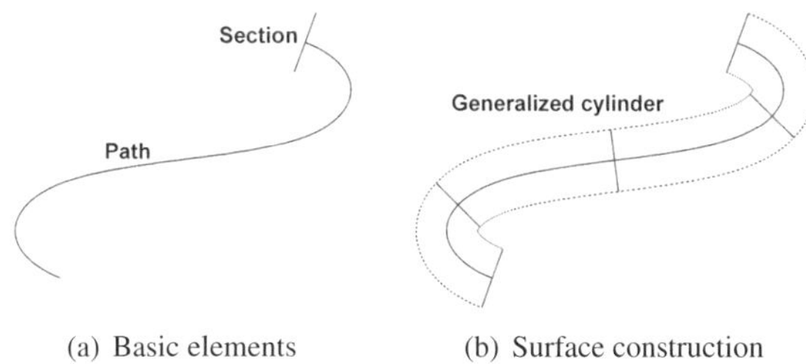

(a) Basic elements   (b) Surface construction

Figure 1. Generalized cylinder construction.

(cf. figure 4). This technique permits to define a smooth surface (figure 1(b)) based on a path (the nodes position of the core model) and a cross section (circle) (figure 1(a)). In addition, new rendering techniques [5] permit to take advantage of the graphics hardware to optimize the rendering speed. Yet, realistic visualization is not enough to simulate the combination of two nested devices. To be able to exhibit realistic behaviors for both objects, special attention has to be placed on the mechanical interaction between the catheter and the guidewire, as illustrated in the following section.

4.2. Catheter / guidewire interaction

When the guidewire is inserted inside the catheter or the catheter moves along the guidewire, the overall shape of both the catheter and guidewire is modified due to a change in the bending stiffness and bending moment in the overlapped portion. The region where the catheter and guidewire are coaxial offers a stiffer resistance to transverse loading. We simulate this meaningful visual cue as a fiber *reinforced* composite material. The transversal stiffness of the overlapped region can be modeled with the well-established empirical expression, the Halpin-Tsai equations [6]:

$$E_{trans} = \frac{E_{cath}(1+\xi\eta f)}{1-\eta f}, \eta = \frac{E_{guide}-E_{cath}}{E_{guide}+\xi E_{cath}}$$

where f is the ratio, in the overlapped section, of the guidewire volume over the volume of the guidewire-catheter combination; ξ is a function of the material properties and geometry of the instruments. Lookup tables describing typical values of ξ under different composition configurations have been published in the literature [6]. The stiffness for the overlapped section can be updated in real-time and the composite physical model reflects this change, accordingly.

5. Stent representation

We propose also to combine our real-time finite element model of wire-like structures with a generic representation of tubular shapes to provide an efficient and flexible way to describe a large range of devices, such as stents, but possibly angioplasty balloons too. The deformation scheme is based on the following idea: a set of beam elements is used to define the skeleton of the device, and is then mapped to a surface representation adapted to the particular device being modeled (see Figure 2). Since the main difference between such devices and wire-like structures is their ability to handle radial deformations, we mostly need to define the relationship between the skeleton and the surface representation.

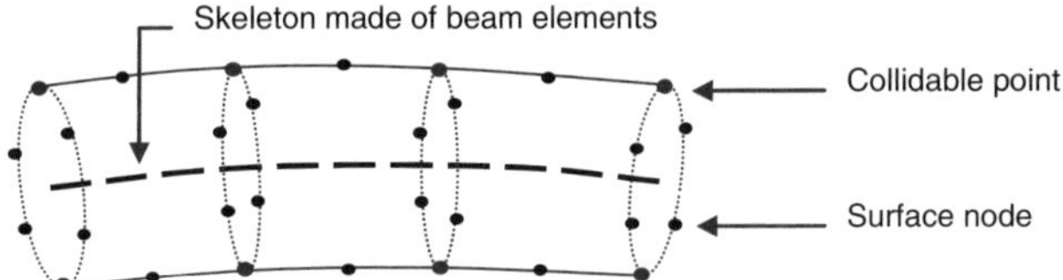

Figure 2. A stent modeled as a skeleton combined with a deformable surface representation.

The displacement $\mathbf{Us}$ of a surface point $\mathbf{Ps}$ is defined as a linear combination of two deformations, one due to the beam deformation ($\mathbf{Us}^b$) and one local deformation ($\mathbf{Us}^l$).

The $\mathbf{Us}^b$ vector is directly obtained from the beam model by interpolation of the displacement $\mathbf{Ub}$ of the n beam nodes, as describe by the following equation: $\mathbf{Us}^b = \sum_{i=0}^{n} w_i U b_i = [\mathbf{H}]\mathbf{Ub}$. The beam model gives the relation between forces $\mathbf{Fb}$ and displacements $\mathbf{Ub}$ of beam nodes: $\mathbf{Ub} = [\mathbf{Kb}]^{-1}\mathbf{Fb}$. Then, the forces $\mathbf{Fs}$ applied on the surface point are distributed to the different beam nodes using the transpose matrix of $[\mathbf{H}]$: $\mathbf{Fb} = [\mathbf{H}]^{\mathrm{T}}\mathbf{Fs}$

Then a local deformation model gives also the relation between local motion displacement $\mathbf{Us}^l$ and forces applied to surface point: $\mathbf{Us}^l = [\mathbf{K}_{\mathrm{local}}]^{-1}\mathbf{Fs}$, where $[\mathbf{K}_{\mathrm{local}}]$ is the local stiffness matrix used to compute $[\mathbf{K}]$ (cf. section 3).

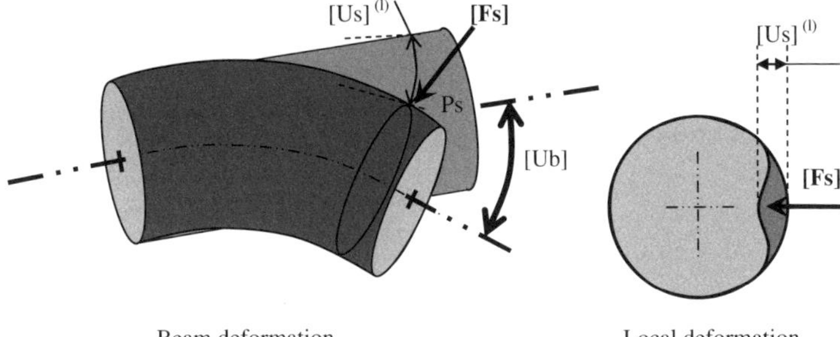

Figure 3. The deformation of a tubular structure is composed of a global deformation (left) included by the deformation of the skeleton and a local deformation of surface (right)).

Using compliance (flexibility) formulation we can combine the two contributions:

$$\mathbf{Us} = \mathbf{Us^b} + \mathbf{Us^l} = ([\mathbf{K_{local}}]^{-1} + [\mathbf{H}][\mathbf{Kb}]^{-1}[\mathbf{H}]^{\mathbf{T}})\mathbf{Fs}$$

Finally, a list of points sampled is distributed on the surface of the device, which will be used for collision detection purpose.

6. Results

The first result (illustrated in Figure 4(a)) show the effectiveness of the physics-based model. In this simulation, the catheter navigates through the vascular network and is simulated with 100 nodes in real-time (about 45 frames per second). The model exhibits a realistic behavior, sliding against the vessel walls and passing through bifurcations.

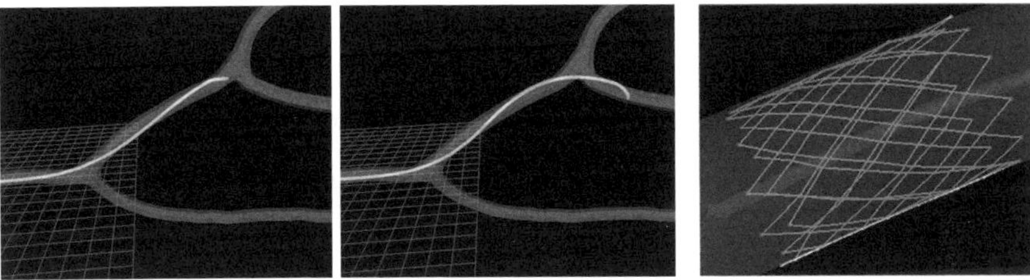

(a) Two step of a simulation in the vessel network.   (b) Stent deployment

Figure 4. Catheter simulation in artery and stent deployment.

The second result (illustrated in Figure 4(b)) shows a stent deployed in an artery. The bending properties as well as the radial stiffness of the stent can be controlled to model a large set of devices. Once released inside the vessel, the stent deploys automatically under the influence of internal forces. Then, the collision detection representation of the stent model is used to handle contact with the vessel wall thus stopping the expansion of the stent.

The last result (illustrated in Figure 5) shows the interaction between two nested devices. In this animation, a straight guidewire is inserted into a curved catheter and, as it is moving toward the tip of the catheter, straightens it, This is a direct result of the use of our composite model, and illustrates both the changes in the visual and bending properties of the combined representation.

7. Conclusion and future work

This paper proposes a unique representation to interactively model various devices required for simulating interventional radiology procedures. While the core model exhibits realistic behaviors typical of wire-like structures, we show how it can be enhanced to

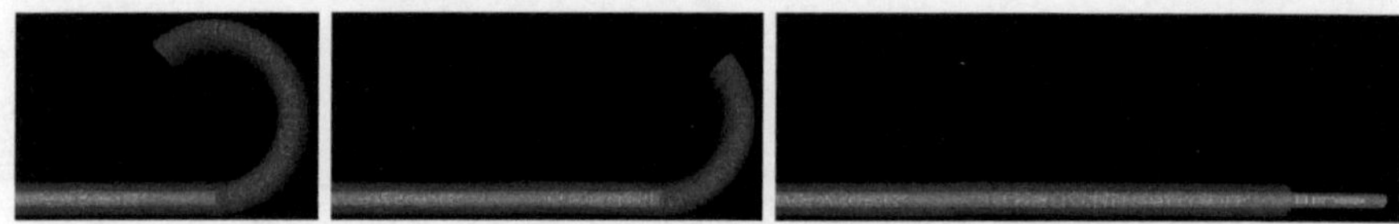

Figure 5. Guidewire deforming a catheter.

represent a guidewire/catheter combination or a stent, for instance. The incremental FEM representation of the core model ensures accurate, real-time, physics-based simulations of devices such as catheters and guidewires. Each additional model based on this representation benefits from its realism (torsion and bending are taken into account) but adds specific levels of modeling or visualization. The composite model of catheter/guidewire combines an optimized visualization technique (that can render both objects from one unified model) with a method that dynamically updates the model's material properties in real-time. Finally, a stent model can also be derived from the core representation, demonstrating its genericity. A surface layer attached to the core deals with the vascular surface interaction.

We would like to enhance our stent model by managing the interaction between the stent surface and the physics core in a finer way. We also would like to generalized the usage of our physics core to other therapeutic devices like angioplasty balloons.

References

[1] T.O. Binford. Generalized cylinder representation. In Shapiro S.C., editor, *Encyclopedia of Artificial Intelligence*, pages 321–323. John Wiley & Sons, 1987.

[2] J. Bloomenthal. *Graphics Gems*, volume 1, chapter Calculation of Reference Frames along a Space Curve, pages 567–571. Academic Press, 1990.

[3] S. Cotin, C. Duriez, J. Lenoir, P. Neumann, and S. Dawson. New approaches to catheter navigation for interventional radiology simulation. In *proceedings of Medical Image Computing and Computer Assisted Intervention (MICCAI)*, Palm Springs, California, USA, 2005.

[4] S. Dawson, S. Cotin, D. Meglan, D. Shaffer, and M. Ferrell. Designing a computer-based simulator for interventional cardiology training. *Catheterization and Cardiovascular Interventions*, 51:522–527, december 2000.

[5] Laurent Grisoni and Damien Marchal. High performance generalized cylinders visualization. In *proceedings of Shape Modeling'03 (ACM Siggraph, Eurographics, and IEEE sponsored)*, pages 257–263, Aizu (Japan), july 2003.

[6] J.C. Halpin and J.L. Kardos. The halpin-tsai equations: a review. *Polymer Engineering Science*, 16:344 – 52, 1976.

[7] U. Hoefer, T. Langen, J. Nziki, F. Zeitler, J. Hesser, U. Mueller, W. Voelker, and R. Maenner. Cathi - catheter instruction system. In *Computer Assisted Radiology and Surgery (CARS), 16th International Congress and Exhibition*, pages 101 – 06, Paris, France, 2002.

[8] J. Lenoir, S. Cotin, C. Duriez, and P. Neumann. Interactive physically-based simulation of catheter and guidewire. In *Second Workshop in Virtual Reality Interactions and Physical Simulations (VRIPHYS)*, Pisa, Italy, 7th november 2005.

[9] J. Lenoir, P. Meseure, L. Grisoni, and C. Chaillou. Surgical thread simulation. *Modelling and Simulation for Computer-aided Medecine and Surgery*, November 2002.

[10] V. Luboz, X. Wu, K. Krissian, C.-F. Westin, R. Kikinis, S. Cotin, and S. Dawson. A segmentation and reconstruction technique for 3d vascular structures. In *proceedings of Medical Image Computing and Computer Assisted Intervention (MICCAI)*, 2005.

[11] M. Manivannan, S. Cotin, M. Srinivasan, and S. Dawson. Real-time pc-based x-ray simulation for interventional radiology training. In *Proceedings of 11th Annual Meeting, Medicine Meets Virtual Reality*, pages 233–39, 2003.

[12] W.L. Nowinski and C.-K. Chui. Simulation of interventional neuroradiology procedures. In *proceedings of International Workshop on Medical Imaging and Augmented Reality (MIAR)*, pages 87–94, Hong Kong, june 2001. IEEE Computer Society, 2001.

[13] D. Pai. Strands: Interactive simulation of thin solids using cosserat models. *Eurographics*, 2002.

Medicine Meets Virtual Reality 14
J.D. Westwood et al. (Eds.)
IOS Press, 2006

311

A Web-Based Repository of Surgical Simulator Projects

Peter Leškovský [1], Matthias Harders [a] and Gábor Székely [a]
[a] *Virtual Reality in Medicine Group*
Computer Vision Lab
ETH Zurich
Switzerland

Abstract. The use of computer-based surgical simulators for training of prospective surgeons has been a topic of research for more than a decade. As a result, a large number of academic projects have been carried out, and a growing number of commercial products are available on the market (see e.g. [1]). Keeping track of all these endeavors for established groups as well as for newly started projects can be quite arduous. Gathering information on existing methods, already traveled research paths, and problems encountered is a time consuming task. To alleviate this situation, we have established a modifiable online repository of existing projects. It contains detailed information about a large number of simulator projects gathered from web pages, papers and personal communication. The database is modifiable (with password protected sections) and also allows for a simple statistical analysis of the collected data. For further information, the surgical repository web page can be found at www.virtualsurgery.vision.ee.ethz.ch.

Keywords. Surgery Simulators, Online repository

1. Introduction

The field of computer-based surgical simulation is rapidly expanding. Keeping track of all existing projects is a tedious task and following the state-of-the-art becomes difficult, due to the fact that the relevant information is shattered across a number of published articles. Moreover, detailed technical information is not always available.

We have set up an online repository of a number of surgical simulators. Included in the database are research projects as well as commercial systems. The used web-engine makes it easy to correct entries or add more data directly via the web-browser. It also makes the addition of new projects simple. For each page describing a single simulator, we give a general overviews including contact information and scientific details consisting of selected categories, such as the intervention area, algorithms used, haptic devices, performance measurements, etc.

---

[1] Correspondence to: pleskovs@vision.ee.ethz.ch

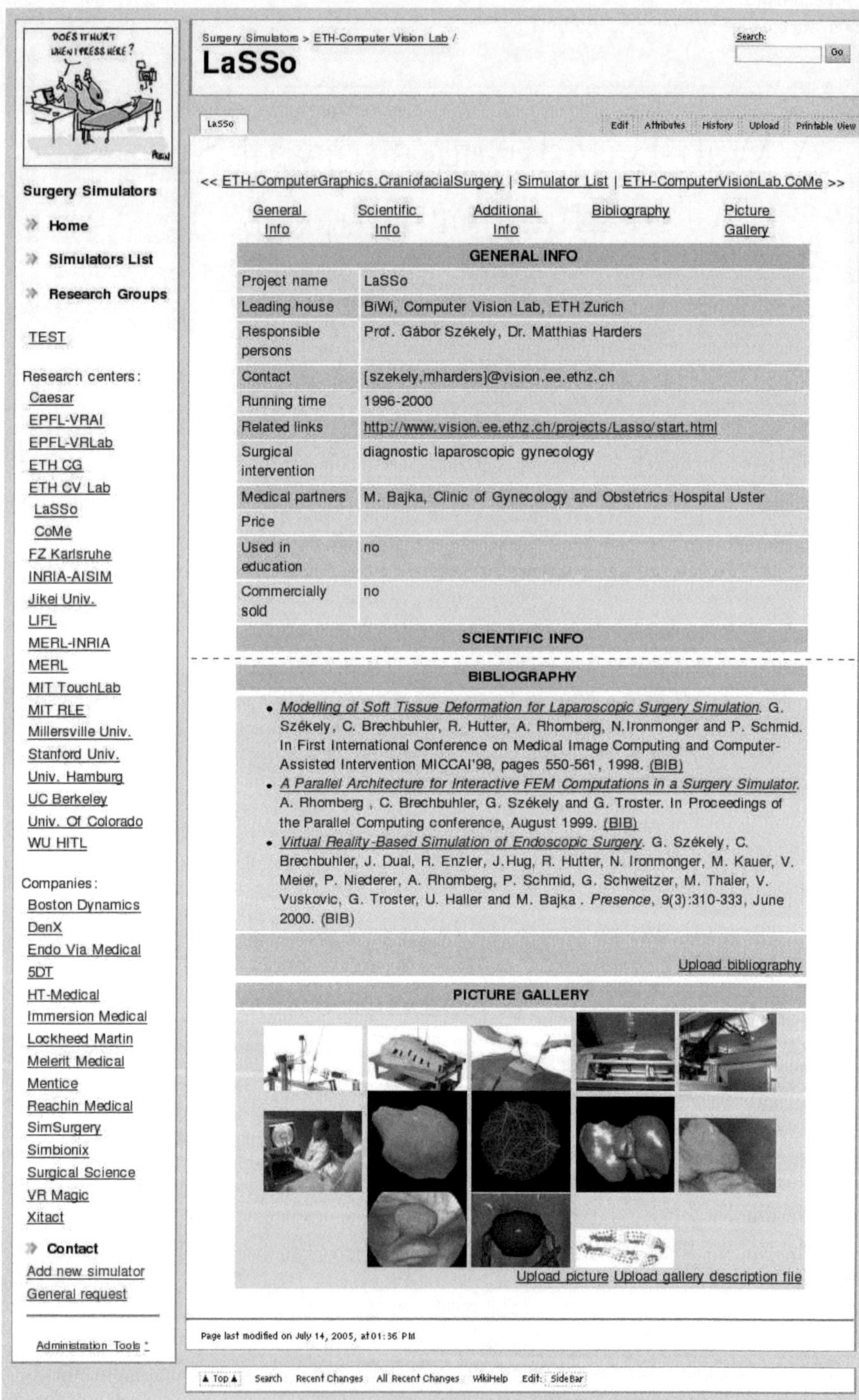

Figure 1. A snapshot of a part of the online repository (the scientific section is cut out).

Moreover, sections with related bibliography and pictures exist (see Figure 1). The database is searchable, and simple statistics of selected categories can be created (see Figure 2).

This project gives a convenient overview of new developments and thus provides useful information for the design of new simulators. In addition, it gives an opportunity for research centers to get known in the community, and to set up new scientific collaborations.

We believe, that having the information about each surgical simulator directly available on one web-page is beneficial for the medical as well as for the research community. However, the success of this projects depends on the cooperation of the sites active in this area. Although the initial data about 45 simulators has been filled in, it will be up to the individual centers to provide and update information relevant to their projects.

2. Tools and Methods

A "Wiki" [2] web page (www.virtualsurgery.vision.ee.ethz.ch) has been created to enable easy modification by individual research groups using intuitive and simple markup language within a user friendly web-based environment. All sections are password protected to ensure that only the respective teams can edit the information.

Table 1. Structure of the scientific information section, with categories listed for each subsection.

Scientific Information

Overview	Overall focus area, the goal of the simulator, medical application area, main contribution and problems encountered.
Hardware information	Operating system, computation engine used and a possible patient mock-up.
Model generation	Medical data source, data generation process and integrated pathologies.
Soft tissue deformation	Deformation algorithm, numerical integration, tissue parameter source, model size and reached deformation update rate.
Tissue cutting	Possibility of cutting the tissue, basic idea of the cutting algorithm and its limitations.
Collision detection	Collision detection algorithm, collision response technique and the reached refresh rate.
Visualisation	Visualisation paradigm, visualisation model size, display technology, visualisation effects added, bleeding model description, the refresh rate and additional teaching hints provided.
Haptic feedbacks	Specification of haptic devices used, haptic rendering algorithm, update rate and surgical tools imitated.
Evaluation	Evaluation studies, performance measurements and medical curriculum integration.
Additional information	Parallelisation techniques used and additional technical information.

The creation of a new simulator page is managed via a request sent to the administrator directly from the web page. The administrator will stay in contact with the new representative while checking the request and denying inappropriate projects and unsolicited requests. After creating a new simulator section, the access passwords and an invitation to fill in the simulator information will be sent immediately.

For each simulator page we list the general information about the project, i.e. name, contact persons, involved institutes, related web-pages and the running time. Detailed scientific information about the technology used follows. The structure of the scientific data, with the subsections and all categories listed, can be seen in the Table 1. The related published articles are listed too, with accessible bibliography data. Finally, a section with screen-shots and other pictures is presented. A place for entering additional technical information, i.e. a new category, is included at the end of the scientific section.

As a part of the "Wiki" engine, all entered data is searchable. In addition, the search capabilities are currently being improved by providing a summary of each category.

3. Results

Because of all information is categorized in a table form (see the category list in Table 1), statistical evaluation of the data is possible (see Figure 2). Since all entries are in text form without any context restrictions, automatic evaluation cannot be offered. Nonetheless, the descriptions given for each category can be listed separately supporting the definition of appropriate queries.

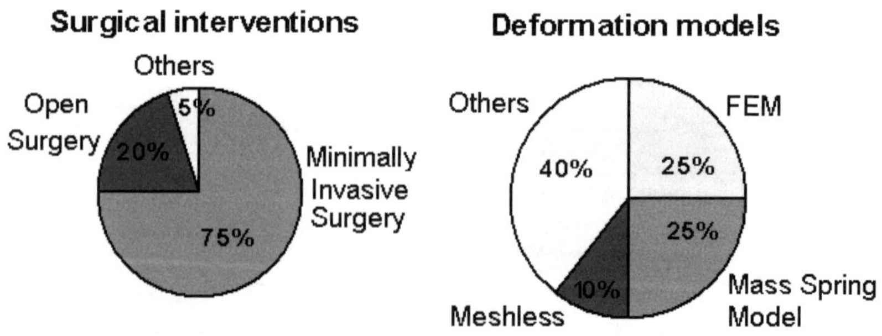

Figure 2. Proportions of different surgical interventions simulated and the deformation models of the soft tissue used nowadays in the surgical simulators.

Examples of our statistical studies follow:

- The majority of the simulators uses surface models based on triangle and polygonal meshes as a visual paradigm. A couple of volumetric-visualisation-based systems exists and a first study using a point-based graphics and haptic rendering was presented.
- Some systems, mainly the commercial ones, provide interactive games for improving the tool manipulation skills of the surgeon.

- 75% of reviewed simulators model minimally invasive surgery scenarios.
- 60% of reviewed simulators use physically based deformation models.
- 82% provide haptic feedback.

4. Conclusion

An online repository of surgical simulator projects has been created, which currently contains 45 entries of different simulators. All relevant information was extracted from published articles and internet resources. Moreover, statistical data of the projects are available. All research groups have been contacted to verify the stored data. In the future statistical analysis will be improved and information retrieval further streamlined.

This project is a living database that relies on the input of the community. To guarantee up to date information, the interaction of other groups is needed. We hereby ask people to contact us and provide further input to the surgical simulators repository. We would also be grateful for any further comments and suggestions concerning web-page improvements.

Acknowledgements

We acknowledge Nicolas Mirjolet and Manuel Wittwer, students at ETH Zurich, for their help in making the collected information publicly available. This project has been supported by the NCCR Co-Me of the Swiss National Science Foundation, and the IST European Program Touch-Hapsys (IST-2001-38040) and IN-TUITION (IST-NMP-1-507248-2) projects.

References

[1] A. Liu and F. Tendick and K. Cleary and C. Kaufmann, A Survey of Surgical Simulation: Applications, Technology, and Education, *Presence, Vol. 12, Issue 6*, MIT Press, 2003.
[2] http://www.pmwiki.org
[3] C. D. Combs and K. Friend, Tracking the Domain: The Medical Modeling and Simulation Database, *MMVR* **13**, 90–93, IOS Press, 2005.

Medicine Meets Virtual Reality 14
J.D. Westwood et al. (Eds.)
IOS Press, 2006

GiPSiNet: An Open Source/Open Architecture Network Middleware for Surgical Simulations

Vincenzo Liberatore [1], M. Cenk Çavuşoğlu and Qingbo Cai
Department of Electrical Engineering and Computer Science
Case Western Reserve University

Abstract. In this paper, we present the design and techniques of GiPSiNet, an open source/open architecture network middleware being developed for surgical simulations. GiPSiNet extends *GiPSi* (General Interactive Physical Simulation Interface), our framework for developing organ level surgical simulations, to network environments. This network extension is non-trivial, since the network settings pose several serious problems for distributed surgical virtual environments such as bandwidth limit, delays, and packet losses. Our goal is to enhance the quality (fidelity and realism) of networked simulations in the absence of network *QoS* (Quality of Service) through the GiPSiNet middleware.

Keywords. Surgical simulation, Virtual reality, Network, Middleware, QoS

1. Introduction

Virtual environments receive increasing interest as a new medium for surgical training. The network extension can substantially amplify the accessibility of surgical virtual environments and enable remote continuing education and advanced training. However, this network extension is non-trivial, since the network settings and realities pose several serious problems for distributed surgical virtual environments such as bandwidth limit, delays, and packet losses due to congestion. These network issues can greatly impair the user-perceived simulation quality (fidelity and realism). Thus, the performance of a networked surgical simulation critically depends on the techniques applied to implement an effective remote interaction.

In our previous work [1,2], we proposed *GiPSi* (General Interactive Physical Simulation Interface), an open source/open architecture software development framework for organ level surgical simulations, to accommodate heterogeneous models of computation and interface heterogeneous physical processes. In our ongoing project, we extend GiPSi to network environments by adding a network middleware module *GiPSiNet*, which acts as an intermediary between simulation applications and the network and takes actions

---

[1]Correspondence to: Vincenzo Liberatore or M. Cenk Çavuşoğlu, Department of Electrical Engineering and Computer Science, Case Western Reserve University, 10900 Euclid Avenue, Cleveland, OH 44106, U.S.A. Tel.: +1 216 368 4088; E-mail: vxl11@case.edu or cavusoglu@case.edu.

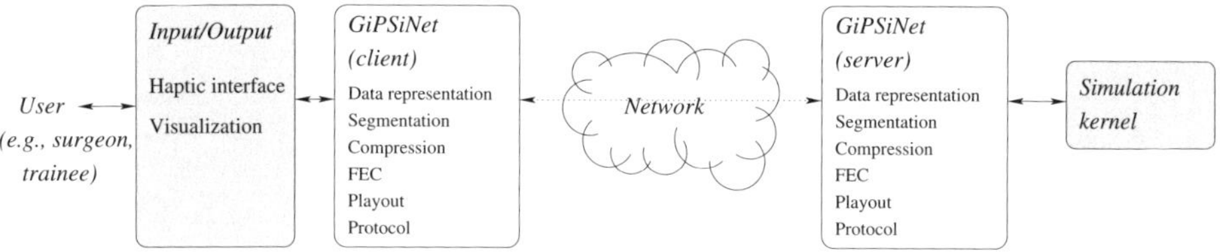

Figure 1. The GiPSiNet middleware architecture. Shaded module are part of the existing GiPSi platform, clear modules are part of the GiPSiNet middleware.

to compensate for the lack of network *QoS* (Quality of Service) [3]. Our goal is to enhance the quality of networked simulations in the absence of network QoS through the GiPSiNet middleware.

Specifically, the design objectives of the GiPSiNet middleware are as follows:

- Providing abstraction to address heterogeneous haptic devices and data representations.
- Ensuring modularity through encapsulation and data hiding.
- Supporting customizability to accommodate various surgical simulations.
- Utilizing network bandwidth and other system resources efficiently. GiPSiNet should be lightweight and efficient for data communication.
- Devising compensation strategies for networks with delay, jitter, and congestion.

In this paper, we present the design and techniques of GiPSiNet, an open source/open architecture network middleware being developed for surgical simulations.

2. GiPSiNet Architecture

In our current implementation of GiPSi, an API is provided between the simulation kernel and I/O (i.e., haptic I/O, visualization, graphical user interface (GUI)). To extend the kernel-I/O API to network environments, we add a middleware layer (GiPSiNet) between the kernel and the I/O module to encapsulate all networking functionality (Figure 1). The resulting simulator has two communication end-points: (1) the *client*, which interacts with the end-user (e.g., surgeon, trainee) through the haptic and visualization interfaces, and (2) the *server*, where the simulation kernel runs and the physical processes are numerically simulated. The GiPSiNet high level client-server architecture and data flow are illustrated in Figure 2.

Accordingly, relevant modules in GiPSi (i.e., haptics I/O and visualization) are restructured so that their functionalities are appropriately distributed over the network. For example, the architecture of the GiPSi haptics I/O module is shown in Figure 3. In this architecture, the Haptic Interface (HI) class provides an abstraction and a uniform API for the physical haptic interface device, and hardware specific low-level function calls. The Haptic Interface Object (HIO) class is the representation of an actual haptic interface in the simulation. Then, the Haptics Server is responsible of creating the instances of the HI class, initializing them, attaching them to the proper HIOs, and when requested by the Simulation Kernel, enabling, disabling, and terminating them. The Haptics Client starts and initializes instances of HIs, starts the real-time schedulers for the physical haptic interface devices, establishes network communication with the Haptics Server, and,

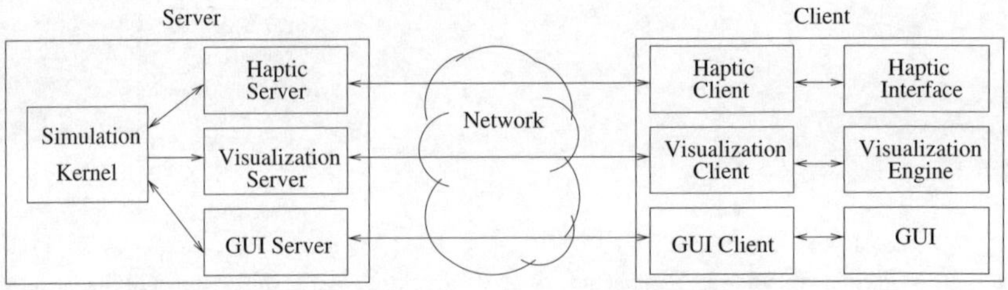

Figure 2. The GiPSiNet client-server architecture and data flow.

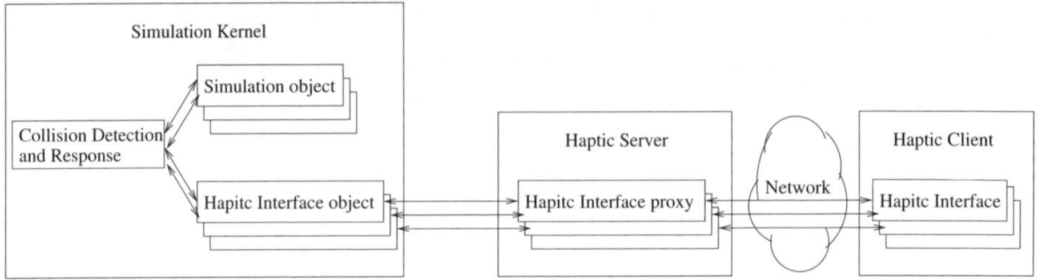

Figure 3. The high level architecture and data flow for GiPSiNet haptics.

when requested by the Haptics Server, enables, disables, and terminates HIs. Each HI at the haptic client side has a corresponding HI Proxy residing at the haptic server which encapsulates the network communications for haptics I/O and consequently is the main API for extending to GiPSiNet.

2.1. Communication Model

GiPSiNet uses the following agreement for the client-server communication. The client sends the server a data unit including: (1) an input x_i, the state of user actions, e.g., a scalpel position, and (2) an integration interval Δt_i. The server computes a linearized approximation V_{i+1} of the system state after the integration interval Δt_i assuming that the input x_i is applied continuously during such interval, and replies to the client with a data unit including the new system state V_{i+1}. GiPSi views such data units as building blocks for its operations. However, for each "unit", several operations are required to make it suitable for network transmission, for example, segmentation and compression as implemented in the GiPSiNet middleware.

Figure 4 shows a canonical simulation client-server communication: the client sends $(x_i, \Delta t_i)$ to the server, and the server replies to the client with the new system state V_{i+1}. The information exchange follows a classical on-demand protocol: the client sends a request $(x_i, \Delta t_i)$ to the server, and the server replies with a response (V_{i+1}). Ideally, the client sends requests at regular intervals of length Δt_i (say, 100ms, as in the GiPSi simulator), and the server reply is delivered to the client before Δt_i. However, in a best-effort network such as the Internet, a server reply may be delayed or lost due to congestion, and cannot be delivered before Δt_i. Therefore, we should take actions to remediate for such network impairments and ensure timely data delivery as discussed in Section 3.

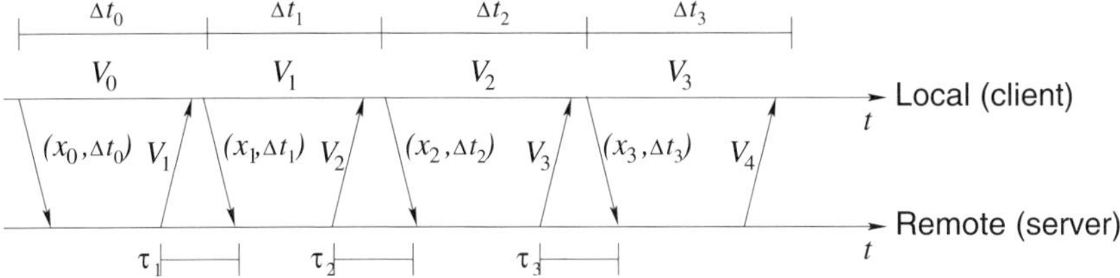

Figure 4. Timeline of data unit exchanges between client and server.

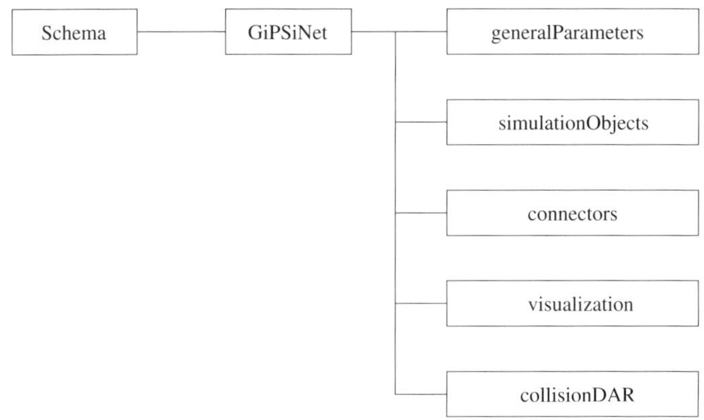

Figure 5. An overview of the XML schema representing the data exchange between a simulation server and a user interface client.

2.2. GiPSiNet Modules

Data representation module. This module implements a format to represent the data exchange implied by the GiPSi kernel-I/O API. For example, we adopt XML, a platform independent and well supported technique, to exploit the data exchange between a simulation server and a user interface client. Figure 5 shows an overview of the XML schema used in GiPSiNet to set up or change the parameters of the simulation environment.

Protocol module. A simulation server should sense clients' input through haptic devices, apply corresponding operations, and respond to clients with haptic feedback and the updated simulation object geometry in real time. Therefore, in the protocol module, we implement a lightweight protocol for efficient communication between the client and server. This protocol is based on User Datagram Protocol (UDP), which incurs much less overhead than Transmission Control Protocol (TCP) and is consequently better suited for real-time traffic.

Segmentation module. The sizes of client and server data unit (i.e., $(x_i, \Delta t_i)$ and V_{i+1}) are currently of the order of 14 and 11,664 bytes respectively. However, the size of packets in the Internet traffic cannot exceed certain limits, typically 1500 bytes (the Ethernet Maximum Transmission Unit). Therefore, a data unit is divided into multiple packets (*segmentation*) if it is longer than the limit. Moreover, in a best-effort network such as the Internet, there is no guarantee of data delivery, i.e., packets can be lost, duplicated, delayed, or delivered out of order. Meanwhile, the light-weight protocol in GiPSiNet is

UDP-based and UDP provides no mechanisms to ensure reliable data delivery. Therefore, segmentation handling is necessary.

Compression module.   Data compression can reduce bandwidth requirements in communication network and the loss probability. Moreover, compressed data has a shorter transmission time given the same end-to-end available bandwidth. However, compression also imposes additional processing at the data source and destination. There is intensive research on devising efficient compression algorithm for various types of data. In GiPSiNet, we implement a data compression algorithm based on the standard Burrows-Wheeler algorithm [4], a simple and light-weight algorithm leading to better compression rates than other widespread techniques. Moreover, this algorithm can compress each data unit independently of others and consequently make the compression resilient to data losses.

Section 3 introduces the rest of the GiPSiNet modules incorporating with the techniques to ensure timely data delivery.

3. Timely Data Delivery

Most of today's networks are unreliable and are based on the best-effort model, which provides low level of QoS. Data delay and losses can greatly impair the realism and fidelity of a networked simulation. An approach to address these issues is to apply techniques to ensure timely data delivery in the GiPSiNet middleware.

Retransmission.   There are three categories of data losses: the client data unit loss, the server data unit loss, and both data unit loss. If a server data unit is lost, the client will fail to receive the updated system state and the simulation will appear irresponsive to the user. On the other hand, if both data units are lost, both the server and the client will wait for data from each other and the simulation will be deadlocked. A solution is to let the client resend its data unit to the server at a regular interval length δ regardless of the client data unit loss. This regular retransmission by the client can support timely data delivery to some extent.

Forward Error Correction (FEC) Module.   FEC is an error control method which adds redundancy to the data transmitted using some algorithm. The receiver only needs a certain portion of the data that contains no errors. FEC does not eliminate packet losses, but it can significantly reduce the data loss probability. Hence, a FEC module is included in the GiPSiNet middleware.

Playout Module.   The round-trip time (RTT) changes over time due to varying network conditions. This variance of network delay (jitter) disturbs the temporal relationships in the visualization and hapic media stream. An approach to address this problem is to buffer the received packets and delay their playout, and the buffering time inteval should be long enough such that most packets can be received before their scheduled playout times. However, this buffering time cannot be too long, since it would effect the realism of a networked simulation. Hence, the appropriate way is to set the buffering time dynamically according to the network conditions (RTT) and the server computation time.

In GiPSiNet, a playout module is included to implement the adaptive playout. We will apply Algorithm 4 from [5], which appears to be effective, simple, and robust for audio applications over the Internet. Accordingly, this dynamically changing playout time is included as Δt_i in the client's request to the server, and is the basis to compute a linearized approximation of the system state V_{i+1}.

4. Conclusion and future work

In this paper, we presented the architectural design of the GiPSiNet middleware, which extends our GiPSi framework to network environments. We also described the techniques applied in GiPSiNet to ensure timely data delivery and enhance the quality of networked surgical simulations. In the future, we will implement GiPSiNet, run experiments to obtain a better perception of the interaction between network and the virtual environments, and evaluate the technical and educational impacts of GiPSiNet.

Acknowledgements

The authors acknowledge Technology Opportunities Program (TOP) of Department of Commerce, NASA NNC05CB20C, NSF CCR-039910, NSF IIS-0222743, NSF EIA-0329811, NSF CNS-0423253, and the Virtual Worlds Laboratory at Case Western Reserve University.

References

[1] T. Goktekin, M.C. Cavusoglu: GiPSi: A Draft Open Source/Open Architecture Software Development Framework for Surgical Simulation, *the International Symposium on Medical Simulation* 2004, 240–248.

[2] M. C. Cavusoglu, T. G. Goktekin, F. Tendick: GiPSi: A Framework for Open Source/Open Architecture Software Development for Organ Level Surgical Simulation, *IEEE Transactions on Information Technology in Biomedicine*, 2005 (In Press).

[3] J. Smed, T. Kaukoranta, H. Hakonen: Aspects of networking in multiplayer computer games, *Proceedings of the International Conference on Applications and Development of Computer Games in the 21st Century* 2001, 74–81.

[4] M. Burrows, D. J. Wheeler: A block-sorting lossless data compression algorithm, Digital Systems Research Center Research Report 124, 1994.

[5] R. Ramjee, J. F. Kurose, D. F. Towsley, H. Schulzrinne: Adaptive Playout Mechanisms for Packetized Audio Applications in Wide-Area Networks, *INFOCOM* 1994, 680–688.

Medicine Meets Virtual Reality 14
J.D. Westwood et al. (Eds.)
IOS Press, 2006

Measurement of the Mechanical Response of Intra-Abdominal Organs of Fresh Human Cadavers for Use in Surgical Simulation

Yi-Je Lim[1], Daniel B. JONES[2], Tejinder P. SINGH[3], Suvranu DE[1]

[1]*Department of Mechanical, Aerospace and Nuclear Engineering,*
Rensselaer Polytechnic Institute, Troy, NY 12180 USA
[2]*Department of Surgery,*
Beth Israel Deaconess Medical Center, Boston, MA 02215
[3]*Department of Surgery,*
Albany Medical College, Albany, NY 12208 USA

Abstract *Determination of soft tissue properties is essential for the realism of the virtual scenarios. The major challenge is that soft tissues exhibit complicated mechanical properties including viscoelastic, nonlinear, inhomogeneous, and rate dependent behaviors. Measurements on live human patients present significant risks, thus making the use of cadavers a logical alternative. Cadavers are widely used in present day surgical training, are relatively easy to procure through excellent donor programs and have the right anatomy, which makes them better candidates for training than the porcine model. To investigate the static and dynamic properties of soft tissue, we have developed a high precision tactile stimulator by modifying an exisitng haptic interface device, the Phantom, and used it to record the force-displacement behavior of intra-abdominal organs of fresh human cadavers at the US Surgical facility in Connecticut and Albany Medical College.*

1. Introduction

Determination of soft tissue properties is essential for the realism of the virtual scenarios. Measurement of soft tissue properties is a well-established research area [1,2]. However, the major challenge in this field is that soft tissues exhibit complicated mechanical properties including viscoelastic, nonlinear, inhomogeneous, and rate dependent behaviors. For surgical simulation, ideally it is necessary to measure, and then model the *in vivo* mechanistic response of the soft tissues operated on. However, the current efforts are either aimed at obtaining *ex vivo* properties [1,2,3], which are grossly different from *in vivo* conditions, or utilizing animal models such as the porcine model [4,5] which have fundamental differences in anatomy and tissue consistency compared to human tissue.

Tissue samples are removed from the organ of interest and tested with devices and procedures similar to those used for engineering materials. However, after removing samples from a body, tissue conditions change drastically from factors such as 1) temperature (changes in viscosity) 2) hydration (drying up might change elasticity and viscosity) 3) break-down of proteins (change in stiffness) 4) loss of blood supply. Moreover, the boundary conditions of a sample are different from *in vivo* states. In general, *ex vivo* steady stiffness of organs are much higher than for their respective *in vivo* measurement [5]. The amount of change is highly dependent on the time after the death of the animal.

It is well known that soft tissue behavior is highly nonlinear. The majority of the non-invasive imaging techniques, such as elastography [6] are good for measuring linear small strain behavior. While static techniques cannot examine the viscoelastic behavior of tissues, the dynamic techniques employ high excitation frequencies [7] which are irrelevant to surgical explorations.

There is a variety of techniques that have been developed to investigate the force-displacement response of tissues by applying deformations to the tissue directly. Indentation test is the most popular technique for determining the biomechanical behaviors of soft tissues. A number of groups have developed instruments that apply a normal indentation to the tissue. Miller *et al.* [8] performed tests on porcine brain, using a spherical indenter and a ramp and hold displacement. Carter *et al.* [9] examined human liver using a hand-held instrument employing a spherical indenter and a larger concentric tube. Zheng and Mak developed an ultra-sound palpation system including a pen-size hand-held indentation probe for the lower limb soft tissue [10,11].

Porcine esophagus and liver have been studied using a Phantom haptic interface as a robot stimulator, in which a 6-axis force-torque sensor records the applied loads and precise position is applied by a robot arm [5].

A number of groups have modified surgical instruments, equipping them with force and position sensors [12], as well as motors [13] for system controls. With these instruments, the response of tissue to grasping can be measured. Brower *et al.* makes use of a pair of opposing graspers, which hold and then stretch tissue between them [4].

The TeMPeST 1-D has been used to acquire data on porcine liver and spleen *in vivo*, as well as a variety of rat tissues *in vitr*o [7]. However, it is designed explicitly to investigate the viscoelastic properties of tissue under small deformations. The Dundee Single Point Compliance Probe is designed to measure force response of organs to indentation stimuli during an open surgery [14].

In vivo material properties of organs were also measured using modified laparoscopic instruments [15]. The force feedback endoscopic grasper - FREG makes use of standard laparoscopic instruments with the tool shaft of the instrument mounted onto the slave subsystem and the tool handle attached to the master subsystem. Rosen *et al.* instrumented a laparoscopic grasper with force/torque sensors to measure force and torque at the surgeon hand/tool interface when the instrument was used to perform laparoscopic surgeries on pigs [16]. Brouwer *et al.* measured the *in vivo* mechanical properties of various abdominal tissues such as the stomach, spleen and liver using a uniaxial tensile machine that grasped the abdominal tissues and measured the forces corresponding to different stretch ratios [4].

The use of fresh human cadavers is a risk-free alternative to live human experiments, and is pursued in this paper. Cadavers are widely used in real life surgical education. Excellent gift programs make them relatively easy to procure and they pose minimal hazards. Of course, depending on the time elapsed after death; they lose the elasticity and consistency characteristic of live human patients. Hence the use of fresh unfrozen cadavers is essential. We have developed a set of experiments to obtain biomechanical properties of intra-abdominal organs of fresh human cadavers at the US Surgical facility in Connecticut and Albany Medical College. The rest of this paper is structured as follow: in section 2 we present the experimental setup and protocols for the measurement of mechanical response of intra-abdominal organs of fresh human cadavers. In section 3 we describe the experimental results.

2. Experimental setup and methods

We have developed a setup for performing *in situ* force-displacement experiments on cadaver internal organs, which we describe in section 2.1. In section 2.2 we discuss the protocol for performing the controlled experiments.

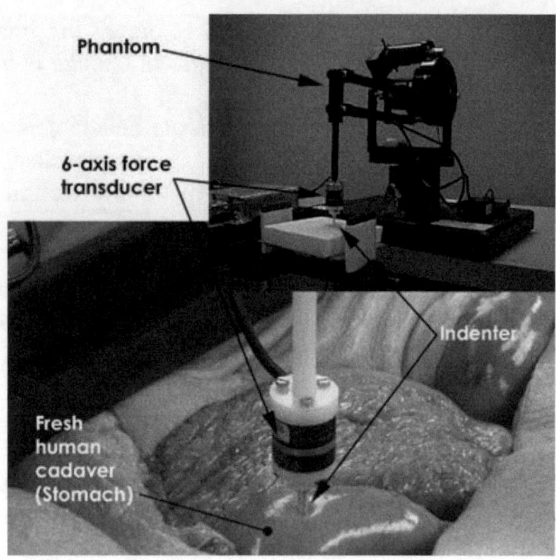

Figure 1. Experiment set up for indentation experiments.

2.1. Experimental setup

For performing *in situ* force-displacement experiments on internal organs, we have modified a Phantom Premium 1.0 (Sensable Technologies) haptic interface device (Figure 1). This device is used to deliver precise displacement stimuli and is fitted with a six-axis force sensor from ATI Industrial Automation (Nano 17) to measure reaction forces. The transducer has a force resolution of 0.78mN along each orthogonal axis and a bandwidth of 10 kHz. The Phantom has a nominal position resolution of 30 μm, a maximum force of 8.5 N and bandwidth exceeding the typical motion frequencies in actual surgery. Flat-faced cylindrical indenters are fitted to the tip of the force sensor to apply the displacement stimuli without introducing significant contact nonlinearities due to change in contact area during deformation. Reaction force and tool displacement data samples are time-coded and recorded 1000 times per second using custom software. Phantom control and data acquisition are performed using a 2 GHz Pentium IV PC.

2.2. Test Protocol

In the indentation experiments, the cadaver is placed on a surgical table in the supine position. A midline incision is performed to open the abdomen and expose the intra-abdominal organs. The Phantom is placed on a rigid stand next to the table, which is adjusted such that the indenter is normal to the organ surface. The indenter is lowered at small increments until it is visually determined to be barely in contact with the organ surface when the stimuli are delivered and the force measurement is started.

It is important to consider the effect of preconditioning on tissue elasticity measurements. When cyclic loading/unloading tests are performed on soft tissues, hysteresis of tissue force-displacement curves occurs [1], indicative of viscoelastic behavior (see Figure 2). The response is not repeatable for the initial few cycles. It is therefore necessary to first precondition the tissue prior to actual measurements. To precondition the tissue, cyclic loading was applied for 1 minute at 2 Hz before actual experiments.

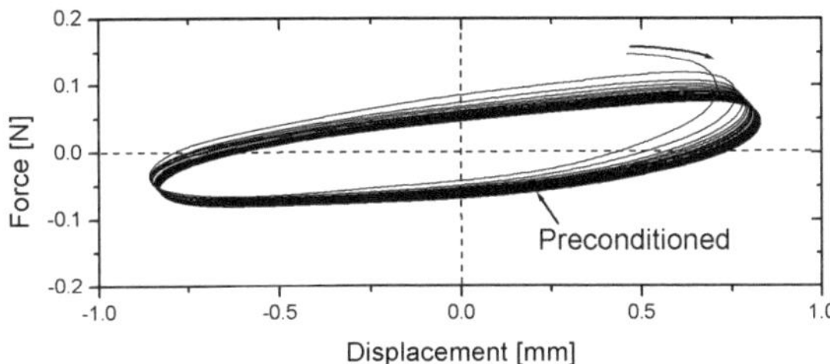

Figure 2. Preconditioning of tissue.

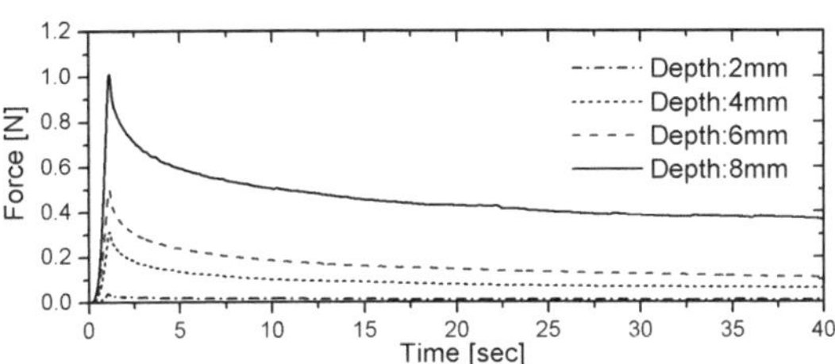

Figure 3. Force response of the liver to ramp-and-hold indentation stimuli.

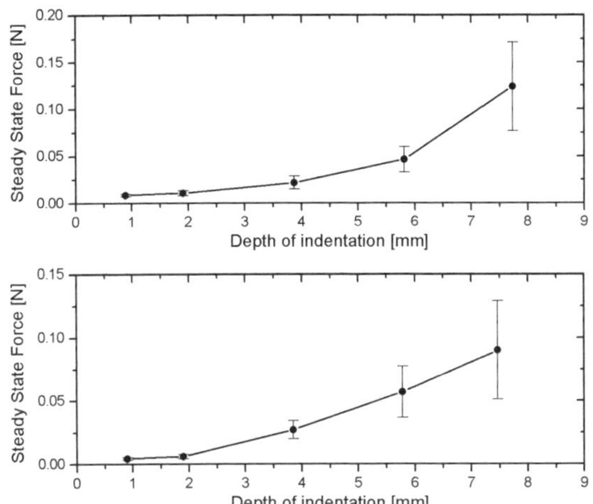

Figure 4. Average steady state force vs. depth of indentation with standard deviation.

The indentation tests comprised of driving the indenter to various depths (1, 2, 4, 6, 8mm) with various velocities (1, 2, 4, 6, 8mm/s) and holding it at each depth for 60 seconds. A 3-minute interval followed each trial to allow the tissue to relax. Each test was performed for a maximum of five trials.

Low frequency sinusoidal indentation stimuli (0.2, 0.5 0.8, 1, 2, 3Hz) were delivered with various amplitudes (0.5, 1mm) superimposed on a pre-indentation of 4mm to ensure that the indenter stayed in contact with the organ over the entire application of the load.

Data analysis was performed using MATLAB® (Mathworks, Inc.) with the noise removed using a unit gain, zero-phase, low-pass, numerical Butterworth filter.

3. Experimental Results

3.1. Ramp-and-hold indentations

The force response of human liver and stomach are plotted in Figure 3 corresponding to the ramp-and-hold loads.

Steady state force as functions of indentation depth are plotted with standard deviations in Figure 4, with the average force value between 38 and 40 seconds after the initiation of the ramp being taken as the steady force value. These curves clearly indicate the nonlinear behavior of the tissue.

3.2. Sinusoidal indentations

Figure 5 shows an example of the response of the cadaver stomach to sinusoidal excitation. When the response force is plotted as a function of displacement, the pronounced hysteresis is observed. The area within the hysteresis curve represents the viscous loss during loading and unloading.

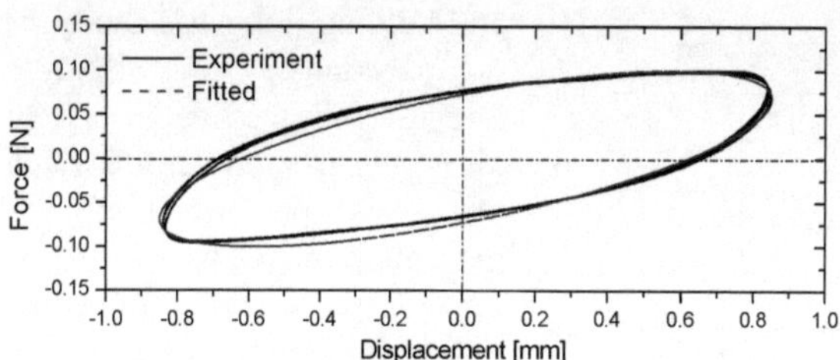

Figure 5. The force-displacement responses of the stomach to sinusoidal indentation at 1.0 Hz.

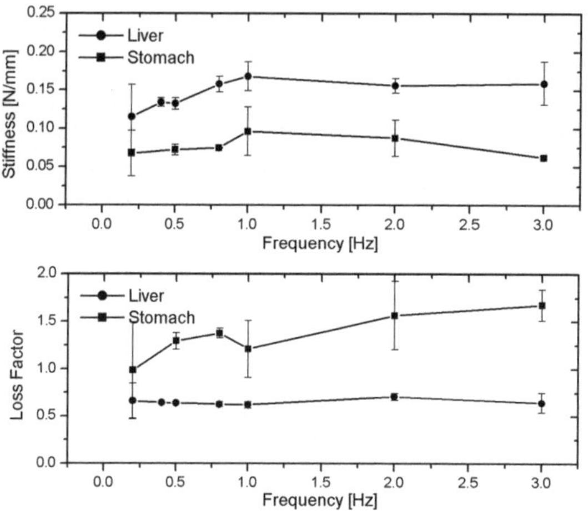

Figure 6. Stiffness and loss factor of cadaver liver and stomach corresponding to sinusoidal indentation at 0.2, 0.5, 0.8, 1, 2, 3 Hz and 1 mm amplitude.

In order to quantify the viscoelasticity of the tissues, we have estimated the stiffness (the amplitude ratio of response force to input displacement) and damping properties (the phase lag between force and input). Figure 6 shows the frequency response of the tissue excited at 0.2, 0.5, 0.8, 1, 2, 3 Hz with 1 mm amplitude. It is found that in general the liver is stiffer than the stomach while the loss factor of stomach is higher than that of the liver. The stiffness and viscoelastic properties of liver and stomach are relatively constant over the frequency range. As is usual of biological tissues, there is significant variability in the response across cadavers.

4. Conclusion

The determination of biomechanical properties and modeling of soft tissue are extremely challenging. Quantitative understanding of the behavior of intra-abdominal tissues is essential to the development of realistic models for surgical simulation. In this paper, we have outlined a measurement system and presented preliminary data on cadaver experiments. Force-displacement data obtained from the indentation experiments on the liver and stomach of cadavers obtained from these experiments shed important light on the fundamental nature of the response of such tissues and are being utilized to develop constitutive models that will be used in our surgical simulation system based on the meshfree point-associated finite field (PAFF) approach [17].

Acknowledgements: Support for this research was provided by grant R21 EB003547-01 from NIH. Special thanks are due to Mr. C. Kennedy and Dr. J. Vlazny of US Surgical, Dr. A. Patel of Beth Israel Deaconess Medical Center and Dr. L. Martino and Dr. D. Conti of Albany Medical Center. Thanks are also due to the Anatomical Gifts Program of the Albany Medical College.

References

[1]   Y.C. Fung, Biomechanics: Mechanical Properties of Living Tissues, 2nd ed. Springer Verlag, 1993.

[2]   H. Yamada, Strength of Biological Materials. SBN: 683-09323-1, Williams & Wilkins, 1970.

[3]   T. Chanthasopeephan, J. Desai, and A. Lau, "Measuring Forces in Liver Cutting: New Equipment and Experimental Results," Annals of Biomedical Engineering, 31(11), pp. 1372-82, 2003.

[4]   I. Brouwer, J. Ustin, L. Bentley, A. Sherman, N. Dhruv, and F. Tendick, "Measuring In Vivo Animal Soft Tissue Properties for Haptic Modeling in Surgical Simulation," Proceedings of MMVR Conference, pp. 69-74, 2001.

[5]   B.K. Tay, N. Stylopoulos, S. De, D.W. Rattner and M.A. Srinivasan, "Measurement of In-vivo Force Response of Intra-abdominal Soft Tissues for Surgical Simulation," Proceedings of the MMVR Conference, 2002.

[6]   L. Gao, K.J. Parker, R.M. Lerner, S.F. Levinson, "Imaging of the elastic properties of tissue - a review," Ultrasound in Medicine and Biology, vol. 22 no. 8, pp. 959-977, 1996.

[7]   M.P. Ottensmeyer, "In vivo measurement of solid organ viscoelastic properties", Medicine Meets Virtual Reality, vol. 85, pp. 328-333, 2002.

[8]   K. Miller, K. Chinzei, G. Orssengo, P. Bednarz, "Mechanical properties of brain tissue in-vivo: experiment and computer simulation", Journal of Biomechanics, vol. 33, pp. 1369–76, 2000.

[9]   F.J. Carter, T.G. Frank, P.J. Davies, D. McLean, and A. Cuschieri, "Measurements and modeling of the compliance of human and porcine organs", Medical Image Analysis, vol. 5, pp. 231-236, 2001.

[10] Y.P. Zheng and A. Mak, "An ultrasound indentation system for bio-mechanical properties assessment of soft tissues in vivo", IEEE Trans Biomed Eng, 43(9):912–8, 1996.

[11] Y.P Zheng and A. Mak, "Effective elastic properties for lower limb soft tissues from manual indentation experiment", IEEE Trans Rehabil Eng, 7:257–67, 1999.

[12] E.P. Scilingo, D. DeRossi, A. Bicchi, and P. Iacconi, "Haptic display for replication of rheological behavior of surgical tissues: modelling, control, and experiments", Proceedings of the ASME Dynamics, Systems and Control Division, pp. 173–176, 1997.

[13] J.D. Brown, J. Rosen, M. Moreyra, M. Sinanan, and B. Hannaford, "Computer-Controlled Motorized Endoscopic Grasper for In Vivo Measurements f Soft Tissue Biomechanical Characteristics", Medicine Meets Virtual Reality, vol. 85, pp. 71-73, 2002.

[14] F. J. Carter, T.G. Frank, P. J. Davies, D. McLean, A. Cuschieri, "Biomechanical Testing of Intra-abdominal Soft Tissues", Medical Image Analysis, 2000.

[15] B. Hannaford, J. Trujillo, M. Sinanan, M. Moreya, J. Rosen, J. Brown, R. Leuschke, M. MacFarlane, "Computerized Endoscopic Surgical Grasper", Proceedings of MMVR Conference, pp. 265-271, 1998.

[16] J. Rosen, M. MacFarlane, C. Richards, B. Hannaford, M. Sinanan, "Surgeon-Tool Force/Torque Signatures – Evaluation of Surgical Skills in Minimally Invasive Surgery", Proceedings of the MMVR Conference, pp. 290- 296, 1999.

[17] S. De, Y.-J. Lim, M. Muniyandi, and M.A. Srinivasan, "Physically realistic virtual surgery using the point-associated finite field (PAFF) approach". Presence: Teleoperators and Virtual Environments, 2005 (in press).

Medicine Meets Virtual Reality 14
J.D. Westwood et al. (Eds.)
IOS Press, 2006

A VR Planning System for Craniosynostosis Surgery

Ching-Yao LIN[a,b], Yen-Jan SU[b,c], San-Liang CHU[a,b],
Chieh-Tsai WU[b,c], Jyi-Feng CHEN[b,c], Shih-Tseng LEE[b,c]
[a]National Center for High-performance Computing, Taiwan
[b]Medical Augmented Reality Research Center, Chang Gung University, Taiwan
[c]Department of Neurosurgery, Chang Gung Memorial Hospital, Taiwan

Abstract The goal of our project is to build a system which could utilize the Virtual Reality (VR) techniques for the pre-operative planning of craniosynostosis. The system includes different modules. We use the tetrahedral volume meshes for the basic structure for the models which surgery is planning on. This paper will describe the procedures of above stages, from the processing of 2D image slices, 3D modeling, smoothing, simplification, and visibility ordering, to volume meshes generation. We have demonstrated the initial results on a variety of stereo devices. The testing results show the processing time is acceptable and the rendering effect is pretty well.

1. Introduction

Virtual Reality (VR) has enormous potential as a technology to enhance teaching and training. In recent years, VR has emerged as a powerful means in medical field, such as surgical simulator, which provides training for a variety of procedures [1].

Craniosynostosis, also called "Craniostenosis" or "Craniostosis", is the premature fusing of the sutures of an infant's head. The infant's skull growth is restricted, which lead to the defect in function of brain. The general method to cure this disease is to perform surgery to release the fused suture. The purpose of surgery is to rebuild cranial shape, and make enough space for brain to grow normally.

We are building a system that utilizes the Virtual Reality (VR) techniques for the pre-operative planning of craniosynostosis surgery. Doctors could use this system to make the planning of the surgery and as a tool to explain the procedures to patients.

2. Methods

2.1 System Design

In the beginning of the project, we have analyzed doctors' requirements and create a "scenario". This scenario specifies the functions that the system needs to provide, the sequences of procedures, and how the user interacts with the system.

The system is made of five major parts according to the processing work flow:
1. Data reading
2. Segmentation

3. 3D reconstruction
4. Surgery Planning
5. Comparison the surgery result

We import the images (DICOM format) and then using the image processing tools provided by the system to adjust the image attributes and perform the segmentation operations. Then we reconstructed the three-dimensional models from images files.

During planning, the system would provide the cutting, bending, and re-arrange functions as mentioned before. Doctors also want to see the transparency effect in this part because transparent objects can provide clearer and detailed information.

In the last stages, comparison, the system should provide an interface to compare the differences before and after surgery. Doctors are able to explain the surgery to patients using this tool.

Table 1 shows the setup of the environment.

Table 1 System setting

CPU	Intel Pentium 4, 2800 MHz
Main Memory	1536MB
Graphics Card	ATI Radeon 9800 Pro, 128MB
Operating System	Microsoft Windows XP Professional
Compiler	Microsoft Visual C++ 6.0
Program Language	C/C++
Library/software	OpenGL, GLUT, TetGen

2.2 Modeling

We use Marching Cube algorithm [2] to build the skull surface model directly. However, the meshes created from Marching Cube need additional process to remove unwanted triangles and to simplify the meshes for the interaction purpose. We smoothed the mesh by Taubin's signal process approach [3], then use Garland's Quadric Error Metrics [4] to simplify the triangles.

To create volume mesh, we used TetGen [5]. TetGen is a program which could generate tetrahedral meshes for arbitrary 3D domains. The program currently generates meshes including exact constrained Delaunay tetrahedralizations and quality meshes. We can set the radius-edge ratios condition to control the mesh quality.

We also built BSP-tree to divide the 3D space. It has many benefits, such as providing visibility order to render transparency effect. It is also useful when we are doing collision detection using Bielser's tetrahedron-based cutting algorithm to detect the surface collision [6] for the detection of volume collision according the adjacency relation.

2.3 Display

We have setup two different display environments, projection screen and LCD display. Both are able to display data in stereoscopic so user will have depth perception. Projection screen is a better platform for demonstration. To simulate the effect of seeing the data in real-life size, we can use LCD screen as our display devices. The screen has a thin micro-retarder plate on it. The user is able to see stereoscopic images through a pair of polarization glasses

3. Results and Discussion

The results and the execution time are shown below (Table 2 and figures). The testing data were from a kid with craniosynostosis. Data are stored in 16 bits DICOM format with size of 512 x 512 x 54. We only have to process the data one time.

Multi-discipline collaborations are required for the success of this project. We have applied different techniques to make the system work; however, the values of the system is not the technology, it is about the better care for the human.

Table 2

Steps	Times (s)
Marching Cube: Threshold=1200, create 1055016 triangles. Show in figure 1.	12
Smoothing: $\lambda = 0.6$, 50 iterations.	10
QEM: Reduce to 50000 triangles. And smooth the meshes again, as shown in figure 2.	98
TetGen: Transform the result of figure 2 to 98816 tetrahedron, as shown in figure 3	6
Build BSP-Tree for transparency effects.	1

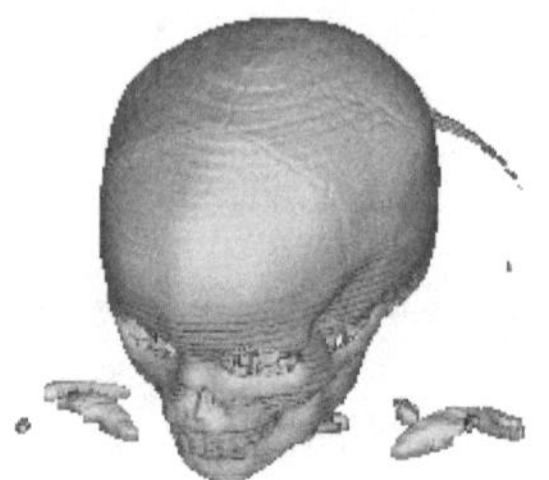
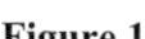

Figure 1

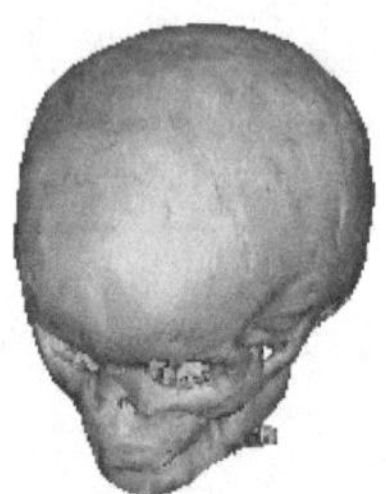

Figure 2

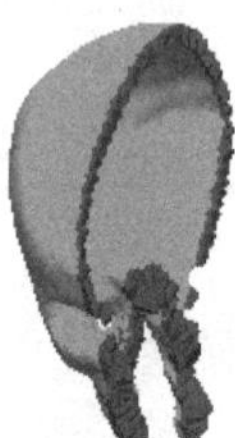

Figure 3

4. Acknowledgement

This work was supported by Ministry of Economic Affairs, R.O.C. under Technology Development Program for Academia (TDPA) in the project of developing a Brain Medical Augmented Reality System with Grant No. 94-EC-17-A-19-S1-035

Reference

[1] Montgomery, K; Stephanides, M; Schendel, S; Ross, M; "User Interface Paradigms for VR-based Surgical Planning: Lessons Learned Over a Decade of Research", Technical Report, Biocomputation Center, Stanford University

[2] Lorenson, W.E.; Cline H.E.; "Marching Cubes: a High Resolution 3D Surface Construction Algorithm", Computer Graphics, 21(4) 163-169, 1987 July.

[3] Taubin, G.; "A Signal Process Approach to Fair Surface Design", SIGGRAPH'95, 351-358, 1995 August.

[4] Garland, M.; Heckbert, P.; "Surface Simplification Using Quadric Error Metrics", SIGGRAPH'97, 209-216, 1997 August.

[5] TetGen : A Quality Tetrahedral Mesh Generator and Three-Dimensional Delaunay Triangulator. http://tetgen.berlios.de/

[6] Bielser, D.; Gross, M.H.; "Interactive Simulation of Surgical Cuts", Pacific Graphics 2000, 116-125.

Medicine Meets Virtual Reality 14
J.D. Westwood et al. (Eds.)
IOS Press, 2006

331

Real-Time Finite Element Based Virtual Tissue Cutting

Alex J. LINDBLAD [a,b,1]; George M. TURKIYYAH [b] Suzanne J. WEGHORST [a]
Dan BERG [c]

[a] *Human Interface Technology Lab., UW, Seattle, 98195 U.S.*
[b] *Dept. of Civil and Environmental Eng., UW, Seattle, WA 98195 U.S.*
[c] *Dermatologic Surgery Dept., UW, Seattle, WA 98195 U.S.*

Abstract. Tool-tissue interaction is most accurately modeled as an imposed displacement constraint, thus augmenting the traditional finite element equation, $\mathbf{Ku} = \mathbf{f}$, to a 2×2 block system. This augmentation does two things: it enlarges the system, and it introduces the Schur complement($\mathbf{S}$) during the solution. This research has focused on efficient methods to update the Schur complement and it's inverse during displacement constraint removal and addition to allow for soft-tissue cutting to occur in real-time.

By taking advantage of how the constraints impact the Schur complement, removal and addition of these constraints are handled by either performing a rank-2 or rank-1 update on $\mathbf{S}^{-1}$, respectively. This greatly reduces the computational load on the CPU; and through use of timing tests shows that the update frequencies are well within an acceptable range for tactile feedback. To further solidify this method as being highly useful, a prototypical simulator has been developed that allows users to haptically perform bi-manual soft-tissue cutting.

Keywords. Finite Element, Real-Time, Soft-Tissue Cutting, Haptics

1. Introduction and Background

Real-time numerical simulation of arbitrary soft-tissue cutting through use of finite element (FE) procedures is inherently difficult because of the continuous change in mesh topology. One solution to this problem is to predefine the cut path, generate a FE mesh that incorporates the dislocation, and use displacement constraints to initially close the gap in the mesh. This method is conceptually seen in Figure 1, where the dark cross bars indicate displacement constraints, and the light lines are the edges of the cut. By using displacement constraints, the typical FE equation of $\mathbf{KU} = \mathbf{f}$ is augmented to form a 2 x 2 block system of equations, which introduces the Schur complement, $\mathbf{S} = \mathbf{CK}^{-1}\mathbf{C}^{T}$, where $\mathbf{C}$ is the displacement constraint matrix and $\mathbf{K}$ is the global stiffness matrix. In this representation, cutting is modeled by a constraint removal, where constraints are automatically removed as a virtual scalpel passes over them; and tool-tissue interaction is modeled by a constraint addition or modification. ›

---

[1]Correspondence to: Alex J. Lindblad, Human Interface Technology Lab, University of Washington, Seattle, WA 98195-2142. Tel.: +1 206.543.5075; Fax.: +1 206.543.5380; E-mail: alex@hitl.washington.edu

Broadly speaking, there are two types of surgical simulators: ons based on mass-spring models and ones based on continuum fi nite element models. Examples of mass-spring soft-tissue cutting simulators include ones by HDilingette et al [1] and CBruyns et al [2]. Previous fi nite element based soft-tissue cutting simulators have employed a separation of elements method [3] while others use condensed methods solved on the GPU [4].

This research has focused on effi cient methods to update the Schur complement and its inverse during displacement constraint addition and removal to allow for soft-tissue cutting to occur in real-time. It has also focused on integrating this solution method in a previously described [5] bi-manual surgical suturing simulator to allow for haptic based soft-tissue cutting.

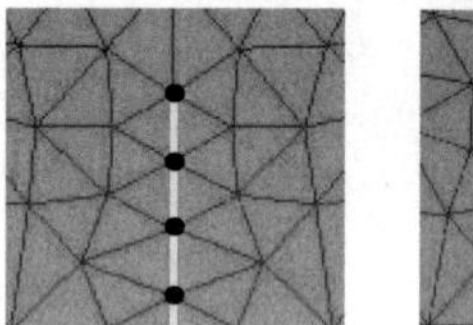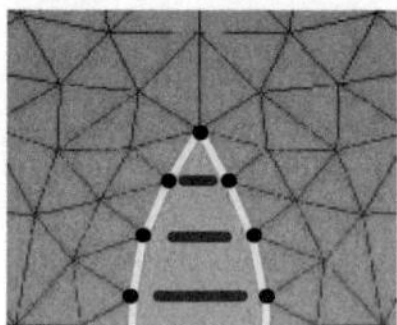

Figure 1. Conceptual images indicating how displacement constraints are used to initially close the wound.

2. Methods

A typical fi nite element system generates the governing equation $\mathbf{Ku} = \mathbf{f}$, however, the addition of constraints, such as those used to model sutures, tool-tissue interaction, and the cut in this simulation, generates a 2×2 block system, where after performing a block Gauss elimination produces the following set of equations (Equations 1):

$$\begin{bmatrix} \mathbf{K} & \mathbf{C}^T \\ \mathbf{0} & -\mathbf{C}\mathbf{K}^{-1}\mathbf{C}^T \end{bmatrix} \begin{Bmatrix} \mathbf{u} \\ \mathbf{v} \end{Bmatrix} = \begin{Bmatrix} \mathbf{f} \\ \mathbf{g} - \mathbf{C}\mathbf{K}^{-1}\mathbf{f} \end{Bmatrix} \tag{1}$$

Where $\mathbf{u}$ is the nodal displacement vector, $\mathbf{f}$ is the vector of external nodal applied loads, $\mathbf{v}$ is the vector of reaction forces, lambda coeffi cients, based on the constraints and $\mathbf{g}$ is the vector of imposed displacements associated with each constraint.

Low-rank updates of the Schur complement are formulated to handle dynamic constraint removal and addition. In our implementation, storage is pre-allocated for the matrix $\mathbf{C}$ to accommodate the largest expected set of cut and tool-tissue interaction constraints. By using this preallocation, the addition and deletion of constraints can be handled algebraically as a change in constraint coeffi cients; therefore, as the tissue is cut and constraints are removed, the inverse of S is changed by a rank-one update using the Sherman-Morrison Woodbury formula:

$$\mathbf{S}_0^{-1} = \mathbf{S}^{-1} + \mathbf{e}_i \mathbf{e}_i^T - \frac{1}{\mathbf{e}_i^T \mathbf{S}^{-1} \mathbf{e}_i} \mathbf{S}^{-1} \mathbf{e}_i \mathbf{e}_i^T \mathbf{S}^{-1} \tag{2}$$

where $\mathbf{e}_i$ is the ith unit vector corresponding to the ith constraint being removed. At the point of initial tool-tissue interaction, constraints are added to the system, where this addition is done using the generalized Woodbury formula:

$$\mathbf{S}_0^{-1} = \mathbf{S}^{-1} - \left[\mathbf{S}^{-1}\mathbf{M}\left(\mathbf{1} + \mathbf{N}^T\mathbf{S}^{-1}\mathbf{M}\right)^{-1}\mathbf{N}^T\mathbf{S}^{-1}\right] \tag{3}$$

where $\mathbf{S}_0 = \mathbf{S} + \mathbf{M}\mathbf{N}$ and both $\mathbf{N}$ and $\mathbf{M}$ are rank-two matrices. It is possible for numerical errors to arise in $\mathbf{S}^{-1}$ through repeated use of low-rank updates, thus it is necessary to re-compute the inverse of the Schur complement periodically during the simulation, such as when the user switches virtual tools.

3. Results

Timings were performed to validate the use of rank-one and rank-two updates. All timings are the average of ten different tests and were performed on a 3.06 GHz Pentium 4 processor with 1 GB of RAM. From these timings it is evident that the update of the inverse of the Schur complement can occur at haptically interactive rates, 200-500 Hz, for usable problem sizes.

m	30	50	100	200	300	500
T_1 (ms)	0.0	0.0	0.0	1.9	4.6	5.0
T_2 (ms)	1.0	0.0	1.0	2.1	5.5	18.4

Table 1. Timing results for rank-one (T_1) and rank-two(T_2) updates of various sized matrices, where m is the number of constraints..

4. Conclusions

This research focused on improving the effi ciency of removing and adding displacement constraints in a fi nite element system in real-time, with the goal of creating a robust framework to haptically demonstrate bi-manual surgical suturing and soft-tissue cutting. Through the use of low-rank updates, performed on the inverse of the Schur complement, perturbations to the system, such as tool-tissue contact and tissue cutting, are accurately handled with solution rates that lie well within acceptable limits for haptic interaction.

References

[1] Herv Delingette and Stphane Cotin and Nicholas Ayache, *A Hybrid Elastic Model allowing Real-Time Cutting, Deformations and Force-Feedback for Surgery Training and Simulation*, Proceedings of the Computer Animation 1999.

[2] C. Bruyns and K. Montgomery, *Generalized Interactions Using Virtual Tools within the Spring Framework: Cutting*, Medicine Meets Virtual Reality 2002 (MMVR2002), Newport Beach, CA, 2002.

[3] Mendoza, C. and Laugier, C., *Simulating Soft Tissue Cutting Using Finite Element Models*, Proc. of the IEEE Int. Conf. on Robotics and Automation, May, 2003.

[4] Wen Wu and Pheng Ann Heng *A hybrid condensed finite element model with GPU acceleration for interactive 3D soft tissue cutting*, Computer Animation and Virtual Worlds 2004, 15: 219-227.

[5] Lindblad, A.J., Turkiyyah, G.M., Sankanaranayanan, G., Weghorst, S.J. and Berg, D.. *Two-handed next generation suturing simulator.*, Proceedings of MMVR 2004, pp. 215-220.

Medicine Meets Virtual Reality 14
J.D. Westwood et al. (Eds.)
IOS Press, 2006

The Design and Implementation of a Pulmonary Artery Catheterization Simulator

Alan LIU [a,1], Yogendra BHASIN [a], Michael FIORILL [b], Mark BOWYER [a] and
Randy HALUCK [b]

[a] *The Surgical Simulation Laboratory*
National Capital Area Medical Simulation Center
Uniformed Services University
http://simcen.usuhs.mil

[b] *Verefi Technologies, Inc.*
http://www.verefi.com

Abstract. Pulmonary Artery Catheterization (PAC) is a commonly performed procedure. It is used when hemodynamic and other cardiac measures must be accurately monitored in seriously ill patients. A flow-directed, balloon-tipped (Swan-Ganz) catheter is typically inserted into a major vein, passed through the heart, and into the pulmonary artery. This procedure is normally not performed under fluoroscopy. Instead, transducer readings from the catheter tip provide a continuous report of local blood pressure. An experienced practitioner can infer the catheter's location from this information, yet several studies have found that physicians and critical care nurses have a wide variability in competency. A simulator for this procedure can address some of the educational and training issues highlighted. This paper describes our ongoing progress in developing a PAC trainer.

Keywords. Pulmonary Artery Catheterization, Medical Simulation, Common Medical Simulation Platform,

1. Introduction

Pulmonary Artery Catheterization (PAC) is a minimally invasive procedure that is performed to accurately measure a range of hemodynamic parameters. These measurements can be made over an extended time period (days). Conditions that may require PAC include heart failure, shock, acute valvular regurgitation, congenital heart disease, burns, and kidney disease. PAC may also be performed to monitor for complications arising from a heart attack, or to monitor the effects of certain heart medication.

A Swan Ganz catheter [1,2] is used for the procedure. This is a multi-lumen catheter approximately 110 cm in length. The catheter is introduced percutaneously into the body. To accomplish this, the Seldinger technique [3] is normally used. A Cordis introducer

---

[1] Correspondence to: Alan Liu, http://simcen.org/surgery.

is inserted in a major vein. Common access approaches include the internal jugular vein and the subclavian vein. A small inflatable balloon is located near the distal (far) end of the instrument. Once the catheter is inserted, the balloon is inflated. Blood flow causes the catheter to be drawn toward the heart, through the right atrium and ventricle until it becomes lodged in the pulmonary artery. Pressure and temperature sensors are located along the catheter. When inserted correctly, additional openings in the catheter permit measurements to be conducted at strategic points in the heart, such as the right ventricle, right atrium, or superior vena cava. Using this catheter, a number of key cardiovascular parameters can be determined, including cardiac output, and central venous pressure. Blood samples can also be retrieved in some versions of this catheter.

The catheter is normally inserted without fluoroscopic guidance [4,5]. Instead, a sensor near the tip provides continuous real-time feedback of local blood pressure. An experienced physician can interpret the pressure trace and determine the location of the tip.

A need exists to provide adequate training in this procedure. Recent studies show uniformly poor performance on multiple choice testing of all aspects of pulmonary artery catheterization given to 535 European critical care physicians [6]. Similar findings have been found with several hundred intensive care physicians in the US and Canada [7]. In this study, 47% of clinicians were unable to correctly derive even the most basic information provided by the PA catheter.

To address the training requirements of this procedure, we are building a computer-based PAC simulator. This paper describes the ongoing work.

2. Methods

Building the PAC simulator involves both hardware and software development. In this section, we briefly describe SimPod, a common hardware platform for medical simulation. The main software components of the PAC trainer are also described.

2.1. Hardware

The PAC simulator is built on the SimPod platform. The SimPod is currently under development at Verefi Technologies. Formerly known as VRDemo, the SimPod aims to provide a common hardware platform for simulation development. Medical simulators have many common hardware elements. They include one or more displays, a computer system, and common input hardware such as keyboards and pointing devices. Each simulator must duplicate these elements and integrate them with procedure-specific components. Often, proprietary interfaces are developed. This approach increases the cost and complexity of bringing a simulator to market.

The SimPod addresses these limitations. The current prototype consists of a central hardware core, containing elements common to all simulation systems. The core includes a single-board computer with a Pentium IV 2.8 GHz processor. This provides the computational power necessary for modeling the physical and physiological aspects of the procedure. High-end graphics hardware provides the rendering capability for visual feedback. The graphics hardware drives a touch-sensitive LCD display, which also serves as an alternative input device in place of the mouse. All procedure-specific tools and hardware plug into the central core via a common USB-based communications bus with a well defined, open standard.

This unified architecture simplifies simulation development. An open interface standard encourages the development new procedures. Hardware developers can focus on building only the devices necessary for a new procedure. By developing on a common platform, the cost of adding new simulations can be reduced. Earlier SimPod prototypes have demonstrated the concept of interchangeable, procedure-specific tools for use in laparoscopy. When complete, PAC will extend SimPod's repertoire of supported simulations.

The PAC simulator uses a catheter tracker specifically developed for this purpose. The tracker plugs directly into SimPod. When in use, the catheter is passed through the tracker, simulating passage of the instrument into the body. The device is completely self-contained. Power for the device is drawn off the USB bus. The tracker consists of an opto-mechanical rotary encoder, a complex programmable logic device (CPLD), and a USB-bus interface. Movement of the catheter rotates the encoder. Fig. 1 illustrates the current prototype. The device is self-calibrating, and can reliably measure catheter movement with an accuracy of $0.001cm$ at speeds of up to $5 \times 10^5 cm/s$. A smaller final version will be developed. The reduced size will make it suitable for embedding within a mannequin, thereby providing greater realism.

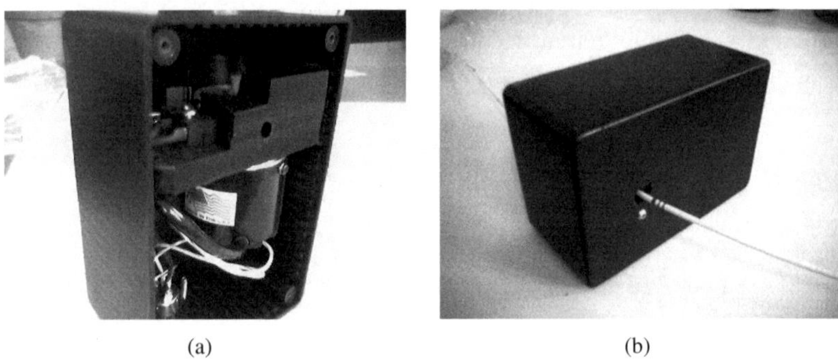

(a)   (b)

Figure 1. The catheter tracking device. (a) Rotary encoder, (b) The assembled device. A catheter can be seen passing through it.

2.2. Software Components

The main software components of the PAC simulator consists of the Graphical User Interface (GUI), and an AI engine for modeling patient physiology and scenario control. We describe each in turn.

2.2.1. The Graphical User Interface

During the simulation, the GUI displays pressure transducer and EKG waveforms. As the catheter is advanced, the waveforms change. The displayed traces are consistent with the present location of the catheter's distal end. The AI module, described in section 2.2.2, controls the nature and type of waveform displayed, depending on the nature of the simulated patient.

In addition to transducer and EKG traces, the user can also retrieve material specific to the present scenario, such as the patient's history, and the hemodynamic measurements to be performed. The GUI also serves as a means for students to receive feedback on their performance. Fig. 2 illustrates.

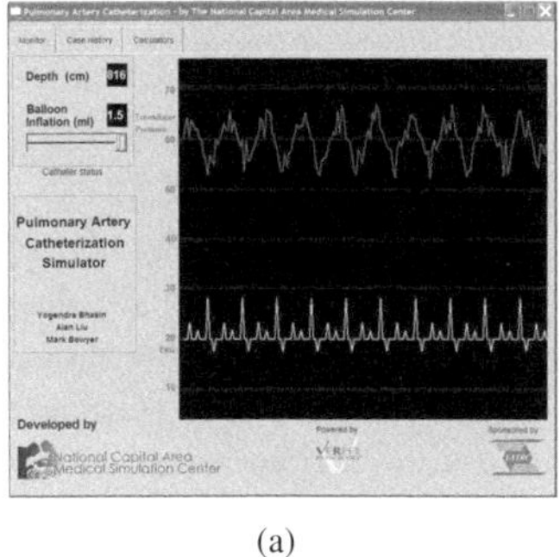
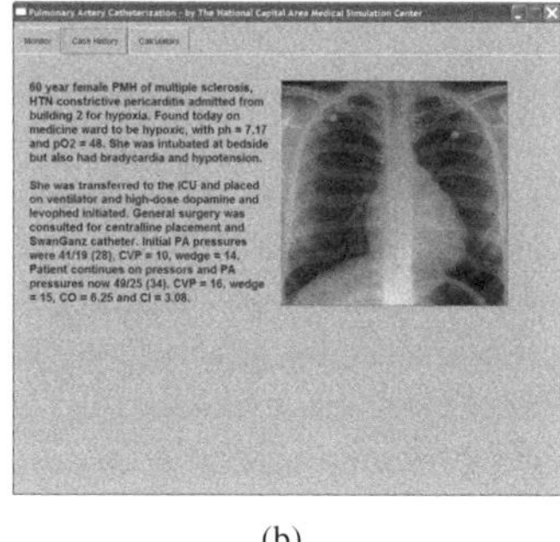

(a)   (b)

Figure 2. The graphical user interface. (a) Displaying pressure and EKG traces. (b) Displaying the patient's history.

2.2.2. The AI Module

The AI module controls the scenario and the physiology of the virtual patient during the course of the simulation. It models a particular scenario as a a finite state automaton (FA) [8]. New cases can be added to the simulator by defining a different FA. In our implementation, the FA consists of a set of states S. Each state $s \in S$ represents a particular combination of the patient's condition, and the catheter's position that may occur during the course of the simulation. The initial condition of the patient is given by the start state $s_0 \in S$. A set of states representing possible final outcomes is given by $S_e \subset S$. Both successful as well as unsuccessful outcomes are included.

Each state s has a set of transitions T_s to other states. A transition consists of a set of conditions c, a set of actions a, a destination state, and the probability p that this transition occurs. Examples of conditions include events such as the catheter balloon inflating, or time intervals. When all the conditions of a transition are satisfied, the AI module executes the set of actions specified in a. Examples of actions include: changing the displayed waveform, alerting the student that an error has been made, and updating the patient's condition.

When the simulation begins, the AI's current state is set to s_0. The student's actions changes current conditions in the simulator. When these conditions match one or more transitions from the current state, a transition occurs and the current state is changed. The patient's condition changes in response. The student notes these changes and proceeds further, which in turn causes the AI to enter a new state. This cycle continues until a final state is entered, at which point the simulation ends. If the student correctly performed the procedure, a successful end state is reached. Otherwise, an unsuccessful end state is reached, and the patient suffers an undesirable result, such as death.

Transitions can also be probabilistic. When conditions for more than one transition are satisfied, a transition is randomly chosen with a probability given by its value of p.

Probabilistic transitions can be used to model different patient responses to treatment. They also permit a range of complications to be simulated with varying frequency. By changing the value of p for different transitions, the same scenario can be made easier or more difficult by allowing complications to occur with different degrees of likelihood.

3. Results

Fig. 3(a) illustrates the current PAC simulator running on a prototype SimPod. This version of the SimPod was designed to be portable, and has been ruggedize for use in austere environments. The entire simulator, including the LCD touch-panel display and computer, is built into a hard-shell carrying case. The catheter tracker fits within the case.

Fig. 3(b) is a graphical illustration of the state machine for a typical case. The scenario includes a number of common complications, such as the catheter looping within the right ventricle.

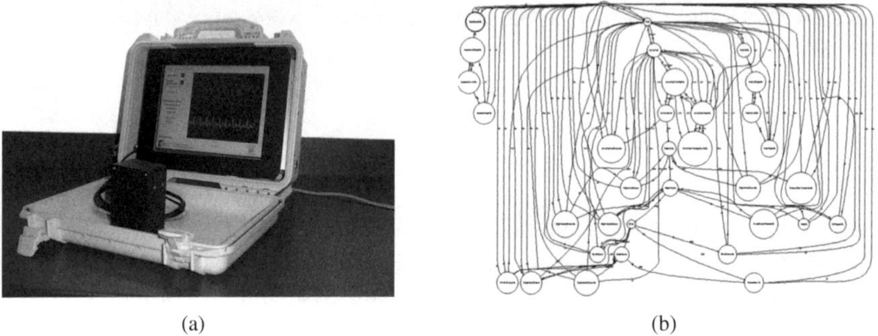

(a)   (b)

Figure 3. (a) The PAC simulator running on a prototype SimPod. (b) A visual representation of a FA for a sample scenario.

4. Discussion

The PAC simulation focuses on imparting cognitive skills. To provide a comprehensive learning experience, it must be capable of presenting a wide range of cases and varying levels difficulty.

A FA is a flexible method for representing medical case content. Both normal outcomes and complications can be modeled. As there can be an arbitrary number of of states and transitions, the detail to which the case is modeled is fully determined by the case author. The instructor can begin with a straightforward case, then add complexity as required to address advanced training requirements. Probabilistic transitions allow for more realistic patient responses to treatment. Complications can occur with varying probabilities, given the nature of the patient. Differences in the patient can cause that individual to behave differently given the same treatment. These variations can also be modeled using probabilistic transitions. By changing relative probabilities, the same scenario can be made easier or more difficult as required based on the student's skill level.

In this way, the same scenario can be revisited multiple times as the student gains experience. Finally, the random nature of such transitions implies that no two simulation experiences are exactly the same, even with the same scenario. This variation challenges the student, and helps sustain the individual's interest.

A disadvantage of using a FA is the large number of states required, even for simple cases. We are currently investigating semi-automated methods for constructing FAs that model case content. One promising approach is to present only relevant portions of the FA in detail, and to collapse non-relevant states for display as aggregate states. An interactive visual editing tool for this purpose is currently being planned.

5. Conclusion

PAC is a procedure that is performed to monitor hemodynamic parameters in seriously ill patients. Proficiency in this procedure requires the ability to correctly interpret blood pressure waveforms during catheter insertion, and the ability to perform calculations of hemodynamic state based on sensor readings. This paper presents the design of a PAC simulator. Development of the simulator is currently ongoing. Our development effort differs from previously developed simulators by adopting a common platform. This approaches permits new hardware development to be minimized. The result is reduced cost and development time. The simulator also includes an AI module that uses a FA to model patient physiology. This approach is both flexible and powerful. The patient's physiology can be modeled with as much or as little detail as desired. The ability to use probabilistic transitions permits the difficulty level of a scenario to be changed without rewriting the case. It also enables the simulation experience to be slightly different every time, even when practicing on the same case.

References

[1] Swan H.J., Ganz W., Forrester J., Marcus H., Diamond G., and Chonette D. Catheterization of the heart in man with use of a flow-directed, balloon-tipped catheter. *N. Engl. J. Med.*, 283:477–51, 1970.

[2] Forrester J., Ganz W., Diamond G., McHugh T., Chonette D. W., and Swan H.J. Thermodilution cardiac output determination with a single, flow-directed catheter. *Am. Heart J.*, 83:306–11, Mar 1972.

[3] Seldinger S.I. Catheter replacement of the needle in percutaneous arteriography (a new technique). *Acta Radiologica, Stockholm*, 39:368–376, 1953.

[4] Swan H.J. The pulmonary artery catheter in anesthesia practice. *Anesthesiology*, 103:890–3, Oct 2005.

[5] Lipper B. Findling R. Femoral vein pulmonary artery catheterization in the intensive care unit. *Chest.*, 105:874–7, Mar 1994.

[6] Gnaegi A., Feihl F., and Perret C. Intensive care physicians' insufficient knowledge of right-heart catheterization at the bedside: Time to act? In *Crit. Care. Med.*, volume 25, pages 213–220, 1997.

[7] Iberti T.J. et. al. A multicenter study of physicians' knowledge of the pulmonary artery catheter. In *JAMMA*, volume 264, pages 2928–2932, 1990.

[8] Hopcroft J.E., Motwani R., and Ullman J.D. *Introduction to Automata Theory, Languages, and Computation (2nd Edition)*, chapter 2. Addison Wesley, 2000.

Medicine Meets Virtual Reality 14
J.D. Westwood et al. (Eds.)
IOS Press, 2006

Flat Maps: A Multi-Layer Parameterization for Surgery Simulation

Qiang Liu and Edmond C. Prakash

School of Computer Engineering, Nanyang Technological Univeristy, Singapore

Abstract. Modeling organs for surgery simulation is a formidable challenge due to two reasons. First, the organs and body parts have not only very complex shapes, but are deformable too. The second challenge is to provide a mechanism for surgeons to interact with these complex anatomical objects. We present a novel multi-layer parameterized representation scheme that addresses the both challenges. In our approach, we use a 2D flat map representation for the 3D geometry of the organ, that can be used for rendering, collision detection, and deformation. The tool-organ interaction can be computed on the 2D flat maps and then mapped back to the 3D geometry of the organs. With this representation, we demonstrate that we can construct a practical and realistic environment for interactive surgery simulation.

1. Introduction

In most of the existing surgery simulation systems, virtual organs are represented as unstructured 3D meshes. The interactions between the surgery tools and the organs are simulated in 3D space. For example, De et al. [1][2] introduced a meshless technique, called the method of finite spheres, for real time deformation of soft tissues. When the collision between the virtual surgery tool and organ model is detected, a collection of sphere nodes are sprinkled around the tool tip. The vertices inside these spheres are deformed with the method of finite spheres. Gu et al. [3] proposed to take advantage of parameterization and remesh an arbitrary surface onto a completely regular structure called *Geometry Image*, which captures rigid geometry as a simple 2D array of quantized points. In our work we introduce a laparoscopic surgery simulation system that extends the conventional geometry image. A series of 2D flat maps are introduced, not only to represent the geometry of the virtual organ, but also for rendering, collision detection, and deformation, as shown in Figure 1 (a). Especially, the tool-organ interaction can be computed on the 2D maps, then mapped to the 3D mesh, which reduced the computational cost. With our methods, realistic simulation can be achieved with user interaction in real time.

2. Parameterization and Resampling

The virtual organ meshes available are usually unstructured with low resolution. To be used for surgery simulation, they are first parameterized, then resampled into a $m \times n$ regular point arrays with high resolution. which is called the *Geometry Map*. The interpolated normal information of all the points is called the *Normal Map*. Each point

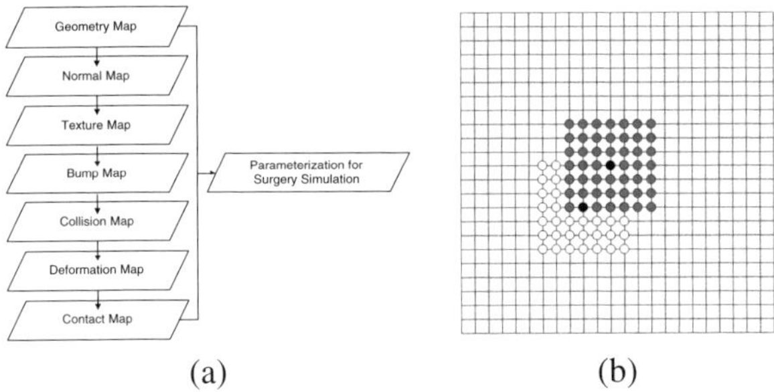

(a)   (b)

Figure 1. (a) The layers of parameterization. (b) The collision map. The grey circles represent points of the collision map at current time step, and the white ones represent points of the collision map at previous time step. The black ones are the collision center at respective time step.

on the geometry map corresponds to a vertex on the 3D space. With geometry map, the 3D mesh of the virtual organ can be reconstructed. For more details about the process of parameterization, resampling, and reconstruction, readers are refered to [4].

3. Tool organ interaction

We implement a grasper surgery tool, which can be controlled by the user interactively to touch, poke, and grasp the virtual organ. The tool is inserted into the abdominal cavity through a hole on the abdominal wall, whose position is fixed. The user can control the movement of the tool tip and the angle of the clamp using the mouse input. Like most surgery simulators, we assume that only the tool tip touches the organ, and only the collision between the tool tip and the organ is checked. Since the organ mesh is resampled at high density, we can assume that the collision happens only at the vertices of the organ mesh. This reduces the computation to a point-point collision detection.

The collision detection is performed on a 2D *Collision Map*, which is a $(2a + 1) \times (2a + 1)$ point array on the parameter space. Before the simulation, the distance between the tool tip and each vertex is calculated. We find the vertex V_n that has shortest distance, whose corresponding point on the parameter space $V_n' = (u_{i_n}, v_{j_n})$ is called *collision center*. The collision map includes the points from $(u_{i_n - a}, v_{j_n - a})$ to $(u_{i_n + a}, v_{j_n + a})$. During the simulation, with the movement of the tool tip in the 3D space, collision center and the collision map are constantly traced and updated. After each time step, the distance between the tool tip and each vertex in the collision map is calculated and compared. The new collision center is the point whose corresponding vertex has the shortest distance. And the new collision map is updated accordingly, as shown in Figure 1(b). Since the movement of the tool in one time step is limited, only points in the collision map need to be checked. The collision detection only involves a small number of point distances calculation, hence fast and efficient.

If a collision is detected, the corresponding 3D vertex of the collision center V_n is bound with the tool tip, and its coordinate is set to be the same as the one of the tool tip, until the collision center changes or when there's no collision. The surrounding vertices are deformed, as described in Section 4. If the clamp angle becomes zero when there is a collision, the collision detection and the updating of collision center stops, until the clamp opens again. During this period, the coordinate of the vertex V_n is set to be always the same as the one of the tool tip, and the organ can be even pulled.

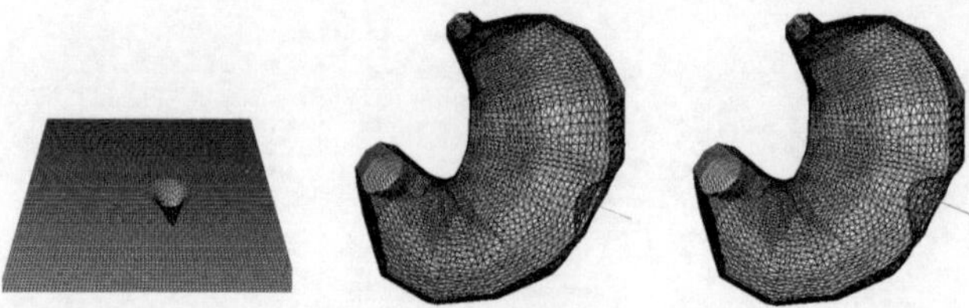

Figure 2. The deformation of the stomach model with free form deformation. Left: the deformation calculated on the 2D plane Center and Right: the deformation mapped onto 3D mesh.

4. Organ deformation

We designed a fast and easy free form deformation method which is based on a 2D map called *Deformation Map*, which is a $(2b+1) \times (2b+1)$ point array on the parameter space, from (u_{i_n-b}, v_{j_n-b}) to (u_{i_n+b}, v_{j_n+b}). When a collision is detected, the displacement of the collision center V_n' is $d_{V_n} = P_{tooltip} - V_n$, where $P_{tooltip}$ is the position of the tool tip. At each point (u_i, v_j) on the deformation map, a gaussian distribution function is evaluated as $g_{ij} = e^{-\frac{(i-i_n)^2+(j-i_n)^2}{\sigma}}$, in which σ is is a parameter that reflects the material property of the organ. The displacement of this point is set to be $d_{ij} = g_{ij}d_{V_n}$. The 3D mesh deformed based on the calculated displacement. As shown in Figure 2, although the scheme is simple, realistic deformation can be achieved.

5. Simulation demonstration

Texture maps and bump maps are used to improve the rendering effect of the virtual organs. Figure 3 whos a few snap shots of the surgery simulation with the interaction between the tool and two organ models.

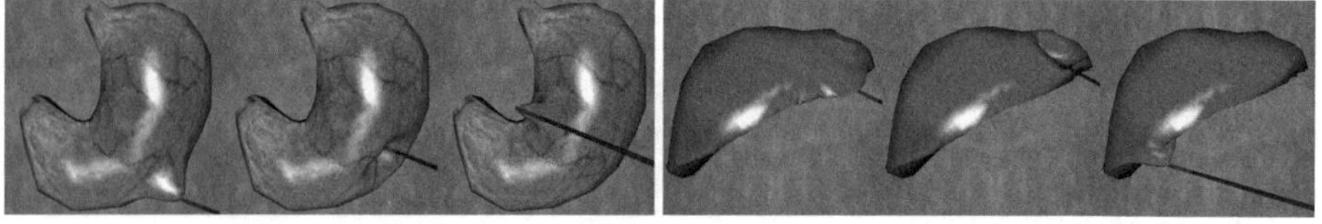

Figure 3. The deformation of the virtual organs with free form deformation. Left: simulation with the stomach model. Right: simulation with the liver model.

References

[1] De, S., Kim, J., and Srinivasan, M. A.: A meshless numerical technique for physically based real time medical simulations. Medicine Meets Virtual Reality (2001) 113–118

[2] De, S., Manivannan, M., Kim, J., Srinivasan, M. A., and Rattner, D.: Multimodal simulation of laparoscopic Heller myotomy using a meshless technique. Medicine Meets Virtual Reality 02/10 (2002) 127–132

[3] Gu, X., Gortler, S. J., and Hoppe, H.: Gometry images. ACM SIGGRAPH (2002) 355–361

[4] Liu , Q., and Prakash, E. C.: Cyber Surgery: Parameterized Mesh for Multi-modal Surgery Simulation. Lecture Notes in Computer Science **3767** (2005) 934 - 945

Medicine Meets Virtual Reality 14
J.D. Westwood et al. (Eds.)
IOS Press, 2006

343

Second Generation Haptic Ventriculostomy Simulator Using the *ImmersiveTouch*™ System

Cristian LUCIANO [a1], Pat BANERJEE [ab], G. Michael LEMOLE, Jr. [c]
and Fady CHARBEL [c]

[a] *Department of Computer Science*
[b] *Department of Mechanical and Industrial Engineering*
[c] *Department of Neurosurgery*

University of Illinois at Chicago

Abstract. Ventriculostomy is a neurosurgical procedure that consists of the insertion of a catheter into the ventricles of the brain for relieving the intracranial pressure. A distinct "popping" sensation is felt as the catheter enters the ventricles. Early ventriculostomy simulators provided some basic audio/visual feedback to simulate the procedure, displaying a 3D virtual model of a human head. Without any tactile feedback, the usefulness of such simulators was very limited. The first generation haptic ventriculostomy simulators incorporated a haptic device to generate a virtual resistance and "give" upon ventricular entry. While this created considerable excitement as a novelty device for cannulating ventricles, its usefulness for teaching and measuring neurosurgical expertise was still very limited. Poor collocation between the haptic device stylus held by the surgeon and the visual representation of the virtual catheter, as well as the lack of a correct viewer-centered perspective, created enormous confusion for the neurosurgeons who diverted their attention from the actual ventriculostomy procedure to overcoming the limitations of the simulator. We present a second generation haptic ventriculostomy simulator succeeding over the major first generation limitations by introducing a head and hand tracking system as well as a high-resolution high-visual-acuity stereoscopic display to enhance the perception and realism of the virtual ventriculostomy.

Keywords. Ventriculostomy, simulation, haptics, neurosurgery, virtual reality

Introduction

Ventriculostomy is a standard neurosurgical procedure for measuring the intracranial pressure (ICP) as well as for providing therapeutic cerebrospinal fluid drainage to lower the ICP [1]. After a small incision is made and a bur hole is drilled in a strategically chosen spot in the patient's skull, a ventriculostomy catheter is inserted

---

[1] Corresponding Author: University of Illinois at Chicago, 842 West Taylor St., 2039 ERF, Chicago, IL 60607, USA; E-mail: clucia1@uic.edu

aiming for the ventricles. A distinct "popping" or puncturing sensation is felt as the catheter enters the frontal horn of the lateral ventricle. Using a pressure transducer system the excess spinal fluid is drained to reduce the ICP.

A twist drill is used to make an opening in the skull perpendicular to the plane of the skull. The surgeon then places the tip of the catheter in the bur hole and orients the catheter based on certain neurosurgical landmarks: the medial canthus of the ipsilateral eye, in the frontal plane (Figure 1), and the tragus of the ipsilateral ear, in the saggital plane (Figure 2). The catheter is slowly inserted through the brain following a straight linear trajectory. After the characteristic "pop" is felt, the tip of the catheter is advanced few centimeters deeper to reach the opening of the foramen of Monro of the ipsilateral frontal horn. The surgeon's goal is to hit the ventricle preferably in the first attempt but most definitely within the first three attempts. Otherwise, intraparenchymal pressure monitoring devices need to be placed because of potential injury to the cerebrum.

Ventriculostomy, commonly employed for treatment of head injury and stroke, is a standard, low risk, but high frequency procedure at the University of Illinois Medical Center with about 300 interventions performed a year. Thus, the sheer number increases the risk profile and the need for an effective training and simulation tool, and standardized evaluation of neurosurgeons.

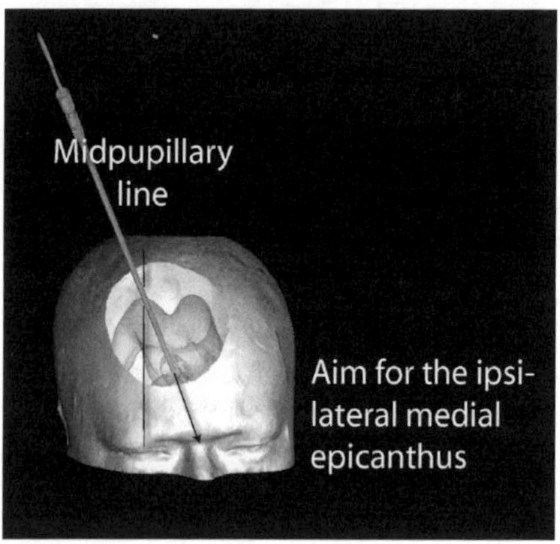

Figure 1. Landmark in the frontal plane

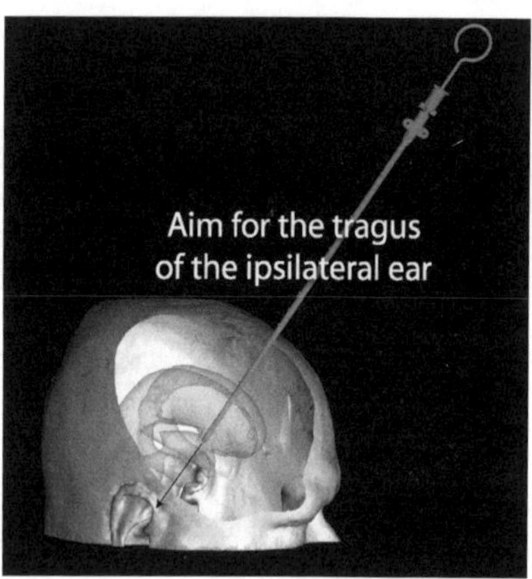

Figure 2. Landmark in the saggital plane

1. Background and previous research

In 2000, [2] developed a cross-platform web-based simulator using VRML, Java and CosmoWorld to simulate a ventricular catheterization. Using this early simulator, the user was able to position and orient the virtual catheter and visualize its trajectory while it was inserted in the 3D virtual head. An auditory cue was played when the catheter pierced the ventricular surface to simulate the "pop". Unfortunately, the catheter manipulation with the mouse was rudimentary and no tactile feedback was provided. Therefore, the effectiveness of the simulator was very limited.

Next came what we term as the first generation of haptic ventriculostomy simulator developed by [3], which concentrated on virtually generating the ventricular entry sensation by the use of a haptic device. This allowed the surgeon to manipulate the virtual catheter with the haptic device stylus in a VR-haptic environment implemented for the Reachin display [4]. While this development created considerable excitement as a novelty device for ventricular cannulation, its usefulness for teaching and measuring neurosurgical expertise was still very limited. The reasons and how we overcome these issues are provided as follows.

During a real ventriculostomy, the patient's head is placed supine (Figure 3). The surgeon places the tip of the catheter in the bur hole facing the horizontal plane and then orients the catheter moving his/her head to one side of the patient's head to another to locate the landmarks in the frontal and saggital planes. Since the Reachin system used by [3] does not provide head tracking, a fixed viewing perspective of the 3D model is displayed, regardless of the actual viewer's point of view. Therefore, the surgeon was unable to visualize the landmarks located in the other planes simply moving his/her head, as s/he would do in the real scenario.

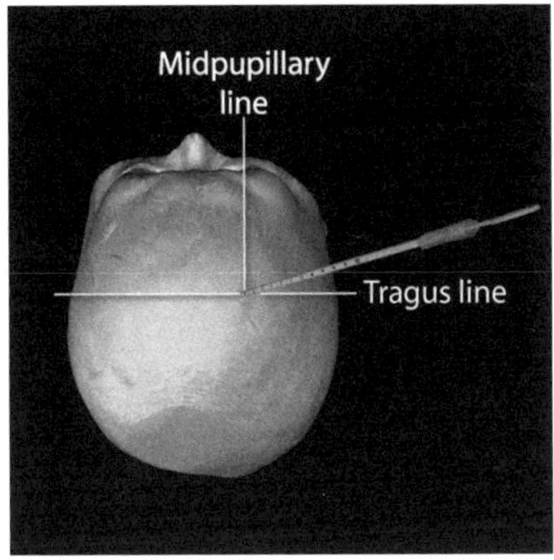

Figure 3. Landmark in the horizontal plane

Moreover, it was very cumbersome to rotate the 3D model back and forth while the surgeon held the tip of the catheter in the bur hole.

Another important requirement is to perfectly overlap the 3D image of the virtual catheter with the haptic stylus (which we term as "real catheter"). While the Reachin display initially can start with a good graphics/haptics collocation, as soon as the surgeon moves his/her head out of the "sweet spot", the virtual and real catheters do not overlap because of lack of head tracking. This created enormous confusion for the surgeon trying to collocate the real and virtual catheter during ventriculostomy; the attention of the surgeon was diverted from the actual ventriculostomy procedure to overcoming the limitations of the first generation haptic simulator. The result was increase in the time and number of trials of the ventriculostomy procedure, attributable primarily to simulator limitation and not surgeon skill limitation. In effect, the device did not adequately reproduce the ventriculostomy procedure.

Since the Reachin API is based on proprietary standards and not open-source, head tracking and viewer-centered perspective cannot be easily incorporated. Moreover, even if head tracking could be incorporated, the Reachin display has a relatively small mirror, so portions of the virtual head could easily disappear from the viewing plane when the surgeon tilts his/her head.

In this paper, we present a first step at conceiving and implementing a second generation haptic ventriculostomy simulator overcoming major first generation limitations by using our *ImmersiveTouch™* system [5].

2. *ImmersiveTouch*™ hardware

ImmersiveTouch™ is the first augmented VR system that seamlessly integrates a haptics device with a head and hand tracking system and a high-resolution high-visual-

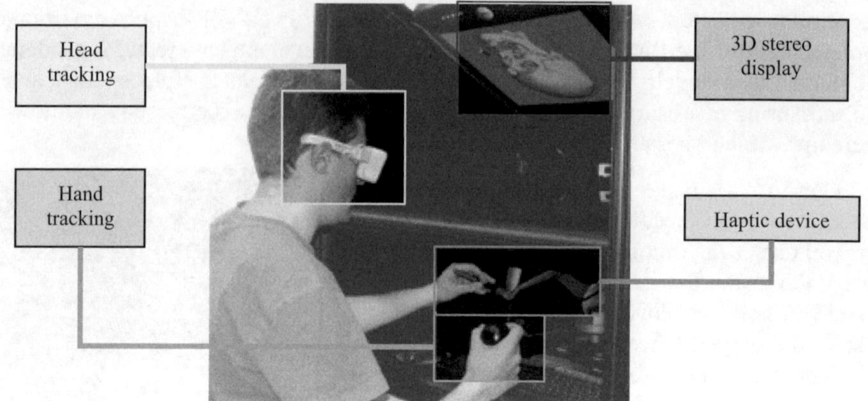

Figure 4. *ImmersiveTouch™* hardware components

acuity stereoscopic display (Figure 4). A translucent (half-silvered) mirror is used to create an augmented reality environment that integrates the surgeon hands, the virtual catheter and the virtual 3D patient's head in a common working volume (Figure 5).

The graphics/haptics collocation achieved by the *ImmersiveTouch™* is maintained at all time as the 3D virtual perspective changes according to the user's point of view because of the use of an electromagnetic head tracking system. In addition, the user can interact with the virtual objects using both hands: the surgeon holds the real catheter (haptic stylus) on one hand, and defines arbitrary 3D cutting planes with the other hand holding a SpaceGrip [6]. A virtual pair of scissors shows the orientation of the cutting plane.

3. *ImmersiveTouch™* software

The ventriculostomy simulator consists of four interconnected modules that are linked against four different APIs (Figure 6):

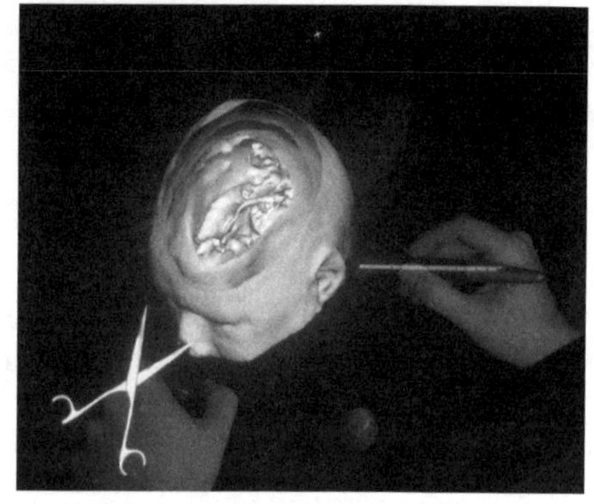

Figure 5. Augmented reality environment created by the *ImmersiveTouch™*

- **Volume data pre-processing** (using VTK 4.5 [7]). During a pre-processing phase, 2D images generated by an MRI or CT scanner are segmented and combined to create a virtual 3D volume of the patient's head. Then, 3D polygonal isosurfaces corresponding to the skin, bone, brain and ventricles are extracted from the 3D volume and exported as VRML files (Figure 7).

- **Head and hand tracking** (using pciBIRD [8]). An electromagnetic sensor attached to the stereo goggles tracks the surgeon's head to compute the correct viewer's perspective while the surgeon moves his/her head around the virtual patient's head to locate the landmarks. Another sensor located inside of the SpaceGrip tracks the surgeon's hand to define the cutting plane and the light source.

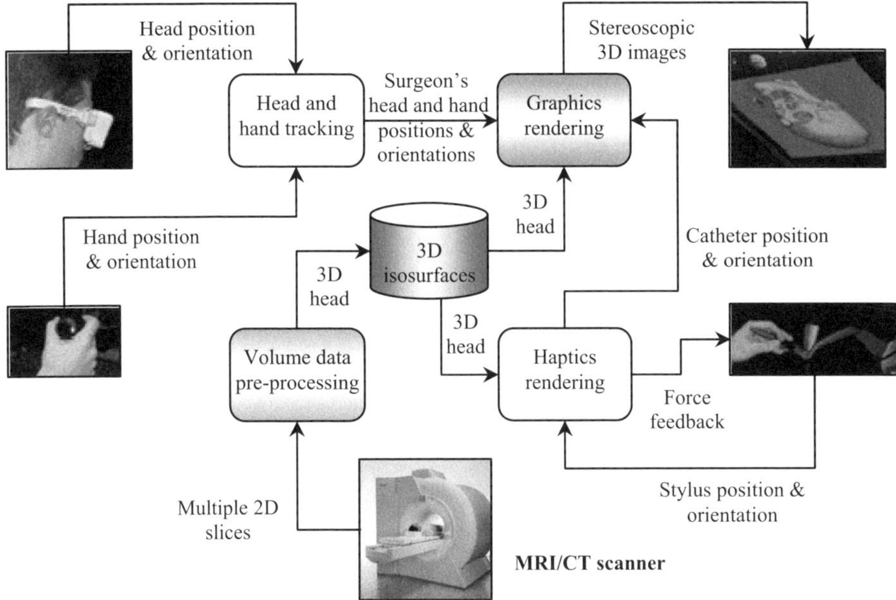

Figure 6. *ImmersiveTouch*™ software components

- **Haptics rendering** (using GHOST 4.0 [9]). The system reads the position and orientation of the haptic stylus, computes the collision detections between the virtual catheter and the imported 3D isosurfaces, and generates the corresponding force feedback. Each isosurface is assigned different haptic materials, according to certain parameters: stiffness, viscosity, static friction and dynamic friction. Therefore, the surgeon can feel the different surfaces and texture of the skin, bone and brain. Certain viscosity effect is felt as the catheter passes through the gelatinous parenchyma of the brain. As soon as the catheter breaks the dense ependymal ventricular lining, the viscosity effect ceases, providing the surgeon the distinct "popping" sensation.

- **Graphics rendering** (using Coin 2.3 [10]). The virtual environment is organized as an Open Inventor scene graph that includes the imported 3D isosurfaces, the light, the cutting plane manipulator, and a special perspective camera node. The camera node displays both perspectives of the surgeon's eyes according to the position and orientation of his/her head. The scene graph is traversed and displayed using a frame-sequential (active) stereo technique on the high-resolution CRT monitor. The *ImmersiveTouch*™ system offers high display resolution (1600x1200 pixels) and high visual acuity (20/24.74), which is important to clearly see the

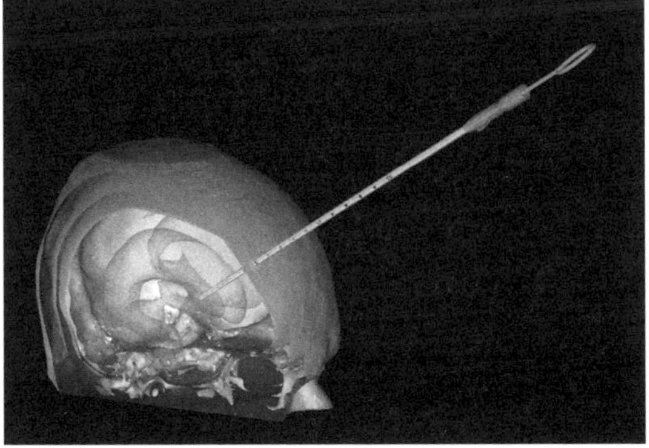

Figure 7. 3D isosurfaces: skin, skull, brain and ventricles

markings of the virtual catheter and small details of the head anatomy, thereby learning the operation with greater efficiency than in the first generation system.

4. Conclusions and future research

We have developed a realistic haptics-based augmented virtual reality simulator for neurosurgical education. A preliminary experiment conducted with neurosurgical faculty, residents and medical students from UIC showed how a learning curve correlated with the neurosurgical educational level of the user. During the experiment, medical students improved their performance from 10%-50% to 100% in fewer than 30 trials showing the potential of the ventriculostomy simulator. More exhaustive assessments will be conducted in future.

Acknowledgements

This research was supported by NSF grant DMI 9988136, NIST ATP cooperative agreement 70NANB1H3014, the Link Foundation Fellowship of the Institute for Simulation and Training at the University of Central Florida, and the Department of Mechanical and Industrial Engineering at the University of Illinois at Chicago (UIC).

References

[1] Winn, Richard H., MD, (2003) *Youmans Neurological Surgery*, 5th edition, Mt. Sinai School of Medicine, New York.

[2] Phillips, N., Nigel, J. (2000) Web-based Surgical Simulation for Ventricular Catheterization, *Neurosurgery*. 46(4):933-937

[3] Cros, O., Volden, M., Flaaris, J.J., Brix, L., Pedersen, C.F., Hansen, K.V., Larsen, O.V., Østergaard, L.R., Haase, J. (2002) Simulating the puncture of the human ventricle. *10th Annual Medicine Meets Virtual Reality Conference*, MMVR 2002

[4] Reachin display, www.reachin.se

[5] Luciano, C., Banerjee, P., Florea, L., Dawe, G. (2005) Design of the *ImmersiveTouch*™: a High-Performance Haptic Augmented VR System, *HCI Int'l Proceedings*

[6] LaserAid, SpaceGrips, http://www.spacegrips.com/spacegrips.htm

[7] Kitware Inc., Visualization ToolKit 4.5, http://www.vtk.org/

[8] Ascension Technologies Corp., pciBIRD API, http://www.ascension-tech.com/products/pcibird.php

[9] SensAble Technologies, GHOST 4.0, http://www.sensable.com/

[10] Systems in Motion, Coin 2.3, http://www.coin3d.org/

Medicine Meets Virtual Reality 14
J.D. Westwood et al. (Eds.)
IOS Press, 2006

349

Hybrid Analysis of a Spherical Mechanism for a Minimally Invasive Surgical (MIS) Robot - Design Concepts for Multiple Optimizations

Mitchell J.H. Lum [a,1], Diana Warden [b], Jacob Rosen [a], Mika N. Sinanan [c] and Blake Hannaford [a]

[a] *Department of Electrical Engineering*
[b] *Department of Mechanical Engineering*
[c] *Department of Surgery*
University of Washington, Seattle, WA, USA
e-mail:<mitchlum, dwarden, rosen, mssurg, blake>@u.washington.edu

Abstract. Several criteria exist for determining the optimal design for a surgical robot. This paper considers kinematic performance metrics, which reward good kinematic performance, and dynamic performance metrics, which penalize poor dynamic performance. Kinematic and dynamic metrics are considered independently, and then combined to produce hybrid metrics. For each metric, the optimal design is the one that maximizes the performance metric over a specific design space. In the case of a 2-DOF spherical mechanism for a surgical robot, the optimal design determined by kinematic metrics is a robot arm with link angles ($\alpha_{12} = 90°$, $\alpha_{23} = 90°$). The large link angles are the most dextrous, but have the greatest risk of robot-robot or robot-patient collisions and require the largest actuators. The link lengths determined by the dynamic metrics are much shorter, which reduces the risk of collisions, but tend to place the robot in singularities much more frequently. When the hybrid metrics are used, and a restriction that the arm must be able to reach a human's entire abdomen, the optimal design is around ($\alpha_{12} = 51°$, $\alpha_{23} = 54°$). The hybrid design provides a compromise between dexterity and compactness.

Keywords. Surgical Robot, Dynamic Optimization, Kinematic Optimization

1. Introduction

Innovations in surgical techniques and equipment allow procedures to beceome more precise, less invasive, and inherently safer. With minimally invasive surgery (MIS), for instance, postoperative hospital stays have been reduced from more than a week (with 'open' surgery) down to just over a day. Integrating robotic systems into the operating

---

[1]Correspondence to: Mitchell J.H. Lum, University of Washington, Dept. of Electrical Engineering, Box 352500, Seattle, WA 98195. Tel.: +1 206 616 4936; ; E-mail: mitchlum@u.washington.edu

room will help this trend in healthcare to continue, and has been a research focus for nearly twenty years. In 1995, Taylor [1] designed some of the earliest surgical robots. Shortly thereafter, Madhani [2] developed the Silver and Black Falcons, which were later adapted to become Intuitive Surgical's Da Vinci system. [3], [4],and [5] have also made important contributions with their designs for robotic systems.

The pivot point constraint imposed by the surgical ports in MIS makes a spherical mechanism ideal for a surgical robot. In a previous study [6], we presented the analysis of a spherical mechanism used as a surgical robot for MIS. Using data collected from the Blue Dragon, a device for tracking the position and orientation of MIS tools during in-vivo animal surgeries [7], we defined the dexterous workspace (DWS) as the workspace in which surgeons spend 95% of their time. Another measurement was also taken on a human patient to determine the workspace required to reach the full extent of the human abdomen. In [6], [8] the spherical mechanism was subjected to a kinematic optimization with a link length penalty as a scoring criteria.

For the case of a square matrix, Yoshikawa's dynamic manipulability measure can be calculated by the absolute value of the determinant of the Jacobian matrix divided by the absolute value of the determinant of the inertia matrix [9]. Broken down, this can be viewed as a *hybrid* of the kinematic manipulability measure with the addition of an explicit dynamic penalty on the inertia matrix. In this study, we changed the methodology of [8] and separated criteria into their individual kinematic and dynamic terms. We show how different performance criteria yield different robot designs for the same task-based optimization problem and discuss the advantages and limitations of each of the resultant solutions.

2. Methods

2.1. Performance Criteria

The two kinematic measures used were kinematic isotropy and kinematic manipulability. Kinematic isotropy is typically defined as the condition number of the Jacobian matrix, which is the ratio of the highest singular value to the lowest singular value [10]. The kinematic isotropy is a measure of directional uniformity, which indicates how easily a manipulator can move in any arbitrary direction. As in [6], we wished to express a bounded scoring criterion. We therefore chose to use the ratio of the lowest singular value of the Jacobian matrix to the highest singular value, or the inverse of the isotropy, as our kinematic measure.

The two dynamic measures used were the link length penalty previously used and the absolute value of the determinant of the inertia matrix. Yoshikawa's dynamic ma-nipulability is defined as the kinematic manipulability divided by the determinant of the inertia matrix [9]. We therefore chose to use the inertia matrix determinant as a dynamic element just as we used the Jacobian matrix as a kinematic element. As in [6], we used a link length penalty, the sum of the link angles cubed, because it is proportional to beam stiffness.

Table 1 lists the eight performance criteria. K_1 and K_2 are purely kinematic mea-sures, D_1 and D_2 are purely dynamic measures, and H_1, H_2, H_3 and H_4 are the hybrid combinations of kinematic and dynamic criteria.

Table 1. Performance Metrics

Denom\Num	1	$|det J|$	$\frac{\sigma_{min}}{\sigma_{max}}$
1	n/a	K_1 (Manpulability)	K_2 (Isotropy)
$|det M|$	D_1	H_1 (Dyn. Manipulability)	H_2
L^3	D_2	H_3	H_4 (Criteria used in [8])

2.2. Optimization Method

Each optimization took into account a performance metric and required workspace. The scoring method uses the average performance of each design over the required workspace as well as the minimum performance within that workspace [11]. Based on previous measurements, we defined the dexterous workspace (DWS) as the workspace in which surgeons spend 95% of their time. The DWS is a conical volume of vertex angle 60°. We also defined the extended dexterous workspace (EDWS) as the workspace required to reach the full extent of the human abdomen. The EDWS is a conical volume of vertex angle 90°.

Based on preliminary mechanical design, we add the constraint that the elbow joint can only close to a minimum joint angle of 20° and extend to a maximum joint angle of 180°. Each design is a pair of link angles, $(\alpha_{12}, \alpha_{23})$, and the design space was the combination of all pairs of link angles, each of which range in 1° increments from 30° to 90°. We sought a design with optimal performance within the workspace that surgeons spend most of their time (the DWS) that could still reach the full extent of the human abdomen (the EDWS). We therefore scored across the entire DWS, and then only considered those designs that contained the EDWS in their workspace.

3. Results

The optimization was performed with respect to each of the eight criteria. When optimized using the DWS as the required workspace for the mechanism, the kinematic measures (K_1, K_2) favored the longest possible links, the dynamic metrics (D_1, D_2)favored shorter links, and the hybrid metrics (H_1-H_4)favored more intermediate results (Table 2).

Table 2. DWS RESULTS Optimal Design of the spherical mechanism with respect to each of the 8 performance metrics. Results for each metric are link angles (α_{12}, α_{23}) in degrees.

Denom\Num	1	$|det J|$	$\frac{\sigma_{min}}{\sigma_{max}}$
1	n/a	K_1:(90°,90°)	K_2:(90°,90°)
$|det M|$	D_1:(33°,39°)	H_1:(34°,39°)	H_2:(40°,35°)
L^3	D_2:(39°,33°)	H_3:(39°,38°)	H_4:(42°,38°)

When the above design space results were further subjected to the requirement that the designs needed to contain the EDWS within the reachable workspace, the smallest possible design was found to be larger (Table 3). This result was expected, since the EDWS is a larger workspace. Interestingly, because the optimal designs over the DWS for the dynamic and hybrid metrics were smaller than could reach the EDWS, those designs were filtered out, leaving similar designs with respect to either the dynamic or hybrid criteria.

Table 3. Results of optimization over DWS suject to the requirement that the design contains the EDWS in its workspace.

Denom\Num	1	$|detJ|$	$\frac{\sigma_{min}}{\sigma_{max}}$
1	n/a	K_1:$(90°, 90°)$	K_2:$(90°, 90°)$
$|detM|$	D_1:$(51°, 54°)$	H_1:$(51°, 54°)$	H_2:$(54°, 51°)$
L^3	D_2:$(53°, 52°)$	H_3:$(53°, 52°)$	H_4:$(58°, 49°)$

4. Discussion

The results have shown eight designs based on different scoring criteria. These scoring criteria take into account well established mechanism analysis methods. However, the optimization does not take into account clinical aspects. Specifically, the mechanism was optimized in isolation of the surgical context. It does not consider multiple manipulators over the patient in the surgical scene. In this section we discuss the advantages and limitations of each of the resultant designs.

When multiple manipulators are placed over the patient in the surgical scene, the manipulators are more likely to suffer from collisions with each other (robot-robot collisions) and with the patient (robot-patient collisions). Damage to the devices could occur from robot-robot collisions, and robot-patient collisions are clearly unacceptable for safety concerns. Robot-patient collisions may be avoided by positioning and orienting the robot so that it is always in an 'elbow up' configuration while operating on the patient. In surgical tasks where the tool tips are moved towards each other, such as running the bowel or tying a knot, robot-robot collisions are not always avoidable. This is particularly true for robots with longer links. Figure 1(a) illustrates this problem, showing two surgical manipulators with $90°$ links that have the tool tips approaching each other inside the patient. Additionally, the longer the link lengths, the more massive the mechanism will be, with greater inertial and gravity loads. This will require larger actuators and higher power consumption.

At the other end of the spectrum, optimization based purely on dynamic criteria yielded designs with very short links. The more compact a device, the less likely is to suffer robot-robot and robot-patient collision problems; however, as the tools reach the edge of the workspace, the manipulator's kinematic performance would suffer from a kinematic singularity at the workspace boundary. A singularity within the surgical workspace would be completely unacceptable. As the link lengths become shorter, the mechanism's mass and inertia decrease, resulting in better dynamic performance and requiring smaller actuators and lower power consumption.

Some of the hybrid cases provide a reasonable compromise between the desire for a compact and lightweight mechanism and good performance throughout the surgical workspace. Optimization over just the DWS leads to link angles ranging from $34°$ to $42°$. When only the designs that contain the EDWS in the workspace are considered,

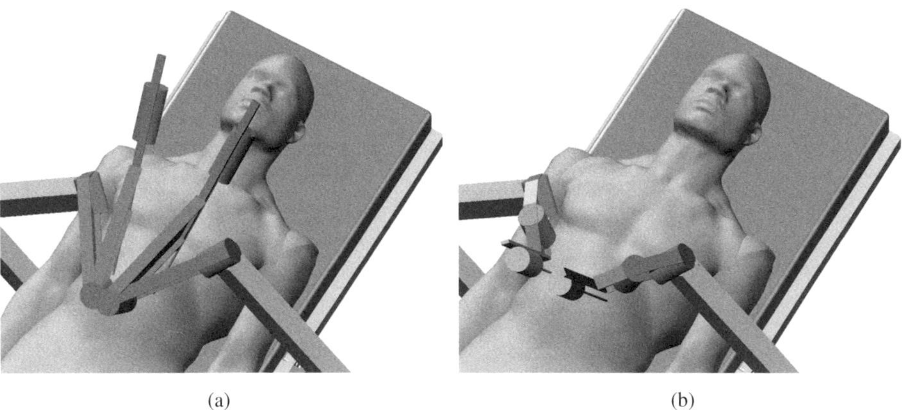

(a)   (b)

Figure 1. (a) Robot arms with long ($90°$, $90°$) links suffer from elbow collisions when performing tasks such as running the bowel. (b) Robot arms with short ($39°$, $33°$) links suffer from kinematic singularities at the workspace boundary.

the link angles range from $49°$ to $58°$. The requirement to reach the EDWS causes a considerable increase in the overall size of the surgical links, but adds the benefit of increased dexterity.

5. Conclusions

Before this study with multiple performance metrics was conducted, we performed a preliminary optimization of the spherical mechanism for MIS applications using the H_4 metric, kinematic isotropy with a link length penalty [8]. Due to differences in the optimization methodology, the previous optimization yielded different results. At that time we determined the optimal link angles to be ($\alpha_{12} = 75°, \alpha_{23} = 60°$). A cable-actuated surgical manipulator based on this result has been designed and fabricated. The surgical manipulator features six degrees of freedom for tool orientation, tool insertion, roll, wrist, and grasp and supports the additon of a second wrist axis. The tool tips are Computer Motion MicroAssist 5 mm tools modified with a quick release system that we developed for interchanging tools with the ability to use a robotic tool changer.

5.1. Future Work

This study has presented the optimization of a spherical mechanism for robotic MIS applications. We have presented eight performance criteria from which designs were generated and discussed the advantages and disadvantages of each. We now understand that the results from our previous study may be overly conservative with respect to the desire for a large reachable workspace. Future development of our MIS robot system may include designing and fabricating new link pieces based on the results of this study. While more compact links will reduce the reachable workspace, it will allow for lower gravity torques on the joints and overall better dynamic performance. Future work will also include clinical trials with surgeons operating on porcine models, in both local and remote teleoperation environments.

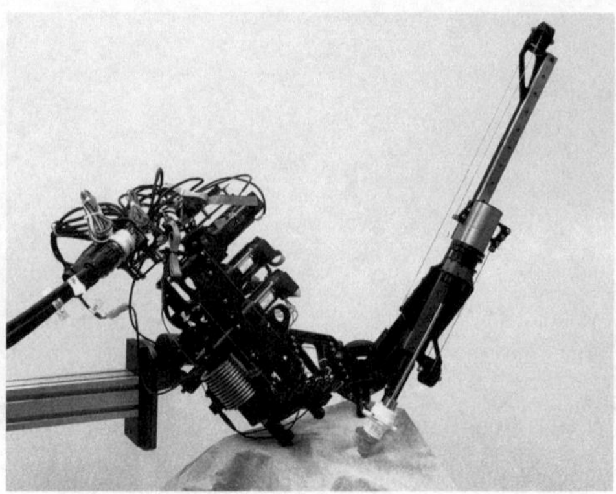

Figure 2. The University of Washington, BioRobotics Lab, 6-DOF Surgical Manipulator

Acknowledgements

This work is partially supported by US Army, Medical Research and Material Command, grant number DAMD17-1-0202.

References

[1] R.H. Taylor and et al. A telerobotic assistant for laparoscopic surgery. *Engineering in Medicine and Biology*, 14, 1995.

[2] A.J. Madhani, G. Niemeyer, and Jr. Salisbury, J.K. The black falcon: A teleoperated surgical instrument for minimally invasive surgery. In *Proceedings of the Intelligent Robots and Systems*, volume 2, pages 936–944, 1998.

[3] S. Sastry, S. Cohn, and Tendick F. Milli-robotics for remote, minimally invasive surgery. In *J. Robot Auton. Syst*, volume 21, pages 305–316, 1998.

[4] T. Li and S. Payandeh. Design of spherical parallel mechanisms for application to laparoscopic surgery. *Robotica*, 20, 2002.

[5] J. Shi and et al. Preliminary results of the design of a novel laparoscopic manipulator. In *Proceedings of the 11th World Congress in Mechanism and Machinese Science*, April 2002.

[6] J. Rosen, M.J.H. Lum, D Trimble, B. Hannaford, and M.N. Sinanan. Spherical mechanism analysis of a surgical robot for minimally invasive surgery - analytical and experimental approaches. In *Medicine Meets Virtual Reality*, volume 111, 2005.

[7] J.D. Brown, J. Rosen, L. Chang, M. Sinanan, and B. Hannaford. Quantifying surgeon grasping mechanics in laparoscopy using the blue dragon system. In *Medicine Meets Virtual Reality 13*, 2004.

[8] M.J.H. Lum, J. Rosen, M.N. Sinanan, and B. Hannaford. Kinematic optimization of a spherical mechanism for a minimally invasive surgical robot. In *Proceedings of the 2004 IEEE Conference on Robotics and Automation*, pages 829–834, New Orleans, USA, April 2004.

[9] T. Yoshikawa. Dynamic manipulability of robot manipulators. *International Journal of Robotics Research*, 4(2):1033–1038, 1985.

[10] J.K. Salisbury and J.T. Craig. Articulated hands: Force control and kinematic issues. *International Journal of Robotics Research*, 1(1):4–17, 1982.

[11] M.J.H. Lum, D. Warden, J. Rosen, and B. Hannaford. Performance metrics for a task-based optimization of a robot: A case study of planar and spherical manipulators. In *Submitted to IEEE/ICRA 2006*, Orlando, FL USA, 2006.

Medicine Meets Virtual Reality 14
J.D. Westwood et al. (Eds.)
IOS Press, 2006

Data Mining of the E-Pelvis Simulator Database: A Quest for a Generalized Algorithm for Objectively Assessing Medical Skill

Thomas MACKEL [1], Jacob ROSEN [1,2], Ph.D., Carla PUGH [3], M.D., Ph.D.
[1] *Department of Electrical Engineering,* [2] *Department of Surgery, University of Washington, Seattle, WA, USA*
[3] *Department of Surgery, Northwestern University, Chicago, IL, USA*
E-mail:{tmackel ,rosen}@u.washington.edu drpugh@northwestern.edu
Biorobotics Lab: http://brl.ee.washington.edu

Abstract: Inherent difficulties in evaluating clinical competence of physicians has lead to the widespread use of subjective skill assessment techniques. Inspired by an analogy between medical procedure and spoken language, proven modeling methods in the field of speech recognition were adapted for use as objective skill assessment techniques. A generalized methodology using Markov Models (MM) was developed. The database under study was collected with the E-Pelvis physical simulator. The simulator incorporates an array of five contact force sensors located in key anatomical landmarks. Two 32-state fully connected MMs are used, one for each skill level. Each state in the model corresponds to one of the possible combinations of the 5 active contact force sensors distributed in the simulator. Statistical distances measured between models representing subjects with different skill levels are sensitive enough to provide an objective measure of medical skill level. The method was tested with 41 expert subjects and 41 novice subjects in addition to the 30 subjects used for training the MM. Of the 82 subjects, 76 were classified correctly (92%). Moreover, unique state transitions as well as force magnitudes for corresponding states (expert/novice) were found to be skill dependent. Given the white box nature of the model, analyzing the MMs provides insight into the examination process performed. This methodology is independent of the modality under study. It was previously used to assess surgical skill in a minimally invasive surgical setup using the Blue DRAGON, and it is currently applied to data collected using the E-Pelvis.

1. Introduction

Inherent difficulties in evaluating clinical competence of physicians has lead to the widespread use of subjective skill assessment techniques. Subjective evaluation techniques lead to inconsistent evaluation by different examiners. Inspired by an analogy between medical procedure and spoken language, proven modeling methods in the field of speech recognition were adapted for use as objective skill assessment techniques. A metric that represents the skill level of a subject was determined by analyzing the subject's performance with respect to the performance of subjects of known skill levels. Previous studies applied the Markov modeling (MM) approach to skill evaluation of Minimally Invasive Surgery [1-6]. Using an approach that is independent of the modality used by the physician, the aim of the current study was to utilize the MM approach in developing a methodology for objectively assessing clinical skills during a pelvic exam using data acquired with the E-Pelvis simulator [7-9].

2. Methods

2.1. The E-Pelvis Simulator and the Acquired Database

The E-Pelvis is a physical simulator, shown in Figure 1, which consists of a partial mannequin (umbilicus to mid thigh) constructed in the likeness of an adult human female [7-9]. The simulator sampled data at 30 Hz from 5 pressure sensors located on key anatomical structures while the subjects performed pelvic examinations (Figure 2). The 41 expert subjects were selected from 362 professional examiners. The 41 novice subjects were selected from a group of 82 students. A different set of subjects, 15 experts and 15 novices, were selected to train the Markov models.

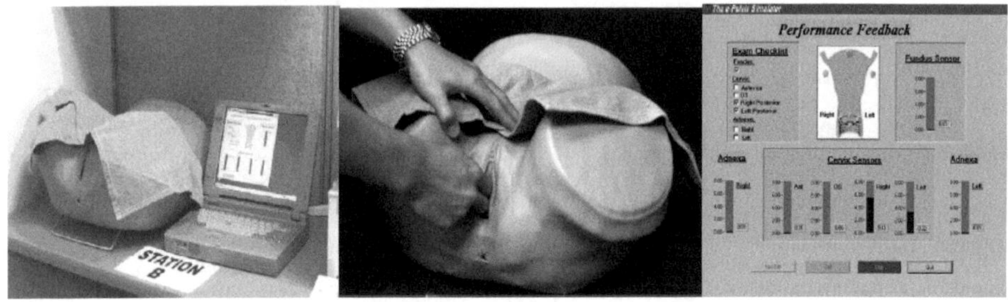

Figure 1.   The Complete E-Pelvis Simulator, a Simulated Pelvic Exam, and the Graphical User Interface.

2.2. Data Analysis

An analogy between the human spoken language and minimally invasive surgery tasks [1-6] was extended to pelvic examination tasks. Based on this analogy, the primary elements, 'words', were the actual states of the MMs. Different 'pronunciations' of each state were observed in the pressure data taken from the E-Pelvis simulator. Data characterizing the performance of two categories of medical examiners, expert and novice, were analyzed using two 32-state fully connected MMs (Figure 2). Within each model certain sequences of state transitions, known as Markov chains, are more probable than others.

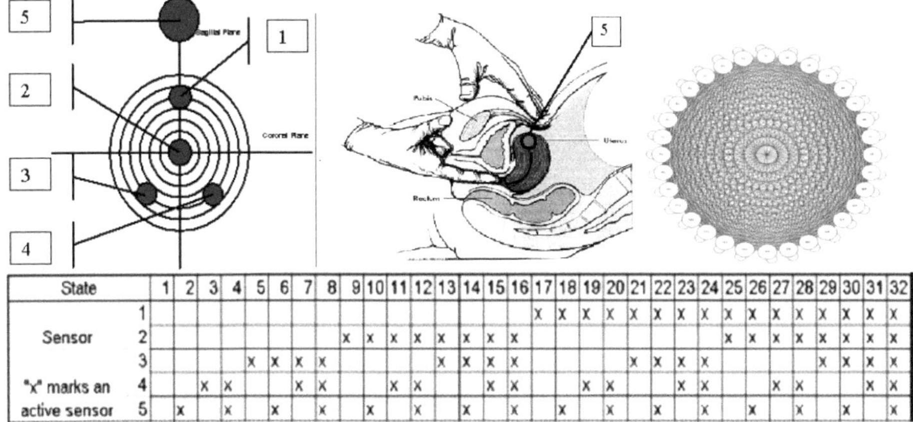

	State	1	2	3	4	5	6	7	8	9	10	11	12	13	14	15	16	17	18	19	20	21	22	23	24	25	26	27	28	29	30	31	32
	1																	x	x	x	x	x	x	x	x	x	x	x	x	x	x	x	x
Sensor	2									x	x	x	x	x	x	x	x									x	x	x	x	x	x	x	x
	3					x	x	x	x					x	x	x	x					x	x	x	x					x	x	x	x
"x" marks an	4			x	x			x	x			x	x			x	x			x	x			x	x			x	x			x	x
active sensor	5		x		x		x		x		x		x		x		x		x		x		x		x		x		x		x		x

Figure 2.   **Top**: Sensor Locations and a 32-State Fully Interconnected Markov Model State Diagram.
Bottom: Active/Inactive Sensor Combinations

Each subject's performance was represented as a 5-dimensional vector of N data points measured from the 5 simulator sensors. A sensor was considered active if the value of the data exceeded a chosen threshold value, and it was considered inactive otherwise. Each state in the MM corresponded to one of the possible combinations (Figure 2) of active sensors. Many states were more commonly used than others, resulting in an uneven distribution of the data points between states.

Each state can be characterized by a mean vector and covariance matrix ([B] matrix – continuous version observation). The frequency transition matrix ([A] matrix) defines the frequency in which transitions occur between the various states. The data points representative of each state were used to compute the 1x5 mean vector, μ, and 5x5 covariance matrix, Σ. To calculate the elements of the [A] matrix the number of state transitions in the training subjects' data were tallied and then normalized to 1.

Bayes' Decision Rule was used to classify an unknown subject as either an expert or novice. If there are two classes, A and B, this rule states to choose class A if P(A) > P(B), choose class B otherwise. Define observation vector O as a sequence of data points x[n]. Let P(A) be the probability of a sequence of data points arising from an expert model, $P(O|\lambda_{ES})$, and P(B) the probability of a sequence of data points arising from a novice model, $P(O|\lambda_{NS})$.

The probability that model λ would generate an observation vector O, $P(O|\lambda)$, is the product of probabilities that each data point x was produced by model λ, $P(x|\lambda)$.

$$P(O \mid \lambda) = \prod_{i=1}^{N} P(\mathbf{x}[i] \mid \lambda) \tag{1}$$

$P(x|\lambda)$ can be defined as the product of the membership probability ('B' matrix) P_M and the transition probability P_T ('A' matrix). The membership probability is defined using the total probability rule.

$$P_M(\mathbf{x}\mid\lambda) = \frac{p(\lambda)L(\mathbf{x}\mid\lambda)}{\sum_{j=1}^{M} p(\lambda_j)L(\mathbf{x}\mid\lambda_j)} \tag{2}$$

where $p(\lambda)$ represents the *a priori* probabilities of each model, $L(x|\lambda)$ is the likelihood of data point x belonging to model λ, and M is the total number of models. Eq. (2) is simplified by assuming identical *a priori* probabilities for each model.

$$P_M(\mathbf{x}\mid\lambda) = \frac{L(\mathbf{x}\mid\lambda)}{\sum_{j=1}^{M} L(\mathbf{x}\mid\lambda_j)} \tag{3}$$

The likelihood is modeled by the multivariate normal probability density function.

$$L(\mathbf{x}\mid\lambda) = \frac{1}{(2\pi)^{p/2}\sqrt{\|\Sigma\|}}\, e^{\frac{-(\mathbf{x}-\mu)^T \Sigma^{-1}(\mathbf{x}-\mu)}{2}} \tag{4}$$

where p is the number of dimensions of data, Σ is the covariance matrix of the model, and μ the mean vector of the model.

The transition probability is given by the transition matrix for the model, A_λ. This probability takes into account the probability of transitioning from the previous state S_1 to the current state S_2, and is found by directly indexing the model's transition matrix. The first data point is a special case, as the previous state is unknown, and P_T is assigned a value of 1 for this case.

$$P_T(\lambda) = \mathbf{A}_\lambda[S_1, S_2] \tag{5}$$

Given a sequence of data associated with a specific subject, the above method can be used to estimate the probability that the MM of a class generated the sequence. The subject can be classified as a member of the class whose model results in the highest probability.

More data is collected during slower examinations. This penalizes both models by increasing the length of the observation vector O, hence increasing the number of factors used to compute P(O|λ). As a result, the P(O|λ) of one subject cannot be directly compared to the P(O|λ) of another. Subjects' behavior relative to one another cannot be measured without the use of a common benchmark. One method uses a third MM trained from the subject's own data samples, P(O|λ_{OS}), which is compared to the novice model and the expert model. Two statistical factors can be defined as:

$$NSF = \log(P(O\mid\lambda_{OS}))/\log(P(O\mid\lambda_{NS})) \tag{6}$$

$$ESF = \log(P(O\mid\lambda_{OS}))/\log(P(O\mid\lambda_{ES})) \tag{7}$$

where O is an observation vector representing the subject's performance, λ_{OS} is a subject model trained by the data O, and λ_{ES} and λ_{NS} are models trained by data from experts and novices respectively.

There are two ways of finding $P(O|\lambda_{OS})$: a competing method and a non-competing method. In the competing method, $P_M(O|\lambda_{OS}) + P_M(O|\lambda_{ES}) + P_M(O|\lambda_{NS}) = 1$ for each observation point. An increase in $P_M(O|\lambda_{OS})$ is accompanied by a decrease in $P_M(O|\lambda_{ES})$ and $P_M(O|\lambda_{NS})$.

In the non-competing method, $P_M(O|\lambda_{OS}) = P_M(O|\lambda_{ES}) + P_M(O|\lambda_{NS}) = 1$ for each observation point. Only the subject transition matrix influences the value of $P(O|\lambda_{OS})$. This method prevents the subject model itself from influencing the classification results.

Given the 'white box' nature of the MM, analyzing the models provides insight into the process in which the pelvic exam is performed. Observing the most probable transitions within each model's transition matrix can identify Markov chains. The most-probable transitions are known as top-level chains. Some top-level chains are distinct to each class, and do not occur even as a subset of a chain of either class.

3. Results

Using the MMs to compute Bayesian classifier probabilities, 40 of the 41 expert subjects (97.6%), and 36 of the 41 novice subjects (87.8%) were correctly classified using this method. Overall, 76 of the 82 subjects tested (92.7%) were correctly classified. These subjects were not used in the training of the MMs. The skill factors computed using the non-competing method is shown in Figure 3.

Analysis of Variance (ANOVA) was performed to compare the data from each novice state with the corresponding expert state. Direct comparison of a set of novice data to a set of expert data showed interaction effects significant at the $\alpha=0.000001$ level for all states except 18, 22, and 27, which were significant at the $\alpha=0.03$ level. Expert data compared with another set of expert data showed interaction effects significant at the $\alpha=0.009$ level or higher for all states, and greater than $\alpha=0.1$ for most states. Novice data compared with novice data showed interaction effects significant at the $\alpha=0.00001$ level for all states, and greater than $\alpha=0.1$ for most states.

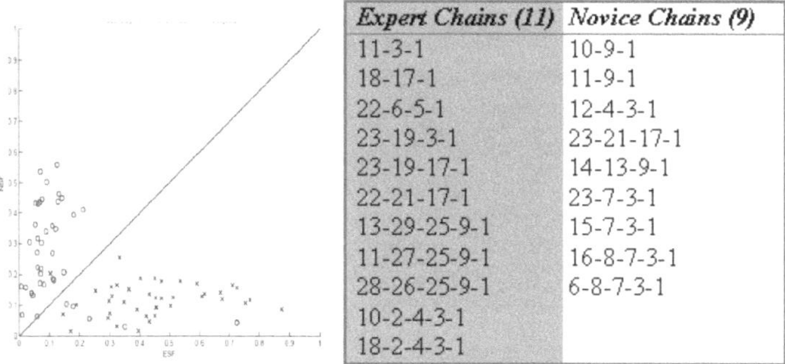

Expert Chains (11)	Novice Chains (9)
11-3-1	10-9-1
18-17-1	11-9-1
22-6-5-1	12-4-3-1
23-19-3-1	23-21-17-1
23-19-17-1	14-13-9-1
22-21-17-1	23-7-3-1
13-29-25-9-1	15-7-3-1
11-27-25-9-1	16-8-7-3-1
28-26-25-9-1	6-8-7-3-1
10-2-4-3-1	
18-2-4-3-1	

Figure 3.   **Left**: Skill Factor Plot with Decision Boundary **Right**: Distinct Top-Level Markov Chains

Observation of the internal structure of the MM indicates that each skill level can be characterized by unique state transitions (Markov chains). 20 top-level chains distinct to only one model are shown in Figure 3.

4. Discussion

The use of MMs for data analysis has been successfully applied to speech recognition. Extension of this concept to objective medical skill assessment has lead to a successful Bayesian dichotomous classification method. Subjects classified in this manner can be compared to one another using their performance indices. The distinct chains identified in the models may help reduce the number of states in the models. The strength of this methodology is that it is independent of the modality under study. It was previously used to assess surgical skill in a minimally invasive surgical setup using the Blue DRAGON, and it is currently applied to data collected using the E-Pelvis as a physical simulator. Similarly, the same methodology can be incorporated into a surgical robot as a supervisory controller that could detect potentially dangerous mistakes by a human or computer operator.

References

[1]   Rosen J, Hannaford B, Richards CG, Sinanan MN. Markov Modeling of Minimally Invasive Surgery Based on Tool/Tissue Interaction and Force/Torque Signatures for Evaluating Surgical Skills. IEEE Transactions on Biomedical Engineering, Vol. 48, No. 5, May 2001.

[2]   Rosen J., M. Solazzo, B. Hannaford, M. Sinanan, Objective Evaluation of Laparoscopic Skills Based on Haptic Information and Tool/Tissue Interactions, Computer Aided Surgery, Volume 7, Issue 1, pp. 49-61 July 2002

[3]   Rosen J., J. D. Brown, M. Barreca, L. Chang, B. Hannaford, M. Sinanan, The Blue DRAGON - A System for Monitoring the Kinematics and the Dynamics of Endoscopic Tools in Minimally Invasive Surgery for Objective Laparoscopic Skill Assessment, Studies in Health Technology and Informatics - Medicine Meets Virtual Reality, Vol. 85, pp.412-418, IOS Press, January 2002.

[4]   Rosen J., J. D. Brown, L. Chang, M. Barreca, M. Sinanan, B. Hannaford, The Blue DRAGON - A System for Measuring the Kinematics and the Dynamics of Minimally Invasive Surgical Tools In–Vivo, Proceedings of the 2002 IEEE International Conference on Robotics & Automation, Washington DC, USA, May 11-15, 2002.

[5]   Rosen J., L. Chang, J. D. Brown, B. Hannaford, M. Sinanan, R. Satava, Minimally Invasive Surgery Task Decomposition - Etymology of Endoscopic Suturing, Studies in Health Technology and Informatics - Medicine Meets Virtual Reality, vol. 94, pp. 295-301, IOS Press, January 2003

[6]   Kowalewski T.M., J. Rosen, L. Chang, M. Sinanan, B. Hannaford, Optimization of a Vector Quantization Codebook for Objective Evaluation of Surgical Skill, Studies in Health Technology and Informatics - Medicine Meets Virtual Reality, vol. 98, pp. 174-179, IOS Press, January 2004

[7]   Pugh CM, Srivastava S, Shavelson R, Walker D, Cotner T, Scarloss B, et al. The effect of simulator use on learning and self-assessment: the case of Stanford University's E-Pelvis simulator. Stud Health Technol Inform 2001;81: 396-400

[8]   Pugh CM, Rosen J., Qualitative and quantitative analysis of pressure sensor data acquired by the E-Pelvis simulator during simulated pelvic examinations, Stud Health Technol Inform. 2002;85:376-9.

[9]   Pugh CM, Youngblood P. Free in PMC, Development and validation of assessment measures for a newly developed physical examination simulator. J Am Med Inform Assoc. 2002 Sep-Oct;9(5):448-60

Medicine Meets Virtual Reality 14
J.D. Westwood et al. (Eds.)
IOS Press, 2006

Segmenting the Visible Human Female

Ameya Malvankar[a] and Bharti Temkin[a, b]
[a]*Department of Computer Science, Texas Tech University*
[b]*Department of Surgery, Texas Tech University*
Bharti.Temkin@ttu.edu

Abstract. Web-based three-dimensional Virtual Body Structures (W3D-VBS) is an interactive image-based anatomical training system over the Internet. It uses segmented low-resolution Visible Human Male (LR-VHM) data to dynamically explore, select, highlight, label, extract, manipulate, and stereoscopically palpate 3D virtual anatomical models with a haptic device. The segmentation results presented in this paper for the Visible Human Female (VHF) and the high resolution Visible Human Male (HR-VHM) have been obtained using our segmentation tools. Segmenting the HR-VHM was an easier task as we use the segmented shapes and label information of existing LR-VHM data, with the same image content. This is not the case for the VHF and we needed to develop a special tool, Segm-VHF, which allows us to integrate the VHF dataset into W3D-VBS.

Keywords: W3D-VBS, Visible Human, Image Registration, Anatomical Models

Introduction

The VHF images must be segmented in order to provide all the features of our current W3D-VBS system [1] [2] for the VHF data set. To develop 3D level features of the W3D-VBS all the structures of interest (SOI) need to be segmented, in all the appropriate slices. For SOI that are common to both male and female we use the existing segmentation and labeling information on axial, sagittal, and coronal images of the VHM. The corresponding VHM and VHF images are viewed side-by-side, see Figs. 1-2, to facilitate accurate segmentation and labeling by a user who may not be familiar with human anatomy. This side-by-side method has also been successfully used to segment structures for the high-resolution Visible Human Male (VHM) images and this has made it possible to integrate HR-VHM dataset into our W3D-VBS system. We demonstrate the use of our segmentation tool, Segm-VHF, for several VHF sagittal and coronal images. We also present a HR-VHM 3D model to demonstrate the level of accuracy that has been obtained when the method is used to segment the HR-VHM dataset.

Segmented VHF images and a 3D model of HR-VHM

Images presenting several segmented structures for the VHF set are shown in Figs. 1-2. The 3D model created using registered and segmented HR-VHM is shown in Fig. 3 [3] [4] [5]. We believe these results validate our approach to segmentation.

 A. Malvankar and B. Temkin / Segmenting the Visible Human Female

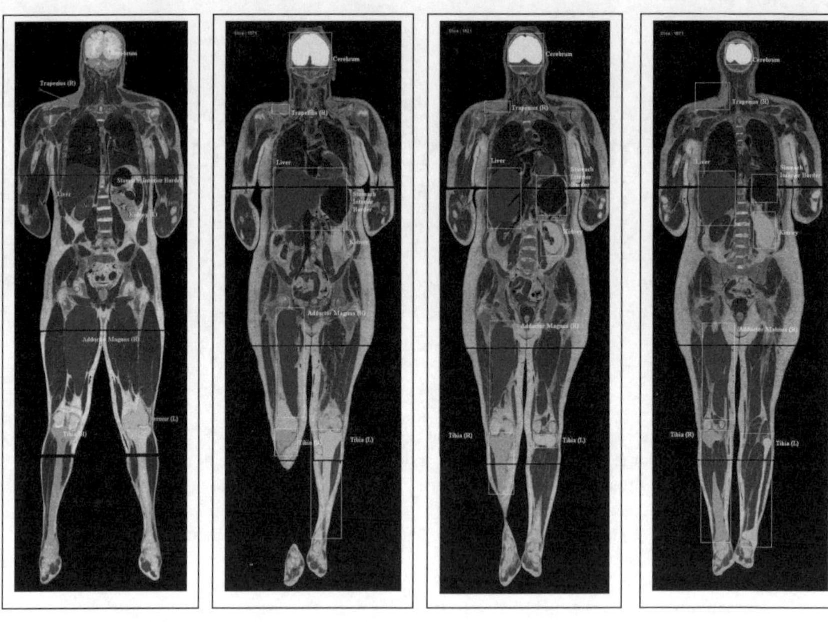

A. LR- VHM (637)   **B.** HR-VHF (571)   **C.** HR-VHF (621)   **D.** HR-VHF (671)

Figure 1. Segmented Coronal Visible Human Female Slices (637, 571, 621, and 671).

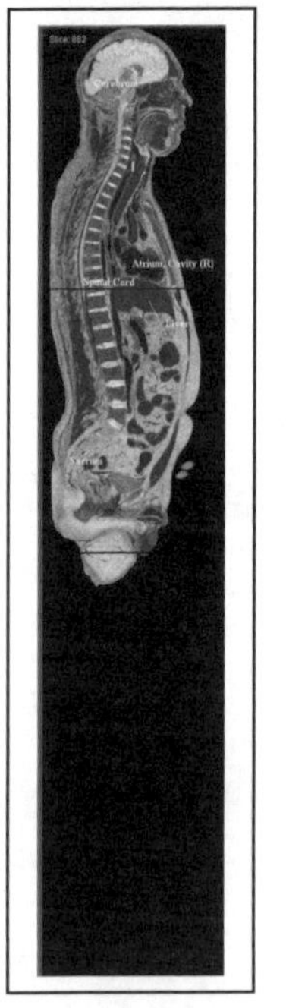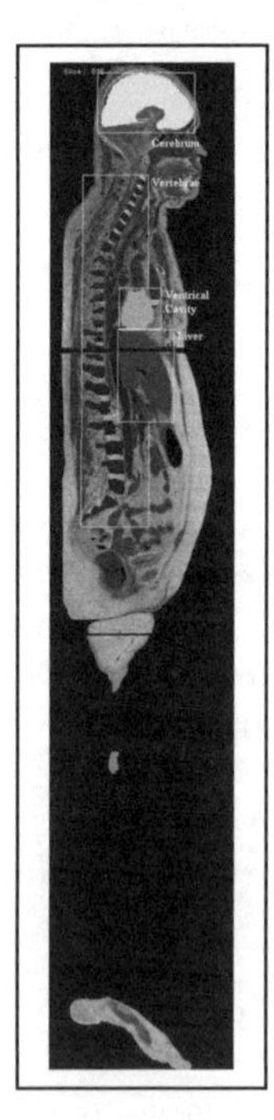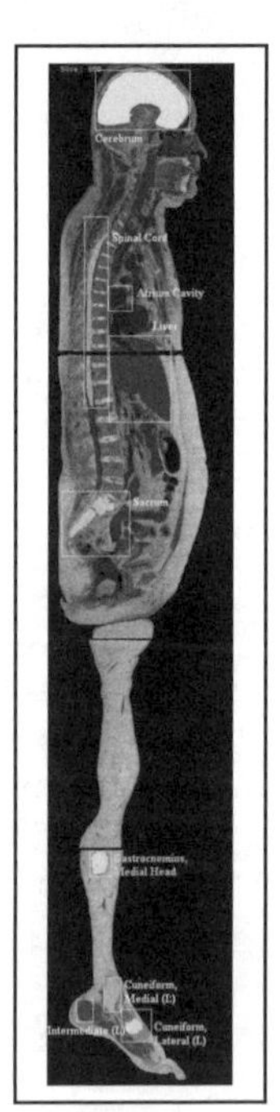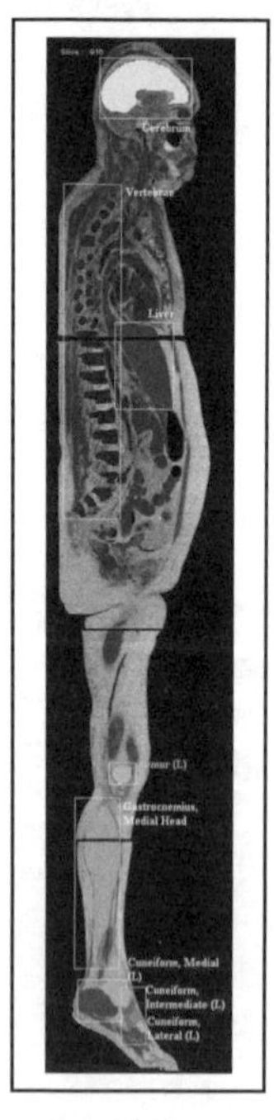

A. LR- VHM (882)   **B.** HR-VHF (816)   **C.** HR-VHF (866)   **D.** HR-VHF (916)

Figure 2. Segmented Sagittal Visible Human Female Slices (882, 816, 866, and 916).

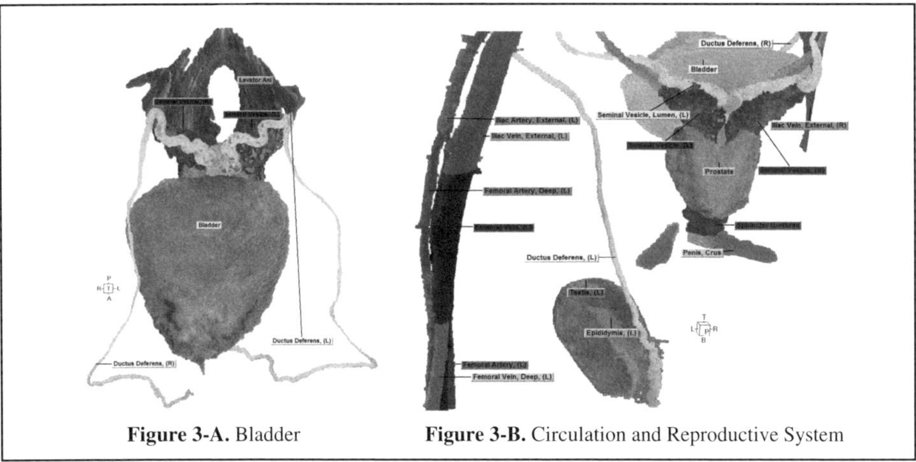

Figure 3-A. Bladder	**Figure 3-B.** Circulation and Reproductive System

Conclusions/Discussions

Figs.1-2, provide a visual verification of the high level of accuracy with which the SOI has been segmented from various regions of the VHF body. Segmented anatomical structures such as kidney, liver, spinal cord, vertebrae etc have been highlighted and labeled using the W3D-VBS. The segmented data produced by Segm-VHF is being integrated into the existing W3D-VBS and the segmented data already produced for the HR-VHM has been used to produce the 3D models. Our side-by-side segmentation approach, with additional assistance of digital atlas images, not only has proven effective in marking accurate shapes of anatomical structures but have helped to correct some of the existing segmentation errors. The automation of this process still remains to be implemented, as a number of algorithmic problems of segmentation, such as over or under segmenting, remain to be solved.

Acknowledgement

We fully acknowledge the contributions of Mr. Eric Acosta and Mr. Sreeram Vaidyanath, whose assistance was instrumental in completing this paper in a timely manner.

References

[1] Temkin B., Acosta E., et al. "Web-based Three-dimensional Virtual Body Structures: W3D-VBS." *Journal of the American Medical Informatics Association. Vol.9:5 (2002).*
[2] Temkin B., Acosta E., et al. "An Interactive Three-dimensional Virtual Body Structures System for Anatomical Training over the Internet." *Accepted for publication in the Journal of Clinical Anatomy.*
[3] Temkin B., Stephens B., et al, "Virtual Body Structures" *The Visible Human Conferences Proceedings, 2000.*
[4] Acosta, E., Temkin, B., "Build-and-Insert: Anatomical Structure Generation for Surgical Simulators," *International Symposium on Medical Simulation*, (ISMS), pp 230-239, 2004
[5] Vaidyanath S. and Temkin B. "Registration and Segmentation for the High Resolution Visible Human Male images" *Accepted for publication in Medicine Meets Virtual Reality 14, January 2006.*

Medicine Meets Virtual Reality 14
J.D. Westwood et al. (Eds.)
IOS Press, 2006

A Discrete Soft Tissue Model for Complex Anatomical Environment Simulations

Maud Marchal [a] [1], Emmanuel Promayon [a] and Jocelyne Troccaz [a]

[a] *TIMC-GMCAO Laboratory*
Grenoble, FRANCE

Abstract. Among the current challenges in human soft tissue modeling for medical purposes, the ability to model complex anatomical structures, their interactions and to accurately simulate them with physical realism are in the forefront of research. This paper describes a discrete soft tissue model which is geared toward solving these challenges. In this model, objects can be described as volumetric or surfacic sets of nodes depending on the level of precision required. Nodes have their own physical properties and a definition of their neighborhood. All these objects are submitted both to internal cohesive forces and to external attractive or interaction forces with other objects. Volume preservation is insured by a constraint. The model is applied to the simulation of the prostate and its surrounding organs.

Keywords. Discrete model, soft tissue modeling, prostate, complex anatomical environments

1. Introduction

Many algorithms have been proposed for interactively modeling deformable objects such as human soft tissues. However very few have attempted to simulate complex organ interactions. Among the existent soft tissue modeling methods, two main approaches are taken[1]: the biomechanical approach, an accurate but often considered as a slow method and the computational discrete approach, a relatively fast method which main drawbacks are unstability, bad physical realism and non-preservation of the volume. For both approaches, there are few examples of the integration of multiple dynamic interactions between soft organs and their environment. In this paper, a discrete soft tissue model is presented. Its originality is to integrate interactions between a given soft organ and the surrounding organs. After a brief description of the model, comparisons with other soft tissue modeling methods are proposed in order to validate the correctness and performances of our model.

2. Model Description

The proposed model is a volumetric evolution of a surfacic model developed in [2]. The components of the model are all derived from a main basis: a set of nodes. A model is described using the Physical Model Language (PML) [3]. Each node description contains a list of its neighbouring nodes and different properties depending on the type of component it belongs to (rigid to model skeleton, deformable to model soft tissues and active deformable to model muscles). Our approach allows to define objects not only with nodes on the surface but also with interior nodes. A new feature of the model allows the user to choose to model each component either with a surfacic description (for example a cavity like a bladder) or a volumetric description (a prostate for example). Components can then be easily stitched together: connections between nodes are defined directly in the neighborhood.

To generate displacements and deformations, forces are applied on the different parts of the model. Three kinds of forces can be used: force fields (e.g. gravitation force), locally applied forces (e.g. forces generated by the user or instruments) and local shape memory forces to model deformable properties. The latter are used to compute the elasticity property thanks to the introduction of a local shape memory on each node of the elastic component. Constraints are added to forces in order to model complex behaviours and to maintain some conditions like non-penetrating volume. Incompressibility is achieved through a constraint for surfacic and volumetric component by controlling the surface. To solve the system dynamics, the forces on each node are summed and the equations of motion are integrated taking into account constraints. Contrary to with classical mass-spring models, our model can insure strict volume preservation. It also presents a better stability, as shown in [2]. The next paragraph presents the first comparaisons of physical realism with other soft tissue modeling methods.

3. Validation

First, the model has been validated by comparing it with Finite Element Method (FEM) taken as a "gold standard" of soft tissue modeling. The Truth cube data [4] have been used as first validation of the physical realism of the model (see Figure 1). With these data, we have been able to compare real data with both our model and FEM. The results of the two approaches are very similar. Differences between real data and FEM in one side and our model in the other side are both less than 0.2 mm for 5% compression for example (mean real displacements of 2.64mm) (see [5] for more details).

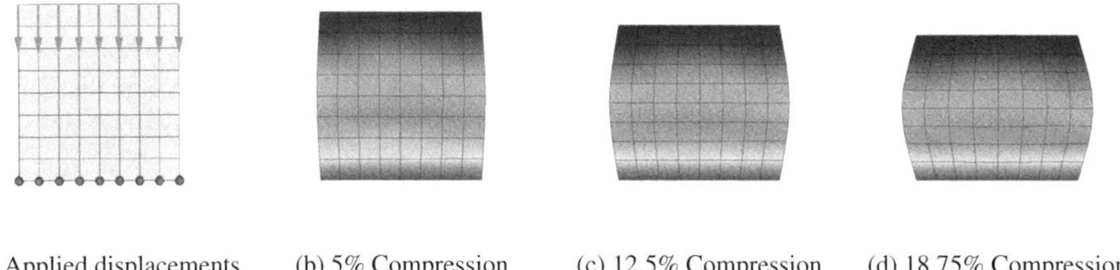

(a) Applied displacements   (b) 5% Compression   (c) 12.5% Compression   (d) 18.75% Compression

Figure 1. Truth cube Experiments: a compression is applied on the top nodes, bottom nodes are constrained to a null displacement

The second stage of the validation deals with the simulation of endorectal echographic probe influence on prostate shape in function of bladder filling (see Figure 2.a for prostate anatomy and your model). Organ shapes are simplified but proportional scales are respected. Prostate has a volumetric description while bladder is represented with surface nodes. Bladder and prostate are stitched together with a limited number of nodes and 12 top nodes of the bladder are fixed for each simulation. An imposed displacement is applied upward inside the rectum, resulting in a compression force that deforms the prostate. Prostate and bladder are both incompressible. Different bladder fillings have been experimented (see Figure 2.b). A mean prostate nodes displacement of respectively 4.52 mm, 4.40 mm and 4.37 mm has been observed for a bladder reference volume of V_0, 2.7 V_0 and 5 V_0 (imposed displacement by the probe was 5 mm). This predicts a linear damping of the prostate deformation relatively to bladder volume decrease.

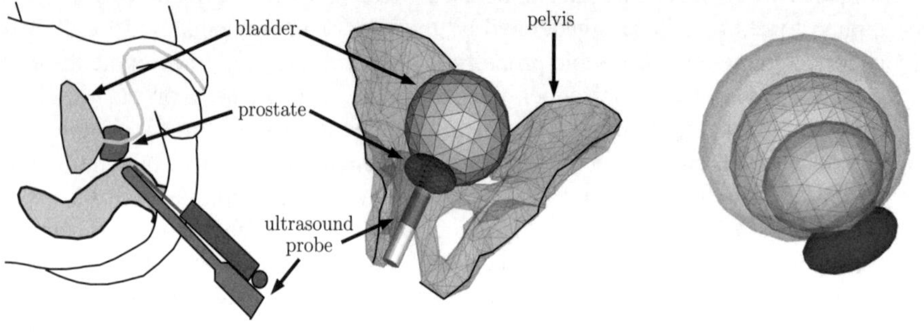

(a) Prostate anatomy during biopsy and our model   (c) Different bladder shapes

Figure 2. Model of the prostate and different bladder fillings

4. Discussion and Conclusion

In this paper, a new approach to soft tissue modeling well-suited to model interactions between organs has been proposed. The presented model allows to show that interacting organs can be simply defined. Our next work is to incorporate the interactions with instruments and to further validate the model with experimental data.

References

[1] Delingette, H.: Towards realistic Soft Tissue Modeling in Medical Simulation. IEEE Special Issue on Virtual and Augmented Reality in Medicine **86**(3) (1998) 512-523

[2] Promayon, E., Baconnier, P., Puech, C.: Physically-Based Model for Simulating the Human Trunk Respiration Movements. In: Proceedings of CVRMed II-MRCAS III (1997) 379-388

[3] Chabanas, M., Promayon, E.: Physical Model Language: Towards a Unified Representation for Continuous and Discrete Models. In: Proceedings of International Symposium on Medical Simulation (2004) 256-266

[4] Kerdok, A., Cotin, S., Ottensmeyer, M., Galea, A., Howe, R., Dawson, S.: Truthcube : Establising Physical Standards For Real Time Soft Tissue Simulation. Medical Image Analysis **7**(2003) 283-291

[5] Marchal, M., Promayon, E., Troccaz, J.: Simulating Complex Organ Interactions: Validation of a Soft Tissue Discrete Model. In: Proceedings of International Symposium on Visual Computing (2005) 175-182

Medicine Meets Virtual Reality 14
J.D. Westwood et al. (Eds.)
IOS Press, 2006

Image-Guided Laser Projection for Port Placement in Minimally Invasive Surgery

Jonathan MARMUREK[1,2], Chris WEDLAKE[2], Utsav PARDASANI[3],
Roy EAGLESON[1,3], and Terry PETERS[1,2,3]
[1]The University of Western Ontario, [2]Robarts Research Institute
[3]Canadian Surgical Technologies and Advanced Robotics (C-STAR)
London, Ontario, Canada

Abstract. We present an application of an augmented reality laser projection system in which procedure-specific optimal incision sites, computed from pre-operative image acquisition, are superimposed on a patient to guide port placement in minimally invasive surgery. Tests were conducted to evaluate the fidelity of computed and measured port configurations, and to validate the accuracy with which a surgical tool-tip can be placed at an identified virtual target. A high resolution volumetric image of a thorax phantom was acquired using helical computed tomography imaging. Oriented within the thorax, a phantom organ with marked targets was visualized in a virtual environment. A graphical interface enabled marking the locations of target anatomy, and calculation of a grid of potential port locations along the intercostal rib lines. Optimal configurations of port positions and tool orientations were determined by an objective measure reflecting image-based indices of surgical dexterity, hand-eye alignment, and collision detection. Intra-operative registration of the computed virtual model and the phantom anatomy was performed using an optical tracking system. Initial trials demonstrated that computed and projected port placement provided direct access to target anatomy with an accuracy of 2 mm.

Keywords. Image-guidance, minimally invasive surgery, augmented reality, tracking systems, validation

1. Introduction

Minimally invasive surgery (MIS), robotic or laparoscopic, is gaining popularity for use in a number of therapeutic procedures. Widespread practice of MIS, however, is limited by the lack of robust and flexible procedures for jointly planning and guiding optimal port placement. Additionally, accurate navigation of surgical end-effectors may enhance current endoscopic guidance techniques. Continuing advances in the quality of medical image acquisition, and developments in remote tracking systems, which can record motions of patients and surgical instruments, afford the opportunity to develop Image Guided Surgery (IGS) systems to assist surgeons. In MIS, systems which guide the surgeon based on patient image data have the potential to optimize the intervention by ensuring appropriate port positions and tool trajectories, in addition to providing real-time virtual navigation of surgical instruments.

Previous work in port placement has focused on the modeling of optimization algorithms to determine the best incision sites for a patient-specific case. Adhami et al. [1] define an optimization problem based on indices of tool dexterity, visibility, target reachability, and surgeon comfort, and have shown successful results on animal trials. Specifically tuned for a Coronary Artery Bypass Graft (CABG) procedure, the optimization problem is refined by Selha et al. [2] such that port configurations attempt to match experimentally determined preset conditions. In addition, virtual environments have been developed [3,4] to display port configurations for robotic cardiac surgery.

Augmented reality (AR) systems designed to superimpose pre-operative planning information on top of the view of the surgical site have been developed to directly assist surgeons in addition to a virtual simulation. Glossop et al. [5] designed and tested an AR laser projection system which displayed pre-computed beam patterns for a simulated cranioanatomy, and Sugano et al. [6] have also used lasers in surgery to guide hip arthroplasty. To our knowledge, however, AR systems have not yet been reported for facilitating port placement.

This paper presents a novel application of augmented reality laser projection for port placement in minimally invasive surgery. Pre-operative image data are used to compute optimal incision sites and tool orientations. We validate the accuracy of the proposed guidance system by comparing simulated and measured port placement trials on a phantom model.

2. Materials and Methods

2.1. Image Acquisition and Visualization

A high-resolution pre-operative volume of a thorax phantom was acquired with helical computed tomography imaging (slice thickness = 1.25 mm, pitch = 1.75, speed = 3.75 mm/rotation, field of view = 40 cm, kVp = 140 and mA = 160, imaging time = 54 sec, resolution = 512 x 512) on a GE Lightspeed Scanner. The thorax phantom volume was visualized using an application based on Visualization ToolKit (VTK). Intensity CT data was examined using an interactive tri-planar display, allowing localization and thresholding of anatomy of interest. The ribs surface was segmented using the marching cubes algorithm.

A foam sphere marked with colored pins indicating assumed positions of target vasculature was used as a phantom organ in an example of a CABG procedure. The test organ was simulated in VTK, and was oriented within the intra-thoracic cavity of the ribs. The computed virtual scene of the thorax phantom and test organ with marked targets was used as a patient-specific model on which to plan the surgical intervention.

2.2. Pre-Operative Optimal Planning

We simulated a generic intra-thoracic MIS procedure in which two surgical tools are used in addition to one endoscope. The port placement objective is to triangulate the

3D virtual coordinates for the three incision sites, in addition to computing and visualizing the required tool orientation for target access. Optimal port placement configurations, specified by port position (x,y,z) and tool orientation (roll, pitch, yaw) for each instrument, were to facilitate and ensure repeatable collision-free access to multiple targets with satisfactory visibility, tool dexterity, and surgeon comfort.

Prior to optimization, a graphical interface was used to allow the user to navigate through 3D surfaces of the patient model, and to select target locations. Next, a grid of potential port locations along the intercostal rib lines was defined (by manually selecting points through the volume). The stored sets of targets and potential ports, along with the virtual geometric descriptions of the patient anatomy were then subject to seeking an optimal port configuration.

The port-placement planning algorithm defined by Adhami et al. [3] was implemented in MATLAB, and was updated to use procedure-dependent preset optimal configurations, as shown by Selha et al. [2]. A discrete optimization problem was posed, to rank all potential configurations of one endoscope and two tools.

For each port configuration, the following geometric parameters were computed: port-to-port distances, port-to-target distances, tool-to-target normal angles, and tool-to-skin normal angles. Configurations were marked as '*admissable*' if the computed parameters lay within the following constraints, respectively: minimum port separation, to avoid placement redundancies, maximum tool shaft length, maximum attack angles to reflecting surgical requirements and tool tip dexterity, and maximum entrance angles to ensure tolerable pressure against the ribs). Port admissibility was also constrained by a collision detection routine which ensures that each tool can reach all targets without obstruction.

Finally, an objective measure was computed for each '*admissible*' port configuration, based on a summation the of least-squares difference between simulated attack angles and optimal preset values (determined experimentally) for all arrangements of surgical tools and target sites. Objective measures for each port configuration were ranked to indicate optimal port positions and tool orientations.

2.3. Intra-Operative Guidance: Registration, Tracking, and Projection

The virtual coordinates of four easily identifiable landmarks on the thorax phantom were recorded. The Polaris optical tracking system (NDI, Toronto, Canada), capable of measuring position and orientation data, was used to measure corresponding positions of physical landmarks by reading the tip position of an active IR-emitting pointer (Traxtal, Toronto, Canada) at each landmark. The spatial transformation mapping the virtual environment to the Polaris (real-world) coordinates was computed by a paired-point registration.

Coordinates of optimal port configurations were transformed to Polaris space, and were displayed on the thorax phantom using the XarTrax (Traxtal) laser positioning system (*Figure 1*). A visible and an infrared laser were displayed by steering two galvanometrically controlled perpendicular mirrors. Laser positions were controlled by specifying angles of rotation for each mirror, using a built-in Application Programming Interface (API), common to both the Polaris and XarTrax control units.

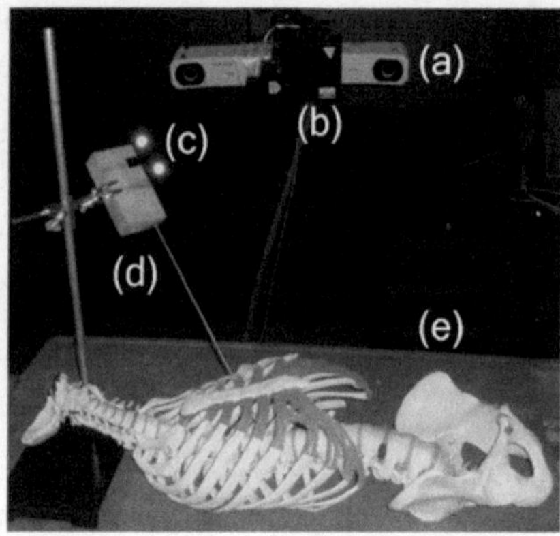

Figure 1 – Experimental setup for port placement and end-effector positioning: (a) Polaris tracking system; (b) XarTrax laser projector; (c) tracking tool; (d) in-lab robotic tool; (e) thorax phantom.

2.4. Experiments

Accuracy validation trials were performed for: 1) port-placement configurations (port-position and tool orientation); and 2) end-effector tracking.

Computed and registered port positions and tool orientations were recorded for each of the five highest-ranked optimal port configurations. For each simulated port position, the location of the corresponding laser projected port (*Figure 2*) was measured by an active IR-emitting pointer with the Polaris optical tracking system. Next, an operating tool was registered to the virtual model and was aligned with computed port configurations. Tool orientations for each simulated port-placement trial were measured with a passive tracking tool attached to the surgical instrument.

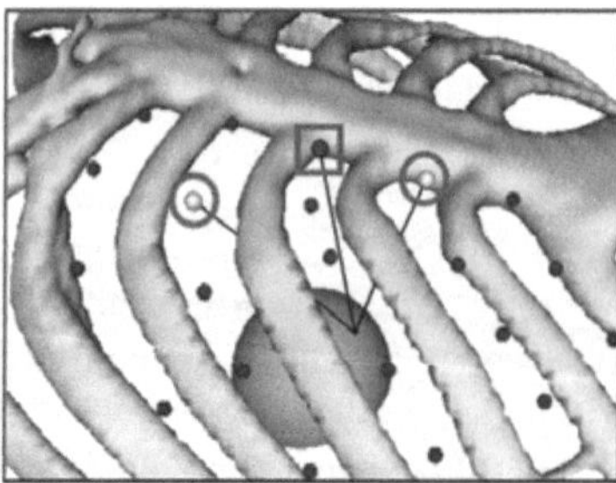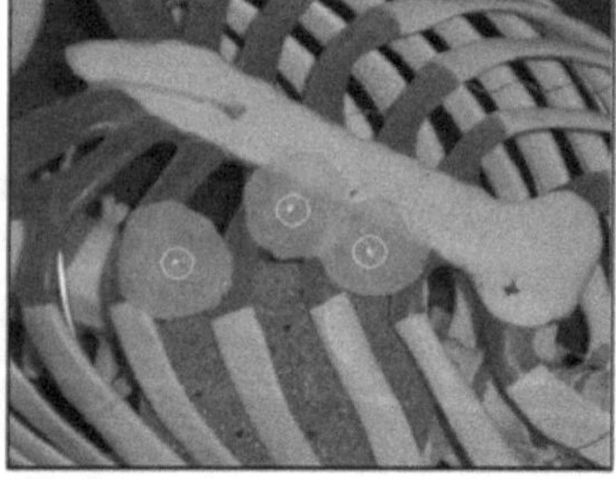

Figure 2 – *Left*: Simulated port configuration showing three highlighted ports which indicate computed optimal port positions for surgical instruments (circles) and an endoscope (square). Computed tool orientation is shown by a line connecting the port and the target. *Right*: Laser projection augmented reality guidance for port placement (outlined bright spot indicates projected incision sites).

Fifteen arbitrary targets were then chosen in the simulated virtual space. The end-effector tool-tip of a registered surgical instrument was placed directly on each of the known physical targets, and simulated tip positions were recorded to measure targeting error.

3. Results

The computed and measured port positions were in agreement with high correlation coefficients in each direction: $R = 0.998$ in x, $R = 0.999$ in y, and $R = 0.992$ in z ($p < 0.001$).   Similarly, measured tool orientations were in agreement with the virtual simulation: $R = 0.994$ for roll, $R = 0.999$ for pitch, and $R = 0.978$ for yaw ($p < 0.001$). Mean error and standard deviations are summarized in *Table 1* for port positions in each direction, and for the three degrees of tool orientation.   Total error for port positions was computed by adding each orthogonal error component in quadrature (calculating Euclidean distance), while total error for tool orientation was computed as the angle between optimal and measured orientation.

Table 1 – Error summary from port placement validations trials

	Port Position Error (mm)				Tool Orientation Error (degrees)			
	x	y	z	Total	roll	pitch	yaw	Total
Mean	1.2	0.6	5.4	5.8	4.3	1.3	6.0	6.4
Std.	0.7	0.4	4.2	3.9	3.1	0.8	5.2	4.9

Port placement results showed lowest accuracy and precision in the z-direction, and about the z-axis (yaw). This anisotropic error was due to the fall-off in tracking and projection precision as the distance increases from the Polaris-XarTrax unit. A single valued t-test was used to determine overall accuracy. The system could provide accurate in-plane port position laser guidance within 1.7 mm and accurate tool orientation within 2.2 degrees ($t_{14} = 1.77, p < 0.05$).

Accuracy of end-effector tool-tip navigation is profiled in *Figure 3* by an ellipsoid indicating the 95 % confidence upper limit in which a tool-tip could be positioned, and by projections showing the bounding error in each plane. Mean error (Euclidean

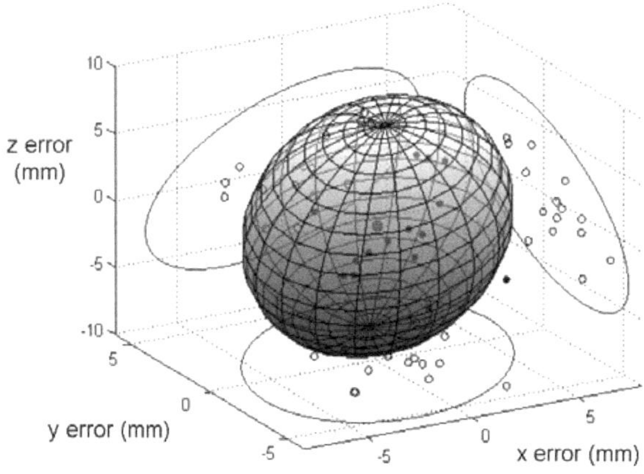

Figure 3 - Confidence ellipsoid for end-effector targeting. Points inside the ellipsoid indicate deviation from target normalized to the origin over fifteen trials. The ellipsoid shown represents the 95 % confidence boundary in which an end-effector tip can be guided ($p < 0.05$).

distance from the tool tip to the target) and standard deviation for the 15 targeting experiments in x, y, and z directions were 1.9 ± 1.4 mm, 1.5 ± 1.0 mm, and 2.5 ± 1.5 mm respectively.

4. Discussion

Intra-operative guidance of optimal port placement in minimally invasive surgery was achieved by superimposing laser projections of incision sites directly onto a test patient. A virtual simulation created from 3D pre-operative image data was used to plan the procedure, and to visualize port positions and tool orientations. Validation tests for port placement and subsequent end-effector navigation showed guidance with accuracy of 2 mm. These encouraging results warrant further developments and improvements on the current implementation. Automation of potential port selection using a centre-line detection algorithm will save planning time by reducing the amount of user input. Additionally, an extensive database defining procedure-dependant preset optimal configurations will be developed through simulated surgical trails.

Clinical use of the proposed procedure will require further validation on case specific models. Opportunity to test the device on porcine subjects will afford assurance that the planning and guidance is sufficiently robust to be used in conjunction with robotic, laparoscopic and telesurgical interventions on humans.

Acknowledgements

We wish to thank Edward Huang from the Robarts Research Institute for providing the CT scan used in this study, in conjunction with the London Health Sciences Centre. Funding for the project was made available by Ontario Research Development Challenge Fund (ORDCF).

References

[1] Adhami, L., and Coste-Maniere, E.: Optimal planning for minimally invasive surgical robots. IEEE Trans. on Robotics and Automation (2003) October Vol 19, no. 5: 854-862.

[2] Selha, S., Dupont, P., Howe, R., and Torchiana, D.: Dexterity optimization by port placement in robot-assisted minimally invasive surgery," 2001 *SPIE International* Symposium on Intelligent Systems and Advanced Manufacturing, Newton, MA, 28-31 October (2001).

[3] Traub, J., Feuerstein, M., Bauer, M., Schirmbeck, E.U., Najafi, H., Bauernschmitt, R., and Klinker, G.: Augmented reality for port placement and navigation in robotically assistive minimally invasive cardiovascular surgery. International Congress Series (2004) 1268: 735-740.

[4] Chiu, A.M., Dey, D., Drangova, M., Boyd, W.D., and Peters, T.M.: 3-D Image Guidance for Minimally Invasive Coronary Artery Bypass. Heart Surgery Forum. (2001) [Online]. Available: http://www.hs-forum.com/vol3/issue3/2000-9732.html

[5] Glossop, N., Wedlake, C., Moore, J., Peters, T.M., and Wang, Z.: Laser Projection Augmented Reality System for Computer Assisted Surgery. MICCAI (2003) 1-8.

[6] Sugano, N., Sasama, T., Nishihara, S., Nakase, S., Nishii, T., Miki, H., Momoi, Y., Yoshinobu, S., Nakajima, Y., Tamura, S., Yonenobu, K., and Ochi, T.: Clinical applications of a laser guidance system with dual laser beam rays as augmented reality of surgical navigation, in: Lemke, H.U. et al. (Eds.). Proc. 16th Int. Congress and Exhibition on Computer Assisted Radiology and Surgery (CARS), Springer (2002): 281.

Medicine Meets Virtual Reality 14
J.D. Westwood et al. (Eds.)
IOS Press, 2006

Planning and Analyzing Robotized TMS Using Virtual Reality

Lars Matthäus [a,1], Alf Giese [b], Daniel Wertheimer [c], and Achim Schweikard [a]

[a] *Institute for Robotics and Cognitive Systems, University of Lübeck, Germany*
[b] *Clinic for Neurosurgery, University of Lübeck, Germany*
[c] *Clinic for Neurosurgery, University Hospital Hamburg-Eppendorf, Germany*

Abstract. Transcranial Magnetic Stimulation (TMS) is a powerful method to examine the brain and non-invasively treat disorders of the central nervous system. Magnetic stimulation of the motor cortex results in the activation of corresponding muscle groups. Hereby, accurate placement of the TMS coil to the patient's head is crucial to successful stimulation. We developed a way to position the TMS coil using a robot and navigate it in virtual reality based on an online registration of the cranium relative to 3D magnetic resonance imaging data. By tracking the head and robotic motion compensation, fixation of the patient's head becomes obsolete. Furthermore, a novel method for motor cortex mapping is presented. The robotized TMS system is used to obtain the characteristic field of a TMS coil. This field is registered to the field of motor evoked potential measurements at the patient's head to yield a prediction of the motoric center of a target muscle.

Keywords. robotized navigated transcranial magnetic stimulation, human brain mapping, hybrid landmark - surface matching registration, robotic motion compensation, characteristic field of a TMS coil

1. Introduction

Transcranial Magnetic Stimulation is a powerful method to examine the brain and treat disorders of the central nervous system non-invasively [1]. TMS works by generating a strong magnetic field in a very short time and thus inducing a current in adjacent nerves. The generated activation depends on the strength of the magnetic field gradient. Modern TMS coils produce very dense and defined fields, which means that small shifts or turns of the coil lead to substantial changes of the magnetic field gradient delivered to a nerve and thus to strong variation in the activation of the target nerves. This explains the urgent need for technologies supporting a precise navigation and position of TMS coils.

Until now work on navigated TMS application relies on tracking the patient's head and the coil, either with optical tracking systems or by joint sensors in mechanical arms carrying the coil, [2]. By registering 3D image data (MRI, fMRI) with the patient's head and by tracking the coil, the site of stimulation can be displayed with respect to the image data, [3]. This method has one major disadvantage: The site of stimulation can be

---

[1] Correspondence to: Lars Matthäus, Institute for Robotics and Cognitive Systems, University of Lübeck, 23538 Lübeck, Germany. Tel.: +49 451 500 5205; Fax: +49 451 500 5202; E-mail: matthaeus@rob.uni-luebeck.de.

determined easily, but exact stimulation at a pre-defined point is hard to achieve. Either head movements must be followed by manually adjusting the coil continuously or the head must be fixed. This results in a loss of accuracy or problems with respect to safety, patient comfort, and durability of the fixation.

Our approach of tracking the head and compensate for its movements by positioning the coil with a robot overcomes these disadvantages. A robot can position and orient the coil much more accurately than a human operator. Furthermore, a robot allows for realtime motion compensation, [4]. Thus, a fixation of the head becomes obsolete. The first part of the article describes the setup of our robotized TMS system and explains the steps necessary for a successful application.

The second part of the paper describes a novel approach to brain mapping using TMS. Navigated TMS systems for motor cortex mapping have already been reported from [5], [6], and [7], but none uses the field information obtained from the coil. In our approach we map the characteristic field of a TMS coil and register this field to the field of MEP measurements obtained from stimulation. The position of the sensor for mapping the field of the coil is then used as a prediction of the responsive site in the cortex.

2. Robotized TMS Application

The system for robotic navigated TMS application is based on the following steps: (1) Creating a virtual reality model of the head, (2) Registering the virtual world with the real world, (3) Planning the stimulation in VR, (4) Moving the robot correspondingly, and (5) evaluating the response to stimulation. The following sections describe each step in detail.

2.1. Creation a virtual reality model

In this first step a virtual reality model of the head is created. First, a 3D MRI dataset of the patient's head is obtained using a standard 1.5 T MR scanner. Second, the open source software VTK [8] is used to segment the cranium surface from the 3D MRI data and visualize the data. The resulting VR model can be seen in Figure 1.

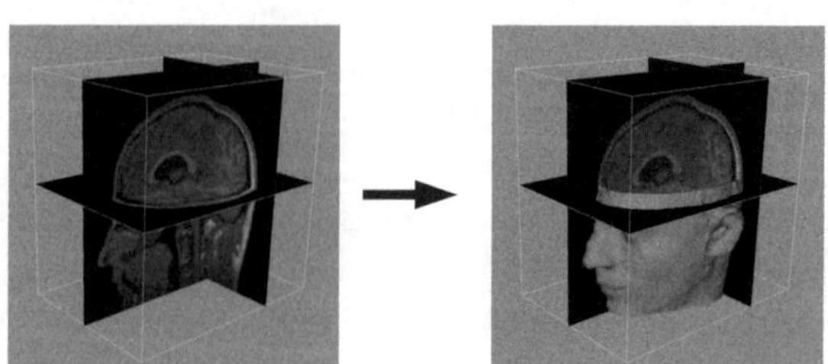

Figure 1. Step 1 - Reconstructing the cranium's surface from 3D MRI data.

2.2. Registration

In a second step the virtual head model is registered to the real head. This is done by a combined landmark and surface matching method. We use the POLARIS optical tracking system (NDI, Ontario, Canada) to acquire three landmark points on the head, e.g. the left and right lateral orbital rim and the tip of the nose, and several hundred surface points. The surface points are taken continuously when moving a pointer over the head's surface, so that the whole process takes less than three minutes. The user marks the landmarks on the virtual cranium surface. Then a coarse registration via point-to-point correspondence is performed. The exact registration is obtained by using the results of the landmark step as start value for an iterative closest point scheme. The process of registering the virtual head to the real head is visualized in Figure 2.

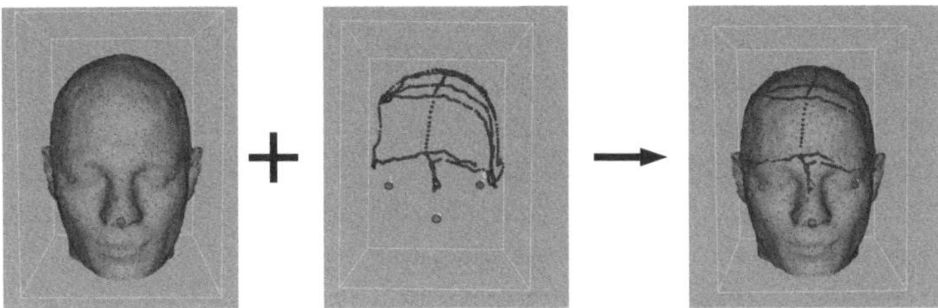

Figure 2. Step 2 - Registering the virtual head to the real head using landmarks and surface points. Left: Surface points and landmarks from the real head. Middle: Virtual head model. Right: VR model registered to the real head.

The registration step already allows for a moving head, i.e. there is no need for a fixation of the head during the acquisition of the landmark and surface points. Before the registration starts, a headband with POLARIS markers is attached to the patient's head. Subsequently, all acquired points are related to the coordinate system defined by those markers, see Figure 3. The patient wears the headband during the whole treatment.

2.3. Coil Calibration

When mounting the Medtronic MC125 TMS coil to the KUKA KR3 robot, a transformation from the robot coordinate system to the coil coordinate system must be determined. For that purpose we developed a calibration tool with POLARIS markers. The calibration tool position and the robot position are measured using the POLARIS system and the robot sensors respectively, see Figure 4. Thus the transformation from the robot coordinate system to the coil coordinate system can be calculated.

2.4. Planning and Delivering the Stimulation

The registration and the head tracking establish a realtime link between the virtual reality and the robot work space. The robot is now used to position the TMS coil after planning in VR. Therefore the user picks a target point on the virtual cranium and chooses the desired distance of the coil from the head and the desired coil rotation, see Figure 5. The virtual coordinates are then transformed into world coordinates taking into account the actual head position.

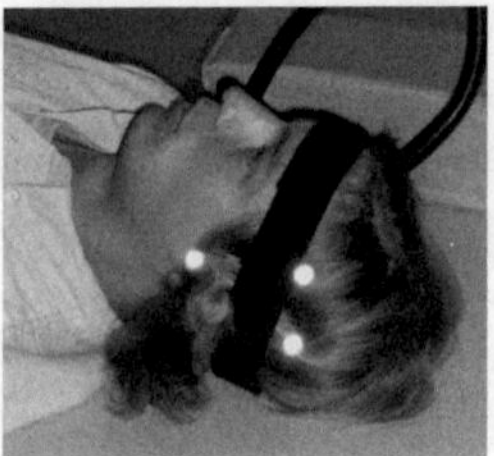

Figure 3. Tracking the head by attaching a head-band with POLARIS markers to it. All points acquired during registration are referenced to the headband coordinate system.

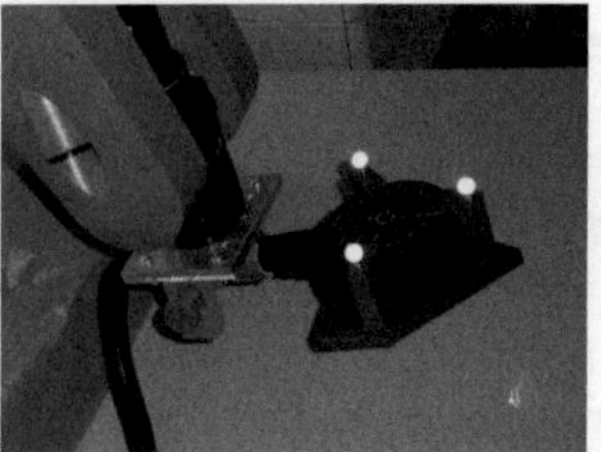

Figure 4. Calibrating the robot mounted TMS coil using POLARIS and KUKA position information. The calibration tool will be removed during treatment.

The robot now moves the coil to the target position. It must be ensured that the trajectory of the robot and the coil are valid, i.e. the transition from one stimulation point to the next must not interfere with the patient's head. Therefore, a module for trajectory planning is included in our system. In short, the coil is moved away from the head, then along an arc around the head over the target region and then towards the head again, see Figure 6.

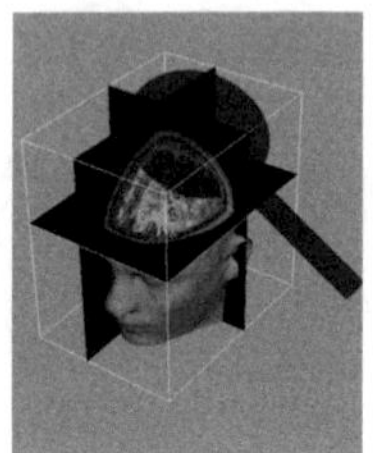

Figure 5. Step 3 - Positioning the TMS-coil at the virtual head.

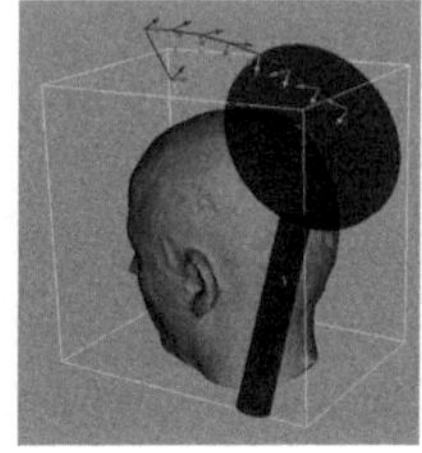

Figure 6. Step 4 - Coil trajectory from one stimulation point to the next.

2.5. Data Handling

All defined target positions are stored relative to the DICOM defined coordinate system in a file. If a TMS session is to be repeated or extended at a later time, the old coil positions relative to the head can be recalled and re-approached by the robot. This is especially useful during a repeated therapy over several days as in the treatment of depressions. Note that by storing the stimulation points relative to the virtual head there is no need for attaching the headband always in the same position.

Furthermore, the physician can assign response values to the stimulation positions. Such values can be measured muscle responses like motor evoked potentials (MEPs) or subjective evaluations from the patients like relief from pain or strength of visual impressions induced by TMS.

3. Brain Mapping

The presented robotized navigated TMS system allows to stimulate and test a large number of target points around the vertex with high precision. It is an open question how to translate the results into exact maps of the cortical function at the brain surface. Several procedures have been described: projecting the stimulation point with the strongest response to the brain surface [7], calculating the center of gravity for all measurements [9], or simulating the propagation of the induced electric field from firing the TMS coil [10]. No algorithm so far uses real field information for the specific TMS coil. We suggest a novel method which incorporates field measurements from the coil obtained in a separate experiment.

3.1. Measuring the Characteristic Field of a TMS Coil

The TMS coil is mounted to the robot as described above. A small wire loop of one centimeter diameter is used as a simple sensor for the local magnet field gradient. By connecting the loop to an oscilloscope and measuring the maximum induced voltage when firing the TMS coil, we obtain a voltage directly proportional to the magnetic field gradient at the sensor[1]. The robot moves the coil over the sensor along a cubic grid. Firing the coil at the vertices of the grid, a total of 20 x 20 x 10 measurements are obtained. The results are displayed in Figure 7, left. It is important that the position of the sensor relative to the grid is known, from measuring it with the POLARIS system.

3.2. Registering the Characteristic Field of the TMS Coil to the Field of MEPs

The MEP field is obtained as follows: The coil is set to different target points around the head, fired, and the measured motor evoked potential at a target muscle is assigned as scalar field value to the coil position. An (artificial) example can be seen in Figure 7, middle. We conjecture that the characteristic field of the TMS coil is in a way similar to the field of motor evoked potentials measured at the head.

Now if both fields are indeed similar, the fields can be registered. We use objective functions from multimodal image registration to define the correct registration. First tests show that Correlation Ratio [11] is much more suited for our application than the better known Mutual Information [12], because it is easier to optimize numerically.

Having registered both fields, the known position of the sensor for obtaining the coil field is taken as prediction for the motoric center for a target muscle, see Figure 7, right.

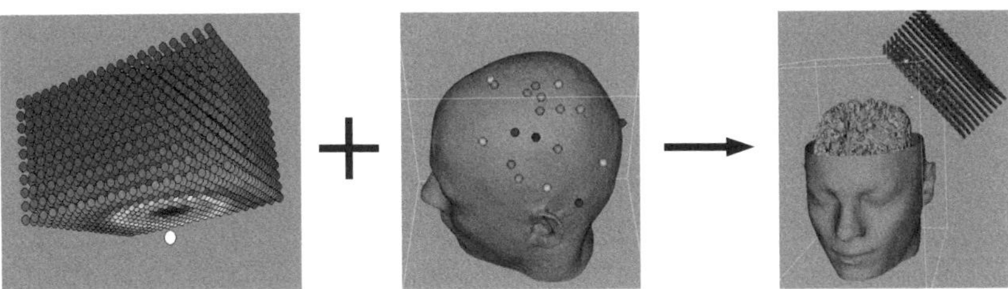

Figure 7. Brain mapping: Registering the coil field (left) to the field of MEPs (middle). The sensor for the coil field (white dot, left picture) predicts the responsive site in the brain (right).

---

[1]Note the physical Law of Induction: $U = \mathbf{A} \cdot \dot{\mathbf{B}}$ for the induced voltage U, the area vector $\mathbf{A}$ of the single wire loop, and the magnetic field gradient $\dot{\mathbf{B}}$.

4. Discussion

We presented a robotized navigated TMS application system, which allows for planning in virtual reality, motion compensation, and repeated stimulation at defined points. First results show that this system provides a save, reliable, and exact way for delivering transcranial magnetic stimulation. The use of the robot prepares the ground for a novel way of mapping the motoric cortex by directly measuring the characteristic field of the TMS coil and registering this field to the field of motor evoked potentials. The evaluation of the correlation of this mapping with other functional mapping methods like functional Magnetic Resonance Imaging (fMRI), Positron Emission Tomography (PET) or direct electrical stimulation will be performed in the near future.

References

[1] A. Pascual-Leone, N.J. Davey, J. Rothwell, E.M. Wassermann, and B.K. Puri. *Handbook of Transcranial Magnetic Stimulation*. Arnold, 2002.

[2] U. Herwig, C. Schönfeldt-Lecuona, A.P. Wunderlich, C. v. Tiesenhausen, A. Thielscher, H. Walter, and M. Spitzer. The navigation of transcranial magnetic stimulation. *Psychiatry Research: Neuroimaging Section*, 108:123–131, 2001.

[3] G.J. Ettinger, W.E.L. Grimson, M.E. Leventon, R. Kikinis, V. Gugino, W. Cote, M. Karapelou, L. Aglio, M. Shenton, G. Potts, and A. Eben. Non-invasive functional brain mapping using registered transcranial magnetic stimulation, 1996.

[4] A. Schweikard, G. Glosser, M. Bodduluri, and J.R. Adler. Robotic motion compensation for respiratory motion during radiosurgery. *Journal of Computer-Aided Surgery*, 5(4):263 – 277, September 2000.

[5] G.J. Ettinger, M.E. Leventon, W.E.L. Grimson, R. Kikinis, L. Gugino, W. Cote, L. Sprung, L. Agilo, M.E. Shenton, G. Potts, V.L. Hernandez, and A. Eben. Experimentation with a transcranial magnetic stimulation system for functional brain mapping. *Medical Image Analysis*, 2(2):133–142, 1998.

[6] E. Fernandez, A. Alfaro, J.M. Tormos, R. Climent, M. Martinez, H. Vilanova, V. Walsh, and A. Pascual-Leone. Mapping of the human visual cortex using image-guided transcranial magnetic stimulation. *Brain research. Brain research protocols*, 10(2):115–124, October 2002.

[7] T. Krings, K.H. Chiappa, H. Foltys, M.H.T. Reinges, G.R. Cosgrove, and A. Thron. Introducing navigated transcranial magnetic stimulation as a refined brain mapping methodology. *Neurosurg Rev*, 24:171–179, 2001.

[8] W. Shroeder, K. Martin, and B. Lorensen. *The Visualization Toolkit An Object-Oriented Approach To 3D Graphics*. Kitware, 3rd edition edition, 2004.

[9] B. Boroojerdi, H. Foltys, T. Krings, U. Spetzger, A. Thron, and R. Töpper. Localization of the motor hand area using transcranial magnetic stimulation and functional magnetic resonace imaging. *Clinical Neurophysiology*, 110:699–704, 1999.

[10] A. Thielscher and T. Kammer. Linking physics with physiology in TMS: A sphere field model to determine the cortical stimulation site in TMS. *NeuroImage*, 17(3):1117–1130, 2002.

[11] A. Roche, G. Malandain, X. Pennec, and N. Ayache. The correlation ratio as a new similarity measure for multimodal image registration. *Lecture Notes In Computer Science, Proceedings MICCAI*, 1496:1115 – 1124, 1998.

[12] W. Wells, P. Viola, H. Atsumi, S. Nakajima, and R. Kikinis. Multi-modal volume registration by maximization of mutual information. *Medical Image Analysis*, 1(1):35–51, 1996.

Medicine Meets Virtual Reality 14
J.D. Westwood et al. (Eds.)
IOS Press, 2006

Medical Student Evaluation Using Augmented Standardized Patients: Preliminary Results

Frederic D. McKENZIE [a]   Thomas W. HUBBARD [b]   John A. ULLIAN [b]
Hector M. GARCIA [a]   Reynel J. Castelino [a]   Gayle A. Gliva [b]
[a] *Old Dominion University*
[b] *Eastern Virginia Medical School*

Abstract. Standardized patients (SPs), individuals trained to realistically portray patients, are commonly used to teach and assess medical students. The range of clinical problems an SP can portray, however, is limited. They are typically healthy individuals with few or no abnormal physical findings. We have developed a functioning prototype that uses sound-based augmented reality to expand the capabilities of an SP to exhibit physically-manifested abnormalities. The primary purpose of this paper is to describe this prototype and report on its use in a study using medical students evaluated in a required annual Observed Structured Clinical Examination (OSCE). Presented is an overview of the prototype, a detailed description of the study, final results from the study, and conclusions drawn about the validity of using augmented SPs as a reliable medical assessment tool.

Keywords: Virtual reality, augmented reality, standardized patients, medical assessment, OSCE

Introduction

To become clinically competent physicians, medical students must develop knowledge and skills in many areas of both the art and science of medicine. Three areas are emphasized in medical students' early clinical training: doctor-patient communication, performing the physical exam involving auscultation, and clinical diagnostic reasoning about patient pathology. Standardized patients (SPs), individuals trained to realistically portray patients, are commonly used to teach and assess medical students in those three areas.

1. Background/Problem

Extensive research on the use of SPs shows this approach to be a reliable and valid teaching and assessment technique [4], with psychometric qualities sufficient for high-stakes professional examinations. The National Board of Medical Examiners and the National Board of Osteopathic Medical Examiners will each require an SP-based exam for licensure of physicians in the U.S. beginning with the class graduating in 2005, as the Medical Council of Canada has done for several years. Additionally, the Education Commission on Foreign Medical Graduates requires graduates of foreign medical schools to pass SP-based exams prior to entering North American medical residency programs.

Actually, SPs have been used as a teaching and evaluation technique in medical education for about 40 years [1] [2], and are used at all levels of medical training [3] [4]. They are also widely used in the other health professions. Their flexibility and adaptability allow SPs to change appearance, provide verbal nuances and non-verbal cues to their communication, and in other ways exhibit the wide range of interpersonal interactions found in real patients. Their realistic presentation of clinical problems has been a major factor in acceptance by medical educators, and allows learners to practice and receive feedback on their clinical skills in a safe context.

The range of clinical problems an SP can portray, however, is limited. They are typically healthy individuals with few or no abnormal physical findings. Augmented reality (AR) can be used to expand the capabilities of an SP to exhibit physically-manifested abnormalities. Augmenting SPs with the ability to simulate abnormal physical findings would expand the opportunities for students to learn more clinical skills, e.g., by finding abnormalities on a physical exam, in a realistic setting with a real person (SP) while practicing their doctor-patient communication skills.

We have developed a functioning prototype of the technology for this augmentation. The prototype allows the listener to hear pre-recorded heart and lung sounds when auscultating the human body. The primary purpose of this paper is to describe this prototype and report on its use in a study using medical students evaluated in a required annual Observed Structured Clinical Examination (OSCE). Using lessons learned from this study, we will test the improved system with students in future required OSCE examinations using an expanded suite of abnormalities. At this future point, we will answer questions relating to the realism as perceived by an experienced clinician of using augmented SPs (ASPs) as a reliable assessment tool.

2. Tools and Methods

Auscultation involves listening for sounds produced by the body at various locations. The primary auscultation tool is the stethoscope. As one might imagine, The SP actor can not normally present abnormal conditions via this ubiquitous medical instrument. During auscultation, the head of the stethoscope placed against the patient's skin and typically has both a diaphragm for detecting high-pitched sounds and a bell for hearing lower-pitched sounds. An examiner listens not only for presence of sound but also its characteristics: intensity, pitch, duration, and quality. Analysis of these qualities leads to an assessment of normal findings or abnormalities suggestive of a pathologic process.

To reproduce sounds that a medical student would hear at various anatomical landmarks probed during auscultation, initial steps were to record normal heart and lung sounds that the system would play when a stethoscope head was touched to any of the 28 "hot zones"[5] on a human (the SP's) torso. Using these anatomical landmarks, 3D hot zones were identified and adjusted for any body morphology using five calibration points.

We adapted an electronic stethoscope so that the examiner hears through the stethoscope earpieces the recorded sound when the stethoscope head (listening piece) is placed against the skin in one of the hot zones. The stethoscope includes a magnetic sensor and a contact switch attached to its head. Figure 1 shows an early prototype [5] of the system. A mannequin is shown for the human SP. In this early prototype we used a plastic stethoscope that has now been replaced with an electronic one. Essentially, the system operates as follows. The medical student would use the stethoscope (3) to place against the ASP and perform auscultation. As the student places the stethoscope head, its position is tracked via (5) using the movement of the attached sensor. When the system software running on the PC (6) detects that the sensor / stethoscope head is placed within an appropriate location, the software triggers the corresponding sound file which plays into the headphones (7), now electronic stethoscope, which the student is wearing.

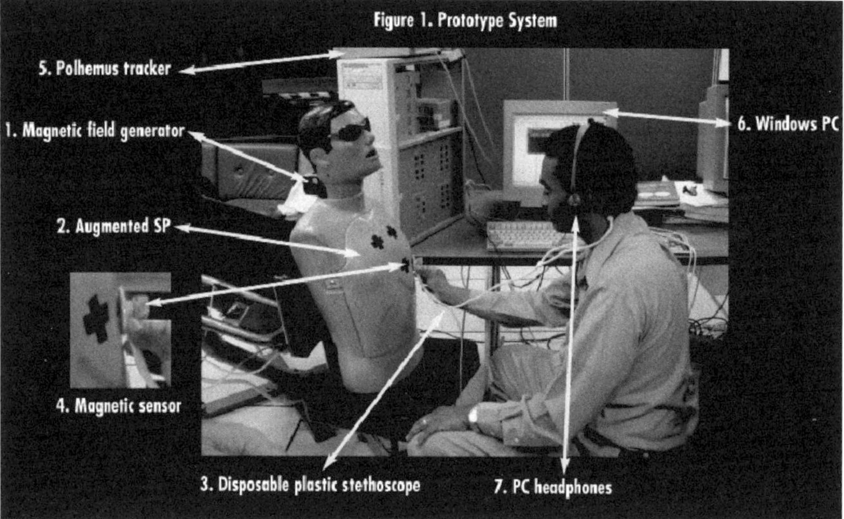

Figure 1: Augmented SP Prototype System

3. Results

In this paper, we report on a study of students testing in a required annual Observed Structured Clinical Examination (OSCE) that are provided an additional assessment using our ASP system. For this study we chose to have our subjects listen for a carotid artery bruit. When auscultating the neck of healthy patients no sounds should be heard. However, in patients with atherosclerosis one often hears a characteristic sound, or bruit, caused by restricted or turbulent blood flow in one or both carotid arteries. For this study we asked subjects whether they detected an abnormal sound as they auscultated the neck areas.

Forth year medical students were the study subjects. The study was completed in two halves with the first half taking place in July 2005 and the second in August 2005 for a total of 105 subjects over approximately 14 different days. The main objective of the study was to determine the validity of using augmented SPs as a reliable assessment tool by presenting abnormal pathology – a bruit.

This sound was chosen because the distinction between normal and abnormal heart and lung sounds is often more subtle than a carotid bruit, and thus may not be distinguished by inexperienced subjects using our current system. The bruit for this study was recorded from a patient. Two SPs were provided with the augmentation in two separate rooms; however, only one SP at a time had an audible bruit to keep students unaware of the purpose of the augmentation. Instead, students were told that we were evaluating a new type of electronic stethoscope and evaluations were performed in addition to normal SP OSCE assessments. Figure 2 shows the configuration of one of the ASP rooms. In the picture, the medical student listens to the neck of the sitting patient with the electronic stethoscope while progress is monitored by a student running the ASP system.

The study was performed at the Theresa A. Thomas Professional Skills Teaching and Assessment Center at the Eastern Virginia Medical School. The Center trains SPs to portray patients providing historical information, nonverbal cues, and physical findings, albeit mostly normal ones.

The students conducted a physical examinations on the augmented SPs, including an auscultation of the left and right side of the ASP's neck and reported whether they heard a carotid bruit or not. Of course, hearing no sound was the normal state for these healthy SPs but a preprogrammed sound of a carotid bruit was played on either the left or right side when desired. Students were instructed on the use of the electronic stethoscope, listened to the SP on both sides of the neck in the areas corresponding to the activated hot zones, and indicated on a form what they had heard.

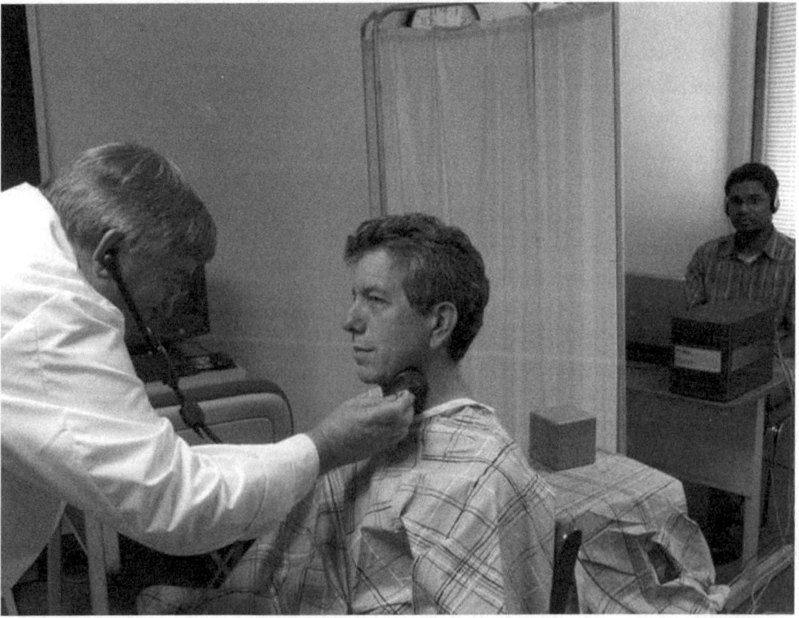

Figure 2: OSCE ASP Assessment Configuration

Assumptions we made include the following:
1. Students would note that a bruit was heard if in fact they heard one in their exam.
2. The students' hearing was normal so they should be able to detect a bruit.
3. The bruit sound was played at an acceptable intensity and that the amplification on the stethoscope was appropriate.
4. That the sound actually played into the earpieces when it was supposed to.

Of the 105 students taking the OSCE, many were excluded for any one of the following criteria:
1. tracker did not indicate a stethoscope sensor in the hot zone,
2. student did not use the electronic stethoscope as the sole instrument for auscultation
3. bruit sound did not play (sound on or off) when sensor was in the hot zone, or the
4. student did not place the stethoscope in a correct anatomic position to listen for a bruit or failed to listen for a bruit (SP scoring)

Upon applying the above exclusions, data from 53 students were used and organized as follows:

Sound on and heard:	16
Sound off and not heard:	19
Sound off and heard:	1
Sound on and not heard:	17

A Chi-Squared test with 1 degree of freedom was performed using a 2x2 table of factors: (sound on, sound off) versus (heard, not heard). The Chi Square test of association gives a value of 10.808 which is equivalent to approximately a tenth of a percent (.00101) chance that the sample distribution can be attributed to randomness. Therefore, we are highly confident that using the ASP system in this case was a valid assessment tool showing that the students could be adequately tested in diagnosing the bruit.

4. Conclusions/Discussion

The study was successful in its attempt to evaluate medical students in their normal OSCE testing environment. Results, however, showed that about 1/3 of the students failed to diagnose the bruit appropriately. This may be because one or more of our assumptions was incorrect for some of these cases. An example may be the presence of partial hearing loss in a few of the subjects due to modern-day headphone speaker usage. Another factor may be the amount of exposure that some 4th year medical students have to carotid bruits. Additionally, comparison of failure rates in other non-augmented portions of the OSCE may shed light on approximately how many students can be expected to not identify such pathology. Nevertheless, the ASP system was shown to be statistically significant in providing a valid assessment tool for carotid bruits.

5. Future Work

Additional studies using more experienced trainees and clinicians as subjects will be done to assess the realism of the Augmented SP system and its continued validity for assessment. The next phase of our work will be: (1) Add additional abnormal sounds to our database, either through collecting them from individuals with abnormalities or modifying normal sounds; (2) Minimize the technology components to increase realism; (3) Explore other ways to augment SPs to display other abnormal physical findings; and (4) test the realism as perceived by an experienced clinician of combining selected abnormal auscultatory findings with pertinent clinical history information to resemble a clinical encounter between doctor and patient.

6. Acknowledgements

This project was a collaborative effort between the Virginia Modeling, Analysis and Simulation Center (VMASC) at Old Dominion University and the Eastern Virginia Medical School. Partial funding was provided by the Stemmler Medical Education Research Fund. Partial funding was also provided by the Naval Health Research Center through NAVAIR Orlando TSD under contract N61339-03-C-0157, and the Office of Naval Research under contract N00014-04-1-0697, entitled "The National Center for Collaboration in Medical Modeling and Simulation." The ideas and opinions presented in this paper represent the views of the authors and do not necessarily represent the views of the Department of Defense.

References

[1] Barrows HS. An overview of the uses of standardized patients for teaching and evaluating clinical skills. *Acad Med.* 68(1993):443-451.

[2] Wallace P. Following the threads of an innovation: the history of standardized patients in medical education. *Caduceus.* 13(Autumn 1997):5-28.

[3] Fincher RE, Lewis LA. Simulations used to teach clinical skills. Ch 16, pp 499-535, in *International Handbook of Research in Medical Education.* Norman GR, Van der Vleuten CPM, Newble DI (Eds.) Dordrecht: Kluwer Academic Publishers, 2002.

[4] Petrusa ER. Clinical Performance Assessments. Ch 21, pp 673-709, in *International Handbook of Research in Medical Education.* Norman GR, Van der Vleuten CPM, Newble DI (Eds.) Dordrecht: Kluwer Academic Publishers, 2002.

[5] McKenzie, Frederic D., Hector M. Garcia, Reynel Castelino, Thomas Hubbard, John Ullian, Gayle Gliva. "Augmented Standardized Patients Now Virtually a Reality." In *Proceedings of the Third IEEE and ACM International Symposium on Mixed and Augmented Reality (ISMAR 2004).* Arlington VA, Nov. 2 – Nov. 5 2004.

Medicine Meets Virtual Reality 14
J.D. Westwood et al. (Eds.)
IOS Press, 2006

385

Direct Volumetric Rendering Based on Point Primitives in OpenGL

André Luiz Miranda da Rosa[a,1], Ilana de Almeida Souza[a], Adilson Yuuji Hira[a] and
Marcelo Knörich Zuffo[a]
*[a]EPUSP - Escola Politécnica da USP – Engenharia Elétrica – LSI (Laboratório de
Sistemas Integráveis)*

Abstract. The aim of this project is to present a renderization by software
algorithm of acquired volumetric data. The algorithm was implemented in Java
language and the LWJGL graphical library was used, allowing the volume
renderization by software and thus preventing the necessity to acquire specific
graphical boards for the 3D reconstruction. The considered algorithm creates a
model in OpenGL, through point primitives, where each voxel becomes a point
with the color values related to this pixel position in the corresponding images.

Keywords. Volume Rendering, OpenGL, Point Primitives.

1.   Introduction

According to Meinzer et al [1], the information acquired from medical images (as
Computed Tomography) strongly depends on the experience and training of the
medical specialist and its knowledge of the current studied object to realize a correct
diagnosis. Therefore, there's a necessity to offer a mechanism that facilitates the three-
dimensional visualization of medical examinations, so volumetric renderization
appeared as a method to project multidimensional data set in a bi-dimensional
visualization plan to gain better knowledge of the structure contained in the volumetric
data.

The aim of this article is to describe a unique volumetric data renderization method
of volumetric data that is simpler than other existing algorithm and that offers a good
performance without the use of special graphical boards. The volumetric data can be
acquired, for example, from archives in TIFF, JPEG, BMP, GIF or DICOM (Digital
Imaging Communication in Medicine - a standard wide used for medical examinations
as Computed Tomography) formats. Particularly, we used the segmented visible human
data [2] because it's commonly used by the scientific community and allows us to
validate and compare this new algorithm.

Our intention is to integrate this visualization technique to the Collaborative
Environment for Second Medical Opinion developed by the Telemedicine Group in the

---

¹ Corresponding Author: André Luis Miranda da Rosa, Av. Prof. Luciano
Gualberto, Travessa 3, n. 158, Prédio de Engenharia Elétrica, Escola Politécnica da
USP, Bairro Butantã, CEP 05508-900, São Paulo-SP-Brasil, E-mail:
amiranda@lsi.usp.br

LSI/EPUSP that allows the remote collaboration between users through the Internet using Chat, Videoconference and Bi-dimensional Collaborative Blackboard.

2.   Implementation

This algorithm was implemented using JAVA language and graphical library LWJGL (Lightweight Java Game Library). As the LWJGL allows the directly call of OpenGL primitives, the use of its high level functions was not necessary and therefore only the OpenGL methods provided by the library was used [3].

The implemented algorithm initially makes a pre-processing loading images in 3D matrices, each one with equal width and height ratios and quantity of images slices. For each image color channel, a matrix is necessary, so there are three matrices to load RGB values of each pixel, each one sequentially stored in its own matrix (R, G or B channels' matrices).

The considered algorithm creates a model in OpenGL, through primitive of points, where each voxel becomes a point with the color calculated by the R, G and B values related to this pixel position in the corresponding images. Therefore, it is possible to visualize a cloud of points placed one to the side of the others, through a distance that allows each voxel to assume the size of one pixel in the users screen. An interaction model with mouse and keyboard was also created, allowing to the user to translate, rotate and scale the model in any direction. Figure 1 show the resulting volume.

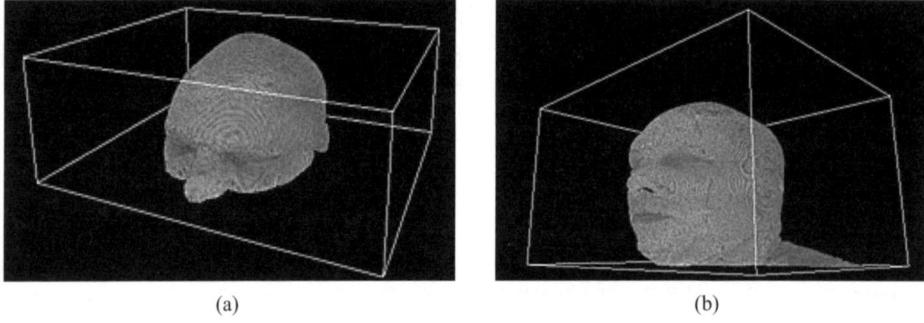

(a)   (b)

Figure 1: Medium resolution Visible Human volumetric renderization: (a) with diagonal cutting plane; (b) without cutting plane.

At some distance the model allows that each voxel may be visualized as pixels accurately side by side, without intervals, therefore the volume may be correctly visualized. But with the scale transformation, the distance between voxels increases when related to the volume and the user visualization point proximity, causing a undesirable effect in the volume visualization. Another bad result is that too much memory is needed to store the volume so it might be impossible to visualize large volumes.

As this direct visualization algorithm only plot the pixels in 3D, transforming them into voxels, it becomes extremely simple. However, he does not offer a good renderization speed (in the case of processing all voxels, without eliminating hidden voxels), with 15 frames/second for low-resolution images (183 x 148 pixels and 150 slices) and 3 frames/second for average resolution (438 x 354 pixels and 150 slices), depending on the processor and the video board used.

Nowadays, there are many graphical boards in the market that perform the volumetric data renderization by means of their hardware. As they're special hardware to accelerate the volumetric renderization, they offer better speed than software based renderization algorithms, but they have the disadvantage to have a higher cost. Therefore, the use of the software based renderization system described here is more appropriate for many situations where we don't want to acquire more expensive component and only want to use components that come with personal computers as accelerating boards that support the OpenGL libraries, becoming very useful for the majority of the population.

3.　　Conclusions

This paper described a software based renderization technique in order to be integrated to the Second Medical Opinion Collaborative Application in current development by the LSI/EPUSP Telemedicine Group. The system supplies the volumetric visualization of DICOM tomographic slices. The application was implemented in JAVA language, using the OpenGL based graphical library.

Currently, we arc optimizing the algorithm so that hidden voxels would not be processed and it would provide faster renderization and will allow its use in real time applications. It is also being added a pixel size control (used to represent each voxel) in relation to the user point of view (so that volume zoom can occur) preventing the undesirable effect of empty spaces originated by the approach of the volume to the user point of view.

Considering the processing speed, the possibility of algorithm parallelization will be studied. It might make the renderization much more fast and efficient but at the same time might increase the cost with new equipment acquisition.

We also intend to implement new collaborative tools, as the volume calculation and the segmentation from slices pre-marked areas, thus allowing the measures extraction to assist future diagnosis.

References

[1]　Meinzer , H., Meetz, K., Scheppelmann, D., Engelmann, U., Baur, H. J. (1991) "The Heidelberg Ray Tracing Model", German Cancer Research Center, Heidelberg. IEEE Computer Graphics & Applications.

[2]　Souza, I.A., Sanches-Jr, C., Binatto, M.B., Lopes, T.T., Zuffo, M.K. (2004). Direct Volume Rendering of the Visible Human Dataset on a Distributed Multiprojection Immersive Environment, Proceedings of II Symposium on Virtual Reality (SVR'04), São Paulo, SP, Outubro, 183-194.

[3]　LWJGL - Lightweight Java Game Library (2005), available in http://lwjgl.org/. Acessed: September, 27th 2005.

Medicine Meets Virtual Reality 14
J.D. Westwood et al. (Eds.)
IOS Press, 2006

A Haptic Device for Guide Wire in Interventional Radiology Procedures

PhD Thomas MOIX [a,1], PhD Dejan ILIC [a], Prof. Hannes Bleuler [a]
and PhD Jurjen Zoethout [b]

[a] *Laboratoire de Systèmes Robotiques, Ecole Polytechnique Fédérale de Lausanne,
1015 Lausanne, Switzerland*
[b] *Xitact S.A., Rue de Lausanne45, 1110 Morges, Switzerland*

Abstract. Interventional Radiology (IR) is a minimally invasive procedure where thin tubular instruments, guide wires and catheters, are steered through the patient's vascular system under X-ray imaging. In order to perform these procedures, a radiologist has to be trained to master hand-eye coordination, instrument manipulation and procedure protocols. The existing simulation systems all have major drawbacks: the use of modified instruments, unrealistic insertion lengths, high inertia of the haptic device that creates a noticeably degraded dynamic behavior or excessive friction that is not properly compensated for. In this paper we propose a quality training environment dedicated to IR. The system is composed of a virtual reality (VR) simulation of the patient's anatomy linked to a robotic interface providing haptic force feedback. This paper focuses on the requirements, design and prototyping of a specific haptic interface for guide wires.

Keywords. Haptic interface, force feedback device, Interventional Radiology

1. Introduction

1.1. Interventional Radiology

Interventional Radiology (IR) is a minimally invasive surgery (MIS) procedure where instruments are steered into the vascular system of the patient. The ongoing intervention is monitored with a real-time X-ray imaging device (C-arm).

Two main categories of instruments are used, guidewires and catheters. Guidewires, either coated wounded wires or bare polymer wires, are very flexible and have tips that can be pre-shaped. Standard guidewires have diameters of 0.035 to 0.038" and lengths of 125 cm to 145 cm.

Catheters are tubular instruments made of polymers (mostly polyurethane, polyethylene, nylon or teflon). Standard catheters have diameters of 4 to 6 F (1 French = 1/3 mm) with lengths similar to guidewires. The tip of a catheter can be pre-shaped to fit in a particular anatomical area. Catheters exist for dedicated tasks. For instance, some catheters have an inflatable balloon at their distal end to perform plastic deformation of

---

[1] Corresponding Author : Thomas MOIX, LSRO, EPFL, Me.H0.559, Station 9, 1015 Lausanne, Switzerland;
E-mail: Thomas.moix@a3.epfl.ch

calcified vessels (a procedure called angioplasty) or are perforated along their distal portion for fluid flushing tasks.

A procedure starts with a palpation to find an entry point in the vascular system. Once a suitable point is found, in most cases in the groin area, a needle is used to enter the vascular system and an entry guide, the sheath, is put in place. Guidewires and catheters can be inserted through the sheath. A guide wire is inserted and driven in the vascular system to the desired anatomical point. Due to their inherent flexibility, guidewires can more easily be steered inside the lumen. Furthermore, their flexible tips help selecting a direction by rotation at branches. Once the guide wire is in place, a catheter can be inserted and driven over the guide wire (i.e. the guide wire is inside the tubular catheter).

The most commonly performed procedure is a diagnostic technique called angiography in which a contrast agent (i.e. liquid that is opaque under X-rays) is injected through a catheter. The resulting X-ray images are recorded and analyzed by the radiologists. Depending on its results the procedure can be extended into therapy. Immediate treatment is possible through techniques including local drug injection, catheter balloon inflation (angioplasty) and stent (implant) placement among others [1].

1.2. Training Methods in IR

IR is especially well suited for simulator-based learning and training: it requires complex understanding of the patient's anatomy from 2D screens and perfect hand-eye coordination. Improperly performed catheterization can lead to extremely harmful consequences. Procedural success is related to the number of procedures that radiologists perform.

Traditionally, IR is taught using a master-apprentice model with additional training on animals or mock models with real medical equipment including X-ray imaging. These methods have several drawbacks including ethical issues, radiation exposure and high costs. Most importantly, there is a risk to patients during the time when physicians begin their specialization. Furthermore, interventions and devices are becoming increasingly complex, while the easier diagnostic procedures used for teaching are replaced by alternate techniques (angio-CT and angio-MRI). These are strong reasons for developing computer-assisted training systems to allow a realistic and adapted training.

2. A Computer-Assisted Training System for IR

2.1. Requirements

This paper focuses on the input interface required in a computer-assisted training system for IR. The requirements in terms of software are not further discussed hereafter.

As previously detailed, IR procedures are performed using thin tubular instruments called guide wires and catheters. Tracking and force feedback have to be applied on rotation and translation of each instrument. Even though passive braking feedback is sufficient for most of the encountered cases, specific occurrences require active force feedback for realistic simulation. An example of such behaviour happens when a pre-shaped guiding catheter gets out of its anatomical steady place and a forward and backward bounce of the catheter is observed.

In IR, forces and torques, estimated for a 5 F (1 F = 1/3 mm) catheter through a series of lab experiments, are in the range of ±1.5 N and ±4.5 mNm [2]. Force and torque resolution shall be of 0.02 N and 0.04 mNm respectively to meet human sensory system [3]. Tracking of a guide wire while inside a catheter should be possible. This configuration is later referred to as "tube in tube".

2.2. The Proposed Interface

The proposed system consists of two haptic devices. The first, that tracks and provides force feedback on a catheter, is fixed at the entrance of the system. The core of the device for catheter is a friction drive arrangement that can be set into rotation. The second device handles a guide wire. The two devices are separated by the desired stroke of the catheter. This architecture found in all reported interfaces for IR solves the "tube in tube" issue but introduces an unrealistic insertion length for the guide wire that can teach wrong habits to trainees [4-8]. This paper focuses on the development of the haptic device for guide wire. The haptic interface for catheters is further described in [9].

The originality of the proposed system is a new approach to solve the inaccurate insertion length of the inner instrument before tracking and force feedback can be applied. The haptic interface for guide wire includes a small gripper mounted at the distal end of a rod. The other end of the rod is attached to the carriage of a linear guide. Diameters of less than 1 mm enable to navigate the rod and the gripper inside a 5 F or bigger catheter. When inserted into the simulator, the guide wire (i.e. the inner instrument) is gripped at the input port. The forces and motion applied to the guide wire are transmitted along the rod to the linear guide even if a catheter is present as depicted in Figure 1. Hence, tracking and force feedback is possible on the guide wire as soon as it is inserted in the simulator.

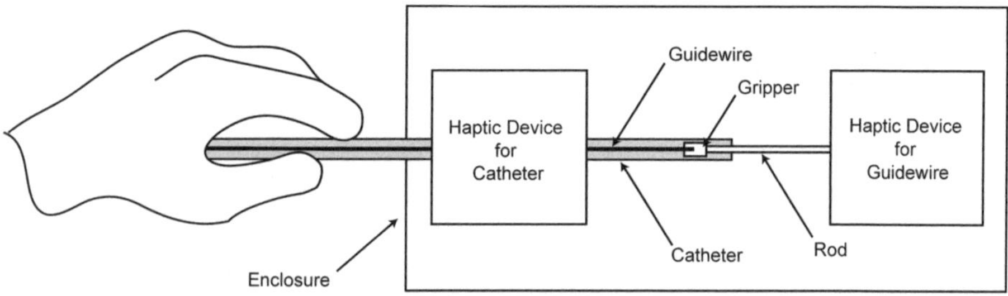

Figure 1. The proposed architecture of haptic interface for IR

3. The Haptic Interface for Guide Wire

3.1. Mechanical Interface

The proposed interface is based on a linear stage actuated by a DC motor and a timing belt transmission. The carriage of the linear stage, illustrated in Figure 2, holds the actuation mechanism of the micro-gripper, optical sensors for tracking and a force sensor for the translational degree of freedom (DOF) of the guide wire.

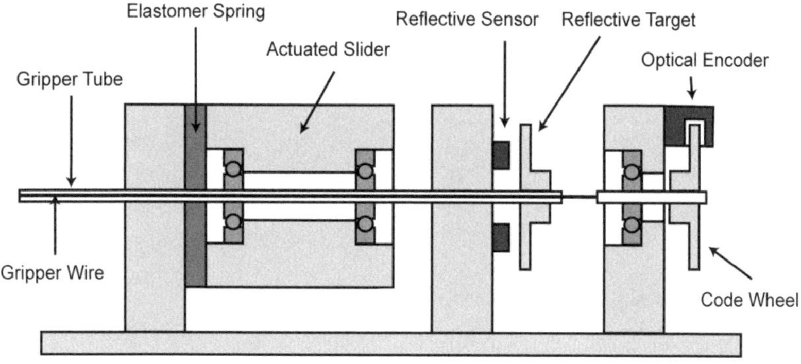

Figure 2. Longitudinal cut view of the linear stage carriage

The actuation principle of the gripper is the relative movement of a tube over a fixed wire. The gripper head, a slotted tube, is glued at the distal end of the wire. The relative movement of the outer tube toward the distal end induces a deformation of the gripper head and thus provides the locking force. A small DC motor and a capstan arrangement are used to move a slider on which the tube is mounted.

The rotation of the rod, corresponding to the rotation of the guide wire, is decoupled from the locking mechanism with an arrangement of miniature ball bearings mounted in the slider. A magnetic particle break provides a braking feedback on the rotation of the guide wire. Two optical code wheel sensors provide the tracking of the guide wire. Figure 3 shows the realized prototype of the haptic device for guide wire.

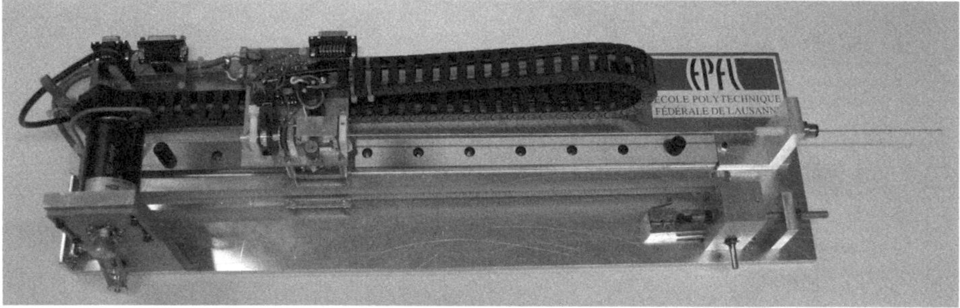

Figure 3. Prototype of the haptic interface for guide wire

3.2. Longitudinal Force Sensing

A 1 DOF force sensor is integrated in the gripper actuation mechanism to measure the applied translational force. When the gripper is closed, the DC motor and capstan arrangement continuously push the slider attached to the outer tube on the frame of the carriage. A piece of elastomer is glued on the surface of the frame, creating a prestressed spring arrangement between the frame and the slider. If a force is applied on the carriage or on the rod, the idle deflection of the spring is modified. This deflection is measured on a reflective target glued at the proximal end of the outer tube by two optical reflective sensors. The two optical sensors are mounted in a mirror arrangement around the outer tube in order to cancel the inherent mechanical unbalance of the measurement setup. Residual angular dependency of the measurement is cancelled by a look-up table compensation.

The calibration procedure of the force sensor displayed a linear measurement range of over ± 3 N with a resolution of 9 mN. The mechanical bandwidth of the force sensor was estimated to be 200 Hz with a spring-mass model. This value was confirmed by the experimental frequency characterization of the realised prototype.

3.3. Force Control Strategy

The measured longitudinal force information is used for friction and dynamic compensation on the translation stage of the device. The proposed control strategy includes a model-based friction compensation and an implicit force controller (PID) that are working in parallel to the impedance force control done by the VR simulation software.

4. Conclusions

The proposed haptic interface for guide wire has been integrated with the existing prototype for catheter into a complete training system for IR procedures.

The software interface of the system is compatible with the commercial CHP platform by Xitact S.A. which enables the use of third party VR simulation software. The next steps of the project include a validation study with medical partners.

Acknowledgements

This research is supported by the Swiss National Science Foundation within the framework NCCR CO-ME (COmputer aided and image guided MEdical interventions) and by the Swiss Innovation Promotion Agency KTI/CTI.

References

[1]   K. Valji, Vascular and Interventional Radiology. Philadelphia, PA: W.B. Saunders Company, 1999.

[2]   D. Ilic, T. Moix, O. Lambercy and al, "Measurement of Internal Constraints During an Interventional Radiology Procedure", IEEE-EMBC'05, 2005

[3]   H. Tan, B. Eberman and al., "Human factors for he design of force-reflecting haptic interfaces," Dyn. Sys. Cont., vol. 55, no.1, 1994.

[4]   G. Aloisio, L. Barone, M. Bergamasco and al., "Computer-based simulator for catheter insertion training," in Studies in Health Technology and Informatics (MMVR 12), vol. 98, 2004.

[5]   S. Z. Barnes, D. R. Morr and N. Berme, "Catheter simulation device," U.S. Patent 6 038 488, 2000.

[6]   G. L. Merril, "Interventional radiology interface apparatus and method," U.S. Patent 6 106 301, 2000.

[7]   B. E. Bailey, "System for training persons to perform minimally invasive surgical procedure," U.S. Patent 5 800 179, 1998.

[8]   J. M. Wendlandt and F. M. Morgan, "Actuator for independent axial and rotational actuation of a catheter or similar elongated object," U.S. Patent 6 375 471, 2002.

[9]   T. Moix, D. Ilic and al., "A Real-Time Haptic Interface for Interventional Radiology", in Studies in Health Technology and Informatics (MMVR 13), vol. 111, 2005.

Medicine Meets Virtual Reality 14
J.D. Westwood et al. (Eds.)
IOS Press, 2006

Computer-Aided Navigation for Arthroscopic Hip Surgery Using Encoder Linkages for Position Tracking

Emily MONAHAN, Kenji SHIMADA
Carnegie Mellon University, Pittsburgh, PA

Abstract. While arthroscopic surgery has many advantages over traditional surgery, this minimally invasive surgical technique is not often applied to the hip joint. There are two main reasons for this: the difficulties of navigating within the joint and of correctly placing portal incisions without damaging critical neurovascular structures. This paper proposes a computer-aided navigation system to address the challenges of arthroscopic hip surgery. Unlike conventional arthroscopic methods, this system uses encoder linkages to track surgical instruments, thus eliminating the problems associated with standard tracking systems. The encoder position information is used to generate a computer display of patient anatomy to supplement the restricted view from a typical arthroscopic camera.

Introduction

Arthroscopy is a minimally invasive surgical procedure used to decrease the necessary incision size for joint-repair surgery. Large operative incisions are replaced by small "portal" incisions. A long, thin camera, called an arthroscope, is placed in one portal to display the joint. Additional portals are employed for the insertion of surgical tools. As shown in Figure 1(a), the surgeon navigates by camera images displayed on an operating room screen.

Despite the benefits of arthroscopic surgery, hip arthroscopy is not a common practice as in knee and shoulder repair [1]. In the hip, arthroscopy can be used for removing loose bodies, smoothing rough bone surfaces, and trimming damaged or abnormal tissue [2]. Unfortunately, the hip joint introduces additional challenges for arthroscopy due to the depth of its location in the body, the tight nature of the ball and socket joint, and the proximity of surrounding neurovascular structures. These challenges have created two obstacles for arthroscopic hip surgery: awareness of spatial orientation during joint navigation; and portal incision placement while avoiding damage to critical anatomical structures. The few surgeons who can perform this procedure rely heavily on intuition gained through experience to overcome these challenges.

This research proposes the use of a computer-aided navigation system to ease the difficulty associated with arthroscopic hip surgery. A linkage of encoders is employed to track the motion of surgical tools during an operation. The real-time motion of the tools is shown relative to the patient anatomy on a computer display. These tools provide additional visual feedback to a surgeon for easier joint navigation and safer portal placement during hip surgery. Ultimately, the proposed computer-aided navigation system can increase the use of advantageous arthroscopic procedures over full-incision operations for the hip joint.

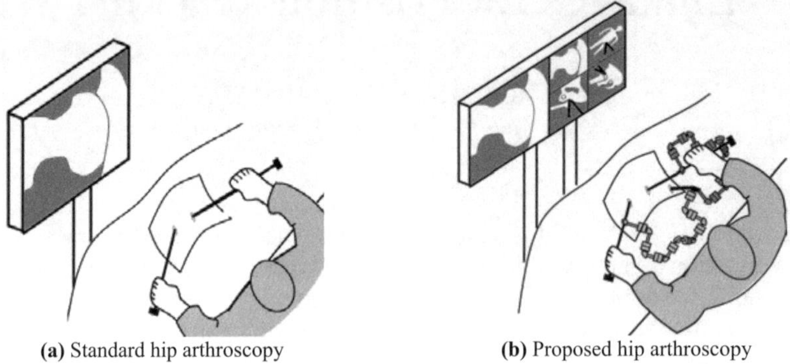

(a) Standard hip arthroscopy   (b) Proposed hip arthroscopy

Figure 1. For current arthroscopy, the surgeon navigates using the arthroscope images only. In the proposed system, encoder chains track instrument position, and an additional screen displays computer images of the instruments and patient anatomy from several viewpoints

2   Previous Work

Although computer-aided tools to assist a surgeon in medical procedures are appearing more frequently, a tool for arthroscopic hip surgery does not exist. Many current computer-aided tools aim to supplement a surgeon's abilities by assisting with accurate and consistent placement of surgical instruments or implants [3-6]. While this research also focuses on the creation of a system to supplement a surgeon's abilities, it addresses the particular issues of portal placement and instrument navigation in arthroscopic hip surgery.

Position tracking is an important component of many computer-aided surgical systems. Although optical and electromagnetic tracking systems are most commonly used, these systems have limitations. An optical system can lose information from its position sensors if the sensor's line of sight to the receiver is broken. Electromagnetic systems are susceptible to distortion or noise from other metallic objects or stray magnetic fields. Due to their associated problems, these typical tracking devices were not employed in the proposed system for hip arthroscopy.

3   System Overview

The basic concept of the proposed navigation system with an encoder linkage is illustrated in Figure 1(b). Instead of a traditional optical or electromagnetic tracking device, a linkage of encoders is introduced as an effective tracking alternative. One end of the linkage is attached to the instrument, while the reference end is attached to a base pin. The base pin is surgically inserted in the patient's pelvis and provides the connection between the linkage and patient. Rotational encoders at each joint location capture the tool motion relative to the patient anatomy.

Given the operative tool positions from the linkage, a real-time display of the surgical instruments relative to the patient anatomy can be generated. The standard arthroscope view of the joint will be supplemented by an additional screen of computer generated images. The additional computer images provide real-time information about the anatomy surrounding the surgical tools as they are manipulated.

For the computer display, a model of the patient's hip joint must be created prior to surgery. Three-dimensional data can be obtained from computerized tomography, magnetic resonance imaging, or a method using x-ray images which has been developed to obtain patient specific models [7]. Also, the position and orientation of the base pin in the patient's hip must be identified for the tracking linkage to correctly locate the surgical tools. The pin will be placed in the pelvis prior to taking x-rays of the patient. Special x-ray markers, like those used in [7], can be employed to determine the camera orientation. The pin can then be located in the model through triangulation with two x-ray images from known view points and orientations.

This paper discusses the tracking linkage and the computer display portions of this arthroscopic navigation system. The design for the encoder chain is outlined. Also, the current computer display and associated features are detailed. Finally, the integration of the arthroscopic navigation system with existing surgical equipment is discussed.

4   System Design and Implementation

The encoder linkage for position tracking is kinematically redundant. While a chain with only six degrees of freedom can reach all desired positions and orientations, the chain may be configured such that it encroaches on the surgeon's workspace in some cases. The current linkage, shown in Figure 2, consists of a chain with eight links, each with one rotational degree of freedom. The two additional degrees of freedom provide sufficient flexibility to prevent chain interference.

The main components of the linkage are the L-shaped links, the US Digital E4 encoders [8], and rotational bearings. The 90° bend in the links place the next joint's axis of rotation perpendicular to the previous one. The encoder resolution is 1,200 pulses per revolution, resulting in an accuracy of +/- 0.3 degrees. Adjacent links are attached via a bearing connection.

The position and orientation of the surgical instruments are determined through two main homogeneous transformations. The coordinate frame attached to the endpoint of the chain must be determined in model coordinates. The first coordinate transformation, calculates the tool position relative to the pelvic pin. The eight encoder angles are used to determine this transformation, and it is recalculated to update the tool position each time the encoder angles change. A data acquisition USB device, the USB1, from US Digital [8] was used to obtain the encoder angles. The second coordinate transformation will move from the pin frame to the model frame. This coordinate transformation will be calculated only once, based on the pin position in the 3-D patient model obtained from x-rays [7].

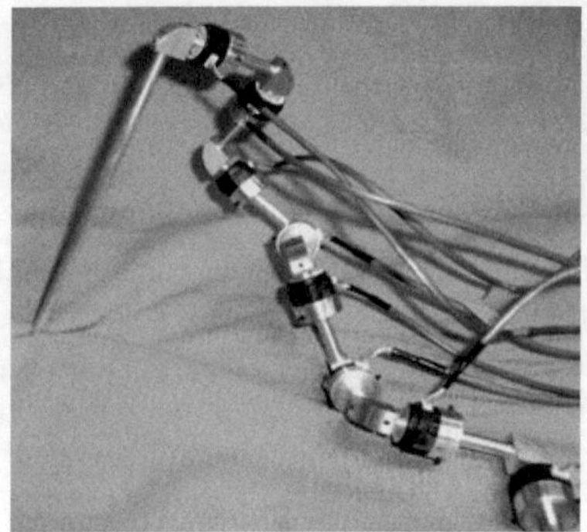

(a) Encoder linkage for tracking

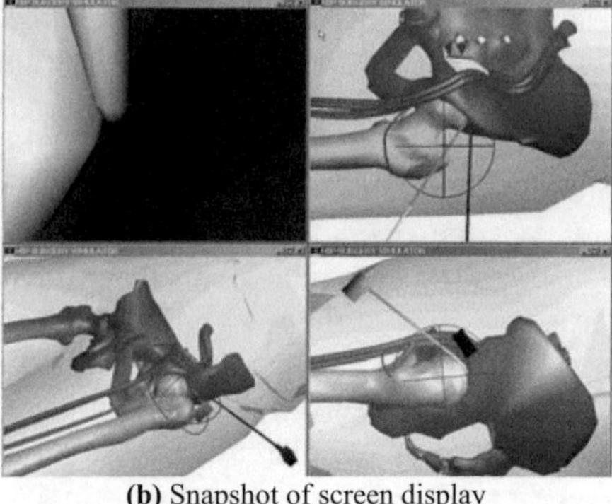

(b) Snapshot of screen display

Figure 2. Components of proposed navigation system

The screen display shown in Figure 2(b) consists of four windows that display different views of the hip joint and surgical tool models. Narrow cylinders, with rounded ends and rectangular handles, are used to represent the arthroscope (red) and a surgical tool (yellow). The upper-left window of the display is a picture of the model as viewed from the simulated arthroscope. This window mimics the actual camera image currently used by the surgeon. The remaining three windows show the model from different perspectives as set by the surgeon.

As the encoder angles change, the screen images are updated to reflect a new instrument position. The screen display update rate is limited by the speed at which the new transformation matrix can be calculated and the graphics can be redrawn. The program currently runs on a computer with a 2.2 MHz AMD64 processor, 1.0 GB RAM and a NVIDIA GeForce 6800 GT video card. With this computer, the screen updates approximately every 78 ms or almost 13 frames per second.

The computer-aided navigation system was integrated with standard arthroscopic equipment on a mockup of the human hip joint as shown in Figure 3. The standard system consists of a Sony video monitor, a 4mm, 70° Video Arthroscope, a Dyonics Xenon light source for the arthroscope, and a Dyonics Vision 325Z Camera System. The video monitor displays the arthroscopic camera images. The arthroscope is connected to the light source by a fiber optic cable, and to the vision system via the camera head. With the addition of the navigation system, the arthroscope also has a connection to the tracking chain.

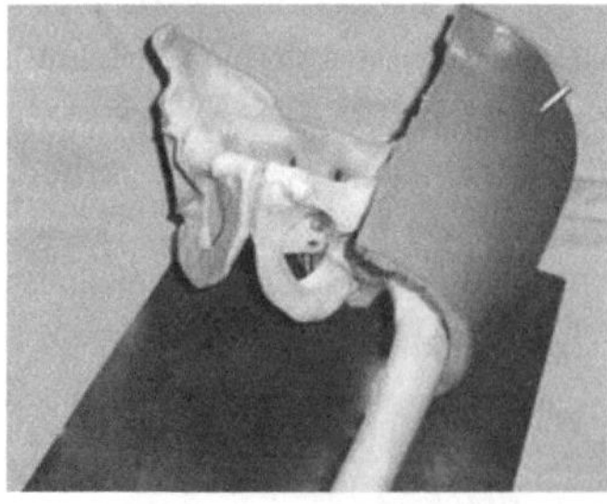

(a) Model of human hip joint

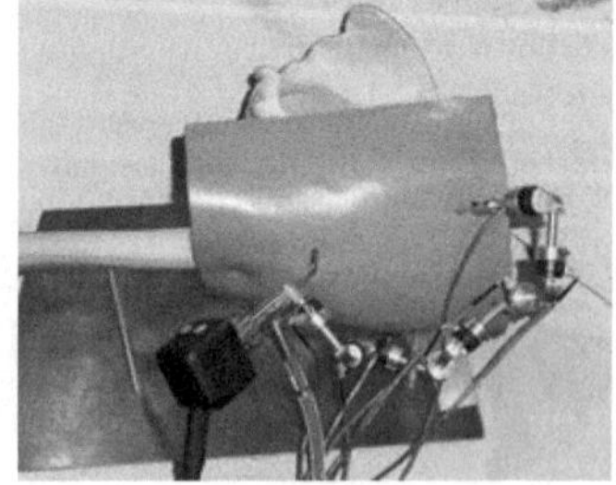

(b) Arthroscope and linkage applied to model

Figure 3. Hip model and arthroscope connections. The arthroscope is connected to both the tracking chain and traditional arthroscopic equipment (camera head and light source).

5   Position Error of Encoder Chain

An accuracy estimation of the tracking system can be observed through the comparison of the camera and computer images. The computer image in the upper left of the display window (Fig. 2(b)) should match the image displayed on the video monitor from the arthroscope. Using both the computer navigation system and the Smith and Nephew equipment on the hip model, simultaneous images were collected from the computer screen and the video monitor for comparison. Figure 4 displays an example of the resulting comparison.

The arthroscope images obtained from the arthroscopic camera and the computer program are very similar, but do not match exactly for several reasons. First, the computer hip model and physical hip model are not identical in the demo system. For an actual procedure, the three dimensional model would be taken from the patient to ensure agreement between the models. Some error is also attributed to the inexpensive encoders used in the current demonstration system. Finally, the initialization method for the chain can contribute to image discrepancies. If the chain is not positioned precisely during the initialization, the calculated transformation matrix for the chain will be incorrect.

Considering error in the encoder readings, the worst case error will occur when the chain is fully extended and all encoders record the maximum error value. The maximum error of $0.3°$ is a result of the encoder resolution. When the chain is fully extended, any error in the measured angles will have the greatest effect since the effective chain length is at its largest. In this worst case, the accumulating error will result in the chain endpoint being approximately 5mm from the reported location. However, the chain has been sized such that it is not frequently in the fully extended configuration for hip arthroscopy maneuvers. Also, the errors in the chain measurements can occur on opposite directions, decreasing the overall endpoint error as the individual errors somewhat cancel. The error can also be decreased by selecting encoders with higher resolution.

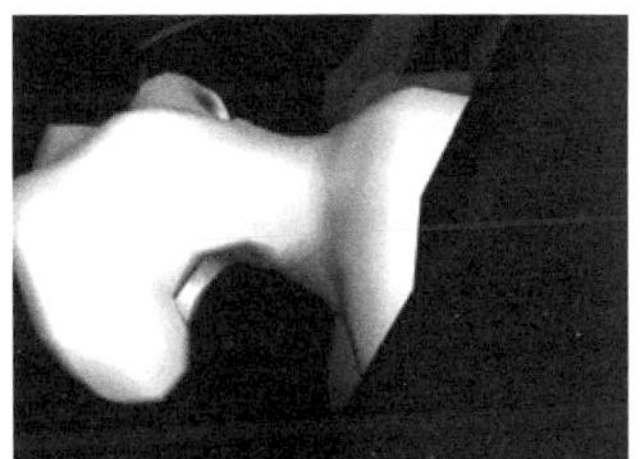
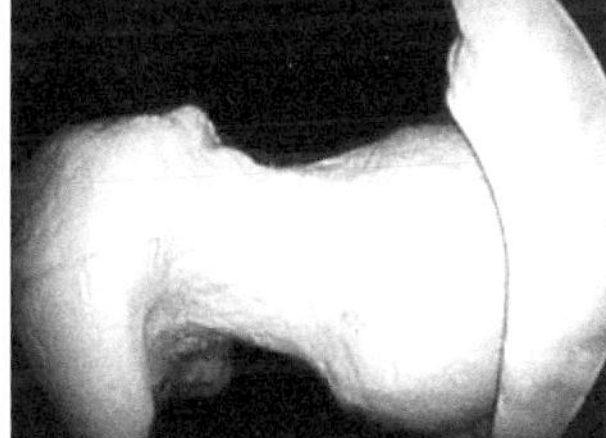

(a) Simulated 70°-arthroscope view   (b) Actual 70°-arthroscope view

Figure 4. Comparison of arthroscope views from the simulated and the actual arthroscope.

6   Conclusions

The navigation system for arthroscopic hip surgery can be used as a tool to address the challenges of joint navigation and portal placement in arthroscopic hip surgery. In the operating room, the system can visually supplement the limited view from the arthroscope. Specifically, a surgeon can view the location of his tools relative to the patient anatomy and be warned when tools enter dangerous regions.

The introduction of a tracking linkage shows significant potential as an alternative to more expensive and often problematic tracking systems. The encoder linkage for position tracking eliminates problems associated with optical and electromagnetic systems in medical applications. The redundant linkage provides the required flexibility for arthroscopic maneuvers while tracking the surgical instrument position. Positive feedback about the completed demo system was obtained from surgeons who perform arthroscopic procedures [9]. The encoder linkage was seen as an acceptable addition to the surgical workspace, and the extra visual feedback was considered valuable.

Next steps of this project include a more rigorous examination of the linkage error, the creation of a new encoder chain, changes to the computer display, and user studies. The chain will use more accurate and smaller encoders. In addition, absolute encoders will be employed instead of incremental encoders. Using absolute encoders will simplify of the linkage initialization and eliminate this source of error. For the computer display, future work involves obtaining matching computer and physical hip models. With identical models, it will be possible to analyze the accuracy of the system in more detail. Finally, feedback about the system will be sought through user studies.

Acknowledgements

This research was supported in part by a National Science Foundation Graduate Research Fellowship. The authors would like to thank Ken Karish and Smith and Nephew Inc. for supplying the standard hip arthroscopy equipment for this project. Finally, input from Dr. Marc Philippon and Dr. Freddie Fu was invaluable.

References

[1]   Scuderi, G. and A. Tria, 2004, *MIS of the Hip and the Knee: A Clinical Perspective*, Springer-Verlag: New York, p. 199.

[2]   Safran, M., D. Stone and J. Zachazewski, 2003, *Instructions for Sports Medicine Patients*, Elsevier Inc.: Philadelphia.

[3]   DiGioia, A., D. Simon, B. Jaramaz, et al., 1995, "HipNav: Pre-operative Planning and Intra-operative Navigational Guidance for Acetabular Implant Placement in Total Hip Replacement Surgery", Comput. Assist. Orthop. Surgery Sym, Bern, Switzerland.

[4]   Taylor, R., B. Mittelstadt, H. Paul, et al., 1994, "An Image-Directed Robotic System for Precise Orthopaedic Surgery", IEEE Trans. on Robotics and Automation, 10(3), p. 261-275.

[5]   Chiu, A., D. Boyd and T. Peters, 2000, "3-D Visualization for Minimally Invasive Robotic Coronary Artery Bypass (MIRCAB)", 22nd Annual EMBS International Con., Chicago IL.

[6]   Taylor, R., 2003, "Medical Robotics in Computer -Integrated Surgery", IEEE Trans. on Robotics and Automation, 19(5), p. 765-781.

[7]   Gunay, M., 2003, "Three-dimensional bone geometry reconstruction from x-ray images using hierarchical free-form deformation and non-linear optimization", Ph.D. Thesis, Carnegie Mellon University, Pittsburgh, PA.

[8]   US Digital Corporation, *http://www.usdigital.com*, March 25, 2005.

[9]   Philippon, Marc J., and Fu, Freddie H., 2004, personal communication.

Medicine Meets Virtual Reality 14
J.D. Westwood et al. (Eds.)
IOS Press, 2006

399

Project Hydra - A New Paradigm of Internet-Based Surgical Simulation

Kevin MONTGOMERY[a], Lawrence BURGESS[b], Parvati DEV[c], Leroy HEINRICHS[c]
[a]*National Biocomputation Center, Stanford University*
[b]*Telehealth Research Institute, University of Hawaii*
[c]*SUMMIT, Stanford University*

Abstract. Computer-based surgical simulation systems have produced tremendous benefits and demonstrated validity as a better method for many areas of surgical skills acquisition. However, despite these benefits, broad proliferation of these systems has continued to be elusive. While in large part this lag in adoption of this technology is due to social factors (organizational momentum, curriculum integration difficulties, etc), the cost of computer-based simulation systems has certainly remained a major deterrent toward broad deployment. Instead, what if it were possible to eliminate the cost of the large computer completely from the system, yet provide a much more extensive and detailed simulation than currently available? Finally, what if a simulation with even greater detail over a wider anatomical area were possible?

This is the genesis of Project Hydra- a shared simulation supercomputer were made available for free and all that is required to access it is a low-end Internet-connected computer and, optionally, interaction/haptics devices as needed for the particular task. This would enable supercomputer-class simulation at every desktop with much greater fidelity than any user could individually afford and provide an online community for simulation research and application. Further, Internet-based simulation provides for many other benefits as well. By the user merely plugging optional, additional hardware into their existing, low-end PC and using the Internet as a means of simulation dissemination, distribution, and delivery means that the user can have immediate access to simulation updates/upgrades and download/access new content (didactic curriculum and cases). Further, this ease of access and use could lead to accelerated adoption and use of simulation within the medical curriculum and this access is provided anywhere in the world 24x7. In addition, once connected, a server-based simulation system would be a natural point for performing easy, automated clinical studies of surgical performance and skills.

Keywords: Surgical simulation, networked haptics, internet, supercomputing.

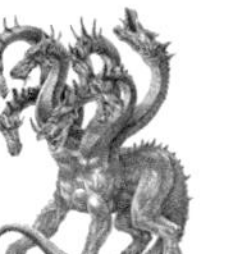

Introduction

Computer-based surgical simulation systems have produced tremendous benefits and demonstrated validity as a better method for many areas of surgical skills acquisition. However, despite these benefits, broad proliferation of these systems has continued to be elusive. While in large part this lag in adoption of this technology is due to social factors (organizational momentum, curriculum integration difficulties, etc), the cost of computer-based simulation systems has certainly remained a major deterrent toward broad deployment.

In short, computer-based surgical simulation systems remain at too high a price point for many surgical education programs to afford. If the cost-per-seat of computer-based surgical simulation could be dramatically reduced to below the discretionary spending limits of most clinical faculty (<$10,000USD), this may enable greater proliferation of this technology.

In analyzing the costs of a typical computer-based part-task training system, the major costs of the system are the haptics device and the computer system used for driving the simulation. As for the haptics device, recent evidence suggests that learning some surgical skills may not require force feedback or a more limited degree than was previously thought. However, the other major cost of the surgical simulation system, a computer powerful enough to drive a surgical simulation with sufficient detail to be useful, remains a major hindrance. Typically, in order to attain a required price point, commercial simulation systems must rely on underpowered computing platforms and make tradeoffs in simulation fidelity to still provide a meaningful training experience. These tradeoffs, such as limiting interaction area, oversimplified models of motion, etc lead to simulators that are unrealistic or greatly limited in scope and utility.

Instead, what if it were possible to break this paradigm and eliminate the cost of the large computer completely from the system, yet provide a much more extensive and detailed simulation than currently available? In short, what if the large simulation computer were eliminated from the ecomonic equation with no impact on the simulation quality? Moreover, what if a simulation with even greater detail over a wider anatomical area were possible?

This is the genesis of Project Hydra- a shared simulation supercomputer were made available for free and all that is required to access it is a low-end Internet-connected computer and, optionally, interaction/haptics devices as needed for the particular task. This would enable supercomputer-class simulation at every desktop with much greater fidelity than any user could individually afford and provide an online community for simulation research and application.

Further, Internet-based simulation provides for many other benefits as well. By the user merely plugging optional, additional hardware into their existing, low-end PC and using the Internet as a means of simulation dissemination, distribution, and delivery means that the user can have immediate access to simulation updates/upgrades and download/access new content (didactic curriculum and cases). Further, this ease of access and use could lead to accelerated adoption and use of simulation within the medical curriculum and this access is provided anywhere in the world 24x7. In addition, once connected, a server-based simulation system would be a natural point for performing easy, automated clinical studies of surgical performance and skills.

Methods

We have ported our open-source mass-spring simulation system ***Spring*** [1,2] to the Maui High Performance Computing Center's (MHPCC) Squall supercomputer. The Squall system is a 2 node x 32 processor IBM SP system. The Squall nodes are 16-way, 375Mhz Nighthawk-2 nodes, each sharing 8Gbytes of shared memory.

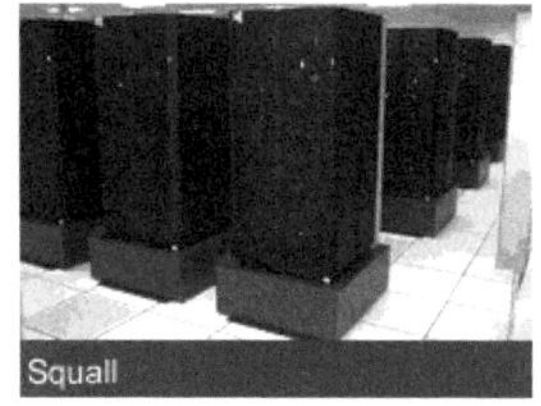

Spring was ported to this platform and to provide a server-based simulation platform for distributed haptics [3] and server-based simulation. Users connect into the server by going to a simple web page. Upon first load, this web page downloads an ActiveX control (ClientServer) to the user's machine which provides for local display and (optionally) haptic device interface. The user then selects the desired training scenario and the ActiveX control connects to the simulation server over TCP/IP. The simulation then receives the current position, orientation, and activation values from the local haptic/interaction device and responds with a reduced

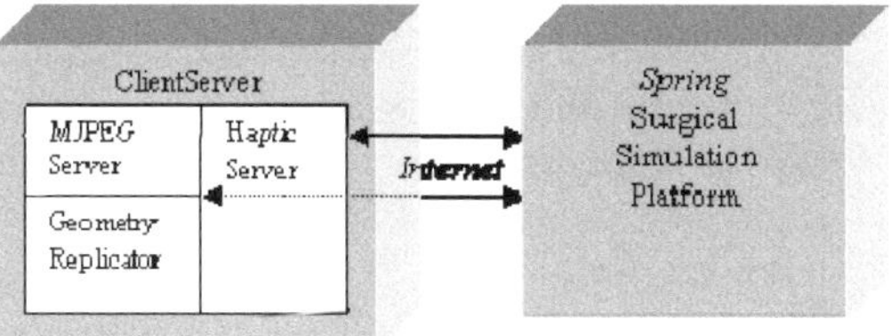

geometric model that the local ClientServer can use to perform simplified local force computation. For display, the simulation server can either stream MJPEG images or geometry information (GeometryReplicator) for local display via the ClientServer as well.

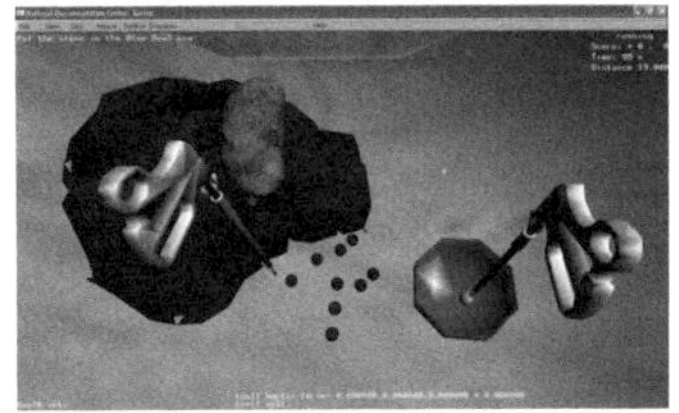

To demonstrate the system, several new training scenarios were developed focusing on simple skills acquisition (manual dexterity task such as dominant and nondominant hand suturing, object extraction and placement tasks, etc). These tasks were demonstrated with near (University of Hawaii colleagues) and far (Stanford University) users.

Preliminary Results

At the time of this abstract, development and refinement of the system continues, but early results of the network performance of the system are presented below:

Test 1: simulation running at MHPCC with haptics at University of Hawaii Telehealth Research Institute (TRI):
Description: simple flat plate for maximum performance
Results:
        Simulation updates per second: 250k
        Haptic device position updates per second: 364k
        Haptic device force updates per second: 96k
Analysis:

This implies that the haptic device was sending 364,000 position values per second, then the simulation was processing 250,000 positions per second (the others are discarded as redundant/old- it uses the most recent values), and the simulator was sending back 96,000 new forces per second. This number is lower because it only is sending forces when the forces actually change (otherwise is a waste of bandwidth). So, this simple simulation server does validate that server-based simulation is possible over a wide area.

Test 2: simulation running at Stanford with haptics at UH TRI:
Description: abdomen dataset with streaming haptics and video
Results:
    Simulation updates per second: 800
    Haptic device position updates per second: 70
    Haptic device force updates per second: 25
Analysis:
    This simulation was much more complex, with full soft tissue modeling, etc. When running, the simulation was performing 800 updates per second and slowed to 650 updates per second when the user grabbed the tissue (aorta) and started distorting it. When he released it, the simulation rate increased again as tissue motion slowed.

These tests validate the technical viability of wide-area networked haptics as a platform for next-generation simulation.

Discussion

These early tests validate that it is technically feasible to construct a Simulation Server and to interact with this server even using haptic interactions over wide-area networking. Moreover, the simulator provided much higher simulation performance than would have been available or affordable locally.

Such a server-based simulation system provides for the lowest entry cost-point possible- only a low-end PC and low-end haptics device are required for accessing and using a simulator of potentially high fidelity. Further, since gaming consoles are typically inexpensive high-performance graphics engines with low-performance computational engines, providing computational power through a distributed processing model outlined here would enable broad use of these platforms as well.

More generally, the distributed processing model allows for a continuum of processing- from more local processing should the local PC be higher performance, to minimal local performance on more computationally limited platforms. Since the system is open standards-based, the local client platform could remain hardware agnostic and use any haptics device from any vendor and use this device with any simulation (just as in the gaming world today where any joystick works with any game).

Even with all these benefits, this distributed, server-based simulator is merely one part of an overall surgical education system- one that provides anatomical information and other curriculum as well as providing for skills-based training, both cognitive and tactile (haptic and non-haptic). The production of a single, centralized surgical education resource at zero cost with little or no capital investment would provide a tremendous benefit to the medical community and could easily integrate all necessary parts of the system, from multimedia curriculum presentation, through cognitive skills training and assessment, through psychomotor skills acquisition and evaluation at an appropriate level of realism to fit the learning tasks desired.

Corollary benefits include centralized administration to ease the logistical support requirements of traditional simulation platforms; the ability for online collaboration, consultation and mentoring; the ability to provide and inexpensively disseminate a standardized surgical education curriculum; the ability to easily conduct large-scale clinical trials to compare surgical skills across groups of distributed individuals and evaluate metrics for surgical performance; and the ability to support a surgical skills authoring system to allow clinical faculty to produce training scenarios with little or no technical assistance. Moreover, to provide all these benefits at little or no cost to the clinical department may be the largest benefit.

Conclusions

As demonstrated above, server-based simulation is a new paradigm in computer-based surgical simulation that is technically feasible and provides many direct and indirect benefits over traditional simulation. Using such a simulation server in the future, clinical faculty may no longer need a team of diverse technical support personnel to enable the deployment of simulation within their department. Providing such a system at no cost and with little or no capital expenditure may allow for the wider and faster deployment of computer-based simulation.

Acknowledgements

The authors would like to thank Chris Aschwanden and Andrei Sherstyuk (UH TRI) and Craig Cornelius and Aneesh Sharma (Stanford) for their hard work on this project. In addition, the ideas put forth in this paper have greatly benefited from discussions with Carla Pugh, Mary Kratz, and many, many others for whom we are profoundly grateful. This work was supported by the Pacific Telehealth and Technology Hui and the National Libraries of Medicine.

References

[1] Montgomery, K; Bruyns, C; Brown, J; Thonier, G; Mazzella, F; Wildermuth, S; Sorkin, S; Tellier, A; Lerman, B; Beedu, B; Latombe, JC, "Spring: A General Framework for Collaborative, Real-time Surgical Simulation", Medicine Meets Virtual Reality (MMVR02), Newport Beach, CA, January 23-26, 2002.
[2] Brown, J; Sorkin, S; Latombe, JC, Montgomery, K; Stephanides, M; "Algorithmic Tools for Real-Time Microsurgery Simulation", Medical Image Analysis, v6(3), September 2002.
[3] Mazzella, F; Montgomery, K; Latombe, JC; "The Forcegrid; A Buffer Structure for Haptic Interaction with Virtual Elastic Objects", 2002 IEEE International Conference on Robotics and Automation, Washington DC, May 11-15, 2002.

Medicine Meets Virtual Reality 14
J.D. Westwood et al. (Eds.)
IOS Press, 2006

Fast Rigid Registration in Radiation Therapy

Ulrich Müller [a,1], Jürgen Hesser [a], Cornelia Walter [b], Barbara Dobler [b],
Frank Lohr [b], Frederik Wenz [b]

[a] *Institute for Computational Medicine, Universities Mannheim and Heidelberg*
[b] *Dept. of Radiation Oncology, Mannheim Medical Center, University of
Heidelberg*

Abstract. Based on a stochastic mutual information type matching and
RPROP as stochastic optimizer, an interactive image-based registration
of a CT volume onto two 2D images provided by a megavoltage system is presented. The matching process is based on semi-automatic pre-
segmentation, an approximate 2D-2D matching with precomputed virtual projections (DRRs) followed by an accurate 3D-2D matching step.
Our sample-based approach requires only a fraction of computed DRRs
for 3D-2D. A simultaneous computation of the DRR rays and their perturbations in 6 dimensions speeds up the rendering process by a factor
of 6.8. The complete registration process takes 5.6 ± 2.3 seconds on a
3 GHz Pentium IV PC, being the fastest non-parallel approach for this
sort of application the authors are aware of.

Keywords. registration, radiotherapy

1. Description of purpose

Image-based navigation during minimally invasive interventions or online registration in radiotherapy is currently of high importance in computer-supported
medicine. Standard imaging systems based on X-ray or ultrasound principles are
used to register the position of a patient in a treatment situation, calculate a possible positioning error and provide a translation vector for position correction. Most
of the systems in current use either need fiducial markers (e.g. Cyberknife^{TM} or
ExacTrac^{TM}) or are still time consuming (volume imaging with cone beam CT).
An image-guided real-time registration would overcome this drawback. Rohlfing
et al. [2] utilize real-time 2D tracking to get 3D-2D registrations within 92 s and
Wein et al. [3] achieve a speed of 1.8-3.2 s with a 12-processor parallel hardware.

Recent developments on an improved version of Viola's *sample-based matching* approach based on *resilient backpropagation* (RPROP) yield fast matching
times provided optimal settings of algorithm parameters. As shown in former
publications [4,5], we are able to find these parameters in interactive time and

---

[1] Correspondence to: Ulrich Müller, Institute for Computational Medicine, B6, 23, 68131
Manheim, Germany; E-mail: ulrich.mueller@ti.uni-mannheim.de

image data dependent. In this paper we concentrate on radiation therapy where we apply 2D-2D and 2D-3D matching in real- or interactive times.

2. Methods

Given a CT volume of size $512 \times 512 \times 48$ with a slice thickness of 10 voxel units and further two 2D projections of size 1024^2 from a megavoltage system with known geometry, an optimal pose $T_{optimal}$ of the projections relative to the volume is searched for.

We apply a two-stage multi-resolution strategy. Images are scaled down to a size of 128^2 pixels, then segmented by a gradient threshold method providing a selection of interesting image pixels for matching, thus reducing the considered data. In addition, an artifact from cross wires used for facilitating manual patient positioning is excluded from that point set. Our registration optimizes the pose T by computing similarity of the greyvalues of the given projections and the digitally reconstructed radiographs (DRRs) of the volume, depending on T. Only pixels of the segmentation point set are considered. This way the two images on the left in Fig. 1 are reduced to sets of 520 and 488 points, mostly being ribcage and sternum pixels. We also downsize the CT volume to size $256 \times 256 \times 48$ voxels.

For the given data, our 3D-2D registration has only a capture range of 5 degrees of rotation and 4 pixels of translation at the smallest image level. To overcome this limitation, we perform a 2D-2D translation matching with precomputed DRRs (see Fig. 1) using normalized mutual information without sampling. Combining the computed 2D translations for each view, we derive the corresponding 3D translation. This way we obtain an initial pose $T^{(0)}$ close enough to $T_{optimal}$ for the 3D-2D matching. Computing $T^{(0)}$ takes 0.22 ± 0.04 seconds.

Starting at $T^{(0)}$, T is updated by the iterative gradient-based stochastic optimizer RPROP. The gradients are computed using the stochastic mutual information (SMI) similarity measure. This means, we use sample sets of image points without the need for computing full DRRs. The optimal sample size for the given data, in this case 100 sample points, is automatically computed once [4]. During each iteration and for every point in the sample seven rendering rays are cast: one for the current 3D-transformation pose, and six for the perturbated rays according to the six dimensions of the rigid search space (three for translation and three for rotation). Casting these seven rays simultaneously significantly cuts rendering time by reducing the memory demand. Since the rays only have subvoxel differences the trilinear interpolation can be done with the same eight vertices around the subvoxel positions, leading to a speedup of factor 6.8 compared to single raycasting.

For each of the two images, an SMI gradient is computed. Due to respiratoy motion the front view images match better than the side view. We account for this by weighting the gradients for the front view. In our experiments, a factor of 3 has lead to the best accuracy of the matching results. The merged gradient serves as input for the RPROP optimizer that updates T. After a registration result on the smallest resolution level is obtained, the registration on the original scale is applied in order to improve accuracy.

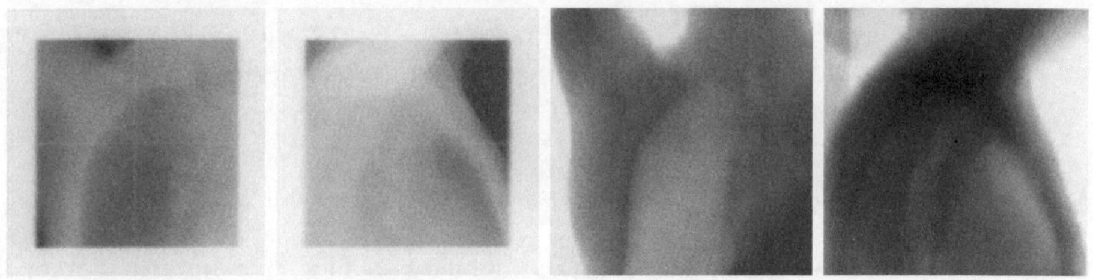

Figure 1. Left: Given projection images, Right: DRRs from the CT volume

3. Results and Conclusion

The evaluation is based on a CT volume of one lung tumor patient and 9 projection pairs of this patient. Automatic selection of optimal optimization parameters for the given data is performed once within 120 seconds. These parameters fit for all 9 registration data sets. After that, matching experiments are performed with randomly chosen initial poses T_{start}.

r_0	good (%)	$d_{xy}(mm)$	$d_z(mm)$	μ_t (s)	σ_t (s)
1	99	1.38	4.94	2.6	0.64
3	95	1.43	5.14	4.7	0.98
4	88	1.51	5.58	6.2	1.76
5	76	1.64	6.73	9.3	3.47
6	53	1.86	8.42	16.7	6.63

Table 1. r_0: angle in degrees for rotation in T_{start}. Results are considered good if the average difference between voxels transformed by T and $T_{optimal}$ is better than 2 mm in the lateral xy-plane of the volume and better than 10 mm along the z-axis. d_{xy}, d_z: voxel accuracy in the xy-plane (z-axis) for good results. μ_t: average matching time on a 3 GHz Pentium IV PC, σ_t: standard deviaton of matching time.

We present an interactive non-parallel PC-based markerless method for 2D-3D matching for radiation therapy data.

References

[1] P. Viola. Alignment by Maximization of Mutual Information. PhD-Thesis, Massachusetts Institute of Technology, 1995.

[2] T. Rohlfing, J. Denzler, D.B. Russakoff, et al. Markerless Real-Time Target Region Tracking: Application to Frameless Sereotactic Radiosurgery. VMV 2004 Proceedings, Stanford, November 16-18, Aka GmbH 2004.

[3] W. Wein, B. Röper, N. Navab. 2D/3D Registration Based on Volume Gradients. SPIE Medical Imaging 2005, Image Processing, Vol. 5747, pp. 144-150.

[4] U. Müller, J. Hesser, R. Männer. Fast Rigid 2D-2D Multimodal Registration. MICCAI 04, LNCS 3216, pp. 887-894, Springer Verlag, 2004.

[5] U. Müller, J. Hesser, R. Männer. Optimal Parameter Choice for Automatic Fast Rigid Multimodal Registration. SPIE Medical Imaging 2005, Image Processing, Vol. 5747, pp. 163-169.

Medicine Meets Virtual Reality 14
J.D. Westwood et al. (Eds.)
IOS Press, 2006

Can Immersive Virtual Reality Reduce Phantom Limb Pain?

Craig D. MURRAY[a], Emma L. PATCHICK[a], Fabrice CAILLETTE[b], Toby
HOWARD[b] and Stephen PETTIFER[b]

[a] School of Psychological Sciences, University of Manchester, United Kingdom
[b] School of Computer Sciences, University of Manchester, United Kingdom

Abstract This paper describes the design and implementation of a case-study
based investigation using immersive virtual reality as a treatment for phantom limb
pain. The authors' work builds upon prior research which has found the use of a
mirror box (where the amputee sees a mirror image of their remaining anatomical
limb in the phenomenal space of their amputated limb) can reduce phantom limb
pain and voluntary movement to paralyzed phantom limbs for some amputees. The
present project involves the transposition of movements made by amputees'
anatomical limb into movements of a virtual limb which is presented in the
phenomenal space of their phantom limb. The three case studies presented here
provide qualitative data which provide tentative support for the use of this system
for phantom pain relief. The authors suggest the need for further research using
control trials.

Keywords Phantom Limb Pain, Amputee, Immersive Virtual Reality

Introduction

Following amputation the amputee commonly experiences the amputated limb as still
intact [1]. The phantom limb is often painful - a problem which can have far-reaching
implications for amputees' lives. For instance, adjustment to amputation is negatively
correlated with levels of phantom limb pain (PLP) [2] and amputees with PLP are less
likely to use a prosthetic limb [3]. Non-prosthesis use often results in the restriction of
normal activities and is associated with higher levels of depression [4,5].

One promising development in the treatment of PLP is the mirror box [6]. This is
created by arranging a mirror in a box in such as way as to allow amputees to view a
reflection of their anatomical upper limb in the visual space occupied by their phantom
limb. For some patients the box is able to induce vivid sensations of movement
originating from the muscles and joints of patients' phantom arms, and to reduce
phantom limb and/or gain control over a paralyzed phantom limb [6-8]. The mirror box
effect may work by providing a means to link the visual and motor systems to help
patients recreate a coherent body image and update internal models of motor control
[9,10]. This suggests that other visual therapies which work in a similar way may also
be of benefit in treating phantom limb pain.

One drawback of the mirror box is that it operates within a narrow spatial
dimension, since it requires the patient to remain in a fairly fixed position with the head
oriented towards the mirror and the body held in mid-saggital plane with the mirror
[11]. It also requires that the user attempts to ignore the intact limb providing the

reflection in order to focus in the image of the phantom limb. These issues make the mirror box a fairly restrictive and tentative illusion. One potential solution to these problems is immersive virtual reality (IVR), which can be used in a similar way to the mirror box whilst allowing far more scope for changes in experimental paradigm [11].

The present research to be described here uses an IVR system which transposes movements of amputee's anatomical limbs into movements of a virtual limb in the phenomenal space occupied by their phantom limb. This gives a similar illusion to the mirror box without the confines imposed by reflection-based work: in the virtual environment (VE) only the virtual phantom limb moves in response to motion of the anatomical limb so the illusion is robust, independent of the orientation or focus of the patient. In the remainder of this paper we outline the preliminary observations of the technology in use and feedback from three participants regarding changes in the phenomenology of their phantom limb or phantom pain. The objectives of the present work are to show proof of principle for the development of this kind of technology for the treatment of phantom limb pain.

1. Description of the virtual environment and virtual tasks

A V6 virtual reality head-mounted display (HMD) is used to present the computer-generated environment to participants and to facilitate immersion. In order to monitor and represent participants' arm/hand/fingers and leg/foot movements movements a 5DT-14 data glove and sensors is used for upper-limb amputees, while sensors alone are used for lower-limb amputees. Sensors are attached to the elbow and wrist joints or the knee and ankle joints. A Polhemus Fastrak monitors head movements and arm and leg movements. A minimal virtual environment (VE) represents the participant within a room, from an embodied point-of-view (see Figure 1).

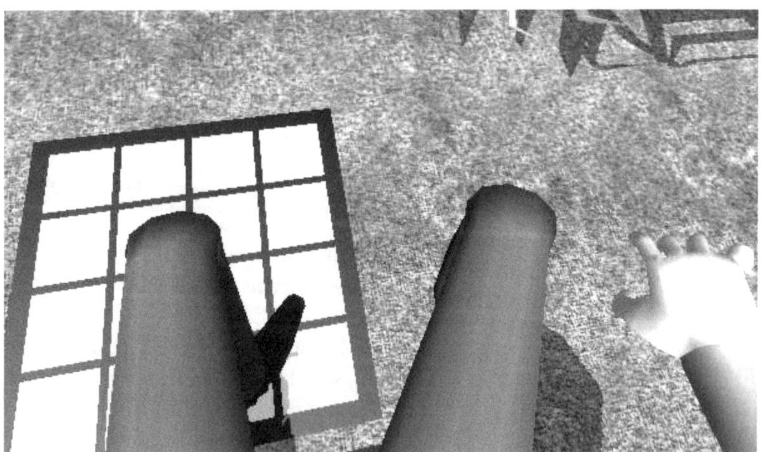

Figure 1. One possible view participants may see when taking part in the experiment

In the present study participants use the IVR system for a period of 30 minutes, completing four tasks in repetitions. A full virtual body representation is provided for participants. A virtual representation of the phantom limb is made available by transposing the movement of the participant's opposite anatomical limb (e.g. their physical left arm) into the phenomenal space of their phantom limb (e.g. their virtual right arm). The tasks are: placing the virtual representation of the phantom limb onto colored tiles which light up in sequence; batting or kicking a virtual ball; tracking the motion of a moving virtual stimulus; and directing a virtual stimulus towards a target.

2. Participants

Participants with severe PLP were recruited through the sub-regional Disablement Services Centre, Manchester. The intensity of the intervention was determined by how often the patients could come for testing since, due to the nature of the equipment, sessions were carried out only at the University of Manchester. All participants are part of an ongoing, longitudinal study which will continue for a minimum of 12 weeks. However, for the purposes of this paper, preliminary indicative qualitative findings are reported here to assess proof of principle for this IVR equipment.

2.1 Case Study One: PK

A 63 year old male left upper-limb amputee (above elbow). He had been an amputee for 12 years and 3 months, as the result of a swimming accident. PK suffered with severe PLP "twenty-four seven – I'm never ever out of pain". His phantom limb was shorter than his anatomical limb in a fixed position with the elbow bent at roughly right angles and the fingers in a cupped position. PK suffered with intense flashes of pain attacks in his phantom which can be very severe; he would often find himself immobilized by the pain. Despite the severity of PK's condition, he insisted on keeping himself busy and, as such, PK came for 5 testing sessions over the 3 week period, with a maximum 5 days in between sessions.

2.2 Case Study Two: WW

A 60 year old male right lower-limb amputee (below knee). He had been an amputee for 12 years and 10 months as the result of a work-related accident. His phantom pain was less severe than PK, but he was still constantly aware of it: "it's always there, like a nagging sensation". The most distressing part of the phantom pain would be the intense flashes of pain he would experience in his phantom foot which felt "as if someone's ramming a sharp knife into the sole". These attacks would vary in frequency but the severity would often interfere with his sleep and his everyday life. WW attended 3 sessions over the course of 3 weeks. The second and third sessions were both carried out two days apart in the same week, two weeks after the first session.

2.3. Case Study Three: DT

DT was a 65 year old female left upper-limb amputee (below elbow). She had been an amputee for 1 year, as the result of a fall. The phantom pain DT experienced is mainly localized to the phantom hand; a constant pins and needles sensation which can vary in severity. DT's phantom hand is immobile with the fingers in a clenched position which is accompanied by a pain she describes as in "…the palm because I think it's like the nails of my fingers digging into my palm." The pain interferes with her sleep on a regular basis. DT has attended only 2 sessions so far in a 3 week period with 2 weeks in between trials.

3. Data Collection

In the present paper we emphasize the importance of achieving a qualitative understanding of patient's phantom limb experience, and of their experience of using the IVR system, in their own words. This is achieved through semi-structured interviews carried out at each session and these interviews provide the core focal point for analysis in this paper, since the authors feel they highlight important aspects of the system which are not encapsulated by quantitative assessment. These interview data are supplemented in the findings reported here, where informative, by pain diaries completed by participants in the interim period between each trial.

4. Indicative Results

During each period of IVR use PK reported a decrease in his phantom limb pain. However, he also reported that this would be accompanied by the pain coming back "with a bit of a vengeance" within a few hours after completion of each testing session. He attributed this to the fact that the pain would be returning after a lull during the sessions which would make the comparative return of the pain seem more severe. During the 3rd session, PK reported vivid sensations of movement in his phantom arm: "During it, I actually felt as if it was my left arm that was doing the work and chasing the ball. My actual phantom arm rather than my right… and that was more like reality than virtual reality." PK commented that "If I could harness that (the movement in his phantom limb) maybe I could open my fingers and ease the cramping pain a little". Interestingly, in the following week to this session, a pain diary measure showed an average rating of 6.8 (out of 10) over the following 3 days, which then increased to an average of 8.3 for the subsequent 3 days. Obviously, this improvement in PLP ratings is short-lived but given the relatively low frequency of testing sessions, this could be considered a promising result. Self-reported evidence from PK suggested a positive change in his sleep patterns after the first session of IVR which has continued throughout the 3 week period: "I've actually been sleeping a little better over the last few days… I'm getting about 5-6 hours of uninterrupted sleep as opposed to 2-3 hours and I'm doing nothing else different in my life except coming here."

WW's results indicate a more variable pattern than PK's. There were no consistent alterations in pain ratings during use of the IVR system for the first two sessions. It is worth mentioning however, that WW did suffer with simulator sickness which meant the first session had to be terminated early. At one point during the second session, his anatomical left leg collided with his stationary prosthetic leg. WW commented that this was an "uneasy sensation… it looks on the thing (HMD) like it's not in the way but then you bang into it and it feels queer." When asked to try and elaborate on this, WW mentioned his phantom pain had increased slightly during this period. This is consistent with research which sites sensory-motor incongruence as a possible source for painful sensations [12]. WW chose to remove his prosthesis for the third session to avoid this situation and consequently, he engaged more in the 3rd session and reported no feelings of nausea for the first time. Interestingly, his pain rating at the end of the session compared to the beginning showed a decrease of 4 points (from a 7 initially to a 3 on leaving). WW also commented that "It feels as though I'm doing something with my right (phantom) leg… It's a queer sensation but it feels good that I'm achieving something with my right leg. That I'm doing the task with my right leg."

DT has attended the fewest number of sessions out of all three participants but interestingly reported a drastic change in her phantom hand after just one session: ".. it's funny… one of my fingers is coming out, sort of pointing out now." When we consider that one of the vivid sensations experienced by DT was that of nails digging into her palm, if this phenomenological change continues, it has the potential to alleviate this pain. DT has also reported vivid sensations of her phantom hand carrying out the tasks and she unconsciously moves the stump of her left arm around whilst carrying out the tasks: "My left arm felt if it was moving… which was quite an odd sensation". She also reports she is tired after sessions and that her left (phantom) arm aches significantly more than her right (the labour intensive arm) after the IVR sessions.

5. Discussion

All participants made some reference to a transferral of sensations into the muscles and joints of the phantom limb. PK and DT support this more vividly than WW and this may indicate the system could potentially be of greater benefit to upper- than lower-limb amputees. This is a tentative claim, however it could be supported by the larger degree of movement afforded by the virtual hand over the virtual foot (i.e. all the fingers move separately whilst for the foot there are no toes – it is represented as if it is wearing a shoe).

DT reports the most drastic change in her phantom limb after just one session. This may indicate that this kind of treatment is more effective for more recent amputees. A speculative hypothesis could explain this in terms of a greater plasticity in the brain for recent amputees as it has had less time to re-define the internal model of the body

All three participants report a decrease in phantom pain during at least one of the sessions. However, another common factor is that they all comment on how they are focused on the tasks which may suggest they are simply distracted from the pain. This evidence stresses the importance of further research using control trials to assess the efficacy of this system over and above any pain relief caused purely by the novelty of the tasks and the concentration required.

Most importantly, the results appear to highlight the necessity for a more intense intervention since the interim pain diaries suggest there is little effect of the sessions beyond a day or two. This is understandable, especially for PK and WW who have suffered with this pain for over 12 years: it would be unreasonable to expect any treatment to have a dramatic effect in such a short space of time.

The authors conclude that these preliminary qualitative findings show sufficient proof of principle to justify further testing with the IVR system using control trials, more intense intervention and a greater number of participants.

Acknowledgement

The work reported in this paper is supported by a grant from Remedi Rehabilitation.

References

[1]   Jensen, T.S., Krebs, B., Nielsen, J. and Rasmussen, P. (1983) Phantom limb, phantom pain and stump pain in amputees during the first 6 months following limb amputation. Pain, 17, 243-256.

[2]   Katz, J. (1992) Psychophysiological contribution to phantom limbs. Canadian Journal of Psychiatry, 37, 282-298.

[3]   Dolezal, J.M., Vernick, S.H., Khan, N., Lutz, D. & Tyndall, C. (1998) Factors associated with use and nonuse of an AK prosthesis in a rural, southern, geriatric population. International Journal of Rehabilitation and Health, 4(4), 245-251

[4]   Murray, C.D. (2005) The social meanings of prosthesis use. Journal of Health Psychology, 10(3), 425-441.

[5]   Ramachandran, V.S. (1993) Filling in the gaps in perception. Part II: Scotomas and phantom limbs. Current Directions in Psychological Science, 2, 56-65.

[6]   Ramachandran, V.S., and Rogers-Ramachandran, D. (1996) Synaesthesia in phantom limbs induced with mirrors. Proceedings of the Royal Society of London, B Biological Sciences, 263, 377-386

[7]   Brodie, E.E., Whyte, A. and Waller, B. (2003) Increased motor control of a phantom leg in humans results from the visual feedback of a virtual leg. Neuroscience Letters, 341(2), 167-169.

[8]   MacLachlan, M., McDDonald, D. and Waloch, J. (2004) Mirror treatment of lower limb phantom pain: a case study. Disability and Rehabilitation, 26, 907-904

[9]   Miall, R.C., and Wolpert, D.M (1996) Forward models for physiological motor control. Neural Networks, 9, 1265-1279

[10] Blakemore, S.J., Wolpert, D. and Frith, C.D. (2002) Abnormalities in the awareness of action. TRENDS in Cognitive Sciences, 6, 237-242

[11] Murray, C.D., Pettifer, S., Caillette, F., Patchick, E. and Howard, T. (2005) Immersive virtual reality as a rehabilitative technology for phantom limb experience. In the proceedings of IWVR 2005: The 4th International Workshop on Virtual Rehabilitation. California. Pp.144-151

[12] McCabe, C.S, Haigh, R.C., Halligan, P. and Blake, D.R. (2005) Simulating sensory-motor incongruence in health volunteers: implications for a cortical model of pain. Rheumatology, 44, 509-516

Medicine Meets Virtual Reality 14
J.D. Westwood et al. (Eds.)
IOS Press, 2006

413

Interactive Simulation Training: Computer Simulated Standardized Patients for Medical Diagnosis

Dale E. Olsen, Ph.D., *SIMmersion LLC*, dale.olsen@simmersion.com
Debbie Sticha, M.B.A., *SIMmersion LLC*, debbie.sticha@simmersion.com

Abstract SIMmersion LLC is a software development company that creates human interactive training simulations. SIMmersion produces PC-based simulations of people with whom trainees are able to hold conversations. Trainees communicate with simulated characters in face-to-face conversations, using voice recognition technology. Topics that would match well with SIMmersion's simulation capabilities include diagnosis of depression, alcoholism, or drug use, grievance counseling, marriage counseling, suicide intervention, and first responder training for biological terrorism. SIMmersion's technology could be integrated with modeling technology to create a speech-interactive, mannequin-based patient simulation system for healthcare training and assessment. Systems currently being developed involve early detection of smallpox as a result of a biological attack.

Problem

SIMmersion LLC, a spin-off of The Johns Hopkins University Applied Physics Laboratory, is a software development company in Columbia, MD that creates human interactive training simulations. The company, in partnership with the National Capital Area Medical Simulation Center and the Henry M. Jackson foundation, was contracted by the Department of Defense to create a medical simulation training module. The contract resulted from the solicitation of the U.S. Army Medical Research and Materiel Command for Training for First Response to Chemical, Biological, Radiological, Nuclear, and Explosive Events.

A prototype simulation was developed to validate the application of SIMmersion simulation technology to the medical training industry and to develop a tool for training complex human interactions, such as those that take place between physicians and patients. Human interactive simulations allow physicians to practice approaching situations that require direct questions that may be uncomfortable, including topics such as a patient's sexual history, history of depression, or drug and alcohol abuse.

The use of highly interactive role-play simulations is known to improve training effectiveness and "boost learning retention rates dramatically"[1]. One common form of experiential learning is human role-playing. One form of training with role-plays is the use of standardized patients in the medical industry. Despite their effectiveness, role-plays demand additional classroom time, and qualified role-players are frequently unavailable. In addition, role-plays do very little to embed the principle being taught because they do not provide repeated practice of skills with consistent, objective feedback to the learner. Since these problems are characteristic of the use of standardized patients, computer simulated standardized patients are being developed to take advantage of their training benefits, and to improve their shortcomings.

Computer-based human interaction training simulations offer several advantages over traditional role-plays since they offers standardized training objectives to all learners in a comprehensive, objective, and uniform manner; they provide immediate and objective feedback to reinforce ideal behavior and correct mistakes for rapid and efficient application of training to real situations; they allow repeated practice to convert newly learned principles into habitual behaviors; and they used vivid characters that make for game-like experiences that hold attention and encourage repeated use.

When developed into a full-featured system, the product will train physicians to accurately diagnose illnesses that could pose a threat to public safety and indicate the presence of bioterrorism agents. Specifically, the simulation will train practitioners to perform efficient and effective exams for the diagnosis of smallpox, chicken pox, Marburg hemorrhagic fever, and Rocky Mountain spotted fever. Future development on a companion system to the current prototype concept may address the differential diagnosis of other bio-terrorism agents. Biological agents under consideration include anthrax, plague, and tularemia, which could initially be mistaken for influenza.

Product

SIMmersion creates PC-based simulations of people with whom trainees are able to hold detailed conversations. These simulations employ human actors in challenging, life-like situations. Trainees communicate with the simulated characters in a face-to-face conversation, using voice recognition technology or a computer mouse to interact. Questions and responses are scripted to emulate what real people would say at any given stage of a conversation. Trainees can select from the scripted questions and the character will respond based on established motives, emotional state, and character state. The result is a nearly free-form conversation that is different with each play of the simulation.

Feedback is available in a variety of ways: an on-screen Intelligent Tutor who provides non-verbal cues, Help buttons that facilitate queries regarding user statements and character responses, numeric scoring, and instant-replay features that enable users to review and analyze portions of their conversation or even the entire dialogue. Since the training simulations are developed based on specific teaching points, it is possible to test the trainee's ability to meet certain lesson objectives; scoring is also built into the system to assess a trainee's proficiency level.

Results

SIMmersion hypothesizes that the computer simulated patients developed in human interactive training simulations will be a superior alternative to the current practice of using standardized patients. The most significant drawbacks to standardized patient training are time and money, specifically, the amount of time required for clinicians to train and the associated expenses. Computer simulated standardized patients also afford consistency over time and allow trainees to practice the simulation an unlimited number of times in a variety of environments. A research study will be conducted once the full multimedia version of the simulation is complete. The study will test the efficacy of the computer simulated patient in comparison with other training methods. The desired outcome is that the computer simulated patient is more effective than standard e-learning or lecture training.

Research conducted on simulation training programs previously developed by SIMmersion indicates improvement in skill level and information retention as well as a high level of user interest. To standardize FBI interview training curriculum for new agents, SIMmersion developed the *Mike Simmen Criminal Investigation* simulation. A study conducted by the FBI on the effectiveness of this simulation found that trainees improved their scores for identification of clues of deception and truthfulness by thirty percent and their overall interview scores by sixteen percent between the first and second simulated interviews. The study found that new agent trainees who were required to conduct only two simulated interviews actually spent their own time conducting an average of five additional interviews with *Mike Simmen*. In all, over sixty percent of the time trainees spent interviewing *Mike Simmen* was voluntary[2].

Discussion

Success in this effort is likely to open the door to many new research projects with the potential to radically change the way that medical education is delivered. Topics that match well with SIMmersion's simulation capabilities include diagnosis of depression, alcoholism, or drug use, grievance counseling, marriage counseling, and suicide intervention.

SIMmersion technology can be integrated with technology available elsewhere to create a speech-interactive mannequin-based patient simulation system for healthcare training and assessment. Trainees will not only be able to practice hands-on assessment skills with the patient and treatment interventions, but also practice their skills in patient interviews through SIMmersion's interactive simulation technology. The mannequin system would emulate human behavior using an interactive computer simulated person in a realistic scenario with a realistic, interactive patient.

1. This work is supported by the U.S. Army Medical Research and Materiel Command under Contract No. W81XWH-050C-0042. The views, opinions, and findings contained in this report are those of the authors and should not be construed as an official Department of the Army position, policy, or decision unless so designated by other documentation.

References

[1]　Boehle, S. Simulations: The Next Generation of E-Learning. *Training.* **42,1** (2005).

[2]　Olsen, D. E, Phillips, R. G., Sellers, W. A. "The Simulation of A Human Subject For Interpersonal Skill Training." Interservice/Industrial Training, Simulation and Education Conference, December 1999.

Medicine Meets Virtual Reality 14
J.D. Westwood et al. (Eds.)
IOS Press, 2006

Soft-Tissue Balance Evaluation System for Total Hip Arthroplasty by Intraoperative Contact Pressure Measurement at the Hip Joint

Yoshito OTAKE[a,1], Naoki SUZUKI[a], Asaki HATTORI[a], Mitsuhiro HAYASHIBE[a], Hidenobu MIKI[b], Mitsuyoshi YAMAMURA[c], Nobuhiko SUGANO[b], Kazuo YONENOBU[d], Takahiro OCHI[e]

[a]*Institute for High Dimensional Medical Imaging, Jikei University School of Medicine*
4-11-1, Izumi Honcho, Komae-shi, 201-8461, Tokyo, Japan
[b]*Department of Orthopaedic Surgery, Osaka Univ. Grad. Sch. of Med.*
2-2 Yamadaoka, Suita 565-0871, Osaka, Japan
[c]*Kyowa-kai Hospital*
1-24-1 Kishibe-kita, Suita 564-0001, Osaka, Japan
[d]*Department of Orthopaedic Surgery, Osaka Minami National Hospital*
2-1 Kidohigasi-machi, Kawachinagano 586-0008, Osaka, Japan
[e]*Sagamihara National Hospital*
18-1 Sakuradai, Sagamihara-shi, 228-8522, Kanagawa, Japan

Abstract. We developed a system for measurement of contact pressure at the hip joint surfaces that enables checking of the artificial hip joint condition during surgery. First, we constructed the pressure sensor that forms the artificial joint. We installed eight small pressure sensors to the spherical head component, a part of the ball-socket joint. Next, we developed software for recording and visualizing the detected pressures that were recorded every 1ms. The pressure distribution was displayed with the 3D computer graphics in real-time. The system enabled intuitive recognition of pressure direction 3-dimensions. Next, using the system, we conducted measurements during total hip arthroplasty. Although it requires some improvements in its measurement accuracy, the system allows real-time acquisition of information on the artificial hip joint in real-time. Further improvements of the calibration method should enable more accurate measurements. As a complete system, it will be a useful tool for selecting an appropriate implant that fits a patient's hip joint or for estimating the risk of complications after surgery.

Keywords. Total hip arthroplasty, Contact pressure, Four-dimensional muscle model, Pressure measurement system.

1. Introduction

Total hip arthroplasty (THA) is a surgical procedure, in which the diseased parts of the hip joint are removed and replaced with new artificial parts. In this surgery, selection of size and type of implant according to anatomical characteristics of an individual patient is important in order to avoid postoperative complications such as dislocation or loosening. In a recent study [1], a 3-dimensional skeletal model made from CT data of a patient was used to select the proper implant with optimal fit, and such system has been applied to clinical use. According to results of a cadaver experiment by Bartz et al.[2], the primary mechanisms of dislocation after THA could be classified into the following 3 groups: impingement of the femoral neck on the cup liner, impingement of the femur on the pelvis, and spontaneous dislocation due to excessive external force against the muscular force. Regarding the first two groups, the surgical planning system using geometric structure data of the hard tissues from CT data allows estimation of proper implant and avoiding impingement. On the other side, as with the last mentioned mechanism, the causes of dislocation do not depend only on the hard tissue alignment (including anatomical structure of bones or position of implants), but also on soft-tissues around the joint. These facts imply that forces induced from the surrounding soft-tissues, i.e. muscles, tendons or ligaments, or condition of the articular cartilage also affect risk of dislocation. Therefore, we considered that if such forces were measured intraoperatively before implant fixation, the measurements would add important information for choosing the best-fit implant for each patient.

The purpose of this study was to develop a soft-tissue balance evaluation system, which would be able to intraoperatively measure contact pressures at the sliding surfaces and evaluate the balance of forces induced by soft-tissues surrounding the joint. By using the system together with preoperative CT-based planning systems, surgeons would be able to select an optimal implant, whose size and type fit each patient and thus, the risk of postoperative complications would be reduced.

2. Methods

First, customized femoral head component was designed using 3D CAD system, in order to embed 8 pressure sensors, including their wirings, under the spherical surface of the implant (Fig.1).

Next, the physical model was manufactured with ABS plastic from the CAD data by using laminate molding technique. Eight subminiature pressure sensors were

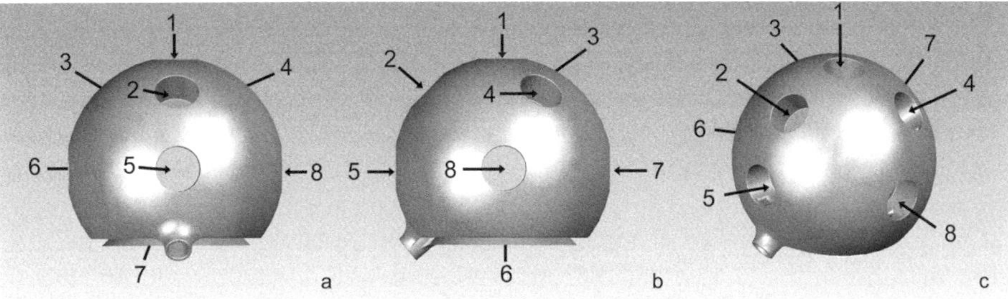

Fig.1 Customized femoral head component, CAD data. The head component was designed using 3D CAD system to embed 8 pressure sensors, including their wiring, under the spherical surface. (a) front view (b) right side view (c) view from an angle. The numbers indicate positions where the sensors were embed.

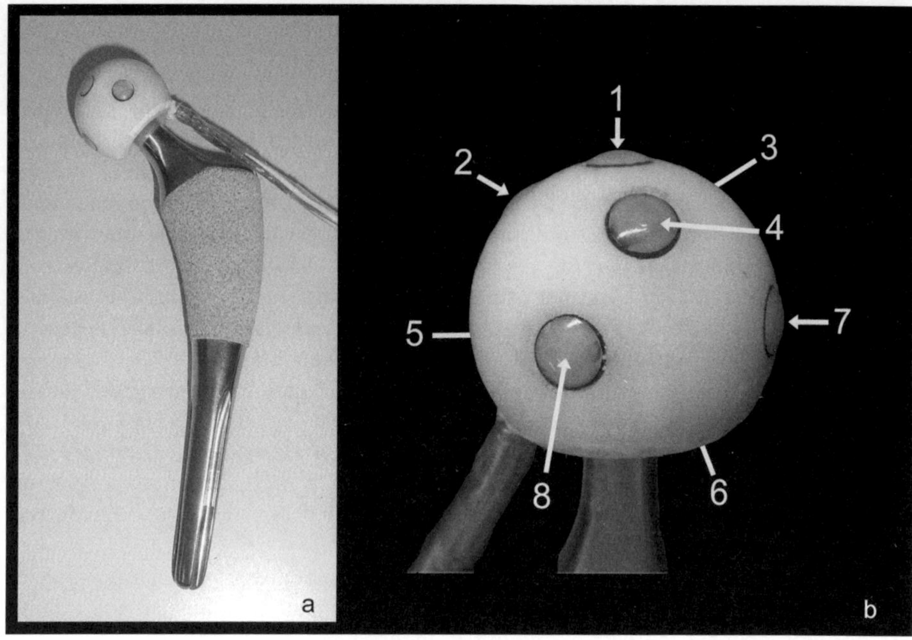

Fig.2. The physical model manufactured with ABS plastic from the 3D CAD data by using laminate molding technique. (a) shows a sensor unit with a stem inserted to the femur. (b) shows a close-up view of the sensor unit. The number in (b) indicates the position of each sensor.

embedded in the customized head and pressure sensing diaphragms covered with spherical ABS plastic parts were used to reduce friction against the cup component during movement (Fig.2). The wirings were assembled to one point on the rim of the head component in order to avoid disturbing the movement during measurements and were waterproofed with silicone and fine poly tube. Similarly, all other sensor parts were waterproofed with silicone and the whole sensor unit was sterilizable. The sensor unit and the other non-sterilizable devices such as personal computer or A/D converter were connected by an easy handling connector for quick connection before measurements during surgery.

The software that controls measurement system, displays the measured data and records them was also developed. The pressure values and 3-dimensional directions were recorded at 1000Hz frequency. Direction of the forces could be intuitively assumed by surgeons with the help of 3D computer graphics. The movie clip which was taken by digital video camera in sync with the pressure data was also recorded by the developed software (Fig.3).

The system was evaluated in a clinical trial. In order to measure soft tissue balance under anesthesia, the pressure sensors were utilized after anesthesia and just before insertion of the implant's femoral head. Pressures at the hip joint surface were measured at 17 hip positions. Since the hip joint angle at each hip position was measured quantitatively by using surgical navigation system, surgeon could evaluate the relationship between the given pressure at the hip joint and the hip position for each patient.

3. Results

Fig.1 shows the CAD data used for design and construction of the customized femoral head component. Fig.2 depicts the manufactured physical model including 8 pressure sensors and waterproofed wiring. Fig.3 shows the display of the operating software.

The results of the clinical trial are presented in Fig.4 and Fig.5. Fig.4 demonstrates a view of an intraoperative pressure measurement. All subminiature pressure sensors were fully operatable during surgery and pressures at the 17 hip positions were recorded. Fig.5 shows the measured pressure at a certain moment. The skeletal structure model constructed from the patient CT data was simultaneously visualized on a computer monitor. The red arrow indicates the direction and the intensity of the pressure. Hip joint angle was measured by surgical navigation system which records in sync with the pressure value.

4. Conclusions

We developed a novel system, which analyses pressure distribution on the femoral head component in real-time during THA. By using the system, surgeons could evaluate the soft-tissue balance around the hip joint and select an implant best fitted for each individual patient from a few alternatives chosen by preoperative CT-based

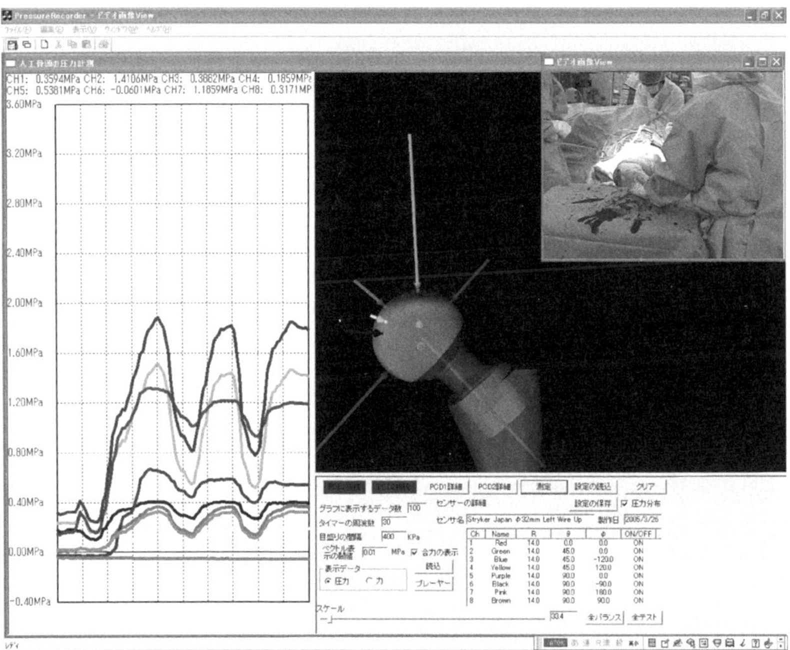

Fig.3 The software that controls the measurement system, displays the measured data and records them. The pressure values and directions were recorded at 1000Hz frequency and 3-dimensionally. Direction of the forces could be intuitively assumed by surgeons with the help of 3D computer graphics.

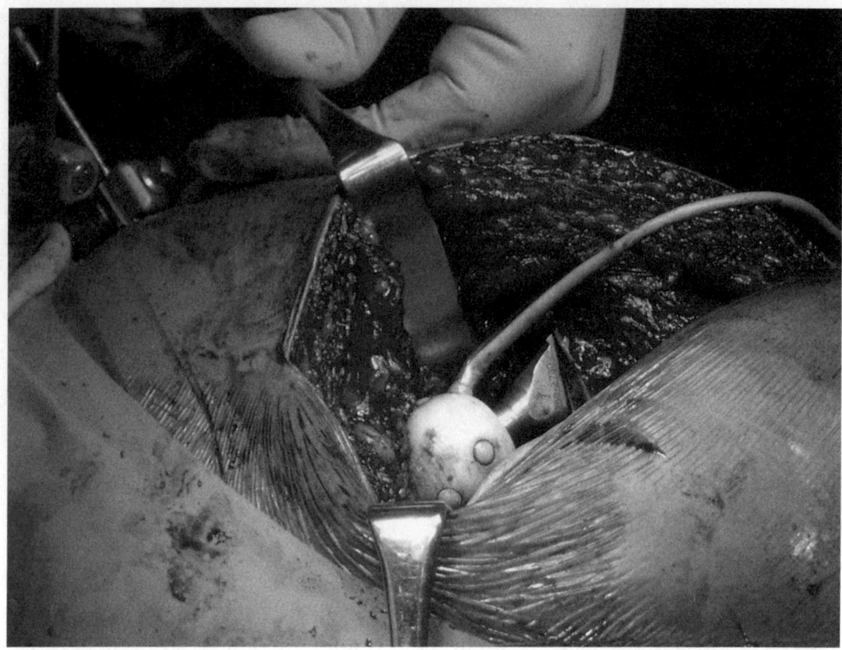

Fig.4 A view of installed pressure sensor during surgery. The sensor parts including wiring were sterilized prior to surgery. The sterilized part and non-sterilized part such as personal computer or A/D converter could be easily connected during surgery.

planning system. Furthermore, we integrated our pressure distribution analysis system with surgical navigation system and simultaneously measured hip joint angles and pressures originating from the joint-supporting soft tissue. In the next step we will integrate this measurement system with a simulation system (now under development) for estimation of post-operative daily motion of a patient after THA [3][4].

Although it requires some improvements in its measurement accuracy, the system acquires information about the installed artificial hip joint state in real-time. Further development of the calibration method should enable more accurate measurements. The improvements will make the system a useful tool for selecting the appropriate implant that best fits an individual patient. Estimation of the risk of complications after surgery and joint dislocation mechanism will be also possible.

References

[1] N.Sugano, K.Ohzono, T.Nishii, K.Haraguchi, T.Sakai, T.Ochi: Computed-Tomography-Based Computer Preoperative Planning for Total Hip Arthroplasty, Computer Aided Surgery, vol. 3, pp. 320-324, 1998

[2] Bartz, R.L., Noble, P.C., Kadakia, N.R., Tullos, H.S.: The Effect of Femoral Component Head Size on Posterior Dislocation of the Artificial Hip Joint, Journal of Bone and Joint Surgery 82-A(9), 1300-1307, 2000

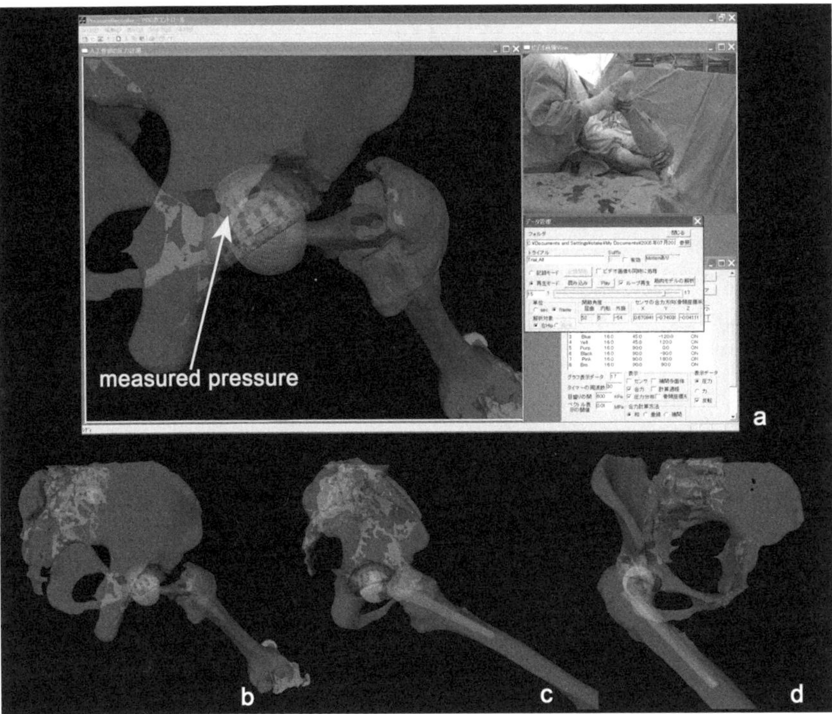

Fig.5 Display of measured pressure at a certain moment. (a) shows the computer display of the software. The red arrow in the left side window indicates direction and intensity of the pressure. (b), (c) and (d) show the 3D view from diagonally backward, right side and diagonally forward.

[3] Y.Otake, K.Hagio, N.Suzuki, A.Hattori, N.Sugano, K.Yonenobu, T.Ochi: Four-dimensional Lower Extremity Model of the Patient after Total Hip Arthroplasty, Journal of Biomechanics, vol.38, pp.2397-2405, 2005

[4] Y.Otake, N. Suzuki, A. Hattori, H. Miki, M. Yamamura, N.Nakamura, N. Sugano, K. Yonenobu, T. Ochi: Estimation of Dislocation after Total Hip Arthroplasty by 4-Dimensional Hip Motion Analysis, Studies In Health Technology and Informatics vol.111, pp.372-377, 2005.

Medicine Meets Virtual Reality 14
J.D. Westwood et al. (Eds.)
IOS Press, 2006

Algorithmically Generated Music Enhances VR Nephron Simulation

PANAIOTIS [a,b], Victor VERGARA [b], Andrei SHERSTYUK [d], Kathleen KIHMM [d],
Stanley M. Saiki [d,e], Dale ALVERSON [c], Thomas P. CAUDELL [b]
Univ. of New Mexico—[a] Dept. of Music, [b] Dept. of Electrical and Computer Eng., [c]
Health Sciences Center
Univ. of Hawaii—[d] Telemedicine and Simulation, [e] School of Medicine

Abstract. While sonification has enjoyed much attention in VR simulation studies, music has generally been incorporated as ambiance. This is partially due to difficulties with manipulating it interactively in real-time while maintaining a sensible musicality. This paper discusses how algorithmically generated music is used to provide ambiance, characterize the visual representation of molecular particle flow, provide orientation cues to the user, and enhance recognition of chemical gradient balances in a reified model of the kidney nephron. The technical obstacles related to the use of music in this context are also addressed.

Keywords. Kidney, nephron, music, virtual reality, medical education, sonfication, musification, algorithmic music, games

Introduction

The medical benefits of VR simulation technologies range from helping teachers explain difficult concepts to assisting surgeons perform difficult procedures. While much of the VR technology research has favored visualization, multi-sensorial systems are currently on the rise. Within these systems, sonification [1] has enjoyed attention in VR simulation development, but music has generally been incorporated only as ambiance. This is partially due to difficulties with manipulating a musically structured system interactively in real-time while maintaining a sensible musicality, and partially due to the tendency for engineers and not trained musicians to be engaged in this research. This paper discusses how algorithmically generated music is used in a kidney nephron simulation to provide ambiance, characterize the visual representation of molecular particle flow, provide orientation cues to the user, and enhance recognition of chemical gradient balances in an educational VR immersion. Some of the technical issues related to the use of music in this context are also addressed.

Project TOUCH (Telehealth Outreach for Unified Community Health) is a multi-year collaboration between the Schools of Medicine at the University of Hawaii and University of New Mexico. A reified kidney nephron served as one of several models for the application of virtual reality and simulation technologies [2].

1. Tools

The development tool used for the Nephron simulation model is Flatland, an open-source visualization and virtual reality application development tool created at the University of New Mexico ([3] and [4]). Flatland provides the facilities for the creation of multi-sensorial virtual environments that enhance human understanding of complex data. It allows software authors to construct and users to interact with arbitrarily complex graphical and aural representations of data. The paradigm is that a user travels through and explores the data, which reveals itself and its derivation with sight and sound (Figure 1).

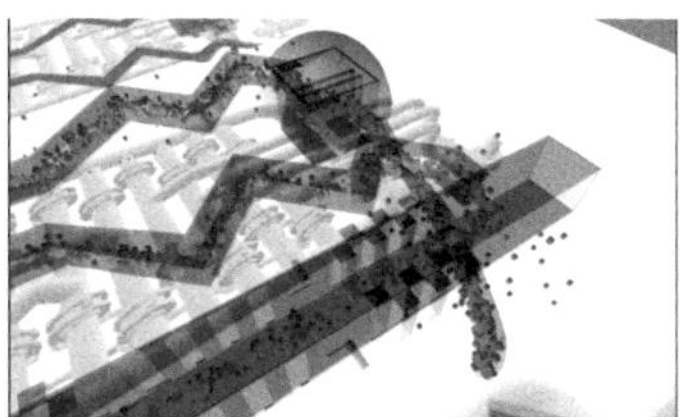

Figure 1. 3D view of the Nephron visualization model within the Flatland environment.

The Flatland sound server is an independent application module designed to handle basic sound-related tasks with a minimum strain on CPU resources [5]. However, some tasks may overburden a single computer, while others require specialized processing. For this reason Flatland's sound server architecture is modular and extensible, providing developers the possibility of using their preferred sound and music generating software and hardware on independent systems, including networked computers and hardware synthesizers.

The preferred sound and music generating software used for the nephron project is Max/MSP [6], a commercially available program designed to create music algorithmically by providing code primitives in an extensible, graphic object-oriented programming environment. Like Flatland, Max/MSP is a run-time engine that allows developers to create their own applications that use it, such as SoundCycler (Figure 2).

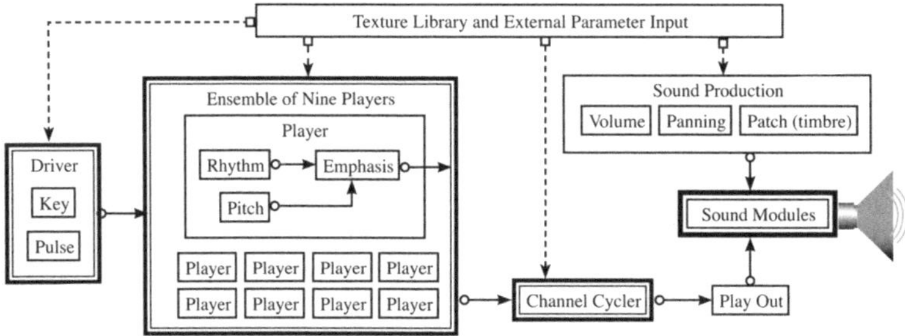

Figure 2. SoundCycler architecture.

SoundCycler, developed by the primary author of this paper, creates algorithmically generated music based on interlocking cycles of independent musical parameters (pitch, rhythm, emphasis, timbre, and space). It can be compared to an ensemble of nine independent players synchronized through a common conductor. Each player has its own cyclic pattern of rhythm, pitch, and emphasis. The result is a music texture that maintains a strong singular identity, but whose details are in constant flux. SoundCycler is capable of creating highly structured, rich music.

Aside from the parameters that govern the musical behavior of each player, some or all players of the ensemble may share global parameters. These include tempo and a common beat, key (pitch level), volume, spatial position and movement, and timbre (instrument). While unusual, it is possible for ten ensembles to play concurrently, providing a virtual orchestra of ninety coordinated players. In the nephron simulation, each ensemble performs an independent and exclusive role.

2. Approach

2.1. Algorithmic music generated in real time

SoundCycler textures are algorithmically generated in real-time, and all parameters are externally accessible and may be manipulated independently of each other (Table 1). This allows subtle and not-so-subtle changes that maintain relevant distinctive features while generating enough continual change to provide freshness.

Table 1. Musical parameters potentially manipulated by external data.

Global Parameters	Texture Component Parameters
• Feel of meter and beat • Harmonic underpinning • Key center • Density	• Melodic contours and patterns • Presence and volume • Density • Rhythmic patterns • Instrumentation

Music has four functions in the nephron VR simulation:
1. Music characterizes the data and components of the environment
2. Music provides an ambience in the listening environment conducive to the task at hand
3. Music provides orientation cues for the user
4. Music provides a means to analyze the data.

The first two of these are a combined consideration. In the case of the first order nephron simulation, it is assumed that the kidney is a healthy example. The music is upbeat and provides ambient music that characterizes particle motion, the level of detail in which the student is immersed.

2.2. Nephron Components

While it is possible to *musify* user activity and choices [7], this project does not call for such treatment. There are three primary components of the simulation that offer the possibility to use sound: individual nephron segments that users put together from a tool chest of nephron parts, various active and passive osmotic pumps, and particles representing chemical activity. The metaphor for the visual design is industrial ductwork. The music that represents the sonic metaphor correlates to this visualization, but also incorporates the particle level of the immersion. Because the chemical gradient activity is the primary educational focus of the model, music representing this activity serves as the basis of the sound and music design.

User manipulation of the nephron pieces are heard as clunks and clinks when they are picked up and put in place. This sonfication provides feedback that users have grabbed, moved, and released objects. Passive chemical pumps are similarly sonified since users directly manipulate them.

The active sodium pumps create an auditory bridge between sonfication and musification. They have a cyclic pattern of sounds that are coordinated with the animation of the pumps, but they are also musically linked to the texture representing the segment to which they are attached. An industrial pump cycle was created using three discrete sounds, each representing different parts of the cycle.

2.3. Nephron Music Textures

Musical textures representing nephron segments are the central sound component of the simulation and provide the ambience and orientation cues that characterize the particle activity and features of each segment. The textures have varying degrees of common elements that unify the overall musical palette.

Each musical texture is created with nine SoundCycler "players." Some of these players represent particular levels of chemicals while others provide a distinct character for a particular nephron segment. There are seven process segments of the nephron: glomerulus; proximal and distal convoluted tubules; descending, lower, and ascending Loop of Henle; and the collecting duct (Figure 3). In addition to these, there is a music texture played when students are not in proximity to any particular segment.

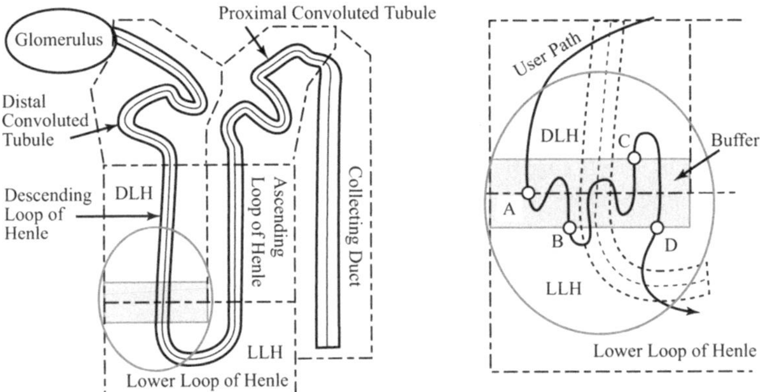

Figure 3. Left: regions (dotted rectangles) representing the nephron segments and region areas. Right: border between two segments and a possible user path.

Features that denote characteristic anatomical concepts with parallel musical ideas provide users with distinct localization cues that assist their orientation within the model. For example, music for the descending Loop of Henle features prominently descending melodic patterns. The same general texture is used for the lower Loop of Henle, but melodic movement is static. Music representing the ascending Loop of Henle is the same as that of the descending loop, except that its melodic patterns ascend.

Information that augments understanding of the chemical gradient activity is also encoded in the music. Particular SoundCycler players represent primary nutrient or electrolyte compositions associated with the filtration process: HCO_3, sodium, potassium, urea, glucose, creatinine, and chlorine. As students explore the nephron, the volume (loudness) of each player is scaled according to the filtration concentration in each segment (Figure 4). Visual elements of the VR simulation parallel this process; duality of sensory data reinforces the experience.

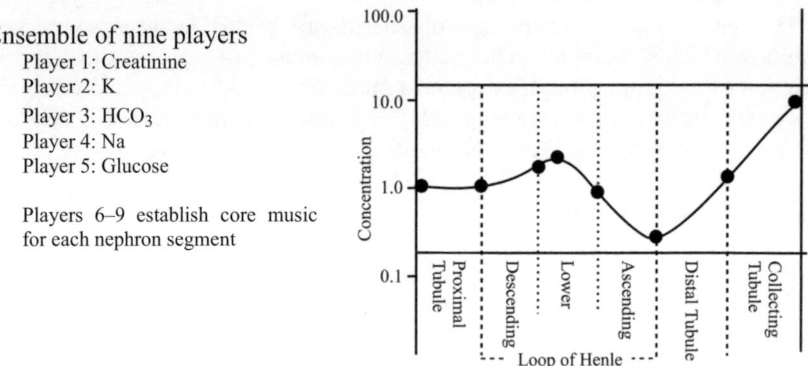

Figure 4. Loudness of each player associated with nutrient or electrolyte composition is scaled according to the filtration concentration in each segment. (Filtration concentrations are adapted from Banasik [8].)

2.4. Transitions

An issue that comes up is the potential difficulty if someone moves rapidly in and out of different regions associated with disparate textures. Such quick or erratic movement can become musically disorienting—even cacophonous, especially if there are many such changes in rapid succession. Two primary software mechanisms address this situation: a delay is imposed before a subsequent music texture begins, and a threshold buffer zone is defined between segment regions (Figure 3).

When a user passes from one region to another, SoundCycler resolves potentially undesirable rhythmic discontinuities between the textures by timing changes to coincide with rhythmic activity. In addition, a five second built-in delay then disables further texture swaps until the new one has been musically established.

Referring to Figure 3 as an example, as long as the user remains in the descending Loop of Henle region, its associated music is played. The music changes to LLH when the user passes through point B, not A. Likewise, as the user continues, the music will change back to DLH after passing point C, and then to LLH after D. However, this is true only if five seconds lapses between points B and C. The switching mechanism is delayed, and appropriate changes are made only after the delay of a previous change and upon evaluating the user's position after the delay. If, for example, the user moves along the path from B through C and D within five seconds, the music will have changed only once: from DLH to LLH. This prevents drastic musical changes from being made if the user is moving quickly or erratically through the environment, or if they are simply straddling the threshold between two regions.

3. Future Work and Conclusion

Music created algorithmically for the nephron suggests how encoding information in musically structured systems may be a powerful tool for analysis and learning. Additional testing is needed to codify and systematize techniques and application of music in VR simulation and modeling. Software that provides musicians and non-musicians the ability to create appropriate music beyond ambiance can facilitate development of VR simulations that encode data. Studies that verify cognitive development and learning using algorithmically generated music may further validate the need for the participation of musicians for virtual environment development.

Acknowledgements

This publication was made possible by Prime Contract No. V549P-4828-02 from the Pacific Telehealth and Technology Hui. Its contents are solely the responsibility of the authors and do not necessarily represent the official views of the Pacific Telehealth and Technology Hui or the US Department of Defense.

References

[1]   Gregory Kramer, ed. *Auditory Display: Sonification, Audification, and Auditory Interfaces*. Reading, MA. Addison-Wesley, 1994.

[2]   Dale C. Alverson, S. M. Saiki Jr., T. P. Caudell, T. Goldsmith, S. Stevens, L. Saland, K. Colleran, J. Brandt, L. Danielson, L. Cerilli, A. Harris, M. C. Gregory, R. Stewart, J. Norenberg, G. Shuster, Panaiotis, J. Holten, III, V. M. Vergara, A. Sherstyuk, K. Kihmm, J. Lui, A. Wang "Reification of Abstract Concepts to Improve Comprehension Using Interactive Virtual Environments and a Knowledge-Based Design: a Renal Physiology Model." *MMVR 14 Proceedings*, IOC Press, The Netherlands, 2006.

[3]   Dale C. Alverson, S. M. Saiki Jr., T. P. Caudell, K. Summers, Panaiotis, A. Sherstyuk, D. Nickles, J. Holten, T. Goldsmith, S. Stevens, S. Mennin, S. Kalishman, Jan Mines, Lisa Serna, S. Mitchell, M. Lindberg, J. Jacobs, C. Nakatsu, S. Lozanoff, D. S. Wax, L. Saland, J. Norenberg, G. Shuster, M. Keep, R. Baker, R. Stewart, K. Kihmm, M. Bowyer, A. Liu, G. Muniz, R. Coulter, C. Maris, D. Wilks, "Distributed Immersive Virtual Reality Simulation Development for Medical Education." *JIAMSE* 2005, Vol. 15, page 19.

[4]   Caudell, T.P, Summers*, K.L., Holten*, J., Hakamata*, T. Mowafi*, M., Jacobs, J., Lozanoff, B.K., Lozanoff, S., Wilks, D., Keep, M.F., S., Saiki, S, Alverson, A., "Virtual Patient Simulator for Distributed Collaborative Medical Education", The Anatomical Record (Part B: New Anat.) V. 270B, pp. 23-29 (Jan., 2003)

[5]   Victor M. Vergara, Panaiotis, T. Eyring, J. Greenfield, K. L. Summers, and T. P. Caudell, "Flatland Sound Services Design Supports Virtual Medical Training Simulations." *MMVR 14 Proceedings*, IOC Press, The Netherlands, 2006.

[6]   Miller Puckette, David Zicarelli, et al., Max/MSP. IRCAM and Cycling74.

[7]   Panaiotis, S. Smith, V. E. Vergara, S. Xia, T. P. Caudell, "Algorithmically Generated Music Enhances VR Decision Support Tool," Science and Technology for Chem-Bio Information Systems (S&T CBIS) Conference, Oct. 2005.

[8]   Jacquelyn L. Banasik. *Pathophysiology: Biological and Behavioral Perspectives*, Chapter 26: "Renal Function," 2nd ed. Philadelphia, W.B. Saunders Company, 2000, pages 626-648.

Medicine Meets Virtual Reality 14
J.D. Westwood et al. (Eds.)
IOS Press, 2006

Haptic Device for a Ventricular Shunt Insertion Simulator

Bundit PANCHAPHONGSAPHAK[a], Diego STUTZER[a], Etienne SCHWYTER[a],
René-Ludwig BERNAYS[b], and Robert RIENER[a,c]
[a]*Automatic Control Laboratory, ETH Zurich, Switzerland*
[b]*Neurosurgical Clinic, University Hospital Zurich, Switzerland*
[c]*Spinal Cord Injury Center, Balgrist University Hospital, Zurich, Switzerland*

Abstract. In this paper we propose a new one-degree-of-freedom haptic device that can be used to simulate ventricular shunt insertion procedures. The device is used together with the BRAINTRAIN training simulator developed for neuroscience education, neurological data visualization and surgical planning. The design of the haptic device is based on a push-pull cable concept. The rendered forces produced by a linear motor connected at one end of the cable are transferred to the user via a sliding mechanism at the end-effector located at the other end of the cable. The end-effector provides the range of movement up to 12 cm. The force is controlled by an open-loop impedance algorithm and can become up to 15 N.

Keywords. haptic display, ventricular shunt insertion, surgical planning simulator

Introduction

Ventricular shunt insertion is a common neurosurgical treatment, which is frequently performed in patients with increased intracranial pressure (ICP) of the brain. The high pressure results from an abnormal accumulation of cerebrospinal fluid (CSF) in the ventricles. A ventricular catheter is a flexible tube that can be inserted into the anterior horn of the lateral ventricle in order to provide a bypass reducing the ICP. A major problem is the misplacement of the catheter tip, often observed when the operation is performed by inexperienced neurosurgeons. The misplacement can result in operation failures, brain tissue damages, and irreversible impairments. To reduce the error rate and to optimize the clinical outcomes, an adequate amount of training and a good preoperative planning are required.

In this article, we present a new 1-dof haptic device that can be used to simulate the ventricular shunt insertion process. The device is intended to be incorporated into the virtual reality (VR) training simulator developed for neuroscience education, neurological data visualization and surgical planning, called BRAINTRAIN simulator [1-2].

The BRAINTRAIN simulator has been developed on the basis of the passive haptic feedback approach, which provides force and tactile feedback to the user via the physical qualities of a tangible interface device between the user and the virtual environment (VE) [3]. The setup of the BRAINTRAIN simulator consists of a plastic model of the brain mounted on a ground-fixed 6-DOF force-torque sensor. Based on a particular real-time force-torque sensing technique [1], the system can detect the position, the orientation, and the amount of force applied by a user, either with a finger or with a medical device such as a ventricular shunt catheter. Although the passive haptic feedback approach can provide satisfactory force and tactile sensations, this approach and the contact sensing algorithm are limited to non-deformable objects and non-destructive applications. This makes the system impractical for simulation of surgical interventions such as a ventricular shunt insertion. To eliminate this limitation, we propose to use a special 1-dof haptic device that produces additional feeling of insertion, when pressing it against the hard surface of the brain model.

1. Methods

The 1-dof haptic device (Figure 1) aims to provide realistic force and position feedback during simulated shunt insertion processes. The design of the device is based on a push-pull cable system. The end-effector of the device comprises four tiny guiding rods and a device holder which slides along these guiding rods. The holder is connected to the actuating cable and is driven by a linear motor mounted at the other end of the cable. While simulating the force and kinematic feedback, forces and movements produced by the linear motor is transmitted to the user via the holder (Figure 1, right).

The rendered force and position are controlled by an open-loop impedance algorithm [4], based on the predefined mechanical properties of the brain tissue. The positions of the holder are recorded by an internal sensor embedded the linear motor. Due to the limitations of the cable system, we can only simulate the insertion process allowing the user only to insert the catheter into the brain.

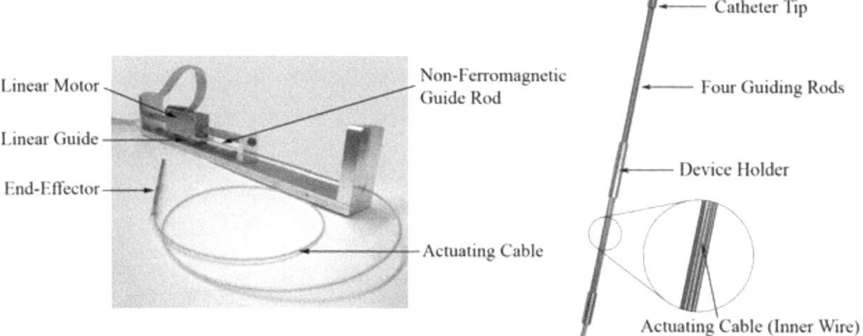

Figure 1. The components of the 1-dof haptic device

2. Results

The maximum range of movement provided by the device is 12 cm and the device can produce feedback forces up to 15 N. While performing the insertion procedure, the user should hold the device and pushes the tip of the device against the brain model. The location of the contact point on the brain model and the spatial orientation of the device are detected by the algorithm inside BRAINTRAIN simulator. All kinematics and geometric data are used to drive a graphical animation of the procedure. The user can see not only the catheter and the brain surface but also internal brain areas such as the ventricles and the catheter tip how it is approaching the anterior ventricular horn (Figure 2). Preliminary tests with this device showed a satisfactory haptic rendering performance. Although the forces produced by the device are deviated from the desired force within 20%, it can provide nice feeling of insertion to the user.

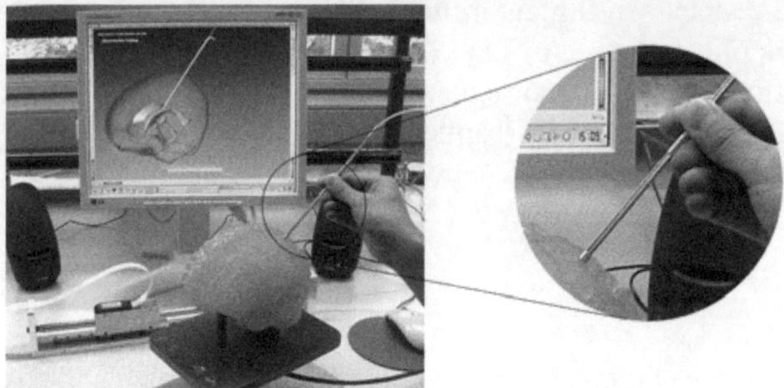

Figure 2. BRAINTRAIN simulator with 1-dof haptic device: The user must hold the device
at the holder and push the tip of the device against the brain model.

3. Discussion

We measured the insertion depth at the end-effector by measuring the position of the linear motor at the other end of the actuating cable. When the user starts pushing the device against the plastic brain model, it can introduce measurement errors up to 5 mm due to the backlash of the push-pull cable. The elongation of the inner wire cable under tensile condition can cause additional errors but much less and can be ignored. Another drawback came from the friction coefficient of the cable which varies according to the bending radius or the shape of the actuating cable. To achieve a better control performance, the shape of the cable should be detected during the simulation and the control parameter must be adjusted according to the current configuration of the cable.

4. Conclusion

In combination with the BRAINTRAIN simulator, the haptic device presented can be used to train ventricular shunt insertions. In the future, a more comprehensive model and a closed-loop impedance controller with an additional force sensor will be required to better simulate the biomechanical properties of the brain tissue. Evaluations with novices and experts will be mandatory.

References

[1]   Panchaphongsaphak, B., Burgkart, R., Riener, R., BrainTrain: Brain simulator for medical VR application, Proc. the 13th MMVR conference, pp. 378-384, 2005
[2]   Panchaphongsaphak, B., Nef, T., Riener, R., A prototype of ventricular shunt insertion simulator (Abstract), Course syllabus the 13th MMVR conference, pp. 184, 2005
[3]   Bowman, D.A., Kruijff, E., LaViola Jr., J.J., Poupyrev, I., 3D User Interfaces: Theory and Practice, Addison-Wesley, 2005
[4]   Carignan, C., Cleary, K., Closed-loop force control for haptic simulation of virtual environments, Haptics-e, vol. 1, no. 2, 2000

Medicine Meets Virtual Reality 14
J.D. Westwood et al. (Eds.)
IOS Press, 2006

431

A Hip Surgery Simulator Based on Patient Specific Models Generated by Automatic Segmentation

Johanna Pettersson [a,1], Hans Knutsson [a] Per Nordqvist [b] and Magnus Borga [a]

[a] *Department of Biomedical Engineering and Center for Medical Image Science and Visualization, Linköping University*
[b] *Melerit Medical AB*

Abstract. The use of surgical simulator systems for education and preoperative planning is likely to increase in the future. A natural course of development of these systems is to incorporate patient specific anatomical models. This step requires some kind of segmentation process in which the different anatomical parts are extracted. Anatomical datasets are, however, usually very large and manual processing would be too demanding. Hence, automatic, or semi-automatic, methods to handle this step are required. The framework presented in this paper uses nonrigid registration, based on the morphon method, to automatically segment the hip anatomy and generate models for a hip surgery simulator system.

Keywords. Surgery simulation, hip, patient specific models, segmentation, registration, morphon

1. Introduction

Cervical hip fractures constitute a problem of increased clinical importance due to an increasing senior population as well as an increased prevalence of osteoporosis. The routine treatment for this kind of trauma is closed reposition and osteosynthesis with screws or nails. The outcome of the operation is highly dependent on how much the surgeon knows about the injury, the skill of the surgeon and, of course, of the complexity of the fracture. Training and planning in simulator systems would be beneficial for this kind of procedure to give the surgeon more experience before starting to work on the real patient. Increased proficiency results in fewer mistakes made during actual surgery as well as a reduction in radiation exposure time, thus increasing the safety for both patient and surgeon. Simulator training has proven efficient for image guided surgical procedures [1] since the physician can develop a technique for and get familiar with the surgical procedure by practicing on a number of virtual models of patients before starting to work on real cases. To fully exploit these systems the virtual models must refer to the anatomy of individual patients. Patient specific models are essential if the systems are to be used as preoperative planning tools. Individual models are important also in the education and training phase as the variety of anatomical cases to practice on is extended.

---

[1]Correspondence to: Johanna Pettersson, Department of Biomedical Engineering, University Hospital, SE-58185 Linkoping, Sweden. Tel.: +46 13 229 445; Fax: +46 13 101 902; E-mail: johanna.pettersson@imt.liu.se.

2. The Hip Surgery Simulator System

The simulator system, shown in fig. 1, gives the user visual, haptic and audial feedback to produce an environment that resembles the real operation room. Input to the simulator is made through real surgical tools that are integrated into the system. Different tools such as guide wires, drills and step reamers are used for positioning and insertion of the nails, and there are also pedals, which are needed to control the use of simulated X-ray to follow the progress of the surgery. The visual feedback is given in form of fluoroscopy images simulated from the virtual data. A snapshot of what this can look like is shown in fig. 1 (right). Furthermore, the system gives sound feedback similar to the one produced during actual surgery.

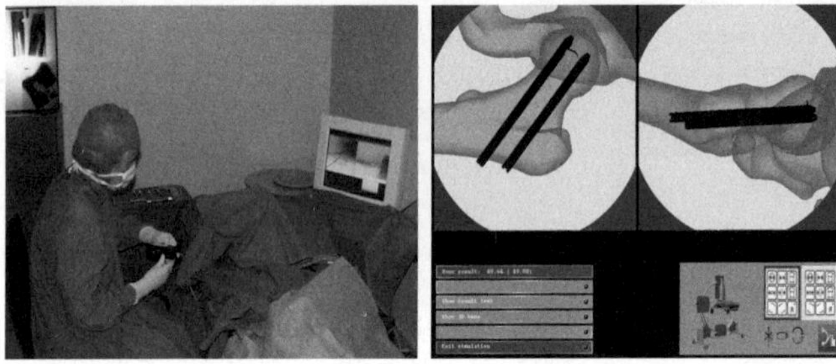

Figure 1. Working in the simulator environment (left). Snapshot of the visual feedback (right).

The haptic instrument makes it possible to manipulate and feel the virtual objects. By connecting the surgical tool to this device the user can interact with the virtual patient in a realistic way. This instrument generates forces based on the location of the tool in the virtual world, providing a natural feeling of resistance when drilling in the bone and inserting the nails. Once the surgery is completed, result of relevant measuring data is presented to the user.

In the original system one hand-made polygon model based on generic data is implemented (the model in fig. 1). This work extends the simulator to include patient specific models, generated from computed tomography (CT) data of different patients.

3. Automatic Segmentation Using Registration

To obtain patient specific surface models of the anatomy a segmentation process is needed. In the segmentation process the bone tissue is separated from the surrounding soft tissue. Once we have a segmented dataset the compact bone surface can be extracted and used as model in the simulator. The most straightforward approach to perform the segmentation is to segment the data from each patient manually and generate a model from that. However, since the data that we are working with are three dimensional CT volumes, with a pixel resolution of 512 and typically around 350 transaxial slices, this would be a very tedious and time consuming operation. A method that could handle this step automatically would be preferable. Especially if the system is used for preoperative planning it is necessary to be able to generate the models quite fast and in an efficient way. To accomplish this a registration method, which is called the morphon method, has been employed [5,6].

3.1. The Morphon Method

The morphon method can be described as a general registration technique. The basic concept of registration is to match one image (or volume), the prototype image, to another image, the target image. The deformation is based on some measure of similarity between the two images. From this measure, an estimate of how the prototype image should be transformed to better match the target image, can be found. The degree of deformation that may be applied to the prototype image is dependent on the application. Sometimes the registration can be done using only a few degrees of freedom, allowing only translations, rotations, scalings or combinations of these (affine transformations). However, for anatomical data these transformation models are often not flexible enough to handle the variations in the datasets. To deal with these more local deformations we utilise a transformation model with more degrees of freedom.

In the morphon method 2D or 3D images are registered based on an iterative deformation process. For each iteration the algorithm passes through three main steps: *displacement estimation*, *deformation field accumulation and regularisation*, and *deformation*. Moreover, the method utilises a multi scale approach, which means that the registration process is initiated on a coarse resolution scale to capture large deformations, and moves on to finer scales where a more detailed matching can be done.

3.1.1. Displacement Estimation Based on Quadrature Phase Differences

The initial step in each iteration is to estimate a field describing the current displacement between the images. This is equivalent to finding the optical flow or the image velocity, which can be done in a number of ways [2]. In the implementation of the morphon algorithm we have chosen a method based on measuring the difference in quadrature phase [3,4]. One main benefit of this technique is its invariance to image intensity.

The output from this step is an image with a vector in each pixel position that describes how the corresponding pixel in the prototype should be moved to decrease the difference in quadrature phase between the target image and the prototype image.

3.1.2. Accumulation and Regularisation

Once we have a displacement estimate for the current iteration the next step is to add this to the accumulated deformation field. The accumulation is needed since we need a field that describes how the original prototype should be deformed. If the prototype is iteratively deformed, and hence iteratively interpolated, this would introduce a blurring effect that would grow continuously until the loop ends. Therefore we generate an accumulated field, that describes the deformation of the original prototype, and update this with the temporary displacement estimates in each iteration.

Since the displacement estimates are found by looking only locally in the image, adjacent estimates can vary quite much. To avoid tearing the image apart when deforming it we would like to have a field that varies smoothly over the image. This means that we should not use the displacement estimates straight off. We need to perform some regularisation of the field first. This is where the degrees of freedom of the deformation is defined. We can choose to fit the field to a global, rigid transformation model to allow only rotations and translations for example, or we can allow a more elastic field by fitting the estimates locally to some neighbourhood function. The local, non-rigid, model is needed for the hip models and is implemented by performing local averaging of the field.

3.1.3. Deformation

The last step in each iteration is to deform the original prototype image according to the accumulated and regularised field. This is done using bi- or trilinear interpolation.

The loop containing this three steps is iterated until the position of the deformed prototype is found adequate. The number of iterations can either be specified beforehand by setting the parameters and then run the application, or by continuously look at the intermediate deformation result and adjust the parameters interactively according to this.

3.2. Morphons for Segmentation

Depending on the purpose of the registration, the target image and the prototype image may vary. One main idea with the morphon method is that it can be used for a wide variety of cases, ranging from registration of images with very similar structures and gray levels, to cases where the prototype image contain a very simple description of the structure that we want to find in the target image. When using the morphon method for segmentation purposes the prototype image can contain an atlas or a labeled model of the data we are working on. In this work the prototype image is a femur and pelvis that has been segmented manually. Here we are working on CT volumes which means that we perform the registration in 3D. Hence, the prototype image is a volume that has been created from an arbitrary patient CT volume in which each voxel has been labeled compact bone, spongy bone, or background (equal to soft tissue). A surface model and a slice from the prototype volume together with corresponding slice from the CT data it was generated from is shown in fig. 2.

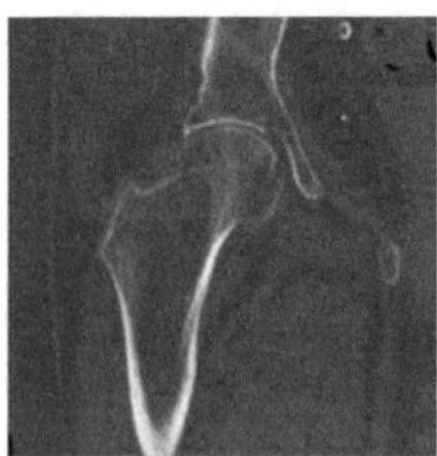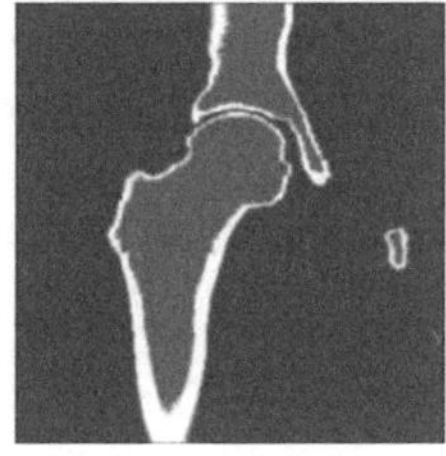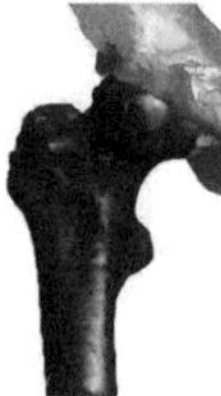

Figure 2. The CT data used as prototype. 2D slices of the original dataset (left) and the manually segmented dataset (middle), and an isosurface of the labeled 3D model (right).

The output from the registration process is a deformed version of the original prototype. This volume contains a labeled description of the shape of the anatomy of the target patient data. From this it is straightforward to generate a surface model for the simulator.

4. Results

The result from the morphon registration is conclusive for the performance of the model generation framework. If this step fails we will not obtain a patient specific model since we have not obtained a deformed prototype that describes the specific patient's anatomy. Therefore it is of utmost importance to study the result from this process. Fig. 3 and fig. 4 show results from one dataset. Note that the registration has been performed in 3D but here we are only looking at 2D coronal (fig. 3 (a)) and axial (fig. 3 (b)) slices of the volumes. The top row in fig. 3 displays the patient specific CT data and the original prototype, which are the input to the registration process. After registration with the morphon method we have obtained a prototype that has adopted the shape of the anatomy in the patient data (bottom row).

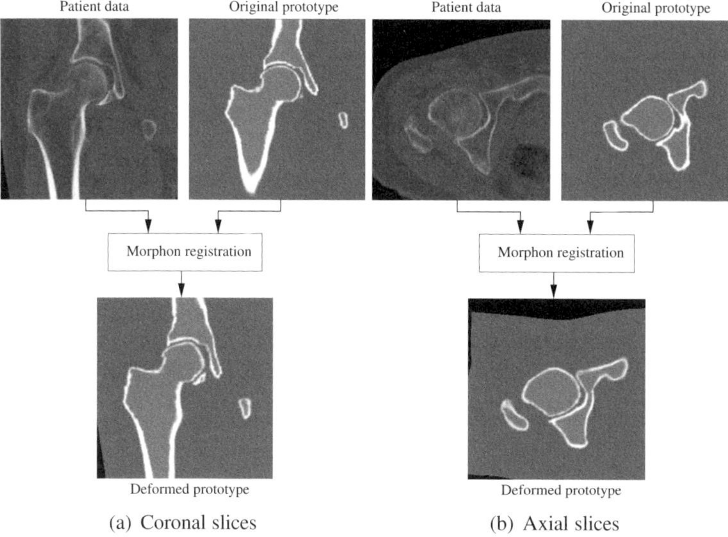

Figure 3. On top are the input to the registration process, the target CT dataset and the original undeformed prototype. These are passed to the morphon algorithm which gives the deformed prototype as output. Results are shown for one coronal slice (a) and one axial slice (b).

The images in fig. 4 contain a black contour that delineates the cortical bone structure in the corresponding prototype slice. The left image in fig. 4 (a) and (b) respectively demonstrate the matching before registration has been done. The contour is placed on top of the target position in the patient CT dataset. The right image show the contour of the deformed prototype on top of the target slice, that is, after the morphing process.

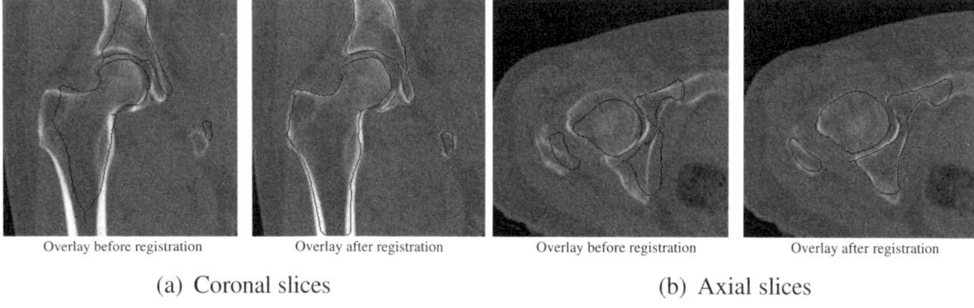

Figure 4. Contour of cortical bone in the prototype on top of the target data, before (left) and after (right) deformation. Results are shown for one coronal slice (a) and one axial slice (b).

Fig. 5 shows two models generated from two different patients using the described method. The left part of fig. 5 (a) and 5 (b) respectively, is an isosurface plot of the model and the right part show snapshots of a person working in the simulator on the model.

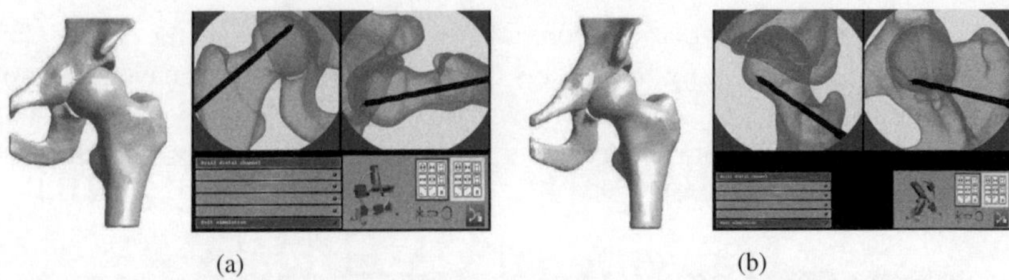

(a)   (b)

Figure 5. Two different patient specific model generated within this project (left and right part, resp.). Isosurfaces of the models and snapshots from the simulator system with these models.

5. Conclusions

The use of patient specific models within surgical simulators is an important step in the evolution of these systems. These models are essential if the simulators are to be used as preoperative planning tools. They are also very important when using simulators for education since the training is then based on a variety of real patient cases. Methods to generate these models is preferably automatic, or at least with minimal user interaction, since the datasets are often large and the shapes complex. The method presented here is based on non-rigid registration using morphons.

Future work involves automatic segmentation and generation of models of bones with cervical fractures. Not until this step has been solved can the simulator be fully exploited as a preoperative planning tool. The hope is also that the simulator in the future can help the user to compute the optimal type, size and position of the implants based on the patient data.

Acknowledgments

This work has been supported by VINNOVA (Swedish Agency for Innovation Systems) and SFS (Swedish Foundation for Strategic Research).

References

[1] G. Ahlberg. *The Role of Simulation Technology For Skills Acquisition in Image Guided Surgery*. PhD thesis, Karolinska Institutet, Stockholm, Sweden, May 2005.

[2] J. L. Barron, D. J. Fleet, and S. S. Beauchemin. Performance of optical flow techniques. *Int. J. of Computer Vision*, 12(1):43–77, 1994.

[3] M. Felsberg. Disparity from monogenic phase. In L. v. Gool, editor, *24. DAGM Symposium Mustererkennung, Zürich*, volume 2449 of *Lecture Notes in Computer Science*, pages 248–256. Springer, Heidelberg, 2002.

[4] G. H. Granlund and H. Knutsson. *Signal Processing for Computer Vision*. Kluwer Academic Publishers, 1995. ISBN 0-7923-9530-1.

[5] H. Knutsson and M. Andersson. Morphons: Segmentation using elastic canvas and paint on priors. In *IEEE-ICIP*, Genova, Italy, September 2005.

[6] A. Wrangsjö, J. Pettersson, and H. Knutsson. Non-rigid registration using morphons. In *Proceedings of the 14th Scandinavian conference on image analysis (SCIA'05)*, Joensuu, June 2005.

Medicine Meets Virtual Reality 14
J.D. Westwood et al. (Eds.)
IOS Press, 2006

Semi-Automatic Segmentation and Tracking of CVH Data

Yingge Qu, Pheng Ann Heng, Tien-Tsin Wong
Dept. of Computer Science & Enginering,
The Chinese University of Hong Kong
{ygqu, pheng, ttwong}@cse.cuhk.edu.hk

Abstract. Construction of speed function is crucial in applying level set method for medical image segmentation. We present a unified approach for segmenting and tracking of the high-resolution Chinese Visible Human (CVH) data. The underlying link of these two parts relies on the proposed variational framework for the speed function. Our proposed method can be applied to segmenting the first slice of the volume data, in the first step; It can also be adapted to track the boundaries of the homogeneous organs in the following serial images. In addition to promising segmentation results, the tracking procedure shows the advantage of less amount of user intervention.

1. Introduction

The *Chinese Visible Human* (CVH) data were acquired in 2002 (male) and 2003 (female). It is the first volumetric data representing a complete normal human of an Asian race [1]. Higher resolution, distinguishable blood vessel, data completeness, and free of organic lesion are the main advantages of this dataset, which make it useful in a variety of research and educational applications. On the other side, it brings lots of difficulties in segmentation due to the high-resolution color details without clear boundaries.

In this paper we describe a new segmentation technique for the volumetric images, which requires little user intervention. It can be used for general segmentation and tracking purpose. The user specifies which region should be segmented, by simply clicking on the *area of interest* (AOI) on the first one of the serial images, instead of describing a precise initial contour (the leftmost image of Figure 1). We use fast marching to expand the initial seeds [5], and to automatically segment the interesting regions from the first of the sequential images. Then the contours are automatically tracked on the subsequent serial images using the proposed level set based tracking method. but also from the following ones by the proposed Level Set based tracking method. This segmentation process is demonstrated in Figure 1. The underlying link of the segmentation and tracking methods relies on the proposed variational framework for the speed function.

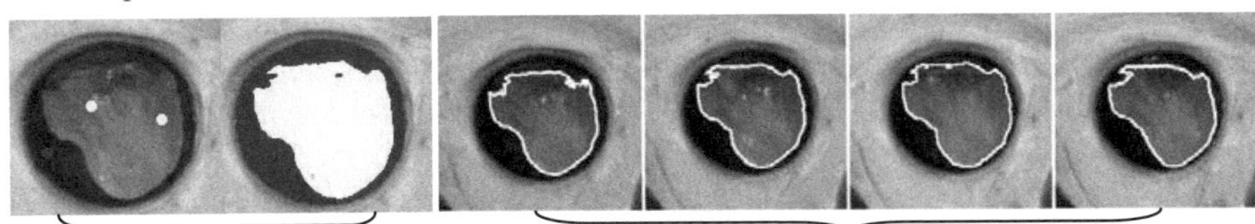

Initial contour segmented in
the first slice by level set

Contours automatically detected in the
subsequent slices

Figure 1. Segmentation in the first image and tracking in the following ones.

Although we only demonstrate the proposed method for segmenting and tracking the CVH data, but it can also be applied to other image modalities such as tagged MRIs.

2. Segmentation

Although the CVH Dataset brings more difficulties to segmentation methods when dealing with high resolution information on one hand, it brings convenience to the tracking-based serial images segmentation on the other hand. For segmenting this volumetric dataset, a two-step scheme based on level set segmentation and tracking is proposed as follows:

1: *Segmentation Step:* This step segments the first slice of a volumetric data (sequence of serial images). In this step, the speed function, which is designed for the segmentation purpose (Section 3.1), incorporates the gradient, texture, and color information. User need to lay the initial seed, by simply clicking on the AOI, as shown in the leftmost image of Figure 1.

2: *Tracking Step:* For the subsequent image slices, after the first segmented step, the level set segmentation is initialized by the evolving the result from the previous image, and propagates the front with a newly proposed speed function, which is designed for tracking (Section 3.2).

3. Speed Functions

3.1 Speed Function for Segmentation

The basic idea in constructing a speed term for segmentation is to make speed F tends to be zero when it is close to the boundary. According to our previously proposed model [2], *BPV* texture feature [3] and gradient feature are incorporated into our speed function:

$$F = K_I(x,y)(\varepsilon K + F_A) + \beta \frac{(\nabla c \cdot \nabla\ )}{|\nabla \phi|} + \gamma(BPV) \tag{1}$$

where εK is to prevent the sharp corner developing; K_I is defined as $e^{-|\nabla G_\sigma \cdot I(x,y)|}$; $\nabla c \cdot \nabla$ proposed by Yezzi et al. [4] is a pull-back stress dependent on the gradient; and *BPV* is to measure the texture feature.

3.2 Speed Function for Tracking

The 0.1mm inter-layer distance of CVH data makes the tracking become possible and reliable for segmentation task. We also extended the speed model in [2] for the tracking problem. Due to the visual consistency constraint between two continuous layers, we can assume the transformation of edge between images I_n and I_{n+1} is between a narrow band with width δ. All the following calculation is done only within the narrow band.

We propose a new speed function to evolve the contour, from image I_n to the next slice I_{n+1}. Taking the segmentation result in I_n as the initial contour in I_{n+1}, the front propagates under the speed function Eq. (2), to attract the front moving to the new AOI boundary. Here, the curvature term K is still adopted to avoid the "swallowtail" during propagation. F_D is the cost function between the two images I_n and I_{n+1}. It can be measured by the sum of square differences between the image intensities in a window, as shown in Figure 2. Eq. (3) tells how to decide the magnitude and the signal of F_D, where $+n$ and $-n$ indicate whether the pixels are outside or inside the zero level set respectively in I_n; C_+^n and C_-^n are the content model of these pixels in I_n. ID represents the pixels in the overlapped in-homogenous areas, see Figure 2.

$$F = KI_{n+1}(\varepsilon K + F_D) + \beta F_C \tag{2}$$

$$F_D = Sig \cdot (I_n - I_{n+1})^2, \quad F_C = Sig \cdot dist(C_n, C_{n+1}) \tag{3}$$

$$Sig = Sign(dist(C_{ID}, C_+^n) - dist(C_{ID}, C_-^n)) \tag{4}$$

Note that F_D, convolved by KI_{n+1}, forces the front to move in the homogeneous area and to stop at the boundaries in I_{n+1}. The sign of F_D decides the curve to expand or shrink.

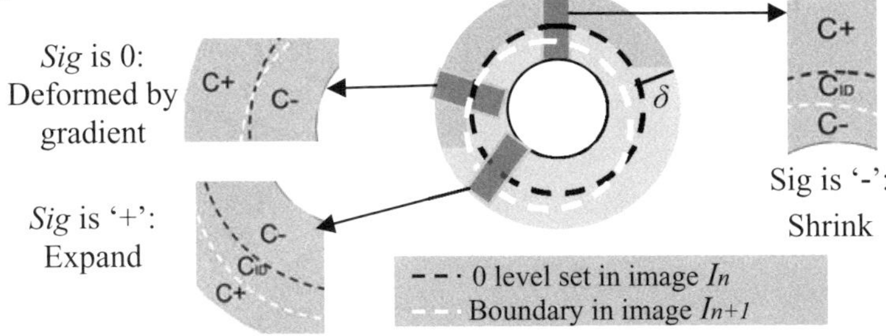

Figure 2. Design of the speed function for tracking: value and signal.

4. Discussion

The newly proposed segmentation method works efficiently because of less amount of user intervention. A two-step scheme is proposed in this paper, starting from segmenting the first image slice. User only need to initialize the first slice by clicking on the AOI. The contours in the subsequent image slices are then automatically tracked.

Acknowledgment

The work described in this paper was supported by a grant from the Research Grants Council of the Hong Kong Special Administrative Region, China (Project No. CUHK4223/04E) and CUHK Shun Hing Institute of Advanced Engineering.

References

[1] S. X. Zhang, P. A. Heng and et al., "The Chinese Visible Human datasets incorporate technical and imaging advances on earlier digital humans," *Journal of Anatomy*, Vol.204, pp.165-173, 2004.

[2] Y.G. Qu, Q. Chen, P.A. Heng, and T.T. Wong," Segmentation of Left Ventricle via Level Set Method Based on Enriched Speed Term". *MICCAI 2004, LNCS3216*, vol. 1, pp. 435-442

[3] C.G. LOONE, *Pattern Recognition Using Neural Network*. Oxford University Press, 1997.

[4] A. Yezzi, S. Kichenassamy, A. Kumar, P. Olver, and A. Tannenbaum, "A geometric snake model for segmentation of medical imagery". *IEEE Trans. on Medical Imaging*, Vol.16, No.2, pp.199-209, 1997.

[5] J.A. Sethian, *Level Set Methods and Fast Marching Methods: Evolving Interfaces in Computational Geometry, Fluid Mechanics, Computer Vision, and Materials Science*, Cambridge University Press, 1999

Medicine Meets Virtual Reality 14
J.D. Westwood et al. (Eds.)
IOS Press, 2006

Tissue Engineering Templates Using Minimal Surfaces

Srinivasan Rajagopalan, Bruce M. Cameron, Richard A. Robb
Biomedical Imaging Resource, Mayo Clinic College of Medicine, Rochester, MN, USA.

Abstract. The status quo of tissue engineering can be summarized as "*a random walk through the design space*". The existing scaffold designs based on computer-aided design (CAD) and solid freeform fabrication (SFF) are anti-biomorphic and mechanically weak cubic partitions with sharp edges. We introduce *minimal surface* based unit cells to create biomorphic scaffolds with optimal stress/strain distribution and superior mechanical strength.

Keywords. Tissue engineering, scaffolds, minimal surfaces, rapid prototyping.

1. Introduction

Tissue and organ loss and defects occur in a wide variety of clinical situations, and their reconstruction to restore structural and functional integrity is a challenging but necessary step in the patient's rehabilitation [1]. Tissue engineering addresses this challenge by integrating the principles of engineering and life sciences toward the design, construction, modification and growth of biological substitutes that restore, maintain, or improve tissue function using scaffolds, cells and growth factors, alone or in combination. In spite of the projected benefits of engineered tissues, their use in transplantation procedures is minimal, partly due to the suboptimal scaffold design [2]. The scaffold fabrication techniques currently employed can be broadly classified into two types: (a) conventional, stochastic techniques, and (b) rapidly emerging, computer-controlled solid freeform fabrication (SFF) techniques. Exploiting the customized design, computer-controlled fabrication, and the reproducibility offered by the SFF techniques, a number of groups have developed novel scaffold architectures. However, the majority of these approaches under-utilize SFF by producing CAD-based scaffolds with straight edges and sharp turns, or those derived from Boolean intersections of geometric primitives such as spheres and cylinders. None of these partitions provide a biomorphic environment suitable for cell attachment, migration and proliferation. A tissue engineering scaffold that best mimics the morphology of extracellular matrix-curved, bicontinuous, and non-intersecting partitions with minimum mean curvature is an ideal construct for viable cell attachment and proliferation. This paper explores the use of triply periodic minimal surfaces (TPMS) as tissue analogue templates. Our premiere physical realization of TPMS constructs demonstrates a viable morphology which when replicated at macro (tissue) level might have profound implications on cell migration and tissue growth and may provide an optimal biomorphic tissue analog.

2. Minimal Surfaces and Triply Periodic Minimal Surfaces

The study of minimal surfaces originated with the problem of determining the characteristics of the surface forming the smallest area for a given perimeter [3]. Meusnier [4] showed that the mean curvature at every point of such a minimal surface is zero and any small patch in it will have the least area of all the surface patches with the same boundary. The shape assumed by soap films is one of the prominent natural examples of minimal surfaces. Triply Periodic Minimal Surfaces (TPMS) are surfaces that are periodic in three independent directions, extending infinitely, and in the absence of self-intersections, partitioning the space into two labyrinths. Figure 1 shows geometry of the Primitive (P) (panel a), Gyroid (G) (panel c) and the Diamond (D) (panel b) TPMS. The natural manifestation of two, continuous, inter-penetrating, non-intersecting networks matches with the preferred porous and solid subspace topology for tissue engineering scaffolds.

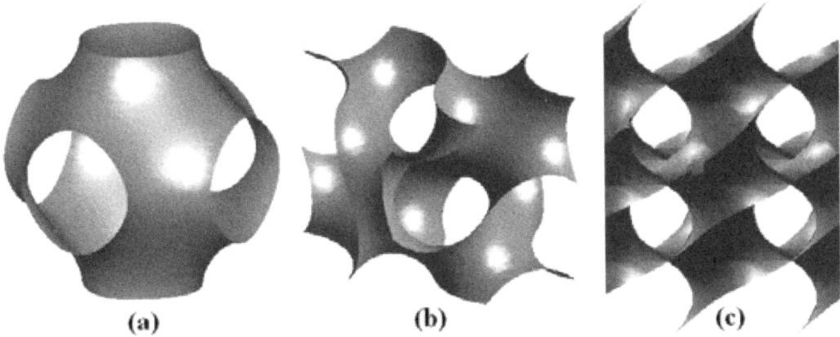

Figure 1. Examples of Triply Periodic Minimal Surfaces. The Schwarz Primitive (panel a) and Diamond (panel c) TPMS was discovered by Schwarz in 1885. Schoen discovered the Gyroid (panel b) in 1967.

3. Biology's preference for TPMS geometry

Given Nature's propensity to adopt curvilinear formations in organic and inorganic phenomena, it is little wonder that the bi-continuous, inter-penetrating, non-intersecting TPMS network has existence in natural biology. It was the seminal work of Donnay et al [5] that unraveled the existence of TPMS in biological forms. Over the next four decades, a number of imaging studies have revealed the existence of D-G-P surfaces, without any obvious restrictions or preferences, throughout all kingdoms, both in natural and pathological or manipulated cells. These studies reveal that the TPMS configurations occur due to unknown but specific demands imposed by the cell machinery during both the normal and pathological development and hence modulate morphogenesis.

4. Geometric Modeling of TPMS

Like any other surface, TPMS can be generated using parametric, implicit or boundary methods. In the parametric method a function maps a region of a plane to a region of the surface. In the implicit method the surface is described as the solution of a single-valued function of three variables. Boundary methods are based on iteratively evolving an initial polygonal model to the final surface model, subject to a variety of boundary and inter-polygonal constraints. The possibility of evolving a straight edged, sharply turning cubic labyrinthine network (reminiscent of the conventionally used topology in CAD based scaffold design) into a smooth, curved, non-intersecting, bicontinuous partition makes the boundary methods an ideal framework to model tissue engineering scaffolds.

4.1. Evolution of a plane into a P-surface patch

To generate the fundamental patch of the Schwarz P-surface, a quadri-rectangular tetrahedron is used as the fundamental region to confine the initial plane and its subsequent evolved surface. Figure 2 shows the evolution of the plane into a P-surface patch. The plane embedded orthogonally with respect to the faces of the fundamental region (panel a) is refined by subdividing each facet to create a finer triangulation (panel b). The triangulated patch is iteratively evolved (subject to volume preservation, surface containment and surface area minimization) to form the P-surface patch (panel c).

4.2. From P-patch to unit P-cell and Scaffolds

To form the unit P-cell, the evolved surface patch is reflected around the fundamental region based on the following properties of minimal surfaces

- If part of the boundary of a minimal surface is a straight line, then the reflection across the line, when added to the original surface, forms another minimal surface.
- If a minimal surface meets a plane at right angles, then the mirror image of the plane, when added to the original surface, also forms a minimal surface.

The quadri-rectangular tetrahedron enclosing the finite minimal P-surface patch provides the plane boundaries about which the evolved patch can be replicated by reflection to yield a TPMS without self-intersection. Six of these pieces combine to form a larger surface piece in the hierarchy of assembly. Further reflections of this piece forms the unit P-cell. Tessellation of the unit-cells produces the bi-continuous network. Figure 3 illustrates this process for both the cubic and P-cell scaffolds.

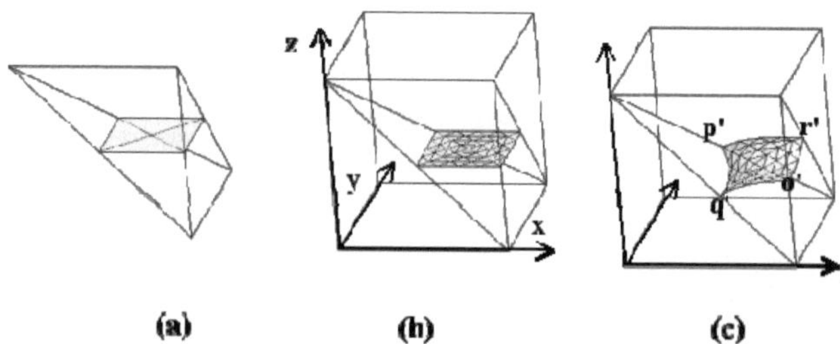

Figure 2. Evolution of finely triangulated plane into a P-surface patch.

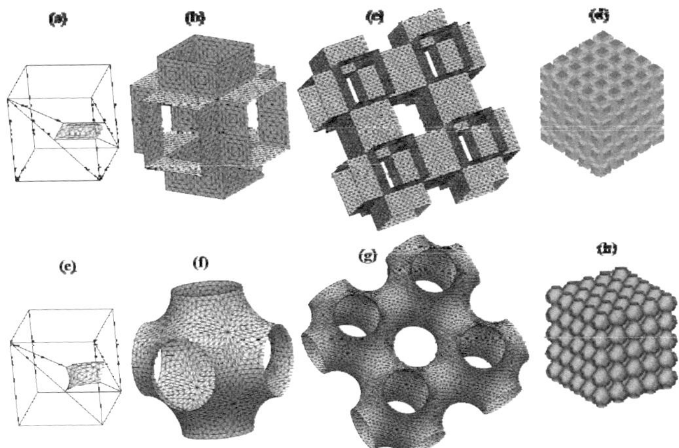

Figure 3. Formation of cubic and P-cell scaffolds and unit cells using tessellations and reflections of the original plane and its evolution.

5. Fabrication and characterization of P-scaffolds

5.1. Fabrication

The unit cells obtained by evolving and tessellating the finely triangulated plane triangulated can be directly converted into the .STL stereolithographic format suitable for fabrication with rapid prototyping devices. Multiple copies of the 5mm^3 scaffolds with strut width and pore diameter of 500 microns were fabricated using a Stereolithography-based rapid prototyping machine (3D systems, Valencia, NH).

5.2. Mechanical Characterization

Mechanical characterization of the unit cells was performed with uniaxial compressive simulation using ABAQUS (HKS Inc, Plymouth, MI). Force of 0.3031 N/ 0.1 N was applied at each of the 32/ 97 face nodes of the open/ closed unit cells. The material properties (material: PMMA; Young's modulus 2.4 GPa; Poisson ratio: 0.375) were set identical for both the cubic and P unit cells. Figure 4 shows the resultant Von Mises stress and Principal strain distribution for the unit cells. It is clearly seen that the stress and strain concentration along sharp edges of the cubic unit cell have been significantly reduced in the unit P-cell. The simulation also reveals the optimal stress distribution and significant strain reduction on the TPMS unit cells.

To further validate the simulations and to characterize the whole scaffold, uniaxial compression of the scaffolds and unit cells was performed on a Dynamic Mechanical Analyzer (DMA: TA Inst., New Castle, DE). Fourteen specimens of both the scaffolds were used for the mechanical testing. The specimens were uniaxially compressed with parallel plates by applying a ramp force of 4N/min for 4.5 minutes. Figure 5 compares the linear modulus of the cubic and P-cell based unit cells and scaffolds. The result correlates with the findings from the finite element simulations.

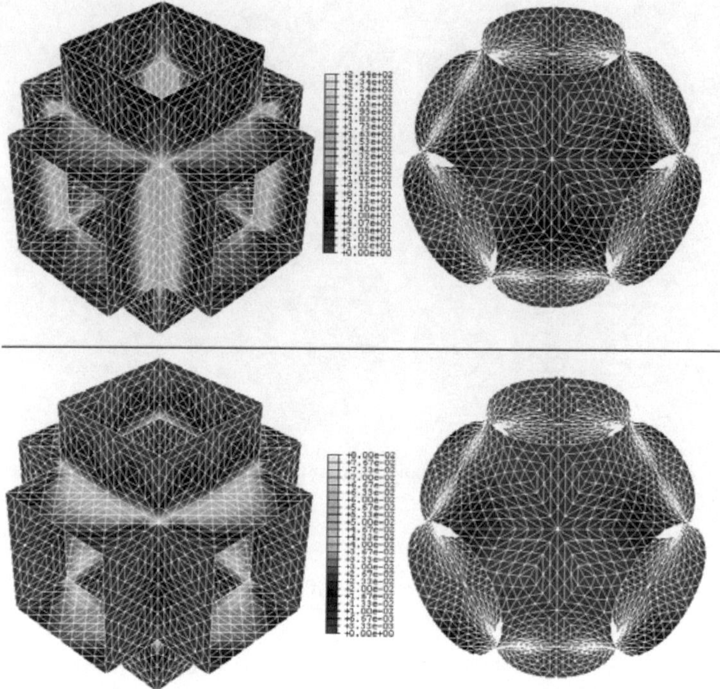

Figure 4. Von Mises stress (top) and Principal strain (bottom) distributions for the uniaxial compression of the open cubic (left) and P- (right) unit cells with identical loading conditions and material properties. These results, reported for the first time, provide insights into the reason behind the natural choice of TPMS forms by biological systems.

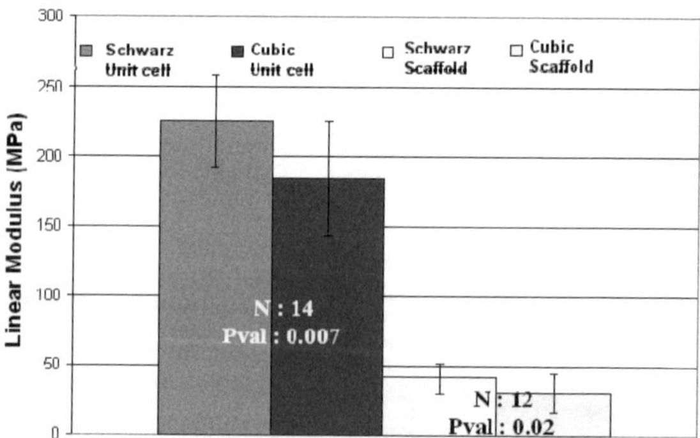

Figure 5. Linear modulus of Schwarz and cubic scaffolds and unit cells based on uniaxial compression on DMA under identical loading conditions (4 N/min. ramp force for 4.5 minutes.

5.3. Cell Seeding

To test the suitability of TPMS morphology in tissue engineering, ATDC cells (mouse chondrogenic cell line) were cultured on the scaffolds and examined for viability after 1 day using Viability/ Cytotoxicity kit. Living cells were stained green and dead cells were red when visualized with confocal scanning microscope. A high viability (>95%) was observed for the adherent cells to the surface of scaffolds. Figure 6 shows the distribution of cells on the surface of the scaffold. The cells are active and well distributed through the edges of the pores. The extended cell processes along the scaffold surface reveals the suitability of the substrate.

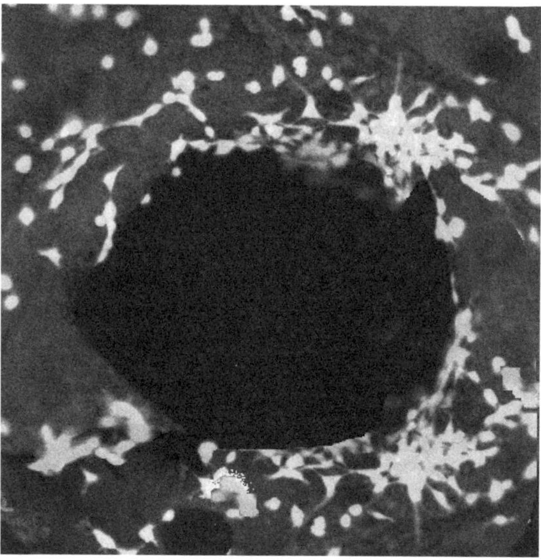

Figure 6. Cell viability study on TPMS scaffolds. The viability results at day 1, shows a high viability (> 95%) for adherent cells.

6. Conclusion

This paper described a first attempt to physically realize and mechanically characterize the scaffolds based on Schwarz TPMS. The preliminary outcomes of our investigation provide the previously elusive justification for the *TPMS-philicity* of plant and mammalian organelles. This viable morphology, when replicated at macro (tissue) level may also have profound influence on cell migration and tissue growth and may provide an optimal biomorphic tissue analog.

7. References

[1]   Yaszemski MJ, Payne RG, Hayes WC, Langer R, Mikos AG. Evolution of bone transplantation: molecular, cellular and tissue strategies to engineer human bone. *Biomaterials,* 1996; 17:175-185.
[2]   Kohn J. Combinatorial and computational approaches can be used for the design of polymeric biomaterials. *In. Proc. Society for Biomaterials 29th Annual Meeting and Exposition,* 2003; Reno, Nevada, USA.
[3]   Lagrange JL. *Miscellanea Taurinensia,* 1760; 2:173-195.
[4]   Meusnier JBMC. *Mem. Mathem. Phys. Acad. Sci. Paris,* 1785; 10: 477-510.
[5]   Donnay G, Pawson DL. X-ray diffraction studies of echinoderm plates, *Science,* 1969; 166(3909):1147-50.

Medicine Meets Virtual Reality 14
J.D. Westwood et al. (Eds.)
IOS Press, 2006

Rendering of Virtual Fixtures for MIS Using Generalized Sigmoid Functions [1]

Jing Ren [a,2], Rajni V. Patel [b,c] and Kenneth A. McIsaac [c]

[a] *Imaging Research Labs, Robarts Research Institute*
[b] *Canadian Surgical Technology & Advanced Robotics (CSTAR)*
[c] *Dept. of Elect. and Comp. Engrg., Univ. of Western Ontario*

Abstract. To avoid undesired collisions and improve the level of safety and precision, artificial potential field (APF) can be employed to generate virtual forces around protected tissue and to provide surgeons with real-time force refection through haptic feedback. In this paper, we propose a potential field-based force model using the generalized sigmoid function, and show that it can represent a large class of shapes. The proposed approach has several advantages such as computational efficiency, easily adjustable level of force reflection, and force continuity.

Keywords. Artificial potential fields, haptic feedback, sigmoid functions

1. Introduction

Compared with open surgery, Minimally Invasive Surgery (MIS) poses new challenges such as poor hand-eye coordination, restricted maneuverability and limited field of view of the surgical workspace. These difficulties may cause accidental damage to critical tissue or collisions between instruments. To avoid these undesired collisions and improve the level of safety and precision, we use artificial potential fields (APFs) to generate virtual forces around protected tissue and to provide real-time force reflection through haptic feedback. Although APFs provide a simple and computationally efficient approach for virtual force reflection via virtual fixtures [3,2], the construction of a potential field based force model which can achieve effective protection for arbitrary shapes without significantly reducing the workspace is still an open problem. The existing potential field models are only capable of generating some simple shapes such as spheres, paraboloids etc. Tissue with a more complex shape can only be approximated with large discrepancies. Even when the resulting potential model can achieve the desired force reflection, it tends to reduce the surgical workspace considerably and therefore limit the surgeon's dexterity during operations.

---

[1]This research was supported by the Natural Science and Engineering Research Council (NSERC) of Canada under grants RGPIN-1345 and RGPIN-249883, by grants from the Ontario Research & Development Challenge Fund and the Canada Foundation for Innovation awarded to CSTAR.

[2]Correspondence to: Jing Ren, Imaging Research Labs, Robarts Research Institute, London, ON, Canada N6A 5K8, Tel.: 01 519 858 5792; E-mail: jren@imaging.robarts.ca

2. Method

In order to generate protective forces that can accurately follow any arbitrary shape with real-time force reflection, we propose a potential field based force model using generalized sigmoid functions. If we define $q = (x, y, z)$, our potential field based on the generalized sigmoid function can be written as,

$$f(q) = \prod_{i=1}^{N} f_{sig}(\varphi_i(q))$$

(1)

where

$$f_{sig}(s) = \frac{1}{1 + e^{-\gamma s}}$$

(2)

with $s = \varphi(q)$, the surface function which is calculated from an implicit function [1] of the surface of the object. On the boundary surface, $s = 0$, and all points on the boundary take a uniform potential value of 0.5. In the obstacle area, $s >> 0$, and all points are associated with a high potential value approaching unity. In the clear area, $s << 0$, and the potential value approaches zero. If we define,

$$F_q = \sum_{i=1}^{N} \left(\prod_{i=1,i\neq j}^{N} f_{sig}(\varphi_i(q)) \frac{\partial f_{sig}(\varphi_j)}{\partial s} \frac{\partial s}{\partial q} \right)$$

(3)

The reflected force is defined as,

$$F = f_q \frac{F_q}{\|F_q\|}$$

(4)

3. Results

Catheter insertion through a blood vessel is a common procedure in surgery and therapy. In this section, we show that the proposed model can generate potential fields for the blood vessel which has low values when close to the vessel center and high values when close to the vessel wall. The resulting forces can constrain surgeon's motions during catheter insertion to prevent the catheter pushing against the vessel wall.

4. Conclusion

We have proposed a potential field based force model for force reflection for MIS. The proposed force model can accurately represent a large class of shapes and has several advantages such as computational efficiency, easily adjustable force softness, and force continuity.

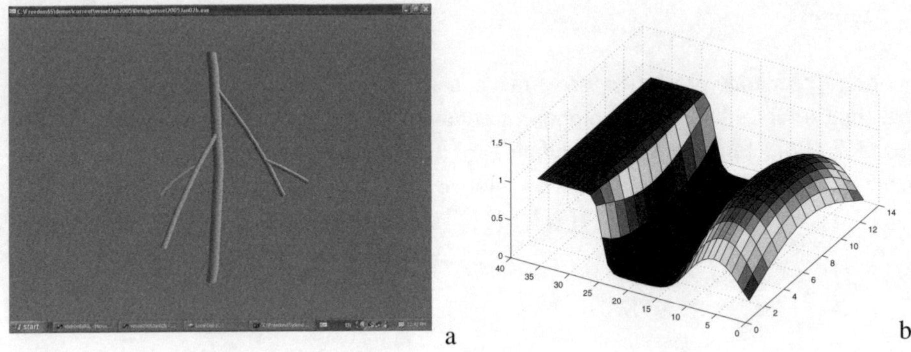

Figure 1. (a) A simulated blood vessel (b) Potential field along the cross-section of the blood vessel

References

[1] J. Bloomenthal *Introduction to Implicit Surfaces*. J. Bloomenthal et al., eds. Morgan Kaufmann, 1997.

[2] M. Li and R.H. Taylor. "Spatial Motion Constraints in Medical Robotics Using Virtual Fixtures Generated by Anatomy". *IEEE Conference on Robotics and Automation,* pp. 1270-1275, 2004.

[3] N. Turro, O. Khatib and E. Coste-Maniere. "Haptically augmented teleoperation". *IEEE Conference on Robotics and Automation,* vol.1, pp. 386-392, 2001.

Medicine Meets Virtual Reality 14
J.D. Westwood et al. (Eds.)
IOS Press, 2006

449

Mobile *In Vivo* Biopsy and Camera Robot

Mark E. RENTSCHLER [a,1], Jason DUMPERT [a], Stephen R. PLATT [a],
Shane M. FARRITOR [a], Dmitry OLEYNIKOV [b]
[a]*University of Nebraska, Department of Mechanical Engineering*
[b]*University of Nebraska Medical Center, Department of Surgery*

Abstract. A mobile *in vivo* biopsy robot has been developed to perform a biopsy from within the abdominal cavity while being remotely controlled. This robot provides a platform for effectively sampling tissue. The robot has been used *in vivo* in a porcine model to biopsy portions of the liver and mucosa layer of the bowel. After reaching the specified location, the grasper was actuated to biopsy the tissue of interest. The biopsy specimens were gathered from the grasper after robot retraction from the abdominal cavity. This paper outlines the steps towards the successful design of an *in vivo* biopsy robot. The clamping forces required for successful biopsy are presented and *in vivo* performance of this robot is addressed.

Keywords. Mobile, Robot, Laparoscopy, *In vivo*, Biopsy

Introduction

Minimally invasive surgery provides the patient with reduced trauma, but limits the surgeon's ability to manipulate the *in vivo* environment directly. The da Vinci surgical robot system has been used to improve surgical dexterity. However, the tools utilized by the da Vinci robot remain constrained by the entry incision. Tool changes still require the removal of the existing tool and the reinsertion of the new one, adding to the overall surgical time and adversely affecting the efficiency of the operation [1-2].

An alternate approach to external surgical robotics is to place the entire robot within the abdominal cavity. These *in vivo* robots are unconstrained by the entry point and can currently provide the surgeon with vision assistance [3]. *In vivo* fixed base camera robots have been developed that can provide the surgeon with additional views of the abdominal environment [4]. These additional views proved helpful for determining orientation and defining depth during a porcine cholecystectomy [3]. To enhance the surgeon's capabilities further a mobile robot was developed [5]. This wheeled robot has provided a mobile platform for an adjustable-focus camera system. This mobile camera robot was used successfully to remove a porcine gallbladder without the aid of a laparoscope [6]. This procedure demonstrates the usefulness of *in vivo* robotics by showing the practicality of a two-port cholecystectomy. The camera port is eliminated by placing the camera inside the patient on an *in vivo* robot.

An *in vivo* manipulator robot could help the surgeon directly manipulate tissue. A family of robots could be placed *in vivo* to perform a task collectively. The camera robot could provide the visual feedback to the surgeon, while a grasper robot retracts the tissue and third robot performs the dissection. To realize the full potential of *in vivo* robotics, robots with grasping capability will be necessary.

1. Robot Design Requirements

There were three sets of design objectives for the biopsy robot. First, the robot would need to provide sufficient clamping forces to sever hepatic tissue. Next, the robot would need to provide sufficient traction to not only traverse the abdominal cavity, but also enough to pull the sample free if not completely severed. Finally, the robot would need to provide effective visual feedback for abdominal exploration and specifically during the biopsy procedures.

The camera system for this robot builds on our previous work using camera systems *in vivo* [6]. The clamping and drawbar forces necessary for successful biopsy were determined experimentally.

1.1. Clamping Force Measured

A biopsy forceps device that is commonly used for tissue sampling during esophago-gastroduodenoscopy (EGD) and colonoscopies was modified to measure cutting forces during tissue biopsy. These forceps, shown schematically in Figure 1, consists of a grasper on the distal end with a handle/lever system on the proximal end. A flexible tube is affixed to one side of the handle and the other end is attached to the fulcrum point of the biopsy grasper. A wire enclosed in plastic inside the tube is used to actuate the grasper. This wire is affixed to the free end of the handle lever and at the other end to the end of the grasper lever arm. Actuation of the handle lever causes the wire to translate relative to the tube and actuate the biopsy graspers. The tip of the forceps is equipped with a small spike that penetrates the tissue during sampling. This normal biopsy device was modified to contain a load cell to measure clamping forces indirectly, as shown in Figure 1. Using this design, the force in the cable was measured.

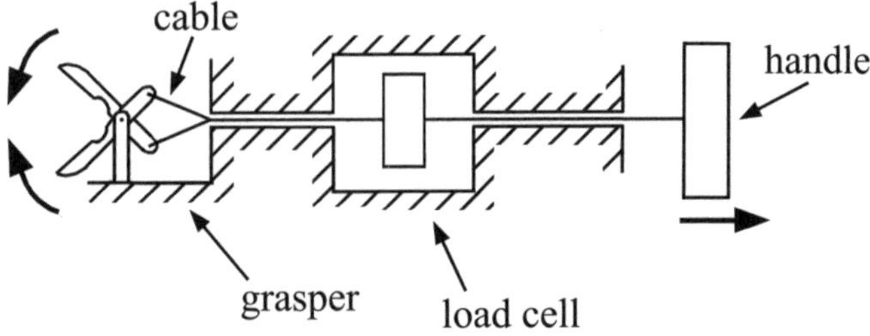

Figure 1. Biopsy tool schematic with load cell in series with the actuation wire

Measurements of cable force were made while sampling liver, omentum, small bowel and the abdominal wall of an anesthetized pig. Representative results for a liver biopsy are shown in Figure 2 (left). The initial negative offset is due to the slight compression in the cable to push the grasper jaws open before biopsy. The average maximum measured force to biopsy porcine liver for three samples was 12.0 +/- 0.4 N. These results are consistent in magnitude with other published results [7] concerning forces sufficient to cut porcine liver.

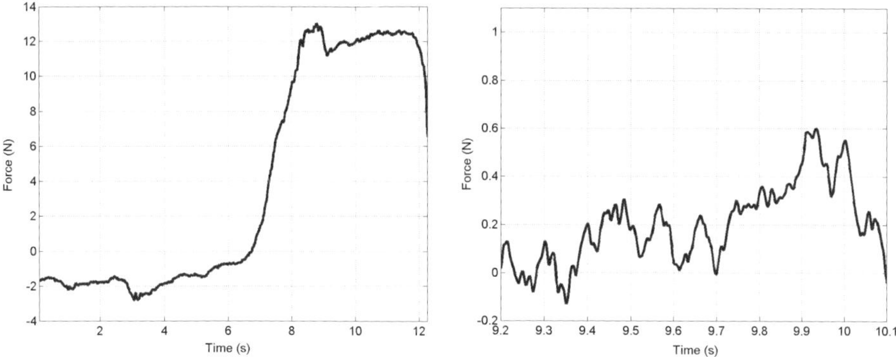

Figure 2. Measured cable force to biopsy *in vivo* porcine hepatic tissue (left) and measured extraction force to biopsy *ex vivo* bovine liver (right)

1.2. Extraction Force Measured

Generally, the biopsy forceps do not completely sever the tissue. In this case, the forceps are gently pulled to free the sample. This extraction force needed to be determined so that a robot could be designed to provide sufficient drawbar force.

A laboratory test jig was built to measure the force needed to free a biopsy sample of bovine liver. After clamping the sample with the biopsy forceps a load cell attached to the handle of the device was gently pulled to free the sample while the tensile force was recorded. Representative results shown in Figure 2 (right) indicate that approximately 0.6 N of force is needed to extract bovine liver tissue with the use of the biopsy forceps.

2. Robot Design

Based on the required clamping force and extraction force a successful biopsy robot was designed, as shown in Figure 3. It provides a mobile *in vivo* platform for visual feedback and for effectively sampling tissue. The wheels are independently controlled by permanent magnet direct current motors to allow for forward, reverse and turning motion. A linkage is used to actuate the biopsy grasper and focusing mechanism for the camera. The robot's grasper is 2.4mm wide and can open to 120 degrees.

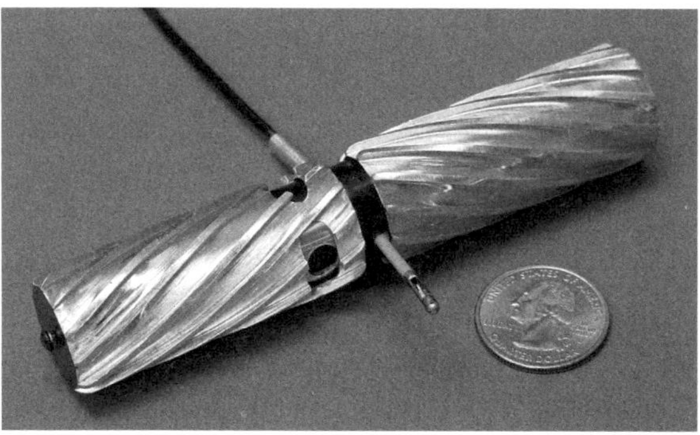

Figure 3. Mobile *in vivo* camera and biopsy robot

3. Results

3.1. Clamping Force Produced

Development of an actuation mechanism to drive the biopsy grasper and the camera was achieved through several design iterations and testing. One challenge was transforming the axis of rotation of the motor, which was perpendicular to the tube of the forceps, to a line of translation parallel with the grasper wires.

The grasper is actuated using a lead screw linkage mechanism as shown in Figure 4. As the motor turns a lead nut is driven up and down. A linkage connects this lead nut to the slider which is actuated horizontally. The grasper wires are attached to this slider. The lead screw linkage mechanism was designed to maximize cable tensile force as the mechanical singularity is reached during the actuation range of motion. The camera lens was attached to this slider too. This provides the camera an adjustable-focus feature necessary in the *in vivo* environment.

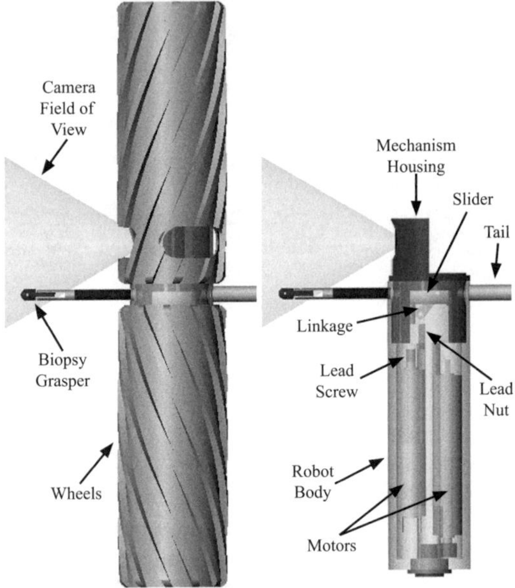

Figure 4. CAD drawing of the robot and actuation mechanism

Force measurements were made in the lab to determine the maximum amount of force that could be produced using the biopsy robot design. Representative results from these tests are shown in Figure 5 (left). The average maximum force produced for three samples was 9.6 +/- 0.1 N. This force is about 16% smaller than the 12 N measured during *in vivo* testing. However, the 12 N merely represents the force that was applied. It does not represent the minimum force required to biopsy the tissue. It is probable that the surgeon performed the biopsy and continued to increase the force and merely "squeezed" the sample. The surgeon applied what he/she knew to be a sufficient force rather than a minimum force. Also, the required force could also be largely reduced by simply taking a smaller biopsy sample. Reducing the contact area by 16% would produce the same applied stress.

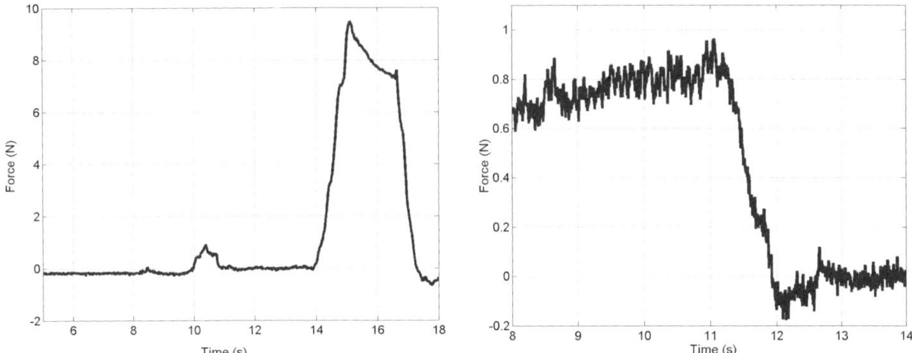

Figure 5. Robot biopsy cable force production measured (left) and robot drawbar force production (right)

3.2. Drawbar Force Produced

As stated earlier a complete severing of the tissue is rarely achieved and some tearing of the sample is usually needed to extract the sample. To be successful the *in vivo* robot needed to produce enough drawbar force to pull the sample free. The biopsy robot shown in Figure 3 was tested *in vivo* and with excised bovine liver to measure drawbar forces. The tail of the robot was attached to a stationary load cell. The robot speed was slowly increased as the drawbar force was recorded as shown in Figure 5 (right). After maximum drawbar force was achieved, around 11 seconds, the robot wheel motion was stopped. Results demonstrate that the robot is capable of producing approximately 0.9 N of drawbar force. This amount of force is 50% greater than the target of 0.6 N in the laboratory measurements (Figure 2, right). This drawbar force is therefore sufficient for sample extraction.

3.3. In vivo Results

In vivo mobility testing with this and other similar prototype robots, suggests that such a wheel design produces sufficient drawbar forces to maneuver within the abdominal environment. Recent *in vivo* porcine tests shows that the helical wheel design allows the robot to traverse all of the abdominal organs (liver, spleen, small and large bowel), as well as climb organs two to three times its height. These tests were performed without causing any visible tissue damage.

The biopsy robot has been successfully tested *in vivo* in a porcine model. The robot was first used to explore the abdominal environment while providing visual feedback to the surgical team.

After exploring the abdominal environment, the biopsy mechanism was used to acquire three samples of hepatic tissue from the liver of the animal. The robot camera was used to find a suitable sample site. The biopsy graspers were opened and the sample site was penetrated with the biopsy forceps' spike. Then the graspers were actuated. This cut nearly all of tissue sample free. The robot was then driven slowly away from the sample site thereby pulling free the tissue sample. This tissue sample was then retrieved after robot extraction through the entry incision. This demonstrates the success of a one-port biopsy and successful tissue manipulation by an *in vivo* robot.

4. Conclusion

Experiments were performed to determine the forces required to biopsy tissue. This data lead to a successful mechanism design that is capable of producing sufficient grasper forces to sample *in vivo* porcine tissues. A successful robot wheel design has led to a robot capable of traversing the abdominal environment without causing tissue damage. This wheel design is also capable of producing sufficient drawbar forces to pull the biopsy sample free during *in vivo* testing. This robot design also incorporates an adjustable-focus camera mechanism capable of providing visual feedback from within the abdominal cavity of the patient.

Current work is focused on wireless developments and modification of the biopsy forceps to provide a clamp capable of clamping shut a severed artery. These developments are important for *in vivo* robotic use in forward environments such as battlefield situations. These achievements in tissue manipulation and visual feedback from within the abdominal cavity will further the development of *in vivo* robotics to assist surgeons in forward battlefield situations and traditional medical centers.

References

[1]   V. B. Kim, W. H. H. Chapman, R. J. Albrecht, B. M. Bailey, J.A. Young, L.W. Nifong, and W.R. Chitwood, "Early Experience With Telemanipulative Robot-Assisted Laparoscopic Cholecystectomy Using da Vinci," Surgical Laparoscopy, Endoscopy & Percutaneous Techniques, vol. 12-1, pp. 33-44, 2002.

[2]   H. Kang, and J.T. Wen, "Robotic Assistants Aid Surgeons During Minimally Invasive Procedures," IEEE Engineering in Medicine and Biology, vol. 20-1, pp. 94-104, 2001.

[3]   Oleynikov, D., Rentschler, M., Hadzialic, A., Dumpert, J., Platt, S., Farritor, S., 2004, "Miniature Robots Can Assist in Laparoscopic Cholecystectomy." Journal of Surgical Endoscopy, 19: 473-476.

[4]   Rentschler, M., Hadzialic, A., Dumpert, J., Platt, S., Farritor, S., Oleynikov, D., 2004, "*In vivo* Robots for Laparoscopic Surgery." Studies in Health Technology and Informatics, 98: 316-322.

[5]   Rentschler, M., Dumpert, J., Platt, S., Farritor, S., Oleynikov, D., 2005, "Toward *In vivo* Mobility." Studies in Health Technology and Informatics, 111: 397-403.

[6]   Rentschler, M., Dumpert, J., Platt, S., Farritor, S., Oleynikov, D., "Mobile In Vivo Robots Provide Sole Visual Feedback for Abdominal Exploration and Cholecystectomy." J. Surgical Endoscopy – In Press.

[7]   T. Chanthasopeephan, J.P. Desai, A.C.W. Lau, "Measuring Forces in Liver Cutting: New Equipment and Experimental Results," *Annals of Biomedical Engineering*, vol. 31, pp. 1372-1382, 2003.

Medicine Meets Virtual Reality 14
J.D. Westwood et al. (Eds.)
IOS Press, 2006

455

An Integrated System for Real-Time Image Guided Cardiac Catheter Ablation

M.E. Rettmann, D.R. Holmes III, Y. Su, B.M. Cameron, J.J. Camp,
D.L. Packer, R.A. Robb

Mayo Clinic College of Medicine, Rochester, MN, USA

Abstract. Minimally invasive cardiac catheter ablation procedures require effective visualization of the relevant heart anatomy and electrophysiology (EP). In a typical ablation procedure, the visualization tools available to the cardiologist include bi-plane fluoroscopy, real-time ultrasound, and a coarse 3D model which gives a rough representation of cardiac anatomy and electrical activity. Recently, there has been increased interest in incorporating detailed, patient specific anatomical data into the cardiac ablation procedure. We are currently developing a prototype system which both integrates a patient specific, preoperative data model into the procedure as well as fuses the various visualization modalities (i.e. fluoroscopy, ultrasound, EP) into a single display. In this paper, we focus on two aspects of the prototype system. First, we describe the framework for integrating the various system components, including an efficient communication protocol. Second, using a simple two-chamber phantom of the heart, we demonstrate the ability to integrate preoperative data into the ablation procedure. This involves the registration and visualization of tracked catheter points within the cardiac chambers of the preoperative model.

Keywords. cardiac ablation, electrophysiologic mapping, EP mapping

1. Introduction

Approximately 6% of the population over the age of 65 suffers from atrial fibrillation (AF) [6], a condition in which the atria of the heart beat rapidly and irregularly [4]. Open-chest surgical procedures, in which incisions are made in the atria to eliminate abnormal electrical pathways responsible for arrhythmias, are highly effective but due to risk, morbidity, and cost, are generally elected as a last option. Cardiac catheter ablation procedures, a minimally invasive alternative to surgical approaches, have become the primary initial choice of therapy over the past twenty years [6]. In this technique, radiofrequency energy is delivered via a catheter to the endocardial surface producing lesions that block aberrant electrical pathways, thereby eliminating arrhythmias. Outcomes for AF ablation therapy have been mixed, with overall success rates between 50% and 70% for single procedures [8]. While these success rates are promising, procedure times are long with significant x-ray exposure. A major limitation of the catheter ablation procedure, as compared with open chest surgery, is the lack of precise visualization and localization of the target heart tissue.

In a typical ablation procedure, the cardiologist uses bi-plane fluoroscopy and real-time ultrasound for guidance of the ablation catheter. Catheter tip tracking technologies can also be used to generate three-dimensional representations of the heart during the procedure. The cardiologist samples a collection of points in the endocardial tissue to gradually build up a coarse 3D model of the left atrium and associated pulmonary veins [3]. Another approach [9] has shown a comparable model of the heart can be generated using non-contact mapping probes. Recent advances also incorporate detailed, patient specific anatomical image data into the procedure [1,2,5,7,10,12,14]. Work is currently underway in our laboratory to develop a prototype system that will incorporate accurate registration and fusion of real-time x-ray fluoroscopy, ultrasound, and pre-acquired patient specific CT data. The addition of real-time mapping of myocardial EP recordings onto cardiac anatomy will result in a fully integrated, 5D mapping system (x,y,z location, time and EP). In this paper, we focus on two aspects of the prototype system. First, we describe the framework for integrating the various system components, including an efficient communication protocol. Second, using a simple two-chamber phantom of the heart, we demonstrate the ability to integrate preoperative data into the ablation procedure. This involves the registration and visualization of tracked catheter points within the cardiac chambers of the preoperative model.

2. Methods

2.1. System Configuration

The overall system configuration is shown in Figure 1(a). The current prototype system consists of three processing/acquisition servers, a user interface, and a database. In addition, our system interfaces to a commercial EP mapping system (Biosense Webster Inc., Diamond Bar, CA) which transmits locations of the tracked catheter to our system via specialized software. Each component of the system is modular and communication between the system components is through the database. This allows for a fast distributed system since the individual components can each run on separate CPUs. Currently, the user interface displays the left atrium and associated pulmonary veins segmented from the preoperative, subject specific CT data. During the procedure, the point server receives coordinate locations from the tracked catheter and the registration server registers these points to the left atrium. The user interface incorporates the most recent registration matrix to provide an updated display of the points acquired during the procedure registered to the preoperative CT data. The streaming video server is designed to capture both fluoroscopy and ultrasound images for integration with the preoperative CT data for real-time display during the ablation procedure.

A photograph of the physical system is shown in Figure 1(b). The system consists of a cluster of four CPU boxes, each containing dual 2.4 GHz Athalons with 2 GB of memory. The point, registration, and video servers each run on separate boxes and the fourth box runs the user interface and database. The

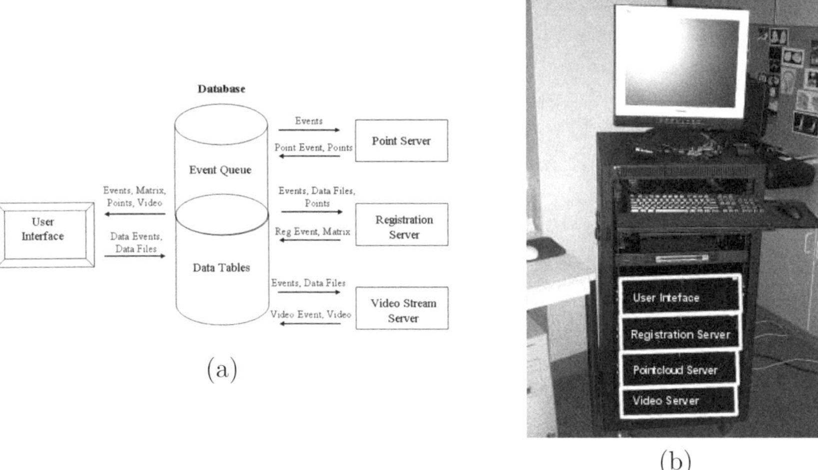

Figure 1. (a) Overall system configuration and (b) a photograph of the physical system.

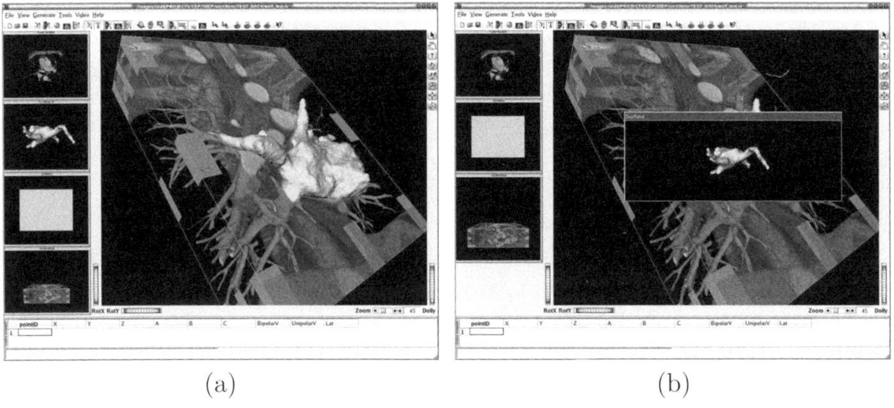

Figure 2. (a) Default layout of the user interface. (b) User interface with one of the specific displays detached.

graphical user interface is shown in Figure 2. This interface provides multiple, independent data visualization windows. A set of "detachable" visualization windows are aligned along the left side of the main interface which allow the user to visualize data from the various image modalities. Each of these windows may be detached from the interface at which point it becomes an independently operating interface that can be resized and repositioned independently of the main window. These mini-interfaces allow the user to perform data set specific tasks such as thresholding, filtering, clipping, etc. Once the user is finished with the window, it can be reattached to the main interface by simply dragging and dropping the detached window back into place.

The communication between the system components is implemented using an SQL database. The communication protocol is currently implemented for the user interface, point server, and registration server; however, due to the modular design of the system, it is straightforward to incorporate additional components (e.g. the video stream server). The database consists of four tables: an Event table, a Data table, a Point table, and a Registration Table. The Event table stores four types of events. A "Data Load" event indicates a new dataset has been loaded into the user interface. A "Point" event indicates a new coordinate location of the tracked catheter has been received by the point server. A "Registration" event indicates that a new registration has been computed between the point cloud and preoperative CT data. A "Quit" event indicates the procedure is finished. Each server reads and writes the appropriate events to and from the database.

A new dataset is loaded via the graphical user interface and the data file is loaded into the database. The point server waits for a Data event and then begins updating the database with coordinate point locations of the catheter as they are received. The registration server waits for a Data event and a catheter point location to be placed in the database. It then automatically registers the point cloud to the segmented left atrium using a downhill simplex method. The resulting registration matrix is updated into the database. When a new registration matrix is loaded into the database, the user interface detects the update and adjusts the visualization accordingly.

2.2. Simulation Study

In this study, we describe a simulation utilizing our physical phantom which demonstrates the functionality of the current prototype system. A photograph of the physical phantom is shown in Figure 3(a) which consists of two chambers representing the left and right atria as well as four rubber tubes for the pulmonary veins. Small markers which serve as landmarks were distributed across the phantom and their three-dimensional position recorded. In addition to the physical phantom, we have also generated an image of the phantom which is used to create our preoperative model. A surface model of the image phantom is shown in Figure 3(b) where the balls represent the landmarks.

In the simulation experiment, the operator used the tracked catheter to collect a point at each of the landmark points. After the selection of each point, the registration is initialized by aligning the centroid of the model from the preoperative data and the centroid of the current set of points. Next, the subset of points are registered to the segmented patient model producing a transformation T. This collection of steps (collecting a point, center of mass alignment, and registration) is considered one iteration in the simulation experiment. The top panel of Figure 4 shows the registration after 5 points have been selected, then 10 points, and lastly, the final regisration with all landmark points. Note the similarity of the registration result with the true landmark locations in Figure 3(b). The bottom panel illustrates the transformation T (computed using only the subset of points at that iteration) applied to all points at various iterations in the simulation. This gives a more intuitive understanding of the accuracy of the registration at each iteration. These images demonstrate that a reasonable registration is achieved after only five points have been collected, and the registration after ten points closely matches the final registration result.

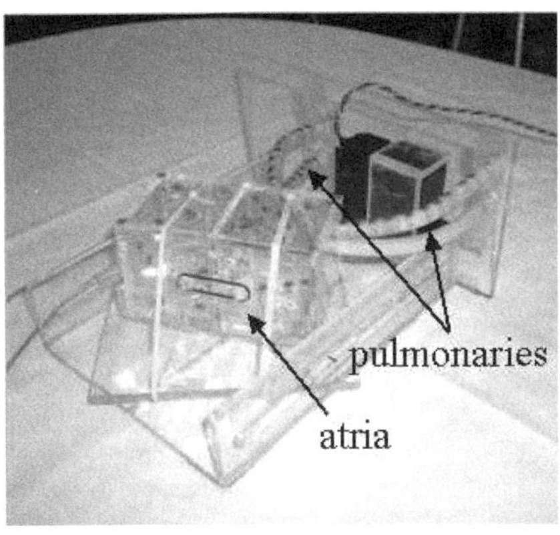

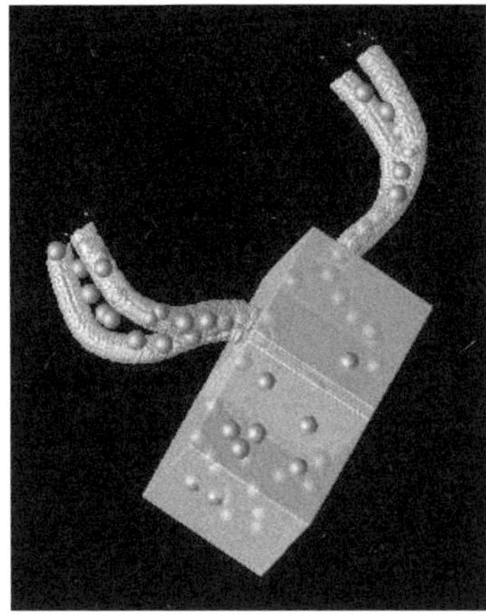

Figure 3. (a) Photograph of physical phantom and (b) surface model of phantom with landmark points.

3. Discussion and Future Work

Real-time cardiac ablation procedures require rapid integration of many different signals. Two features of our system specifically addresses this challenge. First, our system has a flexible, distributed design thereby allowing for easy integration of both existing as well as new signals. Second, we utilize a communication protocol between the servers which is efficient and reliable yet maintains server independence. Improvements planned for the system include models which incorporate physiologic mapping information as well as registration of real-time ultrasound and fluoroscopy provided by the streaming video. Together, these additions will provide a single integrated visualization of real anatomy in real-time for the cardiologist.

Acknowledgements

This work has been supported through NIH/NIBIB grant #EB002834.

References

[1] Dickfield, T. et. al.: Anatomic Stereotactic Catheter Ablation on Three-Dimensional Magnetic Resonance Images in Real Time. Circulation **108** (2003) 2407–2413.
[2] Dickfield, T., Calkins, H., Bradley, D., Solomon, S.: Stereotactic catheter navigation using magnetic resonance image integration in the human heart. Heart Rhythm **2(4)** (2005) 413–415.
[3] Gepstein, L., Hayam, G., Ben-Haim, S.A.: A Novel method for Nonfluoroscopic Catheter-Based Electroanatomical Mapping of the Heart. Circulation **95(6)** 1611–1622.
[4] Green, B.: The Maze III Surgical Procedure. AORN **76** (2002) 133-134, 136–150.
[5] Lacomis, J.M. et. al.: Multi-Detector Row CT of the Left Atrium and Pulmonary Veins before Radio-frequency Catheter Ablation for Atrial Fibrillation. Radiographics **23** 2003 S35–S48.

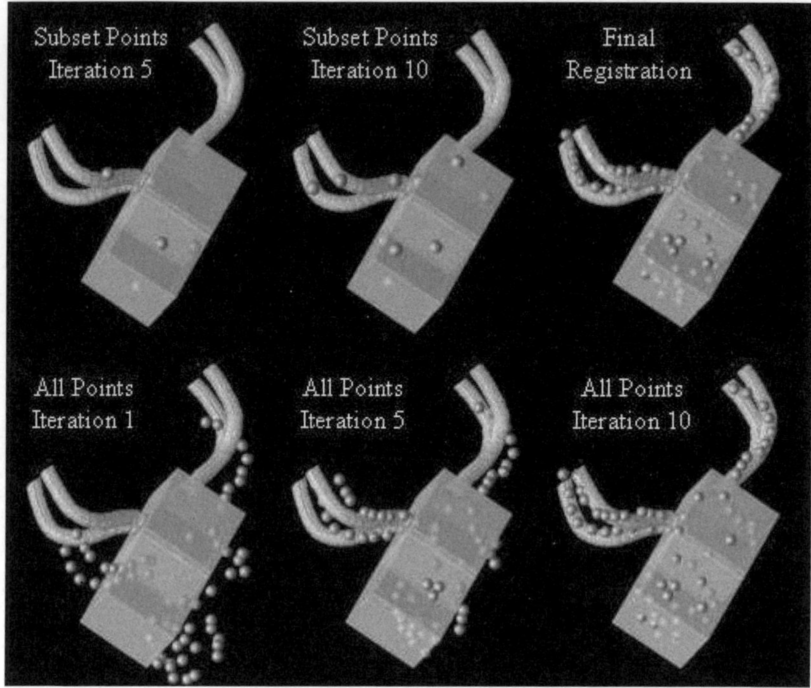

Figure 4. Simulation study with physical phantom. Top panel demonstrates registration on the subset of points after 5 points, then 10 points, and lastly, the final registration. Bottom panel demonstrates transformation matrix computed at each iteration applied to all points.

[6] Lin, D., Marchlinski, F.: Advances in Ablation Therapy for Complex Arrhythmias: Atrial Fibrillation and Ventricular Tachycardia. Curr Cardiol Rep **5** (2003) 407–414.

[7] Mansour, M., Holmvang, G., Ruskin, J.: Role of Imaging Techniques in Preparation for Catheter Ablation of Atrial Fibrillation. J of Cardiov Electrophys **15** 1107–1108.

[8] Packer, D.L., Asirvatham, S., Munger, T.M.: Progress in Nonpharmacologic Therapy of Atrial Fibrillation. Cardiovasc Electrophysiol **14** (2003) S296–S309.

[9] Peters, N.S. et. al.: Human Left Ventricular Endocardial Activation Mapping Using a Novel Noncontact Catheter. Circulation **96(6)** (1997) 1658–1660.

[10] Reddy et. al.: Integration of Cardiac Magnetic Resonance Imaging with Three-Dimensional Electroanatomic Mapping to Guide Left Ventricular Catheter Manipulation. J Am Coll Cardiol **44(11)** (2004) 2202–2213.

[11] Robb, R.A., Hanson, D.P.: ANALYZE: A Software System for Biomedical Image Analysis. Proc. of the 1st Conf on Vis in Biomed Comput (1990) 507–518.

[12] Sra, J. et. al.: Feasibility and validation of registration of three-dimensional left atrial models derived from computed tomography with a noncontact cardiac mapping system. Heart Rhythm **2(1)** (2005) 55–63.

[13] Stewart, S.: Epidemiology and Impact of Atrial Fibrillation. J Cardiov Nurs **19** (2004) 94–102.

[14] Sun, Y. et. al.: Registration of high-resolution 3D atrial images with electroanatomical cardiac mapping: Evaluation of registration methodology. SPIE Medical Imaging **5744** (2005) 299–307.

Medicine Meets Virtual Reality 14
J.D. Westwood et al. (Eds.)
IOS Press, 2006

Stress Management Using UMTS Cellular Phones: A Controlled Trial

Giuseppe RIVA[1-2], Alessandra PREZIOSA [1], Alessandra GRASSI [2], Daniela VILLANI [1-2]

[1] *ATN-P Lab., Istituto Auxologico Italiano, Milan, Italy*
[2] *Dipartimento di Psicologia, Università Cattolica, Milan, Italy*

Abstract: One of the best strategies for dealing with stress is learning how to relax. However, relaxing is difficult to achieve in typical real world situations. For this study, we developed a specific protocol based on mobile narratives – multimedia narratives experienced on UMTS/3G phones – to help workers in reducing commuting stress. In a controlled trial 33 commuters were randomly divided between three conditions: Mobile narratives (MN); New age music and videos (NA); no treatment (CT). In two consecutive days the MN and NA samples experienced during their commute trip 2x2 6-minute multimedia experiences on a Motorola A925 3G phone provided by the "TRE" Italian UMTS carrier: the MN sample experienced a mobile narrative based on the exploration of a desert beach; the NA sample experienced a commercial new age video with similar visual contents. The trials showed the efficacy of mobile narratives in reducing the level of stress experienced during a commute trip. No effects were found in the other groups. These results suggest that 3G mobile handsets may be used as relaxation tool if backed by a specific therapeutic protocol and meaningful narratives.

Keywords: Stress treatment, cellular phones, UMTS, controlled trial

1. Introduction

Health care and mobile phones are usually associated only during debates about the safety of handsets. However, the appearance of smart mobile handsets with advanced multimedia capabilities and high connection speeds may change this situation over the coming years.

Recently Kruger [1] identified three areas where mobile health care services will be applicable within a fully engaged health care scenario: dietary information, fitness and training, and health monitoring. A peculiar application within the fitness and training area is stress management. Stress is the automatic state that results when the body is told to make changes in order to adapt to any demand. When stress is acute or chronic, all parts of

---

[1] Corresponding Author: Prof. Giuseppe Riva, Ph.D., Dipartimento di Psicologia, Università Cattolica del Sacro Cuore, Largo Gemelli 1, 20123 Milan, Italy, e-mail: giuseppe.riva@unicatt.it, web-site: http://www.neurotiv.org

the body's stress apparatus (the brain, heart, lungs, vessels, and muscles) become chronically over- or under-activated. This may produce physical or psychological damage over time.

One of the best strategies for dealing with stress is learning how to relax. However, relaxing is difficult to achieve in typical real world situations. In this study, supported by the Italian MIUR FIRB research project, we developed a specific protocol based on mobile narratives, to be experienced on 3G smart handsets by commuters. Mobile narratives are audio-visual experiences, implemented on mobile devices, in which the narrative component is a critical aspect to induce a feeling of presence and engagement. Through the link between the feeling of presence and the emotional state, mobile narratives may be used to improve the mood state in their users.

2. Sample and Methods

The experimental sample included 17 male and 16 female commuters (N=33) of the Italian regional train line "Milano-Saronno", aged between 20-25 years (M=23.82+/-0.72). The sample was randomly divided between the following three conditions:

- MN - Mobile narratives: the sample experienced four mobile narratives based on a trip in a desert tropical beach (see Figure 1);
- NA - New age videos: the sample experienced four commercial videos with new age music (see Figure 1). The videos were selected for their similar visual content (a tropical beach) to the mobile narratives;
- CT - Control group: no treatment.

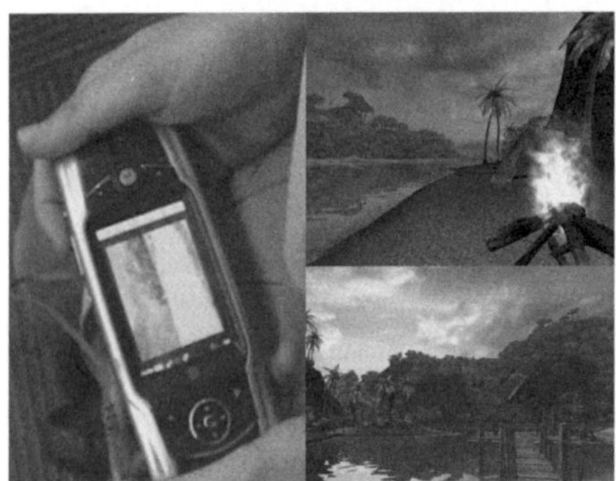 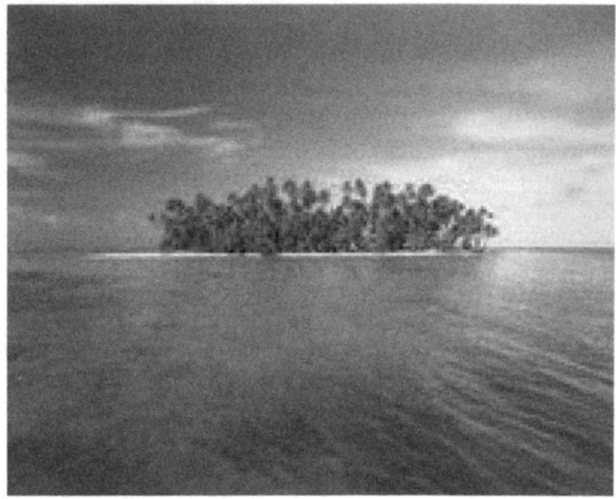

Figure 1. The visual content of the Mobile Narratives (left) and the New Age video (right)

The sample was tracked for two days. During each trip the experimental samples experienced on a Motorola A925 UMTS cellular phone (screen size: 208x320 pixel) the multimedia content. The total length of each experience was 6 minutes. Before and after each trip the subjects were submitted to the following questionnaires: STAI: State-Trait

Anxiety Inventory [2]; VAS: Visual Analog Scale [3]; PANAS: Positive and Negative Affect Schedule [4]; ITC-Sopi: Sense of Presence Inventory [5].

3. Results

The first significant result was the difference in anxiety between the three groups. Only the MN group experienced a significant reduction in the anxiety level (STAI: z=2,943, p<0.01) and an increase in the relax scale (VAS: z=-2,842; p<0.01) at the end of the trial. Also, the anxiety reduction in the MN group was significantly higher than the ones achieved by two groups (STAI: Chi-square: 20.749, p<0.01).

The second relevant result is related to the level of presence experienced by the two experimental groups. The level of "engagement" and "spatial presence" was significantly higher in the MN group. These data suggest that the efficacy of the MN may be related to the higher level of presence induced by mobile narratives.

4. Conclusions

The trials showed the efficacy of mobile narratives in reducing the level of stress experienced during a commute trip. No effects were found in the other groups. These results suggest that 3G mobile handsets, even with their small screens and limited multimedia capabilities, may be used as relaxation tool if backed by a specific therapeutic protocol and an engaging experience.

5. Acknowledgments

The present work was supported by the Italian MIUR FIRB programme (Project *"Neurotiv - Managed care basata su telepresenza immersiva virtuale per l'assessment e riabilitazione in neuro-psicologia e psicologia clinica"* - RBNE01W8WH - and Project *"Realtà virtuale come strumento di valutazione e trattamento in psicologia clinica: aspetti tecnologici, ergonomici e clinici"* – RBAU014JE5).

6. References

[1] Kruger, P. (2004). Mobile Operators – Fully engaged. Herts, UK: Wireless Healthcare.

[2] Speilberger, C.D. (1983). Manual for the State-Trait Anxiety Inventory (Form Y). Palo Alto, CA: Consulting Psychologists Press.

[3] Gift A. Visual analog scales (1989). Measurement of subjective phenomenon. Nursing Research, 38(5):286-288.

[4] Watson, D., & Clark, L.A. (1988). Development and validation of brief measures of positive and negative affect: The PANAS Scales. Journal of Personality and Social Psychology, 54:1063-1070.

[5] Lessiter, J., Freeman, J., Keogh, E., Davidoff, J. (2001). A Cross-Media Presence Questionnaire: The ITC-Sense of Presence Inventory. Presence: Teleoperators & Virtual Environments, 10 (5\3), 282-298.

Medicine Meets Virtual Reality 14
J.D. Westwood et al. (Eds.)
IOS Press, 2006

Structure-Function Relationships in the Human Visual System Using DTI, fMRI and Visual Field Testing: Pre- and Post-Operative Assessments in Patients with Anterior Visual Pathway Compression

Joel Rosiene [a,1], X. Liu [b], C. Imielinska [b], J. Ferrera [c], J. Bruce [d], J. Hirsch [c], and A. D'Ambrosio [d]

[a] *Computer Science Department, Eastern Connecticut State University, Willimantic, CT*
[b] *Department of Biomedical Informatics, Columbia University, New York, NY*
[c] *fMRI Research Center, Columbia University, New York, NY*
[d] *Department of Neurological Surgery, Columbia University, New York, NY*

Abstract. The focus of this project is to improve our understanding of the relationships between brain structure and function in patients presenting with anterior visual pathway compression using functional MRI (fMRI), visual field(VF) maps and diffusion tensor imaging (DTI). Significant visual loss can occur when large pituitary lesions compress the optic chiasm. Surgical resection of these lesions decompresses the chiasm and can lead to visual recovery. In this preliminary study, we selected patients presenting with slowly progressive visual loss secondary to a compressive pituitary region mass. Using preoperative DTI data, we reconstructed white matter projections of the optic radiations and demonstrated a structural correlation with functional vision as quantified by formal visual field mapping and fMRI. The structural data generated through a fiber tracking algorithm may represent a potentially powerful tool to better understand functional visual deficits in patients with anterior visual pathway compression. Furthermore, we believe that specific patterns in preoperative DTI data may predict the likelihood of postoperative visual recovery in a select group of patients.

Keywords. Diffusion tensor imaging (DTI), fMRI, Visual Fields, pituitary tumors,

1. Introduction

The recently developed magnetic resonance technique of diffusion tensor imaging (DTI), [1], can be used clinically to trace the structure of white fiber tracts in the human brain.

---

[1] Correspondence to: Joel Rosiene, Computer Science, Eastern Connecticut State University, Willimantic, CT 06224. Tel.: 1 860 465 0091; Fax: +1 222 333 0000; E-mail: rosienej@easternct.edu.

This novel imaging technique, that derives microstructural and physiological features of tissues, has many potential practical applications. The focus of this paper is to improve our understanding of the structure/function relationships in the human visual pathway in patients presenting with significant visual loss secondary to optic chiasmal compression. Furthermore, we hope to standardize our DTI acquisition protocol to reduce variation in acquired data sets. Large pituitary lesions often cause visual field deficits secondary to their intimate relationship with the optic chiasm. These lesions compress the chiasm from below, often causing a bitemporal field cut secondary to neuronal compromise. If the chiasm is decompressed in a timely fashion, recovery of visual function can occur. This improvement in visual function has been shown to occur in three stages: rapid recovery within minutes to days, delayed recovery over weeks to months, and late recovery in months to years. We hypothesize that, in patients with long-standing chiasmal compression and visual deficits, the preoperative white matter pathways will be abnormal manifesting as fewer connected optic radiation fiber bundles as seen on DTI. Furthermore, in patients who demonstrate functional visual recovery after tumor resection, postoperative DTI studies will demonstrate more robust fiber bundle connectivity when compared to preoperative data.

2. Methods

Preoperative DTI data was obtained according to hospital protocol in conjunction with standard brain MRI acquisition. Automated visual field testing was performed in addition to standard visual field assessment. The functional visual cortex was mapped using fMRI and a reversing checkerboard stimulus with a 30 sec duration. We used an open software application for three-dimensional representation of the optic radiations, [2]

To determine how well the diffusion tensor models the dataset, we calculated the Signal to Noise Ratio (SNR) obtained by comparison of the directions predicted from the model to measured directions. As in [1] the diffusion tensor components $\{DT_{xx}, DT_{yy}, DT_{zz}, DT_{xy}, DT_{xz}, DT_{yz}\}$ are estimated from the sequence of diffusion weighted images DW_i taken at different gradient directions G_i. As a simple check of the quality of the model, the calculated diffusion tensor is used to generate diffusion weighted images $D\hat{W}_i$. The resulting images are used to generate SNRs for each of the gradient images as: $SNR_i = 20\log(D\hat{W}_i/MSE)$ with $MSE = \|DW_i - D\hat{W}_i\|$.

In addition to the Diffusion Tensor, the covariance matrix (Σ) of each voxel over the set of diffusion images is used to obtain the principle components of the voxel $\{\lambda_i = \Sigma e_i : 1 \leq i \leq$ number of DW images$\}$.

3. Results

For the preliminary study, we selected a subject presenting with chronic visual loss in the left eye and subacute loss of visual acuity on the right. Preoperative MRI revealed a large pituitary region mass completely compressing the right optic nerve and chiasm. A preoperative DTI, fMRI, and automated VF map was obtained as previously described. The preoperative functional data demonstrated complete loss of vision in the right eye. Cortical visual mapping correlated well with the patients functional visual by automated

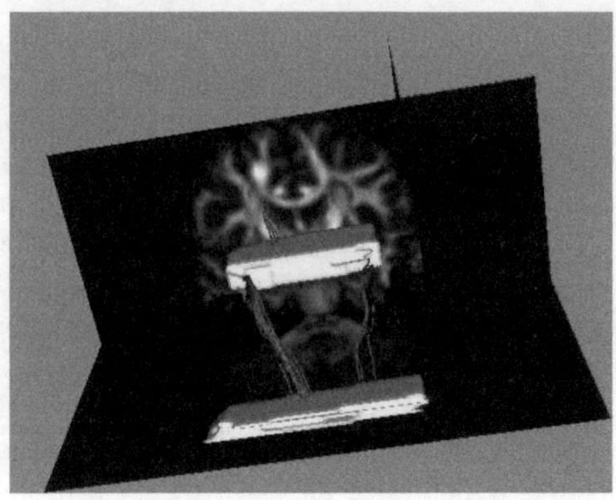

Figure 1. A rendering of the optic nerves and chiasm

assessment. Preoperative DTI fiber tracking demonstrated diminished bundle fiber connectivity to the primary visual cortex responsible for vision in the appropriate distribution, Fig.1.

The preoperative scans and the visual fields have been acquired and seem consistent with the patient's hemianopsia as shown on the visual field testing.

4. Conclusion

We have preprocessed and characterized the estimated diffusion tensor prior to visualization with DTI tracking software developed by Gerig and Fillard [2]. We are also developing in-house software to process DTI images which utilizes pseudo-colored images to visualize nerve bundles, via extraction of the Principle Component. This approach will provide us with a full understanding of the processed DTI data and allow better interpretation of white matter fiber images visualized in 3D. Correlating fMRI, automated VFs and DTI abnormalities may represent a powerful prognostic tool better understand pre- and postoperative functional visual deficits in patients with anterior visual pathway compression.

Acknowledgements

We thank Jeffrey Johnson, Zhizhou Wang and Mariappan Nadar of Siemens's Princeton Laboratory, NJ for helpful discussion regarding the visualization of the optic nerve fibers.

References

[1] P.J. Basser and C. Pierpaoli, "Microstructure and physiological features of tissue elucidated by quantgitative difision tensor mri", *Journal of magnetic Resonanse in Imaging JMRI*, **vol.111**, pp. 209-219, 1996.

[2] Pierre Fillard, John Gilmore, Weili Lin, Joseph Piven, Guido Gerig, "Quantitative Analysis of White Matter Fiber Properties along Geodesic Paths", *Lecture Notes in Computer Science LNCS #2879*, pp. 16-23, Nov. 2003

Medicine Meets Virtual Reality 14
J.D. Westwood et al. (Eds.)
IOS Press, 2006

Estimation of Skeletal Movement of Human Locomotion from Body Surface Shapes Using Dynamic Spatial Video Camera (DSVC) and 4D Human Model

Toshikuni Saito[a], Naoki Suzuki[b], Asaki Hattori[b], Shigeyuki Suzuki[b], Mitsuhiro Hayashibe[b], Yoshito Otake[b]

[a]*Graduate School of Science and Engineering, Waseda University, #61-306 Sota Lab., 3-4-1 Ookubo Shinjyuku-ku, Tokyo, 169-8555, Japan*
[b]*Institute for High Dimensional Medical Imaging, The Jikei University School of Medicine, 4-11-1 Izumihoncho Komae-shi, Tokyo, 201-8601, Japan*

Abstract. We have been developing a DSVC (Dynamic Spatial Video Camera) system to measure and observe human locomotion quantitatively and freely. A 4D (four-dimensional) human model with detailed skeletal structure, joint, muscle, and motor functionality has been built. The purpose of our research was to estimate skeletal movements from body surface shapes using DSVC and the 4D human model. For this purpose, we constructed a body surface model of a subject and resized the standard 4D human model to match with geometrical features of the subject's body surface model. Software that integrates the DSVC system and the 4D human model, and allows dynamic skeletal state analysis from body surface movement data was also developed. We practically applied the developed system in dynamic skeletal state analysis of a lower limb in motion and were able to visualize the motion using geometrically resized standard 4D human model.

Keywords. Dynamic Spatial Video Camera, 4D human model, 4D motion analysis

1. Introduction

Recently, four-dimensional (4D) partial analysis of human locomotion has become possible by using systems like the OpenMRI. Four-dimensional relates to a time-sequential movement of three dimensional structures; until now the 4D analysis of overall human locomotion has been difficult. To overcome the difficulty we adopted an approach based on two main components. First, in order to measure and observe overall human locomotion quantitatively and freely, DSVC (Dynamic Spatial Video Camera) system has been developed[1]. DSVC system is equipped with 65 digital video cameras that are controlled by 33 PCs to collect time sequential digital video images of the subject's motion from multiple angles around the observed subject

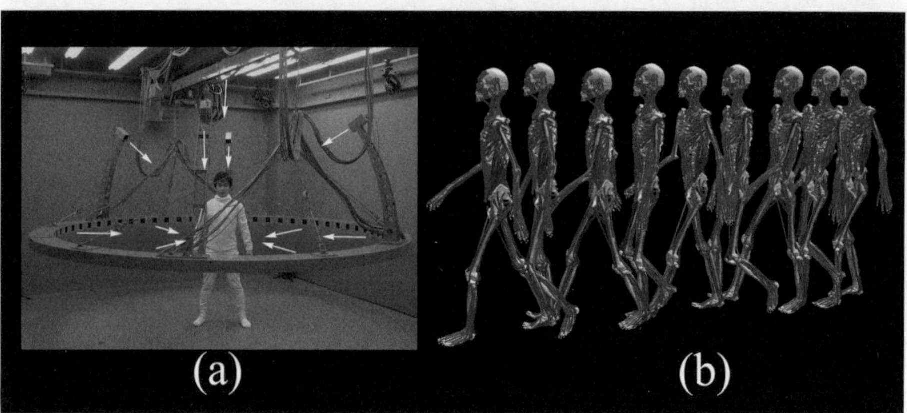

Fig.1 The assembled DSVC system (a) and the standard 4D human model (b).

(Fig.1a). Second, a 4D human model providing a detailed presentation of skeletal structures, joints, muscles, and motor function has been built[2] (Fig.1b). The purpose of the present study was to estimate a skeletal movement of human locomotion from body surface shapes quantitatively and freely by using DSVC and the standard 4D human model. For this purpose, we constructed a subject's body surface model and resized the 4D human model with standard proportions by geometrical features of the body surface model of the subject. Moreover, we practically applied the developed system in dynamic skeletal state analysis of the lower limb in motion and visualized the motion using geometrically resized 4D human model. Such a system would allow accurate diagnosis and facilitate effective treatment in the field of orthopedics and rehabilitation.

2. Methods

Our approach to assess the dynamic skeletal state of a human in motion was based on two parts: construction of a subject's skeletal model and motion analysis of a subject's motion from body surface movement data.

2.1. Construction of a subject's skeletal model

First, a subject's skeletal model for estimation of subject's dynamic skeletal state with his motion was constructed. Our approach was to resize the standard 4D human model data accordingly with on the individual anatomical features of the subject, such as joints center positions. The standard 4D human model with detailed skeletal structure, joint, muscle, and motor function has been previously constructed in our Institute from MRI data of a healthy adult volunteer. The subject's body surface model was constructed using the DSVC system. The DSVC system was set-up in the blue-colored room, so the subject image data could be extracted from the filmed images from each camera by background-image difference and the chroma-key method. Before filming, the location and direction of each camera was calibrated. The subject's 3D body surface model was extracted from the virtual cube by positioning the camera around the object and combining separate 2D contour images from all available angles. The computer calculated the location and direction of each separate image and based on these data, created the 3D surface model of the subject. The constructed body surface model with cube assemblage method was later polygonized and colored using filmed images. Thus, the anatomical feature markers of subject's body surface model were compared with the corresponding points of the standard 4D human model, and resizing parameters were decided based on the obtained difference. The standard 4D human model was resized and a subject's skeletal model with rendered subject's anatomical features was obtained.

2.2. Motion analysis of a subject from body surface movement data

First, motion data from movement of subject's body surface shapes were obtained. Then, time sequential subject's body surface models were constructed from the filmed images of the subject in motion. Generally, a method of construction of the subject's body surface model followed that described above at *2.1*. Time-series of body surface movement were tracked by aligning the geometric features of the constructed body surface models. For improvement of tracking accuracy, we set constraint conditions that limited tracking target area by joint positions of the subject's skeletal model. Position and rotation of joints of the subject's skeletal model were calculated based on tracking data. Finally, the subject's dynamic skeletal state was visualized by driving the constructed subject's skeletal model data on tracked body surface movement data. Software that enabled observation of the results of all model construction processes was developed.

3. Results

Data of a subject in standing position was used to construct the subject's skeletal model. Fig.2 shows the construction process. A body surface shape of the standard 4D human model based on MRI data of a healthy adult volunteer is shown in Fig.2a-1. The constructed subject's body surface model from DSVC system images is shown in Fig.2a-2. Geometrical parameters of selected body parts (colored correspondingly in the figure) of the standard 4D human model and the subject's body surface model were calculated (Fig.2b). A standard 4D human model (Fig.2c-1) was resized to match the subject's body surface model, and the subject's skeletal model was obtained (Fig.2c-2). Next, for motion analysis, we captured a foot swing motion of the subject and tried to estimate a dynamic skeletal state of the lower limb in that motion. Fig.3 shows captured images of the foot swing motion collected by the same camera. The captured images could be observed freely from any viewpoint and any time. Then, time-series of subject's body surface models of foot swing motion were constructed (Fig.4a). The body surface movements in motion were tracked based on geometrical changes of body surface shapes (Fig.4b). The dynamic skeletal state of the foot in swing motion was visualized by applying tracking results and constructed subject's skeletal model data (Fig.4c,d). Observations could be made from any viewpoint and at any time. An example of simultaneous observation of subject's dynamic skeletal state from multiple viewpoints is shown in Fig.5.

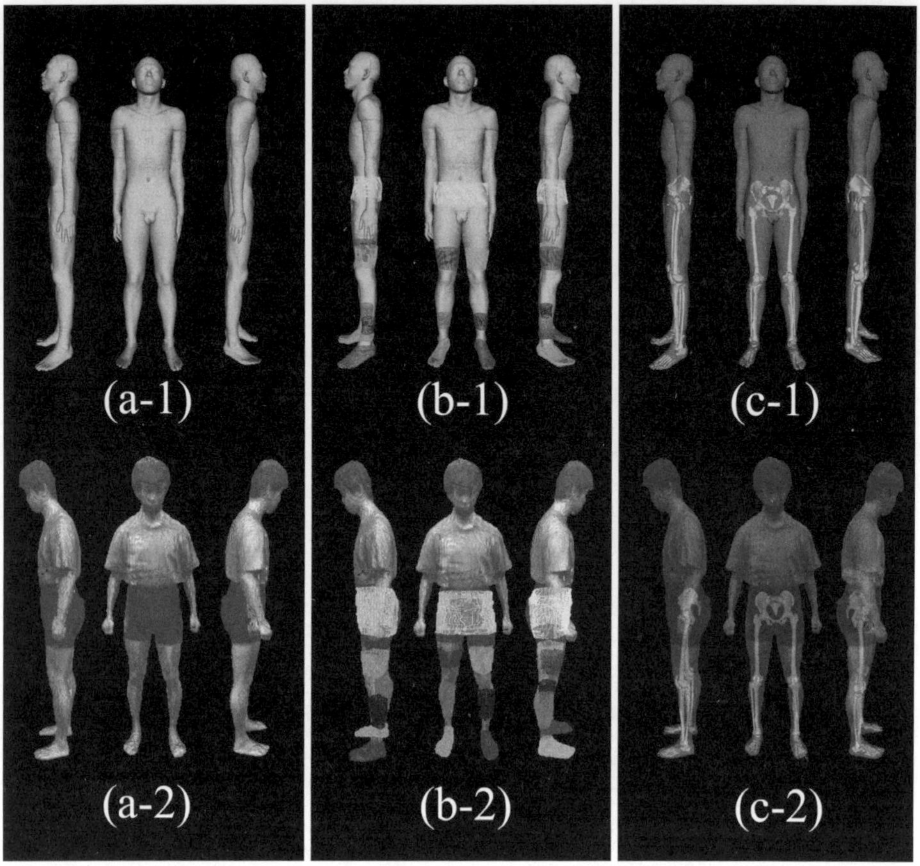

Fig.2 Construction of subject's skeletal model (a: the body surface shapes of the standard 4D human model and constructed subject's body surface model by DSVC system, b: corresponding body parts between the 4D human model and the standard 4D human model, c: resizing of the skeletal structure of the standard 4D human model to construct the subject's skeletal model).

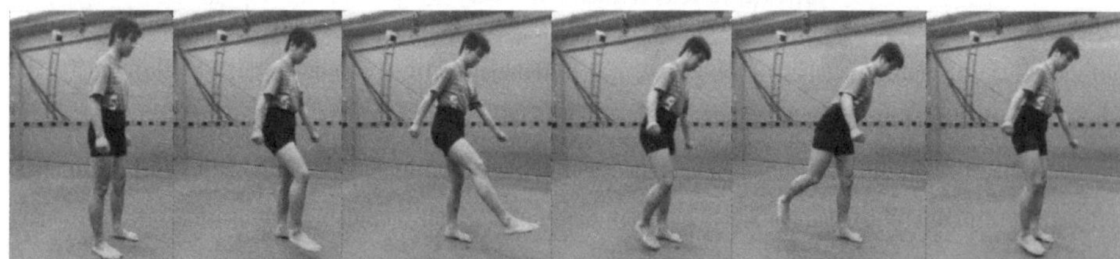

Fig.3 Captured images of foot swing motion using DSVC system.

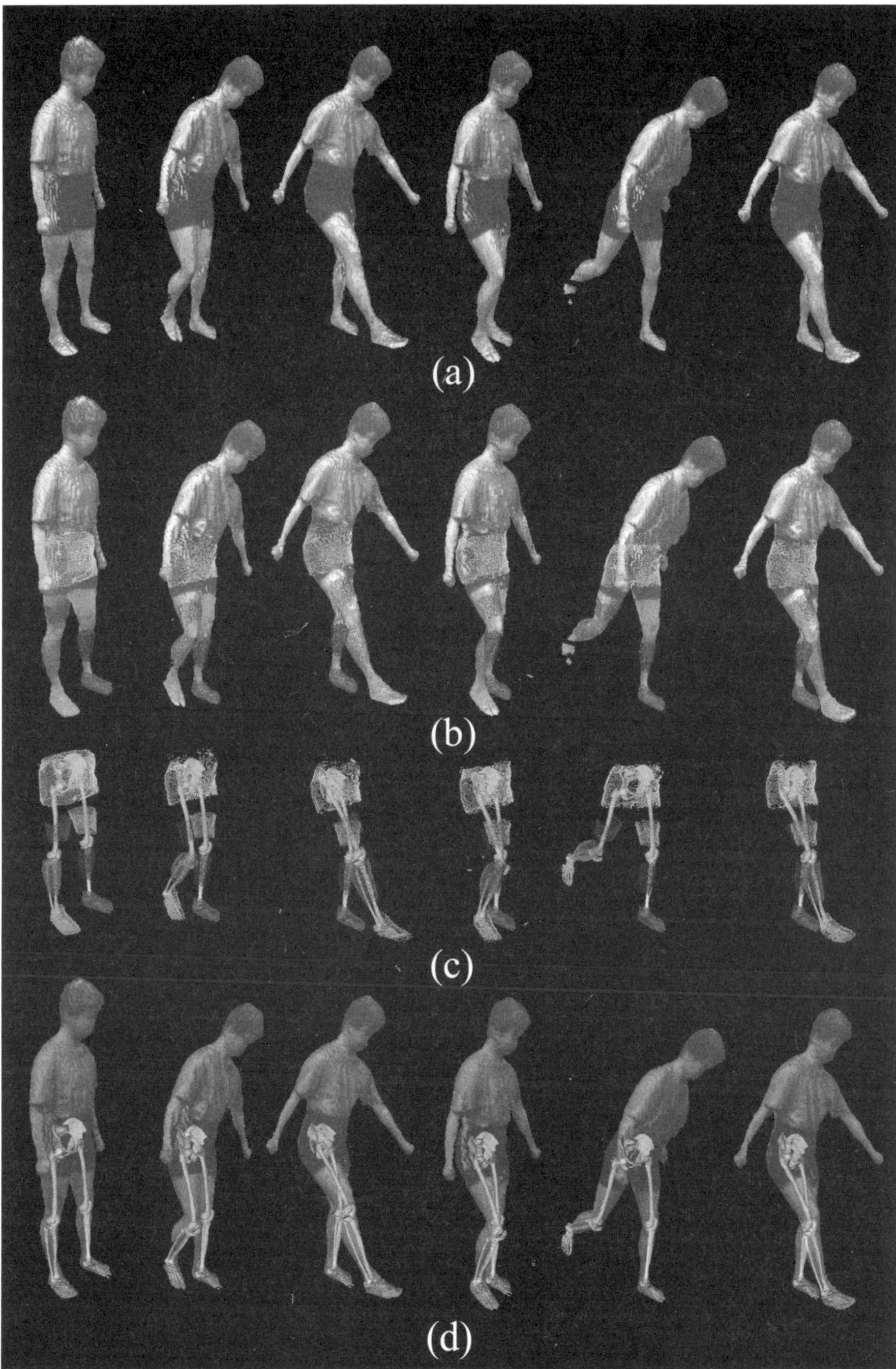

Fig.4 Estimation of subject's dynamic skeletal structure in foot swing motion (a: constructed time-series of subject's body surface model by DSVC system, b: tracking the body parts movement from changes of body surface shapes, c: driving the subject's skeletal model on tracking data, d: superimposed dynamic skeletal state on constructed subject's body surface models).

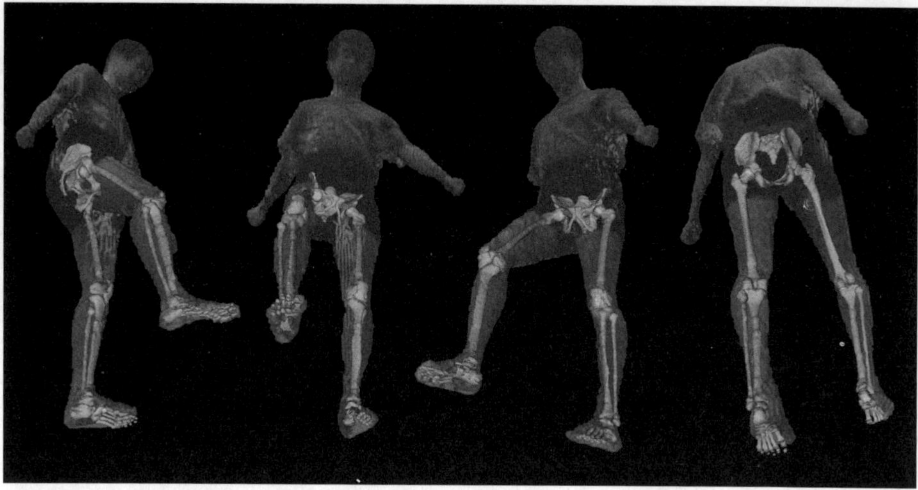

Fig.5 Observation of the dynamic skeletal state in foot swing motion was possible from multiple viewpoints at different stopping times.

4. Conclusions

A body surface model that enables estimation of inner anatomical features has been constructed by using the DSVC system. We estimated a subject's dynamic skeletal state during a lower limb motion without body surface marker or sensors by tracking the movement of subject's body surface shapes. The subject's dynamic skeletal state in motion was visualized based on the resized standard 4D human model and tracking data. The estimation results have been promising and we are planning to validate them quantitatively. We also plan to expand the analysis area to the whole body and optimize our algorithm to make the system applicable for accurate diagnosis and effective treatment in orthopedics and rehabilitation.

References

[1] N. Suzuki, A. Hattori, M. Hayashibe, S. Suzuki, Y. Otake: "Development of Dynamic Spatial Video Camera (DSVC) for 4D observation, analysis and modeling of human body locomotion", Medicine Meets Virtual Reality 11, pp.346-348, 2003
[2] Y. Otake, N. Suzuki, A. Hattori, S. Suzuki, M. Hayashibe: "4-Dimensional Whole Body Human Model for Dynamic Analysis of Human Locomotion", World Congress on Medical Physics and Biomedical Engineering 2003, pp.121, 2003

Medicine Meets Virtual Reality 14
J.D. Westwood et al. (Eds.)
IOS Press, 2006

Validation of Open-Surgery VR Trainer

A.J.B Sanders[1], J.M. Luursema[2], P. Warntjes[1], W.J.B. Mastboom[3], R.H.
Geelkerken[3], J.M. Klaase[3], S.G.J. Rödel[3], H.O. ten Cate Hoedemaker[4], P.A.M.
Kommers[2], W.B. Verwey[2], E.E. Kunst[1]

[1] *Kunst & van Leerdam Medical Technology bv, Enschede, the Netherlands;*
asanders@kvlmt.nl; [2] *Department of Behavioral Science, University of Twente,*
Enschede, NL; [3] *Department of Vascular Surgery, Medical Spectrum Twente,*
Enschede, NL;
[4] *University Medical Center Groningen, Groningen, NL*

Abstract

VREST (Virtual Reality Educational Surgical Tools) is developing a universal and
autonomous simulation platform which can be used for training and assessment of
medical students and for continuing education of physicians. With the VREST -
Virtual Lichtenstein Trainer, simulating the open surgery procedure of the inguinal
hernia repair according to Lichtenstein, the validation of the simulator is ongoing.
Part of this trajectory is the evaluation of the transfer of training of the virtual
incision making. One group of students trained incision making on the VREST
platform where the control group did not. In an experiment both groups has to
perform several incision tasks on a manikin. The results are not available yet but
will be presented at the MMVR14 conference.

1. Background / Problem

VREST developed a Platform for Virtual Medical Training [1] in which in
principle all kinds of surgical techniques can be practiced. On the VREST platform a
resident is educated in knowledge and skills based on 'touch' and 'vision' and
'decision' in a VR environment. The VREST platform is used prior to the first
operating room surgery of the resident. Most work on transfer of surgical skills from
simulator training to the operating room has been done using laparoscopic simulators [2,
3, 4, 5].

The current study aims to validate that the VREST platform will contribute to a
more efficient and effective training trajectory of the resident. Increasing efficiency
will lead to a lower number of operating room procedures needed to become a qualified
and skilled surgeon.

The transfer of the virtual hernia repair training to the operating room is
investigated in this validation.

2. Tools and Methods

Based on the VREST Platform for Virtual Medical Training [1] a Lichtenstein repair of inguinal hernia trainer is developed. This Virtual Lichtenstein Trainer (VREST-VLT) has several features. Bimanual surgery with haptic feedback is enabled by means of two Phantom® devices. To provide the user a high quality three dimensional perception, the virtual operation scene is rendered in stereo, and synchronized with shutter glasses. Co-location of the hand and the virtual world is satisfied with a monitor–mirror system. Together this creates a good 3D perception which is needed to mimic real surgery. Interactive models of the groin area can be manipulated using the haptic devices. An objective virtual teacher replaces the real 'master' surgeon. The virtual teacher can give instruction and gives feedback on the resident's actions with text, speech, literature and video.

Three levels are built in the VREST-VLT. In the first level the resident is guided through the procedure of the Lichtenstein repair technique performing all the tasks the teacher tells him to do. In the second level the resident can perform whatever he likes within the VREST-VLT. In the third level the resident is being assessed while doing the complete hernia repair operation. The third level will end with a VREST-VLT-certificate upon completion of the virtual training. The validation of the VREST-VLT is ongoing in the Medical Spectrum Twente, Enschede, NL and the University Medical Center Groningen, Groningen, NL. Twelve residents are divided into two groups, the VREST-VLT-group and a control group, based on a pre-test for visio-spatial ability, perceptual motor skills and sensitivity to stress. The control group follows their training in the normal way by starting in the operating room and learns by doing with feedback from the 'master' surgeon. The VREST-VLT-group starts to train on the VREST-VLT till they receive their VREST VLT-certificate which allows them to complete their training in the operating room.

The trial ends after completing three real operations. Objective criteria such as the number of errors and the time needed to complete parts of the operation to judge the residents are formulated. Video recordings of all the operations are examined by an independent expert panel of skilled and experienced surgeons. The expert panel judges each resident on the criteria formulated without knowing which resident followed the normal or the VREST-VLT trajectory.

Part of the validation is the evaluation of the transfer of training of the virtual incision making.

30 participants are tested for perceptual motor abilities. Based on the results of this test, participants are randomly matched over two groups of equal ability.

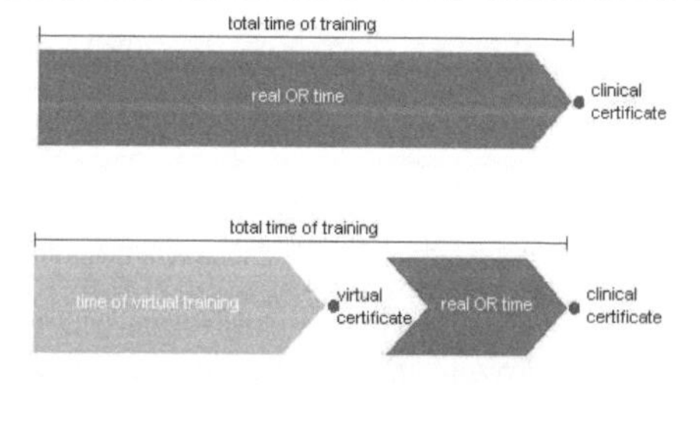

Figure 1: Time of training, present and future

One group experiences a virtual incision making lesson on the VREST platform, the other group experiences no training. Over the whole course of the training sessions, four versions of the same virtual incision-making task are offered. Each participant concludes four training sessions of half an hour spread over four consecutive days.

After the training sessions and a day of rest, transfer is measured by having the participants execute the same task on a manikin. This is videotaped and assessed by experts who are blinded to the participants' identity. Two weeks later the participants again complete a session on the manikin, which again is videotaped and assessed by experts to evaluate not only transfer, but also retention.

3. Results

At the time of this report the validation was not completed. Parts of the validation will be presented during the MMVR14 Conference.

4. Conclusions / Discussion

VR training prior to OR training are expected to enhance both effectivity and efficiency of the surgical training process. The transfer of the training to the operating room can be measured at different stages, each with a different impact. The results after three operations will give a clue of the immediate efficiency of the VREST-VLT. However the results, including the number of operating room procedures needed, after completing the whole training until the resident has gained a sufficient professional level according to the 'master' surgeon will show the over-all efficiency. Furthermore, this validation study aims to indicate the gain in efficiency of the overall surgical training in hernia repair in establishing an expected difference in number of clinical procedures necessary to become a skilled hernia repair surgeon with or without VR training.

5. References

[1]　Kunst EE, Geelkerken RH, Sanders AJB. The VREST learning environment, MMVR13 Proceedings, 2005; 270-272.

[2]　Gallagher, A. G., Hughes, C., Reinhardt-Rutland A. H., McGuigan, J., & McClure, N. (2000): A case-control comparison of traditional and virtual-reality training in laparoscopic psychomotor performance. Minimal Invasive Therapy & Allied Technology, 9(5), 347-352.

[3]　Hyltander, A., Liljegren, E., Rhodin, P. H., & Lönroth, H. (2002). The transfer of basic skills learned in a laparoscopic simulator to the operating room. Surgical Endoscopy, 16(9), 1324-1328.

[4] Korndorffer, J. R., Jr., Seirra, R., Dunne, J. B., & Scott, D. (2004). Simulator training for laparoscopic suturing using performance goals translates to the OR. Journal of the American College Of Surgeons, 199(3), S73-S74.

Medicine Meets Virtual Reality 14
J.D. Westwood et al. (Eds.)
IOS Press, 2006

Open Surgery in VR: Inguinal Hernia Repair According to Lichtenstein

A.J.B. Sanders[1], P. Warntjes[1], R.H. Geelkerken[3], W.J.B Mastboom[3], J.M. Klaase[3], S.G.J. Rödel[3], J.M. Luursema[2], P.A.M. Kommers[2], W.B. Verwey[2], F.J.A.M. van Houten[4], E.E. Kunst[1]

[1] Kunst & van Leerdam Medical Technology bv, Enschede, the Netherlands; asanders@vrest.nl; [2] Department of Behavioral Science, University of Twente, Enschede, NL; [3] Department of Vascular Surgery, Medical Spectrum Twente, Enschede, NL; [4] Department of Design Production and Management, University of Twente, Enschede, NL

Abstract

VREST (Virtual Reality Educational Surgical Tools) is developing a universal and autonomous simulation platform which can be used for training and assessment of medical students and for continuing education of physicians. A workstation consisting of two haptic devices and a 3D vision system is part of the VREST platform. Another part of the platform is a generic software environment in which lessons can be built by the teacher and performed by their students. Using the platform one can see, feel and decide as in reality. With the assessment tool the progress and skills of the students can be supervised.

The first lesson build on the VREST platform is an inguinal hernia repair according to Lichtenstein. This is an open surgery procedure. The VREST platform is used prior to the first operating room surgery of the resident. Interactive models and case dependant feedback is used to enlarge the residents' cognition. This should reduce the training time in the operating room.

1. Problem

The demand for proper health care is a hot issue. With time the expectation of the quality and capacity of medical treatments rises. The number of surgeons has to grow and for the quality issue, new innovative techniques and instruments arise. This results in a situation in which more surgeons need to be certified in lesser time. Besides they have to be able to cope with techniques with a fast growing complexity. Patients expect to be treated by an experienced physician, who is trained with the last insights. The development of an effective education system for surgeons is inevitable to meet these demands.

2. Tools and Methods

VREST (Virtual Reality Educational Surgical Tools) is developing a universal and autonomous platform which can be used for training and assessment of medical students and for continuing education of physicians [1, 2, 3, 4]. Unlike existing virtual trainers, our workstation is capable to load different operations of varying types. With a webbased interface the surgeon as a teacher can build and adjust operation lessons and protocols. The software will translate it to a set of measurable parameters in a clear structure.

Next to the content management system the software comprehends a virtual reality surrounding in which an operation can be simulated in a realistic manner. With the usage of haptic devices, the student is able to navigate in the virtual world and feel his actions due to accurate force feedback. To generate a sense of touch which suits the natural behavior of tools and organs, spring meshes and finite element algorithms are used. With the usage of fast calculating collision detection and a fast force rendering algorithm, we are able to touch and manipulate highly complex organs. The meshes can be cut, pulled aside and sutured afterwards with the graphics and physics. To provide the user a high quality three dimensional perception, the virtual operation scene is rendered in stereo, and synchronized with shutter glasses. Furthermore we have integrated a mirror in the platform to present the virtual patient a natural way; lying on a table in front of the user. Analyzing the information from the virtual surgery room and the information gathered from the haptics, the system is able to train and judge the students' skills.

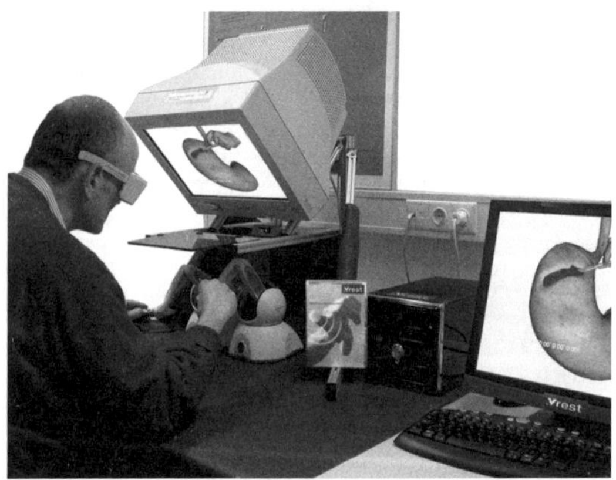

Figure 1: VREST platform

3. Results

In order to validate the system the trainer is filled with an inguinal hernia repair operation according to the Lichtenstein Procedure.

The user is able to use different surgical tools and has to make decisions about how to treat the patient correct. In order to meet the reality the system is supplied with different patients who vary in injury complexity and anatomy. The amount of the feedback is based on the level of the student. During the surgery, the student may consult a database filled with medical media. After an operation the procedure of the student will be matched with the actual surgery protocol and the result is sent to the surgeon. Once the student has reached sufficient competence a virtual certificate can be handed.

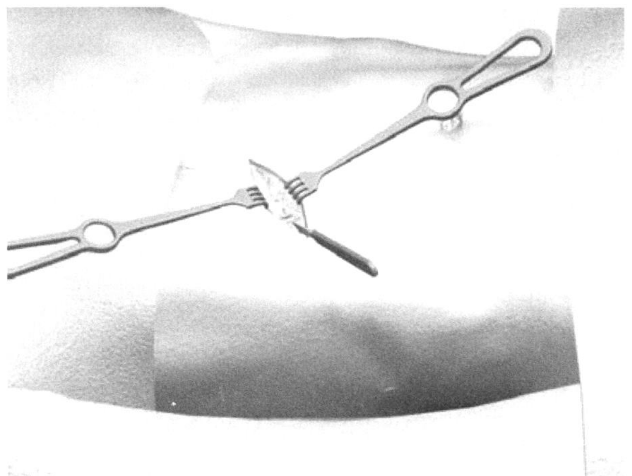

Figure 2: VR incision in inguinal hernia repair training.

4. Conclusion

With the usage of an autonomous teaching and assessing workstation the efficiency of the educational side of medicine will increase. More students can be educated at the same time, while the teaching surgeon has more time available for his normal clinical work. At this moment the workstation is used at a local hospital and the effectiveness is validated by comparing the results with a reference group. We are convinced that, in order to meet medical capacity demands, the usage of autonomous virtual trainers is insuperable in medicine.

5. References

[1]   Kunst EE, Geelkerken RH, Sanders AJB. The VREST learning environment, MMVR13 Proceedings, 2005; 270-272.
[2]   Scott DJ, Valentine RJ, Bergen PC, et al. Evaluating surgical competency with the American Board of Surgery In-Training Examination, skill testing and intraoperative assessment, Surgery 2000; 128(4): 613622.
[3]   Grantcharov TP, Kristiansen VB, Bendix J, et al. Randomized clinical trial of virtual reality simulation for laparoscopic skills training, Br J Surg 2004; 91(2): 146150.
[4]   Ahlberg G, Heikkinen T, Iselius L, et al. Does training in a virtual reality simulator improve surgical performance? Surg Endosc 2002; 16(1): 126-129.

Medicine Meets Virtual Reality 14
J.D. Westwood et al. (Eds.)
IOS Press, 2006

Pneumothorax Influenced 3D Lung Deformations

Anand P Santhanam[1], Cali M Fidopiastis[2], Jay Anton[4], Jannick P Rolland[3]
[1]School of Computer Science, University of Central Florida
[2]Institute of Simulation and Training, University of Central Florida
[3]College of Optics/FPCE, University of Central Florida
[4]METI Corporation, Sarasota FL

Abstract: In this paper we propose a method to simulate morphological changes caused by both closed and tension pneumothorax. We consider a clinical parameter, the pneumothorax-index (i.e., the degree of lung collapse), as the input to the simulation. Specifically, such an index constitutes a key parameter to the computation of the changes in size and shape of the affected lung. Once the index is obtained, the increase in ventilation rate and the change in the pressure-volume relationship of the affected lung are then computed. For tension pneumothorax, the air continuously flows into the pleural cavity and thus every exhalation is followed by the changes seen for a closed pneumothorax, until the affected lung collapses. The subsequent closure of pulmonary veins and resulting hyper expansion of the apposing lung is also presented. Results show a real-time visualization of closed and tension pneumothorax using a high-resolution 3D model obtained from a normal human subject.

1. Introduction

Medical visualization is a critical component to planning procedural interventions and predicting patient outcomes.[1] Current physically based simulation techniques, such as Finite Element Modeling (FEM) and Finite Difference Modeling (FDM), extend the utility of visualizing the complex anatomy and physiology into both 3D space and the fourth dimension of time.[2] The success of such medical simulations is evidenced by the fact that over one third of all medical schools in the United States augment their teaching curricula using patient simulators.[3] In this paper, we describe such a simulation, which illustrates the complex medical condition of pneumothorax, the presence of air in the pleural cavity of the lung, including its time course and different classifications. The two mechanistic variants of pneumothorax are open (hole in the chest wall) and closed (hole in the viscera pleura or chest lining) pneumothorax, which lead to different symptoms and treatment methods.   The visualization is currently presented for 3D lungs and the mathematical component shows scope for including the effect of changes in cardio-vascular functions. The simulation parameters in this paper are currently set to experimental values obtained from the medical literature.

2. Proposed Method for 3D Lung Deformation

In this section we outline the methodology adopted for the dynamic simulation of 3D lungs deformation. This method is sub-divided into two stages. In the first stage we used the method discussed in [4] to parameterize the change in lung volume for a change in pressure (referred to as trans-pulmonary pressure). In the second stage we used the method discussed in [5] to estimate the change in the global lung shape for an increase in lung volume. This is obtained using a physically based deformation method. Within the context of computer animation, a Green's function based deformation was chosen since it has been observed that lung deformations do not undergo vibrations.[6] Fig 1a shows the shape of the normal human lungs before inhalation and Fig 1b shows the shape at the end of inhalation. The PV curve used for this simulation is as shown in Fig 2b.

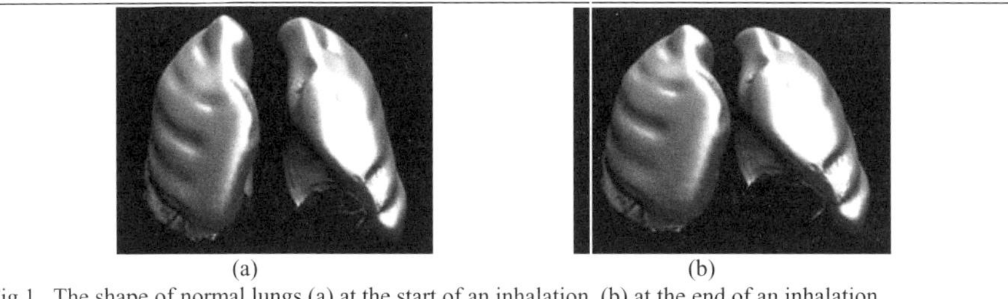

(a)   (b)

Fig 1. The shape of normal lungs (a) at the start of an inhalation. (b) at the end of an inhalation.

2.1 Closed Pneumothorax

The 3D deformable lung models under normal breathing lung conditions are driven by the normal human pressure-volume (PV) curve.[4] A ventilation rate of 12 breathing cycles per minute is taken as the normal breathing rate. We use a pneumothorax index, P as input, which conveys a degree of lung collapse. The value of this index ranges from *0* to *1*. We assume that the volume of air in the pleural space is considered to be proportional to the ratio of the difference between the radius of hemithorax and the lungs, and the radius of the hemithorax. The change in the volume of air inside an affected lung, *dV* (in the range from *0* to *1*) for a given index value, *P*,[7] is given as

$$dV = (P)^{0.33}.\tag{1}$$

This corresponding change in lung shape for the change in volume *(dV)* is obtained by scaling down the 3D surface points of the model along their normals from the hilum, which is the entry point for air into the lungs. The modified 3D model is now displaced vertically from the apex so that it sits on the diaphragm.[8] We also assume that in an upright position, the vertical displacement is proportional to the lateral displacements of the lungs described in [8]. This vertical displacement *(A)* was shown (in [8]) to be

$$A = \frac{(P \times 100 - 4.2)}{4.7 \times 2}.\tag{2}$$

Let T_i and T_e be the time taken for a single cycle of inhalation and exhalation respectively. The subsequent decrease in the time taken for one breathing cycle of the lungs (*dT*),[7] can be given as

$$dT = T \times dV \quad,\tag{3}$$

and $$T'_i = T_i - dT \quad , \tag{4}$$

and $$T'_e = T_e - dT \quad , \tag{5}$$

where T_i' and T_e' are the modified time for a single cycle of inhalation and exhalation respectively, and T is the normal time taken for one breathing cycle.[7] The tidal volume of air flow into the affected lung (V_1) during inhalation in one breathing cycle is set to be

$$V_1 = V_1 \times (1 - dV) . \tag{6}$$

The tidal volume of the unaffected lung *(V_2)* is set to be

$$V_2 = V_2 + \alpha \quad , \tag{7}$$

where α is a constant that refers to the increase in volume due to the extra effort in breathing. The range of values for α can vary for every human subject between (0-2500 millilitres) and clinically accurate range is yet to be determined. The subsequent changes in the PV curve caused by the additional work during inspiration and the decrease in work during expiration ([10]) are modeled using a method discussed in [7]. Such a PV relation allows modeling any degree of lung collapse. The PV relation during inhalation and exhalation is represented using a second-order differential equation with a variable parameter. This parameter is further computed as a linear summation of products of a set of control parameters and trigonometric basis functions that represents the summary muscle resistance. The values of control parameters are extracted from patient's specific clinical data.[11] Fig 2a shows the values of a set of control constants used for generating a normalized PV curve of a normal subject as shown in Fig 2b. We simulate a PV curve that represents pneumothorax by varying the normal control constants. One key property of the control constants that we use is that the values as a sequence converge to zero and the rate of convergence is observed to be faster under higher drive conditions. We thus increased the rate of convergence of control parameters during exhalation since the presence of air in the pleural cavity increases the drive to exhale. Similarly we decreased the rate of convergence during exhalation. Multiplying every parameter with its logarithm and dividing it by the logarithm of the first parameter yields an increase in the rate of convergence during inhalation. Similarly, multiplying every parameter with its exponent and dividing it by the exponent of the first parameter yields a decrease in the rate of convergence during exhalation. Let c_i^{inh} and c_i^{exh} be the array of control constants during inhalation and

exhalation and let d_i^{inh} and d_i^{exh} be the modified control constants respectively. For a

dV amount of air entering the pleural cavity, a method to vary the control constants is given by

$$d_i^{exh} = C_0^{exh} \times \frac{e^{C_i^{exh} \times \varphi \times dV}}{e^{C_0^{exh} \times \varphi \times dV}} , \tag{8}$$

$$d_i^{inh} = C_0^{inh} \times \frac{\log\left(C_i^{inh} \times \varphi \times dV\right)}{\log\left(C_0^{inh} \times \varphi \times dV\right)} , \tag{9}$$

where φ is a proportionality constant that relates the change in control constants to the amount of additional work. Experimental results are shown for small degrees of lung collapse ($P < 0.01$). For an experimental analysis the value of φ is set to 0.1. Fig 2a shows the value of modified control constants used for a dV of 50 ml ($P = 0.008$). The PV curve generated for the modified control constants is shown in Fig 2b. PV curve variations can thus be meticulously modeled in order to model even small degrees of lung collapse.

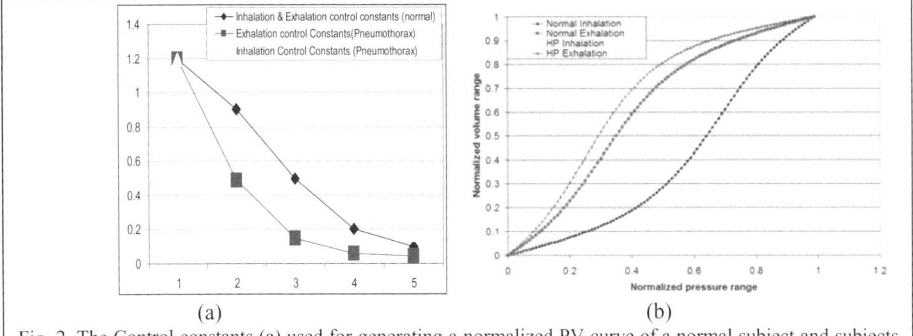

(a)   (b)

Fig. 2. The Control constants (a) used for generating a normalized PV curve of a normal subject and subjects with pneumothorax and the resulting PV curves (b).

2.2 Tension Pneumothorax

Tension Pneumothorax is a condition where the air enters into the pleural cavity but does not leave the cavity. Let t be the number of breathing cycle since the onset of pneumothorax. We now represent dV^t as the volume of airflow into the pleural cavity at the tth breathing cycle. The inflow of air into the pleural cavity for an inhalation is set as

$$dV^t = dV \times e^{-\tau t} , \tag{10}$$

where τ is a constant which controls the rate of air-flow inside the pleural cavity. The negative exponential component represents the decrease in the rate of airflow caused by the decrease in the trans-pulmonary pressure range. The subsequent decrease in the time taken for the inhalation and exhalation are given by replacing dV by dV^t in equations (3), (4) and (5). The change in 3D lung shape is obtained as explained for closed pneumothorax. We now introduce dV_{Sum} which represents the volume of air in the pleural cavity. After a few breathing cycles dV_{Sum} reaches a volume V^1_{max} after which the affected lung cannot inhale or exhale. In order to model the lateral movement of the affected lung we introduce the parameter q^t_i which represents the percentage volume of the bounding box of the left $(i=1)$ and right $(i=2)$ lungs which is inside the respective lungs. Let b_x^{it}, b_y^{it} and b_z^{it} be the dimensions of the bounding box of the ith lung in X, Y and Z at the end of the tth inhalation, respectively. We can now represent q^t_i as

$$q^t_1 = \frac{V_1^t}{b_X^{1t} \times b_Y^{1t} \times b_Z^{1t}} . \tag{11}$$

The magnitude of the global displacement in volume is equal to the volume of air directly entering the pleural cavity and is computed as follows. The displacement of the bounding box of the affected lung $(i=1)$ towards the mediastinum (along the X-axis), denoted by db_X^1 is given by the relation,

$$dV^t = db_X^{1t} \times b_Y^{1t} \times b_Z^{1t} . \tag{12}$$

The displacement of the lung towards the mediastinum can now be represented by replacing $db_X{}^{lt}$ with $q_1{}^t \times dX^{lt}$ in the above equation and simplified as,

$$dX^{lt} = \frac{dV^t}{q_1{}^t \times b_Y{}^{lt} \times b_Z{}^{lt}}.$$ (13)

Let β a cardiovascular factor that represents the maximum global displacement by the lung in the state of arrest at which the superior vena cava closes. The closing of vena cava leads to the collection of blood in lungs and its hyper-expansion until its volume V_2 reaches $V^2{}_{max}$, after which it attains the state of arrest. Thus both lungs have reached a state of arrest.[12,13] The value of β is set to be equal to the average diameter of the vena cava (i.e. 18 mm) for simulation purposes. We now discuss the simulation of closed pneumothorax influenced on a patient's left lungs. For simulation purposes, the value of P and α are set to 0.1 and 100ml, respectively. Fig.3a shows the shape of lungs in an upright position before inhalation. It can be seen that the patient's left lung is lower in volume and is shorter than the right lung. Fig 3b shows the shape of lungs at the end of exhalation. It can be seen that the patient's right lung is more expanded as compared to the normal lung in Fig.2b, which is caused by the value of a. An illustration of hyper expansion during tension pneumothorax is as shown in Fig.3.c In this case the patient's left lung is at *Vmin* and the right lung is at a volume of *Vmax*. The lungs have reached a state of arrest.

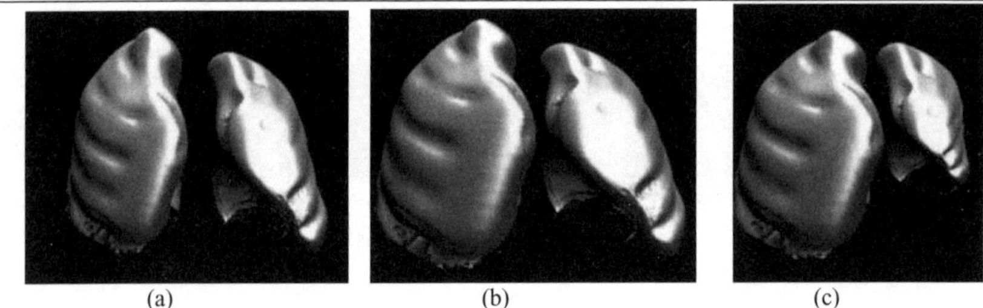

| (a) | (b) | (c) |

Fig. 3. Pneumothorax influenced lung breathing. (a) The shape of lungs influenced by closed pneumothorax before the start of an inhalation. (b) The shape of lungs at the end of an inhalation. (c) The hyperexpansion of the right lung influenced by the lateral movement of the left lung during open pneumothorax.

3. Conclusion

A method for successfully modeling closed and tension pneumothorax has been presented. The proposed method can simulate lung deformations in a physically accurate manner in real-time. Such deformations can be visualized using advanced visualization environments for effective training and visual guidance in clinical maneuvers. Future work will involve a clinical validation of this method, and will help determine the value of the constants α, φ and β for normal and abnormal human subjects.

Acknowledgement

This work was funded by METI Corporation, Sarasota FL. We thank Dr.Paul W. Segars from the Department of Bio-medical Imaging at John Hopkins Medical Institute for providing us with High-resolution 3D lung models. We thank Dr. Raj Karunakara from the Respiratory Critical care at Ocala Regional Health Center for providing us with constructive comments on our work. We thank Claire Balgeman for her contribution in technical editing.

References

1. Nye, L.S., "The minds' eye," *Biochemistry and Molecular Biology Education*. 32 (2) (2004). 123-131.

2. Robb, R.A., *Three-dimensional visualization in medicine and Biology*, in *Handbook of medical Imaging: Processing and Analysis*, I.N. Bankman, Editor Academic Press: San Diego,CA (2000).

3. Good, M.I., "Patient simulation for training basic and advanced clinical skills," *Medical Education*. 37 (2003). 14.

4. Santhanam, A., Fidopiastis, C., and Rolland, J.P., "An adaptive driver and real-time deformation algorithm for visualization of high-density lung models."*Medical Meets Virtual Reality 12*. Newport, CA IOS Press (2004). 333-339.

5. Santhanam, A., Fidopiastis, C., Hamza-Lup, F., Rolland, J.P., and Imielinska, C., "Physically-based deformation of high-resolution 3D lung models for augmented reality based medical visualization."*Medical Image Computing and Computer Aided Intervention, AMI-ARCS*. Rennes,St-Malo Lecture Notes on Computer Science (2004). 21-32.

6. Mead, J., "Measurement of inertia of the lungs at increased ambient pressure," *Journal of Applied Physiology*. 2 (1) (1956). 208-212.

7. Murray, "Textbook of Respiratory Medicine," (1995).

8. Kircher, L.T. and Swartzel, R.L., "Spontaneous pneumothorax and its treatment," *JAMA*. 155 (24-29) (1954).

9. Berger, A.J., *Control of Breathing*, in *Textbook of Respiratory Physiology* (1995).

10. Visaria, R. and Westenkow, D., "Diagnosis of pulmonary complications based on airway pressure-flow waveforms."*Proceedings of the Second Joint EMBS/BMES Conference*. Houston,TX IEEE (2002). 1481-1483.

11. Takeuchi, M., Sedeek, K.A., Guilherme, P., Schettino, P., Suchodolski, K., and Kacmarek, R.M., "Peek pressure during volume history and pressure-volume curve measurement affects analysis," *American Journal of Respiratory Critical Care*. 164 (2001). 1225-1230.

12. Kaye, J.M., Primiano, F.P.J., and Metaxas, D.N., "A Three-dimensional virtual environment for modeling mechanical cardiopulmonary interactions," *Medical Image Analysis*. 2 (2) (1998). 169-195.

Medicine Meets Virtual Reality 14
J.D. Westwood et al. (Eds.)
IOS Press, 2006

Documentation and Teaching of Surgery with an Eye Movement Driven Head-Mounted Camera:
See what the Surgeon Sees and Does

Erich Schneider [a,1], Klaus Bartl [a] Thomas Dera [a] Guido Böning [a] Philipp Wagner [b] and
Thomas Brandt [a]

[a] *Hospital of the University of Munich, Department of Neurology, D-81377 Munich*
[b] *Institute of Applied Mechanics, Technical University of Munich, D-85748 Garching,*
Germany

Abstract. A first proof of concept was developed for a head-mounted video camera system that is continuously aligned with the user's orientation of gaze. In doing so, it records images from the user's perspective that can document manual tasks during, e.g., surgery. Eye movements are tracked by video-oculography and used as signals to drive servo motors that rotate the camera. Thus, the sensorimotor output of a biological system for the control of eye movements evolved over millions of years is used to move an artificial eye. All the capabilities of multi-sensory processing for eye, head, and surround motions are detected by the vestibular, visual, and somatosensory systems and used to drive a technical camera system. A camera guided in this way mimics the natural exploration of a visual scene and acquires video sequences from the perspective of a mobile user, while the oculomotor reflexes naturally stabilize the camera on target during head and target movements. Various documentation and teaching applications in health care, industry, and research are conceivable.

Keywords. Camera motion device, eye tracking, calibration, image stabilization, vestibulo-ocular reflex

1. Introduction

Head-mounted camera systems are widely known and can be used for visualizing manual tasks during surgery, e.g., for teaching and documentation purposes. These cameras give an image of the visual scene that a user can see, but since they are head fixed they are not able to always look where the eyes are looking. They can therefore easily miss crucial events when the head is pointing in another direction than the eyes. In contrast, an eye movement driven head-mounted camera can always record what the surgeon is actually seeing, provided that the system is accurately calibrated. In addition, image stabilization

---

[1]Correspondence to: Erich Schneider, Center for Sensorimotor Research, Marchioninistr. 23, D-81377 Munich, Germany. Tel.: +49 89 7095 4830; Fax: +49 89 7095 4801; E-mail: eschneider@nefo.med.uni-muenchen.de

is an inherent feature of such a camera because it uses the whole range of oculomotor behavior which evolved over millions of years in biological systems to compensate for head and visual target motions.

The head mounted gaze camera system (see Figure 1) uses a video eye tracker to detect eye motions of the user. From these eye motions the gaze direction of the user is calculated and used as an input signal for the camera motion device. Thus the optical axis of the camera is kept parallel to the human's gaze direction. Assuming a sufficiently small latency, the human gaze stabilization based on the vestibulo-ocular, optokinetic and smooth pursuit reflexes can be used to stabilize the camera image. In this camera setup the biological equilibrium organ – the inner ear labyrinth – controls a technical system, hence rendering a technical stabilization by inertial measurement obsolete.

The focus of this work is on a first prototype that offers easy and accurate calibration as well as a sufficiently low latency between eye and camera movement, thereby serving as an experimental platform as well as a possible solution for a head camera system for the surgeon and possibly even for subsequent consumer products.

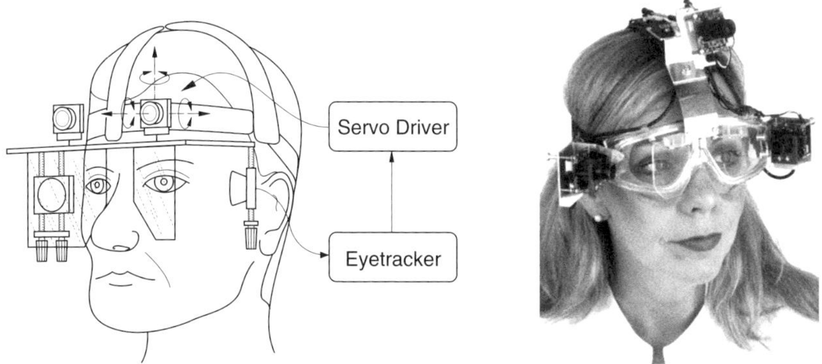

Figure 1. Schematic setup (left) and real implementaion (right) of a gaze camera. An eye tracker that consists of laterally attached infrared video cameras, transparent hot mirrors (one for each eye), and a computer acquires and processes video images of the eyes and calculates servo driver signals from the eye movement data. The servo drivers align one or two (stereo) gaze camera(s) mounted above the forehead to parallel gaze. In doing so, this camera records images from the user's perspective.

2. Tools and Methods

The first demonstrator of our eye movement driven head-mounted camera consists of five main modules (see Figure 1):
1. lightweight head mount
2. eye tracker
3. wearable computer
4. servo driver
5. gaze camera mount with gimbal

Our demonstrator uses video-oculographic image processing algorithms for eye tracking with typical resolutions beneath 0.1 deg [1]. Eye tracking techniques are a thoroughly researched field (see [2,3,4,5]), and therefore the implemented details are not described in detail. In short, rough estimates of the (dark) pupil center coordinates are calculated from the 1st momentum of an eye image that is binarized with an intensity threshold operation. Intermediate results of these operations are schematically drawn in the small inset plot of Figure 2 that shows an image of an eye. Numerical differentiation along the pupil edges and a subsequent ellipse fit [6] deliver an improved pupil center estimate with subpixel resolution.

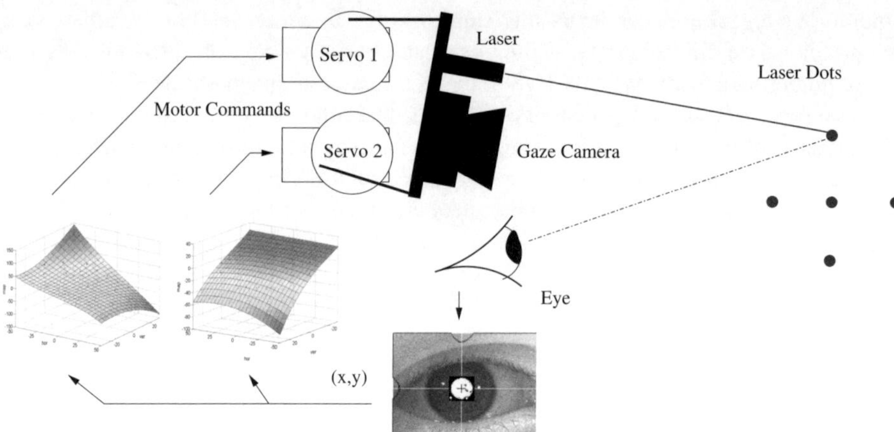

Figure 2. Schematic setup of the calibration technique. The user fixates a laser dot that is moved together with the pivotable camera. The mapping between measured eye positions in image coordinates and corresponding motor commands is achieved by 3rd order polynomial fits. Intermediate results of the image processing algorithms are shown in the inset image from the eye tracker (bottom). Detected pupil pixels are artificially colored with white.

The transformation between the different coordinate systems of the eye tracker and the pivotable camera is based on a new calibration method. A small laser pointer is rigidly mounted on the camera module. During the calibration procedure a small laser pointer that is rigidly mounted on the head camera module projects a bright dot that appears centered in the head camera image. The user is asked to fixate it as it jumps to predefined positions with known servo motor commands. The eye position values are then linearly fitted by two 3rd order 2D-polynomials to the corresponding motor commands.

Free user mobility and low latency are two major goals for the design of this device. The whole setup is powered and controlled by a single off-the-shelf laptop with a total weight of 1.3 kg (Acer TravelMate 382TMi, Pentium M725 processor, 1.6 Ghz, 400 Mhz FSB, 2 MB L2 cache, 512 MB DDR RAM). The main reason for using this type of laptop was its 6-pin IEEE1394 connector that integrates a power supply for external devices. By connecting IEEE-1394 digital cameras (Flea, Pointgrey, Vancouver) for the eye tracking part to this port, there was no need for an additional power supply. These cameras can typically be operated at a frame rate of 100 Hz when the image resolution is restricted to 320x240 pixels by pixel binning. Compared to other standard video cameras the increased frame rate helped to reduce latency.

The actuators must be able to reach high velocities and accelerations to move the selected camera with a performance similar to the human oculomotor system [7]. Other important requirements are low weight, small dimensions and high reliability. Therefore, electric DC motors with reduction gears have been chosen. The most appropriate actuators turned out to be servo actuators for model aircrafts. A major advantage of these actuators is the fact that DC motor, gear and a position control are all integrated in a common package making the complete actuator extremely compact. For the prototype, Graupner DS 3781 actuators have been chosen which are amongst the fastest servo actuators (1000 deg/s) still having a reasonable size and weight (28 g). In contrast to other servo actuators this type can be operated at signal input rates of up to 400 Hz, which significantly reduces over-all latency. With these components a camera motion device was developed with dynamic properties that come close to or even excel those of the human eye [7].

A microcontroller (PIC18F4431) was used as an interface between the laptop and the actuators. This servo controller was connected via an USB-RS232-adapter (Manhattan products Part 205146) to the laptop's USB port and operated at 115200 kBaud. The controller board additionally serves as a power supply system for the actuators, the calibration laser and the head mounted camera. It is assembled together with a FireWire-hub in a small plastic case that is attached to the backside of the head mount.

A parallel kinematics setup was used to pivot the head-mounted video camera. The most important part of the system is a Cardan module. This joint allows rotations around vertical (pan) and around horizontal (tilt) axes. With this design two degrees of freedom are realized for the motions of the gaze camera. Two servo actuators move the camera module using push rods and universal joints.

3. Results

The first tested criterion was wearability. The over-all weight of the head-mounted system is 600 g. Subjects were asked to perform every-day activities like descending a stair or even play tennis with this system and to assess its comfort (see Figure 3). An experienced tennis player was able to play a match with only moderate restrictions of visual field and mobility while wearing the head-mounted camera system. Stair negotiation was possible with no difficulties.

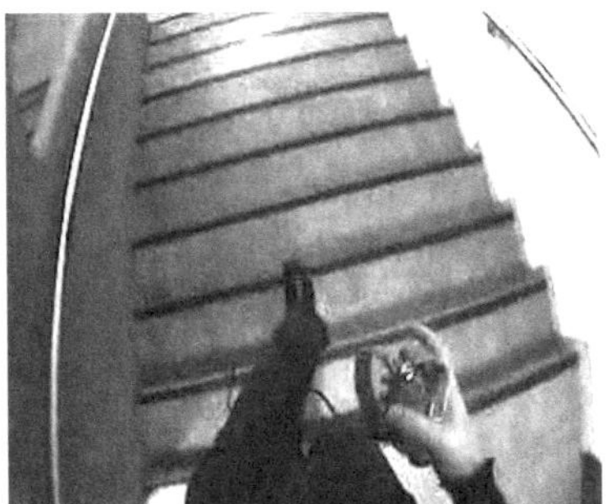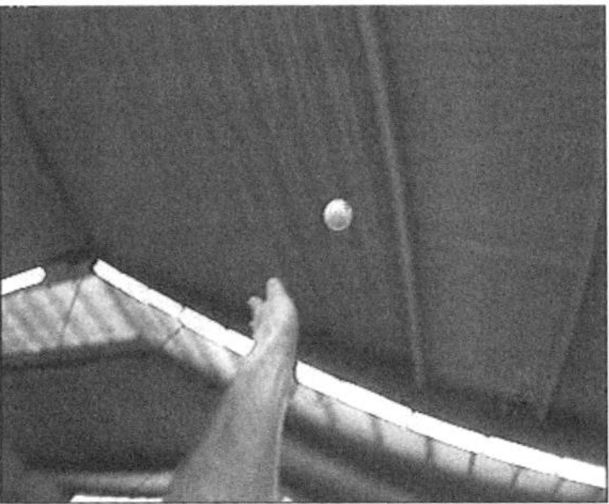

Figure 3. Descending a staircase (left) and a tennis serve from the player's perspective (right).

The latency of the system was measured by attaching an artificial eye to an additional actuator that was moved sinusoidally. We used 5 frequencies ranging from 1Hz to 10Hz. The eye tracking system detected the artificial pupil as it would do with a real eye. The detected position served as input to control the head mounted camera. Both the angular velocities of the artificial eye and of the head mounted camera were synchronously measured by attached gyroscopes, yielding an over-all latency of 36 ms. This latency is greater than but still on the order of the 10–15 ms latency of the biological image stabilizing vestibulo-ocular reflex [7].

In order to test the accuracy and resolution of the system, a subject was asked to sequentially fixate dots arranged in a 5x5 matrix on a poster after calibration. Both the fixation dots and the laser projection were visible in the recorded video stream of the head camera and their distance (in deg) served as the measure of positioning accuracy. A mean deviation of 0.5 deg and a resolution (standard deviation) of 0.25 deg were measured, which was well within the 2 deg of foveal vision.

Visual inspection of the images showed a good reproduction of smooth pursuit eye movements. However, high frequency head movements were not compensated very well, due to the latency of 36 ms and due to the eye tracker slippages that were mistaken for eye movements.

4. Discussion / Conclusions

Video recordings from the subjective perspective of a mobile user were possible in this first demonstrator of a gaze-driven camera. The camera proved to be usable with lower-frequency head movements and with ocular following tasks. A new calibration procedure significantly reduced the complexity of both the implemented algorithms and the required user interactions. Such a camera system can already be used for documentation and teaching purposes in, e.g., health care, quality assurance, and even sports. Future developments will concentrate on the compensation of eye tracker slippage, on further reductions of the over-all latency and on the reproduction of the whole range of 3D eye movements by 3D eye tracking and by implementing a three-degree-of-freedom camera motion device.

Acknowledgements: This work was supported by the Bavarian Research Foundation (FORBIAS) and the Deutsche Forschungsgemeinschaft (GL 342/1-1).

References

[1] E. Schneider, S. Glasauer, and M. Dieterich, A comparison of human ocular torsion patterns during natural and galvanic vestibular stimulation, *J Neurophysiol* **87** (2002), 2064–2073.

[2] L.R. Young, B.K. Lichtenberg, A.P. Arrot, T.A. Crites, C.M. Oman, and E.R. Edelman. Ocular torsion on earth and in weightlessness. *Ann NY Acad Sci* **374** (1981), 80-92.

[3] T. Haslwanter and S.T. Moore. A theoretical analysis of three-dimensional eye position measurement using polar cross-correlation. *IEEE Trans Biomed Eng* **42** (1995), 1053–1061.

[4] S.T. Moore, T. Haslwanter, I.S. Curthoys, and S.T. Smith. A geometric basis for measurement of three-dimensional eye position using image processing. *Vision Res* **36** (1996), 445–459.

[5] D. Zhu, S.T. Moore, and T. Raphan. Robust pupil center detection using a curvature algorithm. *Comput Methods Programs Biomed* **59** (1999), 145-157.

[6] A.W. Fitzgibbon, M. Pilu, and R.B. Fisher. Direct least squares fitting of ellipses. *IEEE Transactions on Pattern Analysis and Machine Intelligence* **21** (1999), 476-480.

[7] R. J. Leigh and D. S. Zee. The Neurology of Eye Movements. *Oxford University Press*, New York, Oxford (1999).

Medicine Meets Virtual Reality 14
J.D. Westwood et al. (Eds.)
IOS Press, 2006

491

A Simulation-Based Training System for Surgical Wound Debridement

Jennifer SEEVINCK [a]   Mark W. SCERBO [a]   Lee A. BELFORE, II [a]
Leonard J. WEIRETER, Jr. [b]   Jessica R. CROUCH [a]   Yuzhong SHEN [a]
Frederick D. McKENZIE [a]   Hector M. GARCIA [a]   Sylva GIRTELSCHMID [a]
Emre BAYDOGAN [a]   Elizabeth A. SCHMIDT [a]
[a] *Old Dominion University*
[b] *Eastern Virginia Medical School*

Abstract. A simulation-based training system for surgical wound debridement was developed and comprises a multimedia introduction, a surgical simulator (tutorial component), and an assessment component. The simulator includes two PCs, a haptic device, and mirrored display. Debridement is performed on a virtual leg model with a shallow laceration wound superimposed. Trainees are instructed to remove debris with forceps, scrub with a brush, and rinse with saline solution to maintain sterility. Research and development issues currently under investigation include tissue deformation models using mass-spring system and finite element methods; tissue cutting using a high-resolution volumetric mesh and dynamic topology; and accurate collision detection, cutting, and soft-body haptic rendering for two devices within the same haptic space.

Keywords. Surgical debridement, wound debridement, training, virtual agent, multimedia, debris modeling, prototype, augmented reality.

Introduction

In 1999, The Institute of Medicine issued a report estimating that as many as 98,000 people die from errors in hospital settings each year [1]. Subsequently, the AMA's Accreditation Council for Graduate Medical Education limited the time that residents can be required to work to 80 hours a week. Although this action was intended to improve patient safety, it also reduced the number of patient-contact hours needed to train residents. Thus, medical educators are looking for alternative methods to provide residents with meaningful learning experiences. Many are turning to simulator-based training to meet that need [2, 3].

In many high risk domains (e.g., aviation, military training, nuclear process plant control, etc.), simulators are often used to allow trainees to acquire and practice skills in a safe and controlled environment [4]. One of the important benefits of this approach is that trainees can acquire much of the fundamental knowledge and skills needed to perform elementary activities largely on their own without the need for constant supervision by an instructor. Accordingly, that approach was adopted as the guiding principle behind the development of the surgical wound debridement simulator system.

1. Wound Debridement

Wound debridement refers to the process of removing necrotic, devitalized, or contaminated tissue and/or foreign material to promote healing [5]. In surgical debridement, a scalpel or scissors is used to cut away the necrotic tissue. Wound debridement is a minor surgical procedure, but one that is performed by surgeons, physicians assistants, surgical assistants, nurses, and military medics and corpsmen. At present, this procedure is typically learned with actual patients under the guidance of a more experienced physician.

2. The Simulation-Based Training System

A simulation-based virtual reality (VR) training system for surgical wound debridement was developed to provide trainees with the fundamental knowledge and skills to perform the procedure through self-instruction and practice, thereby eliminating the need for one-on-one instruction. The system comprises a multimedia introduction, a surgical simulator (tutorial component), and an assessment component.

2.1 Multimedia Training Component

The multimedia training component describes varieties of wound categories (e.g., burns, lacerations, etc.); methods of debridement (e.g., sharp, mechanical, etc.), and equipment/materials used in the procedure. This module provides the pedagogical context for skills training and assessment, linking together all of the required elements for mastering the procedure. Pedagogical material and methodologies have been researched (e.g., [5]) and the system design stems from training requirements and iterative development obtained through consultation with domain experts.

Modules are arranged in sequential order to support educational advancement of the novice; however, the navigational menu design permits all items to be accessible at any time thereby also supporting the experienced user. Further, freedom to run the multimedia component on a platform other than the one used for the skills training makes it possible to support multiple users simultaneously.

2.2 Virtual Agent

A software virtual agent is included and performs the role of an instructor by providing verbal guidance and assessment feedback (see Figure 1a). Designed to be comprehensive in order to reduce the need for a more senior instructor, the software addresses the patient's condition, initial description of the injury, and provides instruction on operation of the simulator. Specific instructions cover the removal of foreign objects with forceps, scrubbing with a brush, rinsing with saline solution, and the maintenance of sterility. The trainee is prompted to move on when the current stage is satisfactorily completed. The current software implementation for the agent uses Haptek®[1] and NeoSpeech[2].

2.3 The Simulator: General Description and Technical Implementation

A prototype of the wound debridement trainer has been developed using the Derivative, Inc., API[3], for fast initial testing of user and design requirements (see Figure 1b).

---

[1] Haptek®, *PeoplePutty, Haptek Player SDK, Haptek® Player* viewed 10-17-05, http://www.haptek.com
[2] NeoSpeech, *Kate,* viewed 10-17-05, http://www.nextup.com/neospeech.html
[3] Derivative Inc. *Touch Designer,* viewed 10-17-05, http://www.derivativeinc.com/

OpenHaptics™ Toolkit (SensAble, Inc.) interfaces with a Phantom® haptic device (Omni™ or Premium) for wound interaction while viewing it on a Reachin display device [4,5]. A parallel research effort with an open architecture uses OpenSceneGraph alongside an FEM physics approach for increased flexibility and realism in the training application (see Section 3.2).

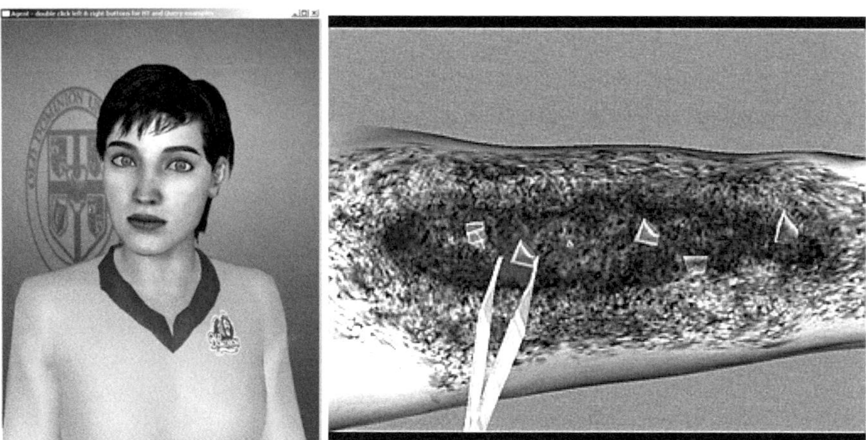

Figure 1a, b. Simulator system for surgical wound debridement: a) virtual agent tutor shown on the left and b) prototype system for removing glass shards from thigh laceration shown on the right.

2.3.1 The Anatomy and Wound

The simulator provides training on a shallow laceration wound to the thigh caused by a motorcycle accident. Our wound research focuses on the extremities and the leg model is derived from the National Library of Medicine's Visible Human Project [6]. Axial anatomical imagery is manually segmented, registered, and triangulated polygonal surface meshes of relevant objects are constructed. Subsequent to viewport culling, the skin mesh, as used in our prototype, is approximately 1000 polygons.

Foreign material embedded in the wound is modelled both geometrically and as surface texture. It is possible to render a high degree of dirt without an increase in computational expense as would be the case if debris implementation were pursued solely as geometry. Currently the majority of the debris (dust, dirt) is rendered as texture on the wound surface geometry while larger objects are polygonal meshes.

The simulation uses several textures for a range of the debridement processes (see Figure 2). Each polygon in the mesh is handled separately in terms of texture image while texture coordinates remain constant. The intersection between an instrument and surface polygon results in a substitute texture being called for that polygon.

Bleeding is implemented using a particle system. Particles are created only when instruments intersect with polygons within the wound area. Small amounts of gravity and randomness are added to particle motion. Upon collision with the wound surface, a particle's reflecting vector is reduced normal to the collision. These implementations contribute to a realistic rendering where particles slow down and approach the wound surface geometry over the duration of their lifespan.

[4] SensAble Technologies *OpenHaptics™ Toolkit, Phantom® Premium,, Omni™*, viewed 10-17-05, http://www.sensable.com
[5] Reachin Technologies *Reachin Display*, viewed 10-17-05, http://www.reachin.se/

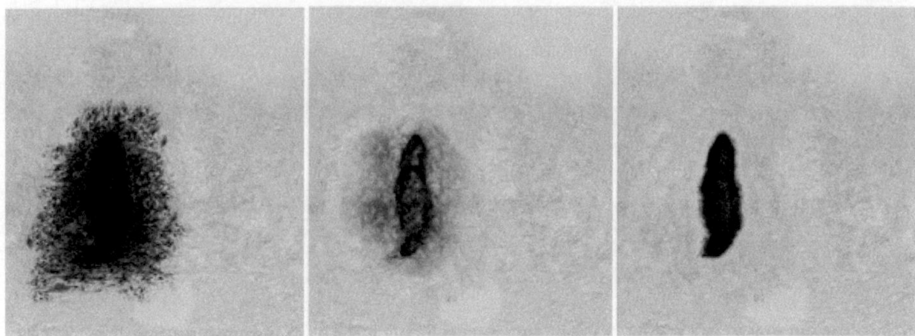

Figure 2. The concept of using textures to model debris around the wound.

2.3.2 Graphics and Haptics Simulation within the Prototype Application

A mass-spring simulation implemented within the prototype application and Derivative API drives graphics deformation. Approximately 200 nodes are deformed to restrict the simulation to those that fall inside the wound area (the remainder are fixed). All nodes have the same mass and drag and the spring is kept fairly stiff for stability.

A haptic model that does not update topological changes from the deforming mass spring model in Derivative has been implemented. Users do not readily perceive the limited synchronicity between the graphics and haptics implying an effective and economic implementation. The haptic rendering also supports grabbing points on both the deforming graphic and the haptic meshes (e.g., with forceps, see Figure 1b). Force is subsequently applied and the user feels tension through the haptic device. Releasing the tissue updates the graphical points back to their starting position. Both graphics and haptics applications of the simulator will run on a single laptop computer (i.e., with 3.2 GHz CPU; 1GB RAM; GeForceFX Go 5700). Running in parallel, the applications average 60Hz for graphics and 300Hz for haptics.

3. Ongoing Research and Development

3.1 Assessment

At present, assessment is limited to the amount of foreign material successfully removed from the wound and the time needed to perform the procedure. The next generation will include assessment modules for the didactic content addressing preoperative and postoperative care, performance-based feedback during the tutorial, summative feedback at the end of the tutorial, and assessment information for either the trainee or instructor. Performance-based assessment will target two types of errors. One set of errors is intended to be "recoverable". For example, removal of a very large shard of glass from the wound could cause a significant amount of bleeding. It would then be necessary for the trainee to stop the bleeding and proceed with the debridement. The second type of error is intended to be "unrecoverable". For instance, the trainee might damage a major blood vessel or nerve. At this point the simulation would terminate and feedback would be provided that describes the seriousness of the error, why it occurred, and how to avoid it in the future.

3.2 Development Platform

There are many fundamental challenges to developing a simulation system for an open procedure like surgical debridement. To address the issues in the current prototype using the Derivative API, a new solution employing more capable and flexible technologies is currently under research and development. The following briefly describes several major components under research and development:

- Object oriented software design and development are employed to ensure software quality, ease of component integration, future extension, and maintenance. Major classes of the simulator include tissue and instrument supporting the simulated objects and mass spring and finite element models underlying the physics-based models. Some auxiliary classes are also developed to facilitate computation, such as topology processing. In addition, the software components are not tied to a specific operating system specific and facilitate portability to other platforms.
- OpenSceneGraph, an open source high performance 3D graphics toolkit, is utilized for developing the visualization component of the debridement simulator. Utilizing scene graph technology and the latest OpenGL® 2.0 graphics, OpenSceneGraph has strength in performance, productivity, portability, and scalability. A variety of models are utilized for different computations. Volume mesh is used by tissue deformation and cutting simulation, while surface mesh used by irrigation simulation and collision detection. For computational efficiency, instruments are represented by a line segment(s) enclosing them for collision detection purposes.
- Removing necrotic or contaminated tissue with a scalpel or scissors is a critical procedure that differentiates between surgical debridement and other debridement approaches. Thus, simulation of tissue cutting in a surgical debridement simulator is essential. To effectively model and simulate the cutting procedure, a volume mesh is utilized to represent the wound region on the thigh. A surface mesh is extracted from the volume mesh to render the thigh graphically. Tissue cutting is simulated by deleting volume elements in contact with the cutting instruments, with color images from the visible human data set rendered as 3D textures.
- Mass-spring system and finite element method (FEM) approaches are implemented to simulate soft tissue deformation. Research is underway to build fast computational schemes to improve real-time performance for fast FEM computational methods, rapid neighborhood construction, and a hybrid structure of Mass-spring and FEM.
- XML, a simple and very flexible markup language, is selected as the file format to store the graphical and physical properties of the thigh model, including geometry, texture maps, topology, and FEM parameters. XML writer and reader programs have been developed to create and parse XML files.

The finite element code developed for the wound debridement application computes the 3D volumetric deformation of the leg model based on the displacement of a few surface nodes as determined by the collision detection module. The current model assumes all materials are either linear elastic or rigid. Rigid materials, (e.g., bones), can be represented by applying 0-displacement boundary conditions to an appropriate subset of the model's nodes. The stiffness of elastic tissues in the model can be varied according to segmented tissue type.

The finite element code was written specifically for the purpose of interactive simulation. It makes use of sparse matrix data structures and efficient LASPACK sparse matrix solution routines. Incremental updates to the stiffness matrix are made as the model mesh is cut during the simulation. The finite element code provides as output: (1) the displacement of every node in the model, and (2) the force vector in effect at every node. The force vector that is computed at the point of contact between a surgical instrument and the deformable model defines the force that should be haptically displayed to the user. Currently, the finite element code computes a deformation solution at a rate of 60-70 Hz for a model with 400 elements and 20-30 Hz for a model with 1100 elements which is sufficient for graphics. Further optimization of the code to improve efficiency and a parallel implementation is planned.

4. Conclusion

A simulator-based training system was developed for surgical wound debridement. The goal was to create a system that would allow health care providers to acquire the fundamental knowledge and skills to perform the procedure through self-instruction. The current system contains a multimedia component for didactic material, a tutorial, and a VR-based simulator with haptic feedback. Trainees can learn to clean to a wound and remove foreign objects. However, many technical challenges remain to improve the realism of the graphical and haptic displays. These include: 1) more realistic tissue deformation using mass-spring and finite element models, 2) better collision detection, 3) incorporating tissue cutting, and 4) adding two-handed haptics because debridement is typically performed using both hands. It is expected that solutions to these challenges will not only help to refine the physics-based models underlying the anatomy and physiology represented in the system, but will also expand the variety of wounds that can be included in the set of training cases.

5. Acknowledgements

This project was a collaborative effort between the Virginia Modeling, Analysis and Simulation Center (VMASC) at Old Dominion University and the Eastern Virginia Medical School. Partial funding was provided by the Naval Health Research Center through NAVAIR Orlando TSD under contract N61339-03-C-0157, and the Office of Naval Research under contract N00014-04-1-0697, entitled "The National Center for Collaboration in Medical Modeling and Simulation". The ideas and opinions presented in this paper represent the views of the authors and do not necessarily represent the views of the Department of Defense.

The authors would like to acknowledge and thank the following efforts toward this surgical simulator: R. Bowen Loftin for his guidance in a variety of technical and design discussions; Dwight Meglan for early contributions to design discussions; Wesley Taggart and Daniel Spence, for CAD modelling and multimedia training development; and Joe Bricio for his early assistance with the virtual agent software.

References

[1]   Kohn, L. T., Corrigan, J. M., & Donaldson, M. S., Eds. (1999). *To err is human: Building a safer health system*. Washington, D.C.: National Academy Press.

[2]   Dawson, S. L. (2002). A critical approach to medical simulation. *Bulletin of the American College of Surgeons, 87*(11), 12-18.

[3]   Healy, G. B. (2002). The College should be instrumental in adapting simulators to education. *Bulletin of the American College of Surgeons, 87*(11), 10-11.

[4]   Swezey, R. W., & Andrews, D. H. (2001). *Readings in training and simulation: A 30-year perspective.* Santa Monica, CA: Human Factors and Ergonomics Society.

[5]   Lammers, R. L. (2004). Principles of wound management. In J. R. Roberts & J. R. Hedges (Eds.), *Clinical procedures in emergency medicine, 4th Ed.* (pp. 623-654). Philadelphia, PA: Saunders.

[6]   U.S. National Library of Medicine (NLM).
        http://www.nlm.nih.gov/research/visible/visible_human.html

Medicine Meets Virtual Reality 14
J.D. Westwood et al. (Eds.)
IOS Press, 2006

Achieving Proper Exposure in Surgical Simulation

Christopher SEWELL[a], Dan MORRIS[a], Nikolas BLEVINS[b], Federico BARBAGLI[a],
Kenneth SALISBURY[a]

*Departments of [a] Computer Science and [b] Otolaryngology, Stanford University,
Stanford, CA, USA*

Abstract. One important technique common throughout surgery is achieving proper exposure of critical anatomic structures so that their shapes, which may vary somewhat among patients, can be confidently established and avoided. In this paper, we present an algorithm for determining which regions of selected structures are properly exposed in the context of a mastoidectomy simulation. Furthermore, our algorithm then finds and displays all other points along the surface of the structure that lie along a sufficiently short and straight path from an exposed portion such that their locations can be safely inferred. Finally, we present an algorithm for providing realistic visual cues about underlying structures with view-dependent shading of the bone.

Keywords. Surgical simulation, metrics, visibility, exposure, mastoidectomy

Introduction

In addition to providing the obvious advantages of low-cost, easily-accessible training opportunities, computerized surgical simulators are in position to take advantage of complete knowledge of the virtual environment and of the user's actions to analyze performance with regards to a wide range of elements of good surgical technique and to afford the trainee with valuable constructive criticism. Although some existing simulators report rudimentary metrics such as time to completion and collisions between instruments and objects that should not be touched, the development and generalization of metrics for a wide variety of surgical procedures remains an important open problem in the field.

In close collaboration with an otolaryngologist, we have developed a visuo-haptic simulator for mastoidectomy, a surgical procedure in which a portion of the temporal bone is drilled away in order to access the inner ear [1]. A data file is recorded when a user runs the simulator, and this file can be read and played back in a program that allows performance to be visualized and analyzed. We have devised, and are continuing to develop, a number of metrics for use with this simulator, including comparisons of the trainee's force profiles, velocity profiles, and bone removal characteristics to those of "model" mastoidectomies performed on the simulator by expert surgeons.

One important technique common throughout surgery is achieving proper exposure of critical anatomic structures so that their shapes, which may vary somewhat among patients, can be confidently established and avoided. In the context of this procedure, achieving proper exposure involves drilling until only a thin layer of bone remains over vulnerable structures (such as the facial nerve, sigmoid sinus, and dura). When the layer of bone is sufficiently thin, the structure can be seen, due to the partial transparency of the bone. Although it is not necessary to expose the entire structure, many, such as nerves and blood vessels, twist and turn in unpredictable ways, so it is imperative to expose enough of it such that the entire shape of the structure (within the surgical field) can be confidently inferred.

A few simulators, such as 5DT's Upper GI Endoscopy Simulator, track percentage of surface area visualized with the scope [2]. We have previously reported on a related metric that determines whether bone was within the user's field of view when drilled away, since it is essential to maintain proper visibility of the drilling region [3]. This enables the surgeon to avoid vulnerable structures just below the bone surface. If instead some bone is removed by "undercutting" (drilling beneath a shelf of bone that obscures visibility), there is increased risk of damaging these structures.

In order to accurately measure a trainee's ability to properly expose critical structures, the simulator must provide the user with realistic cues as to the structures' locations. In temporal bone surgery, the most important cues are visual, as a thin layer of bone is sufficiently translucent to make out underlying structures. This visual effect must therefore be provided in the simulator in order for our exposure metrics to be meaningful.

1. Direct Exposure

In our simulator, soft tissue structures are modeled using triangulated meshes, while the bone is represented using a hybrid data structure that allows computation of appropriate drill forces using rapid collision-detection in a spatially-discretized volumetric voxel representation while graphically rendering a smooth triangular mesh that is modified in real-time as the voxels are drilled away.

A given point on a structure is considered fully exposed when the ray from the given point to the viewpoint does not intersect any bone voxels nor any other soft tissue structures. Intersection between this ray and the other meshes is checked using an axis-aligned bounding box hierarchy [4], and collision detection between the ray and the bone is performed by sampling the ray at small increments (proportional to the voxel grid resolution) and directly indexing into the voxel array for each sample position to determine if there is a bone voxel at that location. This method does not guarantee that all ray-voxel intersections are found; the ray may cut through a corner of a voxel between samples. This could be remedied by sampling at increments equal to the voxel resolution and performing a box-ray intersection test for all existing voxels in the twenty-seven neighbor slots in the voxel grid for each sample point, but in general this is not necessary because the bone is partially transparent and we are primarily concerned with rays that intersect reasonably thick layers of bone. Points along the ray beyond the maximum extent of bone (which, for computational simplicity, can be represented by a primitive bounding volume) need not be tested.

In reality, a structure should not be fully exposed; instead, there should remain a layer of bone thin enough such that the underlying structure can be seen (due to the partial transparency of the bone) but thick enough such that the drill does not touch the structure. Thus, samples closer to the given point than some user-specified threshold distance are not considered in the bone collision tests. See Figure 1A.

Each vertex on a selected structure is tested to determine whether it is directly exposed. Since this depends on the viewpoint, it must be recalculated whenever the viewpoint changes. In our simulator, the viewpoint can be repositioned by the user using the camera tool. It is not good practice to attempt to identify the subtle visual cues needed to determine a structure's location while in the midst of moving the camera, so the visibility checks are only needed at the beginning and end of a camera movement. (Since bone is only removed and not replaced, exposure cannot decrease for a constant viewpoint, so the need for a check at the end of one movement is obviated by the check at the beginning of the next movement.)

The run-time for the voxel collision detection is proportional to the product of the number of vertices, the voxel grid resolution, and the number of camera movements. Ray-mesh collision detection is also run once for each vertex on the structure of interest after each camera movement; each call could involve checks against up to m triangles (where m is the total number of triangles in all meshes in the simulation), but the bounding volume hierarchy usually reduces this closer to O(log m) operations.

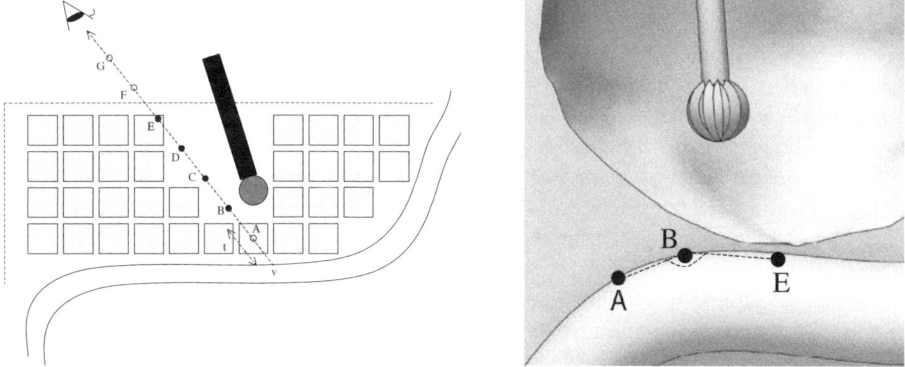

Figure 1A. At left, a given point (v) on a vulnerable anatomic structure (curved tube) is tested for direct exposure by tracing a ray from it to the viewpoint (eye). Points (A through G) at regular increments along the ray are tested for intersection with the bone voxels (light gray squares). Points (A) less than some threshold distance (t) from the given point are ignored, since proper exposure allows for a thin layer of bone to remain. (In fact, the trainee could be penalized for removing bone in this region, too close to the structure.) Points (F and G) beyond the bounding volume (large dashed rectangle) of bone need not be checked. Here points B, C, and D are checked and found not to intersect, but a collision is detected at Point E, so point v is not yet exposed. **Figure 1B.** At right, a point (E) is considered directly exposed if the overlying bone is sufficiently thin, as shown in Figure 1A. The position of another point (A) on the structure may then be safely inferred if the path distance along the surface (AB+BE) and "curvature" (the angle ABE along the surface through path midpoint B) are less than specified values.

2. Inferred Exposure

Having directly exposed some points along a structure, a surgeon may be able to confidently infer the location of other nearby points along the structure, provided that the structure is relatively straight in the vicinity. An expert may be able to establish a set of inferred points that includes all points of the structure within the surgical field by directly exposing only a small number of points in optimal locations; thus, the ratio of the sizes of the inferred and directly exposed sets, in addition to the absolute sizes of these sets, may be useful for determining a user's level of expertise.

Given a set of directly exposed points, as determined by the algorithm described in the preceding section, we make use of Dijkstra's algorithm [5] to determine the set of points whose locations can be safely inferred. The surface of the structure's mesh can be viewed as a graph (with the edges defined by the triangulation), and we attempt to find vertices for which there exists a path along the surface of sufficiently short length and sufficiently small curvature from a directly exposed point. Distance between two points along the surface is a more meaningful measure of their proximity than absolute distance because many structures (such as nerves and blood vessels) may twist and turn unpredictably. The mesh triangulation needs to be sufficiently fine and well-conditioned (i.e., no sliver triangles) so that the distance between any two points along edges of the triangulation closely approximates the shortest possible distance along the surface (although extremely high accuracy of distances is not necessary for this metric).

Dijkstra's algorithm is run once for each directly exposed vertex, which serves as the source. The algorithm repeatedly selects the vertex from the priority queue with the smallest shortest path estimate, and considers all outgoing edges from this vertex. For one such edge (v_1, v_2), where v_1 is the vertex just returned by the priority queue, if v_1's shortest-path estimate plus the distance between v_1 and v_2 is less than v_2's current shortest-path estimate, the edge may be "relaxed". Relaxing an edge involves adding v_2 to the queue and to the set of inferred points and updating its shortest-path estimate. However, the edge is not relaxed (and thus v_2 is not added to the set of inferred points) if v_2's new shortest-path estimate is greater than some user-specified distance threshold, or if its curvature relative to the source exceeds another specified threshold. Curvature is calculated as the deviation from 180^0 of the angle formed by the source, the midpoint along the path from the source to v_2, and v_2. (The curvature is only calculated for paths longer than some minimum threshold, since the curvature of very short paths is heavily influenced by the triangulation topology.) Thus, only vertices for which there exists a sufficiently short and straight path along the surface from a directly-exposed vertex are added to the set of inferred points. See Figure 1B.

The asymptotic running time of Dijkstra's algorithm is $O(E \log V)$, where E is the number of edges and V the number of vertices in the graph. If, as is almost always the case with a mesh, $E = O(V)$, (or, if the priority queue is implemented as a Fibonacci heap), this reduces to $O(V \log V)$. Since edges and vertices beyond the distance and curvature thresholds are never touched, V can actually be much less than the total number of mesh vertices if only a small region has been directly exposed and the distance and/or curvature thresholds are tight. This algorithm is called once for every directly exposed vertex after each camera movement.

3. View-Dependent Shading

In order to mimic the partial transparency of bone that enables structures to be seen without removing all overlying bone, we shade bone voxels near structures with appropriate colors or texture maps. A straightforward way of implementing this effect is to pre-compute the distances of all bone voxels from the underlying structures and then to interpolate between the shading color and natural bone color for each voxel in proportion to its distance. The distance between a voxel and a mesh is determined as the minimum distance between the voxel's (center) position and any triangle of the mesh. The distance between a point and a triangle is calculated by projecting the point onto the plane of the triangle, as described by Jones [6].

However, this has the effect of making the structure appear thicker all the way around. For example, in Figure 2A, if a viewer looks along the dotted line, he/she will think the dark structure (with gray shading) is directly along his/her line of sight, when in fact it is not. This effect is unrealistic and misleading.

Instead, a ray can be cast from the viewpoint through each voxel, as shown in Figure 2B. If and only if this ray intersects the structure is the voxel shaded, with intensity inversely proportional to the distance along the ray between the collision point and the voxel. As in Section 1, collision detection between this ray and the mesh is performed using an axis-aligned bounding box hierarchy. Rather than trace a ray through every voxel in the entire array, only those with a distance from the mesh (pre-computed as described above) less than a user-specified shading radius threshold need be considered. As in Section 2, these calculations depend on the viewpoint, but the rays are recast only at the end of every camera movement, since this visual effect is too subtle to be of great concern while actually moving the camera.
+
For each camera movement, ray-mesh collision detection is called once for each of m voxels, where m depends on the shading radius. Again, the bounding volume hierarchy usually reduces the potential checks against up to n triangles (where n is the number of triangles in the mesh for which the bone is being shaded) for each call to close to O(log n) operations.

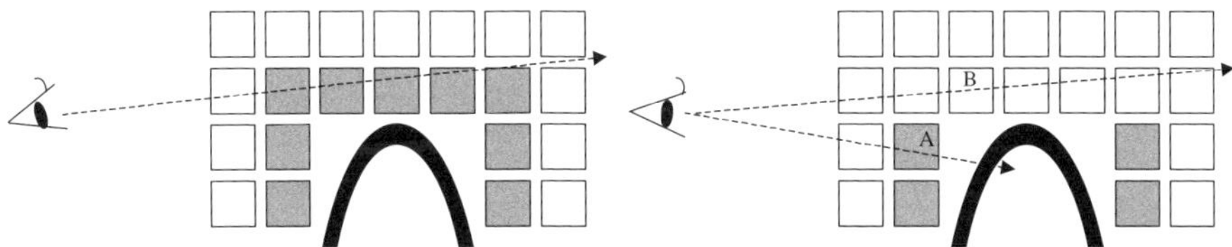

Figure 2A. At left, all voxels (squares) within a small radius of an underlying structure (black arc) are shaded. When the user looks along the ray shown, he/she sees shaded voxels, making it appear that the structure is along this line of sight, when in fact it is not. **Figure 2B.** At right, rays are cast from the viewpoint (eye) through each voxel within a small radius of the structure, and only those for which this ray intersects the structure are shaded. Thus, voxel A is shaded while voxel B is not.

4. Discussion

View-dependent shading has been incorporated into our interactive simulator, and an analysis of direct and inferred exposure has been added to our metrics console, which can replay runs of the simulator in real-time while providing visual and quantitative feedback, as shown in Figure 3A. While the simulation replays in the left panel, regions of selected structures shown in a cut-away view in the right panel are shaded based on whether proper exposure has been achieved. An example of shading the bone in the interactive simulator using a texture map is given in Figure 3B.

We are beginning a user study in which we will attempt to establish construct validity for several of our metrics, including those discussed in this paper. We intend to begin looking more closely at metrics related to force and velocity profiles, but some work remains for visibility-related metrics, including accounting for view obstruction by bone dust. Most of our work on metrics thus far has been related to temporal bone surgery, but we believe that many of these ideas are fundamental throughout surgery and plan to extend them to other procedures.

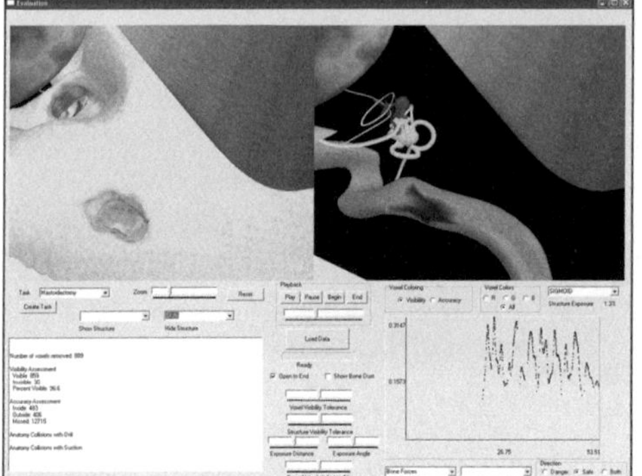 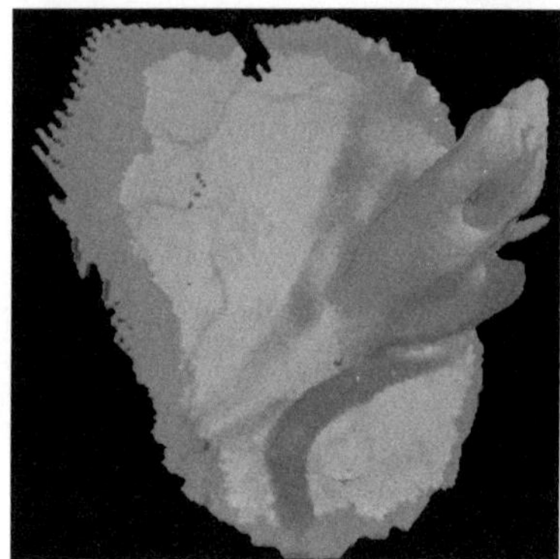

Figure 3A. At left, our metrics console, playing back a run of the simulator. In the left panel, shading of the bone is visible as the sigmoid sinus is approached. In the right panel, underlying structures are shown. The directly exposed portion of the sigmoid is shaded in one color, while the portion that can be safely inferred from the exposed region is shaded in another color. **Figure 3B.** At right, the back of the temporal bone, shaded in the proximity of the sigmoid sinus and of the dura, using a texture map applied to the voxels.

Acknowledgement and References

We would like to acknowledge NIH Grant R33 LM07295 for funding this work.

[1] Morris D, Sewell C, Blevins N, Barbagli F, Salisbury K: A collaborative virtual environment for the simulation of temporal bone surgery. *Proc of MICCAI* 2004, Vol. II, pp. 319-327.

[2] Bloom MB, Rawn CL, Salzberg AD, Krummel TM: Virtual reality applied to procedural testing: the next era. *Annals of Surgery* 2003, 237(3): 442-448.

[3] Sewell C, Morris D, Blevins N, Barbagli F, Salisbury K: Quantifying risky behavior in surgical simulation. *Proc of MMVR* 2005, pp. 451-457.

[4] Cohen JD, Lin MC, Manocha D, Ponamgi MK: I-COLLIDE: an interactive and exact collision detection system for large-scale environments. *Proc. ACM Interactive 3D Graphics Conf.*, 1995, pp. 189-196.

[5] Dijkstra EW: A note on two problems in connexion with graphs.*Numerische Mathematik*, 1959 1: 269-71

[6] Jones MW: 3D Distance from a point to a triangle. Technical Report, Department of Computer Science, University of Wales Swansea, 1995.

Medicine Meets Virtual Reality 14
J.D. Westwood et al. (Eds.)
IOS Press, 2006

Structural Flexibility of Laparoscopic Instruments: Implication for the Design of Virtual Reality Simulators

SHANG, D.[a], CARNAHAN, H.[a], and DUBROWSKI, A[b]
[a] Department of Kinesiology, University of Waterloo
[b] Surgical Skills Centre at Mt. Sinai Hospital, Department of Surgery, University of Toronto, Toronto, ON, Canada
(Corresponding author's e-mail: daniel.shang@gmail.com)

Abstract. Laparoscopic training, under simulated settings, benefits from high fidelity models of the actual environment. This study was aimed at reducing uncertainty in the displacement and loads experienced by a laparoscopic instrument during surgical training. Infrared tracking of laparoscopic instruments is ineffective when real tissues attenuate the infrared signals. Incorporating the use of strain gauges for tip deflection measurements allows for online motion and load tracking during a procedure. Strain gauge voltages and infrared markers indicating displacement were both linear with respect to loads up to 700 grams. The resultant strain gauge voltage was equated to deflection values with a calibration constant. The results serve two purposes. First, it may enable the tracking and analysis of the skill level of novice surgeons using bench models. Second, the mechanical model of each instrument can be quantified and incorporated into virtual simulations, thus increasing model fidelity, effectively leading to better learning.

1. Introduction

Minimally invasive surgery (MIS) has become a staple and necessary technique to learn for surgical residents. However, the visual-motor skills involved in MIS deviate from traditional surgery and the necessary investment to acquire expertise is often limited by the amount and quality of practice available [1].

Skills acquisition can be characterized by the minimization of instrument movement and loads [2]. It is of particular interest that by examining the deflection at an instrument's tip, it is also possible to analyze the dynamic load experienced by the instrument. Furthermore, the common trends in instrument dynamics can be observed during particular tasks and procedures and across expert surgeons. For example, transverse loads on the instruments are minimal during laparoscopic suturing, and they are substantial in cholecystectomy or small bowel passing [3].

This type of data can also be utilized in virtual reality simulations, which have promised accessibility beyond traditional live procedures but have not yet resolved inherent issues of model fidelity [4]. To this point, the deflection of laparoscopic instruments under load has been often neglected despite obvious discrepancies between the simulated and actual environments [5].

Previously, instrument dynamics have been examined by Hughes et al. for a selection of instruments by monitoring their behavior under load with optoelectric motion tracking system [5]. However, when working inside animate or inanimate training models signal attenuation from surrounding tissues may pose a serious disadvantage to this data acquisition system, limiting its usage. Presently, we propose a more robust system based on analog voltage from strain gauges to capture instrument dynamics.

2. Method

2.1 Equipment

Instrument: A needle driver (Stryker) of 5 mm bore and 30 cm length was instrumented with strain gauges and infrared sensors to detect deflection and instrument rotation.

Measurement systems: An optoelectric position and 3D motion tracking system using infrared markers (IREDs) and cameras was used for motion tracking (OPTOTRAK 3020; Northern Digital Inc., Waterloo, ON, CA).   OPTOTRAK is capable of measuring to an RMS accuracy of 0.1 mm.   Sampling frequency of the system was set at 200 Hz.   Deflection at the instrument tip (bending in the shaft) was defined and measured with respect to the reference established at the collar of the instrument. Ten infrared sensors were mounted around the shaft near the base of the instrument and one at the tip near the grasper (see Hughes et al, 2005 for details). Continuous signals from at least 3 unique markers provided the minimum Cartesian representation of the instrument which was used to extrapolate an overall instrument model when sensor signatures were compared to a static reference model of the needle driver.   Dynamic rotational and deflection data were extrapolated in the same manner without signal attenuation.

Strain gauges mounted in a full-bridge, dual-channel formation allowed for extrapolation of the transverse load on the needle driver.   Load orientation was calculated from resultant voltage contributions from both channels.

2.2. Experimental Design

Static loading: A test bench allowed for static transverse loading of the needle driver. Deflections under specified loads ranging from no load up to 700 grams (by 100 gram increments) were quantified and calibrated by comparing strain gauge voltage output to actual deflection measured by infrared sensors.

Dynamic loading: Rotation of the instrument produced measurements at various angles.   It was expected that there would be equal magnitude deflections in all directions.   Voltage contributions from both channels encode resultant loads with respect to one of the four quadrants is then compared to the directional data produced by the optoelectric system.

3. Results

Figure 1 demonstrates linearity between load and output during unidirectional static loading.   Resultant voltages in Figure 2 show directional output with a 500 gram load.

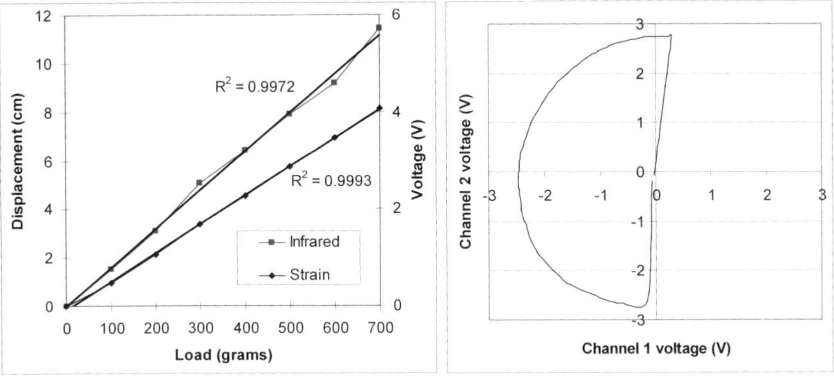

Figure 1 (Left). Strain gauge voltage output closely resembles that of the positional measurement provided by the infrared system. Correlations between line of best fit and the infrared data and strain gauge voltages ascertain linearity up to the maximum deflection load of 700 grams. Furthermore, the ratio between the slopes of the strain gauge and infrared plots provide a calibration value to calculate voltage-based deflection values.

Figure 2 (Right). Semi-rotation of the instrument at the 500 g load showed close approximation to static voltages, thus demonstrating equal magnitude deflection in all directions.

4. Conclusion

When practicing on inanimate and animate models, tracking motions of the laparoscopic instruments by using strain gauges allows for real time monitoring of instrument dynamic without signal attenuation due to surrounding tissues. In this study we have demonstrated that magnitude and directional values for the deflection of the instrument can be quantified based on the dual channel strain gauge system. It is expected that further analyses of the data during actual procedures should yield task or procedure dependent strategies and commonalities needed to establish criteria for evaluating expertise [6].

In accordance with the Practice Specificity Theory, training on models that closely resemble real life scenarios is most beneficial to learning [7]. Testing individual instruments and establishing a library in the virtual environment will ultimately improve virtual reality model fidelity and consequently the rate of skills acquisition when training using this modality.

[1] Fraser SA, Feldman LS, Stanbridge D, Fried GM. Characterizing the learning curve for a basic laparoscopic drill. Surg Endosc. 2005 (in press)

[2] Rosen J, MacFarlane M, Richards C, Hannaford B, Sinanan M. Surgeon-tool force/torque signatures--evaluation of surgical skills in minimally invasive surgery. Stud Health Technol Inform. 1999;62:290-6.

[3] Rosen J, Chang L, Brown JD, Hannaford B, Sinanan M, Satava R. Minimally invasive surgery task decomposition--etymology of endoscopic suturing. Stud Health Technol Inform. 2003;94:295-301.

[4] Reznick RK. Virtual reality surgical simulators: feasible but valid? J Am Coll Surg. 1999;189:127-8.

[5] Hughes S, Larmer J, Park J, Macrae H, Dubrowski A. Structural flexibility of laparoscopic instruments: implication for the design of virtual reality simulators. Stud Health Technol Inform. 2005;111:201-3.

[6] Rosen J, Brown JD, Barreca M, Chang L, Hannaford B, Sinanan M. The Blue DRAGON--a system for monitoring the kinematics and the dynamics of endoscopic tools in minimally invasive surgery for objective laparoscopic skill assessment. Stud Health Technol Inform. 2002;85:412-8.

[7] Schmidt RA, Lee TD. Motor control and learning: A behavioral emphasis. Champaign, IL: Human Kinetics. 2005.

Medicine Meets Virtual Reality 14
J.D. Westwood et al. (Eds.)
IOS Press, 2006

Selective Tessellation Algorithm for Modeling Interactions Between Surgical Instruments and Tissues

Yunhe SHEN[a,1], Venkat DEVARAJAN[a], Robert EBERHART[b], Mark WATSON[b], Jitesh BUTALA[a]

[a] *Virtual Environment Lab, University of Texas at Arlington*
[b] *Department of Surgery, University of Texas Southwestern Medical Center at Dallas*

Abstract. We present a selective spatial tessellation algorithm that is specifically optimized for instrument-to-tissue and instrument-to-instrument collision detection cases, which are the essential part of interaction modeling in surgery simulation with haptic feedback. Virtual surgeries demand haptic rate collision solutions only when instruments are involved in collisions. Other collision cases can be processed at slower rates. The proposed selective tessellation algorithm is capable of differentiating among various collision cases and assigning different priorities to their processing. Without making assumptions about any object movement, the algorithm derives clipping volume as collision detection regions which tightly enclose the objects of interest. Results of implementation of the algorithm in a surgical simulation are provided.

Keywords. Collision detection, collision response, object modeling and virtual reality

Introduction

Virtual patient modeling and interaction modeling: A virtual reality based surgical simulator can be divided into two major parts: a virtual patient and the interaction with that patient [8]: The virtual patient part consists of computer-simulated soft or rigid tissue models of human organs. Generally, these models are physically based and driven by external input such as displacement and force. The interaction part simulates surgeon's interactions with these virtual models; interaction modeling gives input to the virtual patient model. Interaction modeling requires collision detection and collision response solutions to simulate the interactions between a surgeon and a virtual patient. The task of collision detection is to locate contacts or intersections among all the objects in a scene. Collision detection gives input to the virtual patient module, as well as collision response, which then adjusts the interaction among deformable or rigid objects. These physically based adjustments are applied in forms of forces, velocities and displacements.

Instrument-involved collision: A virtual laparoscopic surgery demands haptic rate collision solutions only when surgical instruments are involved in collisions. Tissue-to-

---

[1] Corresponding Author: Yunhe Shen, Virtual Environment Lab, University of Texas at Arlington, Arlington, Texas, 76010; Tel: 817-272-5719; E-mail: Yunhe.shen@gmail.com.

tissue collision cases can be processed at slower rates, or merely ignored in some scenarios. Such applications may demand that their collision detection modules have the ability of differentiating instrument-involved collisions among various collision cases and accordingly, assigning different priorities to their processing. In this research, we propose a new selective tessellation method which derives clipping volume as selected collision detection regions without making assumptions about object movement.

1. Method

1.1. Add "Instrument-First" Feature to Collision Detection

Previous tessellation work: Spatial tessellation algorithms [1-6] represent a workspace with uniform cells, rasterize all primitives (e.g. polygon, particle, or voxel) of every geometric object into the cells, and maintain object and primitive information in every cell with tessellation data structures. After this so called construction phase, intersection tests are applied within each of the non-empty cells to determine any inside collisions. The previous algorithms handle a pair of objects, or they divide the environment into background objects and a foreground object such as a surgical instrument. These algorithms tessellate the background and the foreground into two sets of cells. Once a foreground cell is derived, querying the existence of the same cell in the background dataset (background – foreground (B-F) query) may trigger further detection work on the primitives in the cell. Data structures employed in these algorithms are of a two-level hierarchy: cells and primitives inside each of the cells. This method is extended to multiple-objects environments and self-collision detection in [5], which includes all objects in both background and foreground tessellation.

A generic solution: We had proposed a three-layer OHC data structure (see [9] for details), which organizes the tessellated space into three levels of information, i.e. non-empty cells, objects contained in each of the cells, and primitives of each object in each cell. Figure 1 shows the cell-object-primitive (COP) cascades in the OHC structure. The boxes in figure 1 represent certain types of data structure or container in which information on cell, object and primitive is maintained; the arrows represent mappings between every data pairs.

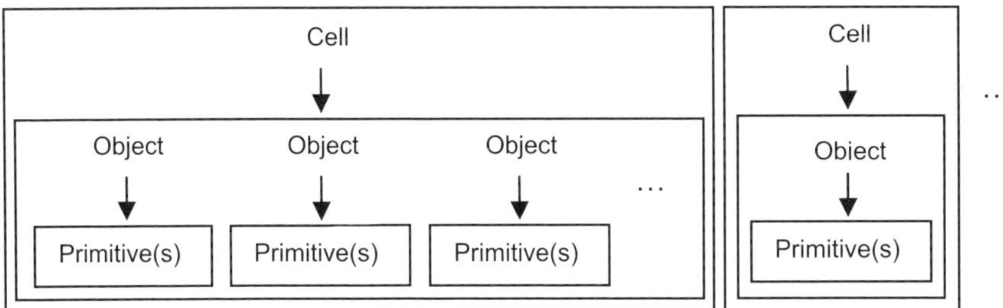

Figure 1. Cell-object-primitive cascades in the OHC data structure

The addition of the object layer adds flexibility and efficiency to tessellation based collision detection strategies. This algorithm does not inherit the concept of B-F query mentioned above; instead, once all the objects and primitives are tessellated, the algorithm traverses the OHC structure guiding further intersection tests to those cells containing more than one object, or a single object that requires self-collision detection.

Selective tessellation for instrument-involved collisions: The general purpose of the selective tessellation is to derive a solution that subdivides the total collision detection work and assigns priority levels to the subdivisions. Each priority level is associated with certain objects and can be dynamically changed during the simulation. For instance, an interaction module may assign the highest priority to the detection of instrument-involved collisions to match with its haptic rendering rates.

We propose a collision detection algorithm which rasterizes selected objects, e.g. surgical instruments, to define an area of interest, and then apply different processes within and out of the area. This approach can be described as follows:

- The "Instrument-First" detection thread first rasterizes instruments into cells.
- Only those cells occupied by the instruments are created in the three-layer tessellation data structure.
- Tessellation of the other objects are then limited within the existing cells. All primitives mapped into new cells are recognized apart from the instruments, and are excluded from further processing in this detection thread.
- The processing exempted in this collision detection thread is the construction of cells with no instruments, and the intersection tests performed for them.
- Excluded data: Cell spaces excluded by the above approach may have tissue-to-tissue collisions inside. If an application prefers not to ignore these collisions, then the excluded data are stored in another tessellation dataset, which can be processed with slower rates.

The procedure is summarized in figure 2.

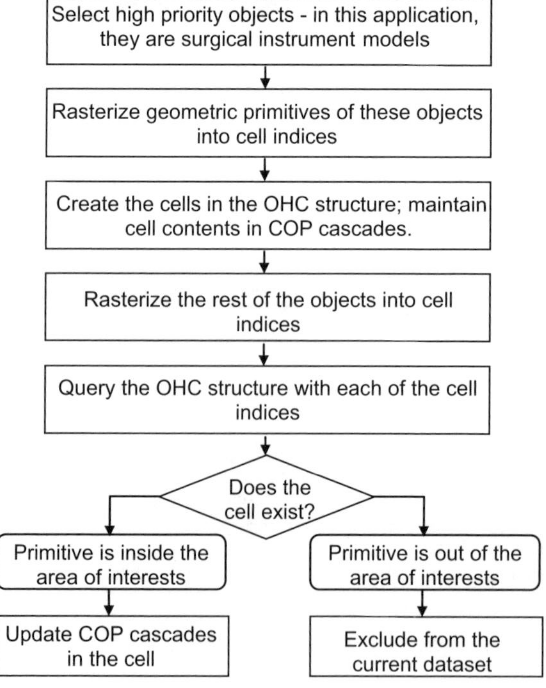

Figure 2. Subdividing the OHC dataset with selective tessellation

1.2. Collision Response

Once any collisions among virtual objects are detected, a collision response solution imposes some adjustments to the behavior and status of the involved objects, in order to approximate their collision response in the real world. For physically based simulation, collision response solutions are generally determined by conservation laws, impulse dynamics, or constraint methods, etc. [7]. For real time surgical simulators, their collision response modules are expected to offer fast, interactive and realistic visual or haptic feedback.

In our approach, the collision detection module calculates intersection between each pair of colliding primitives, and forwards their positions, velocities and intersection status as input to a collision response module. When soft tissues are involved, output such as force, velocity or displacement from the collision response module is taken by the deformable modeling module as input. When instruments are involved, collision response output is also sent to a haptic rendering module. In our surgical simulator, surface mass-spring-damper mesh and elastic volume constraint model have been adopted for deformable modeling [8], and the primitives processed by the collision detection and response modules are triangles. Collision response cases are studied respectively between instrument to instrument, instrument to rigid tissue, instrument to soft tissue, soft tissue to soft tissue, and soft tissue to rigid tissue. Conservation laws and impulse dynamics are applied in calculating the response adjustments [7].

2. Implementation

This selective tessellation algorithm has been utilized in our inguinal herniorrhaphy simulator, as shown in figure 3. In the soft-real time system, interaction and soft tissue deformation servo loops are implemented as three threads in the framework - collision detection and response thread, deformation thread, and haptic rendering thread. Graphic rendering is with the main thread of the simulation program.

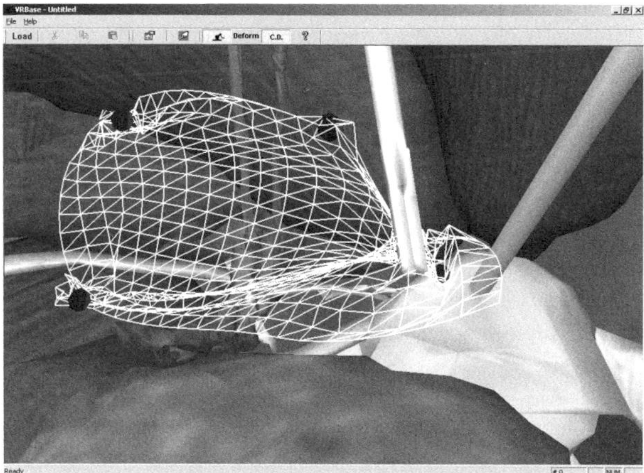

Figure 3. Simulation of laparoscopic inguinal hernia repair

3. Results

The selective tessellation algorithm is tested on a 2.8GHz dual-processor computer. Deformation thread is running above 700Hz. Force feedback thread is at 1 KHz. The entire virtual environment consists of 4K-8K triangles, including some objects without collision detection or deformation concerns. When 2 surgical instrument models (904 triangles) and 11 deformable tissue models (3836 triangles) are passed to this selective collision detection and collision response thread (figure 4), the processing time is about 4ms per cycle, in contrast to 12 ms (an improvement by a factor of 3) for our previous general collision detection and response algorithm (OHC). Collision response time averages 0.03ms per pair.

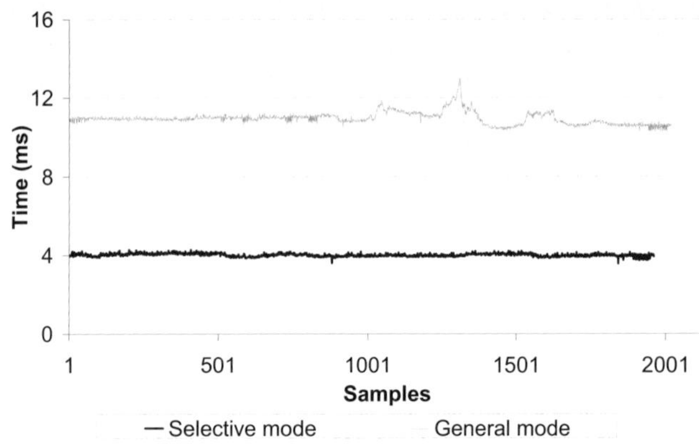

Figure 4. Performance of Selective and general OHC tessellation algorithm

4. Conclusion

Selective tessellation separates instrument-involved interaction modeling from other collision detection and response work, so that the haptic rate processing load in this surgery simulation can be significantly reduced. The overall simulation achieved close to haptic feedback rates.

5. Discussion

This scheme can be extended to handling collision detection work with multi-level priorities in order to break down the real time work load. High priority objects are tessellated before the lower priority objects. In this situation, the OHC data will be constructed into a set of subdivisions with their total number equal to the number of priority levels. Furthermore, GPU based rasterization power can be explored for spatial tessellation approaches [10].

In the following we compare the proposed selective algorithm with previous tessellation based approaches: In the B-F query approach, background and foreground datasets are queried for common cells between them. In this selective OHC approach, two sets of data have no common cells. Therefore, separating them will not cause any missed collisions, and there is no cell query applied after constructing them. In B-F query, each object is to be tessellated twice – in the background pass and then the foreground pass, otherwise self-collisions will be ignored. The OHC algorithm tessellates each object once during construction phase, traverses its data structure and gives self-collision option to every object.

Because computer simulation programs run in discrete time domain, their collision detection algorithms are executed in a sampling instead of continuous manner. This discrete feature suggests instances in which an interaction model misses the exact moment of collision during sampling intervals, even if its detection algorithm is implemented as conservative detection, which guarantees no missed collision when it is executed. The effect on the simulation could be, for example, encountering unexpected deep penetrations before any collision response adjustments have been applied. In this case, penetration depth could be helpful in recovering the virtual objects from any unwanted interceptions or penetrations. Generally, objects modeled with surface mesh require more effort to determine penetration depth than those modeled with a volumetric mesh. Backtracking and reducing simulation time step approach the exact contacting moment, at the cost of interrupting the real time iteration of the simulation.

Acknowledgements

Useful consultation with Robert Rege MD at UTSWMC is gratefully acknowledged. This research is supported in part by Texas Higher Education Coordinating Board.

References

[1] S. Frisken-Gibson, "Using linked volumes to model object collision, de-formation, cutting, carving and joining," IEEE Trans. Visualization and Computer Graphics, 5(4), pp. 333-348, 1999.

[2] M. Overmars, "Point location in fat subdivisions," Information Process-ing Letter, 44, pp. 261-265, 1992.

[3] A. Gregory, M. Lin, S. Gottschalk, R. Taylor, "Fast and accurate collision detection for haptic interaction using a three degree-of-freedom force-feedback device," Computational Geometry: Theory and Applications, 15(1-3), pp. 69-89, 2000.

[4] S. Cotin, H. Delingette and N. Ayache, "Real-time elastic deformations of soft tissues for surgery simulation," IEEE Trans. Visualization and Com-puter Graphics, 5(1), pp. 62-73, 1999.

[5] M. Teschner, B. Heidelberger, M. Mueller, D. Pomeranets, M. Gross. "Optimized spatial hashing for collision detection of deformable objects," in Proc. Vision, Modeling, Visualization VMV'03, pp. 47-54, 2003.

[6] B. Joshi, B. Lee, D. Popescu and S. Ourselin, "Multiple contact approach to collision modeling in surgical simulation," in Proc. Medicine Meets Virtual Reality'13, pp. 237-242, 2005.

[7] J. Butala, "Collision response for virtual laparoscopic surgery," Master thesis, Dept. of Electrical Eng., Univ. of Texas at Arlington, Arlington, Texas, 2005.

[8] Y. Shen, "Real time collision detection and soft tissue deformation for haptic simulation of laparoscopic surgery," PhD dissertation, Dept. of Biomedical Eng., Univ. of Texas at Arlington, Arlington, Texas, 2005.

[9] Y. Shen, V. Devarajan and R. Eberhart, "Haptic herniorrhaphy simulation with robust and fast collision detection algorithm," in Proc. Medicine Meets Virtual Reality'13, pp. 458-464, 2005.

[10] N. Govindaraju, M. Lin and D. Manocha, "Fast and reliable collision detection using graphics processors," Symposium on Computational Geometry, 384-385, 2005.

Medicine Meets Virtual Reality 14
J.D. Westwood et al. (Eds.)
IOS Press, 2006

Realistic Irrigation Visualization in a Surgical Wound Debridement Simulator

Yuzhong Shen [a,1], Jennifer Seevinck [a] and Emre Baydogan [b]

[a] *Virginia Modeling, Analysis, and Simulation Center, Old Dominion University, USA*
[b] *Department of Electrical and Computer Engineering, Old Dominion University, USA*

Abstract. Wound debridement refers to the removal of necrotic, devitalized, or contaminated tissue and/or foreign material to promote wound healing. Surgical debridement uses sharp instruments to cut dead tissue from a wound and it is the quickest and most efficient method of debridement. A wound debridement simulator [1,2] can ensure that a medical trainee is competent prior to performing a procedure on a genuine patient. Irrigation is performed at different stages of debridement in order to remove debris and reduce the bacteria count through rinsing the wound. This paper presents a novel approach for realistic irrigation visualization based on texture representations of debris. This approach applies image processing techniques to a series of images, which model the cleanliness of the wound. The active texture is generated and updated dynamically based on the irrigation state, location, and range. Presented results demonstrate that texture mapping and image processing techniques can provide effective and efficient solutions for irrigation visualization in the wound debridement simulator.

Keywords. Surgical simulation, medical modeling and simulation, texture mapping, image processing,

1. Introduction

Wound debridement refers to the process of removing necrotic, devitalized, or contaminated tissue and/or foreign material to promote healing. At present, this procedure is typically learned with actual patients. Our surgical wound debridement simulator [1] allows debridement to be performed on a virtual patient, promoting knowledge and skill acquisition. The simulator currently uses a shallow laceration wound to the thigh with embedded shards of glass, dirt, and debris. Trainees are instructed to remove the glass shards with forceps, scrub with a brush, rinse with saline solution, and remove devitalized tissue [1]. Wound irrigation is performed at different stages of wound debridement in order to remove dirts and debris and reduce the bacteria count through rinsing the wound. During irrigation, normal saline is used with gentle pressure via syringe to enhance wound cleansing but avoid trauma. This paper presents techniques to achieve realistic irrigation visualization in a wound debridement simulator. The reminder of this paper is organized as follows. Section 2 describes the proposed method and Section 3 gives the implementation results.

---

[1]Correspondence to: Yuzhong Shen, Virginia Modeling, Simulation and Analysis Center, Old Dominion University, Norfolk, VA 23529. Tel.: +1 757 683 6366; Fax: +1 757 686 6214; E-mail: yshen@odu.edu.

2. Proposed Method

We utilize a particle system based approach to model saline and texture mapping techniques to simulate the irrigation process. Texture mapping is a standard and powerful rendering technique used in modern computer graphics and it enhances realism and details in a scene with only a modest increase in computational complexity. In the proposed approach, the wound cleanliness is modeled by a series of images, simulating a variety of debris on the contaminated wound; however, at any time, there is only one texture active over the whole mesh. The active texture is initialized to be the dirty image and updated dynamically at different stages of the surgical debridement, as a result of combination of several different images.

Denote the active texture as T, and the images representing dirty state and clean state as I_d and I_c, respectively. The steps in the irrigation are as follows:

1. At the beginning of irrigation, let $T = I_d$.
2. During irrigation, detect possible intersection between the wound and the prolonged syringe outline. Compute the intersection point P and the triangle that contains P. Assuming the three vertices of the intersected triangles has geometrical coordinates $\mathbf{v}_1, \mathbf{v}_2, \mathbf{v}_3 \in \mathbb{R}^3$ and texture coordinates $\mathbf{t}_1, \mathbf{t}_2, \mathbf{t}_3 \in \mathbb{R}^2$, the texture coordinate $\mathbf{t}_P \in \mathbb{R}^2$ of the intersection point P can be computed as follows:

$$\mathbf{t}_P = \frac{\sum_{i=1}^{3} a_i \mathbf{t}_i}{\sum a_i}, \tag{1}$$

   where $a_i, i = 1, 2, 3$, are the barycentric coordinates of P, expressed as a convex combination of $\mathbf{v}_1, \mathbf{v}_2, \mathbf{v}_3$.
3. Assuming that the sizes of the texture and the images have been normalized into the range of $[0, 1] \times [0, 1]$, the texture T is updated as follows:

$$T(\mathbf{t})_{\|\mathbf{t}-\mathbf{t}_P\| \leq r} = (1 - c)I_d + cI_c, \tag{2}$$

   where r is the range of irrigation and c is a coefficient that determines the thoroughness of the irrigation.

OpenSceneGraph [3], a high-performance 3D graphics toolkit, is utilized for developing the visualization component in our surgical wound debridement simulator. OpenSceneGraph provides a basic collision detection capability between a surface mesh and a line segment. To determine the area being irrigated, the intersection between the surface mesh representing the thigh and the line segment representing the syringe is computed by using the IntersectVisitor class in OpenSceneGraph. The range of irrigation r can be determined by computing the distance between the syringe and the thigh.

3. Results

The irrigation results are shown in Fig. 1. The triangular mesh for the thigh used in the wound debridement is shown in Fig. 1(a); Fig. 1(b) shows the dirty wound as a result of applying a dirty texture image to the mesh in Fig. 1(a); the dirty wound is being

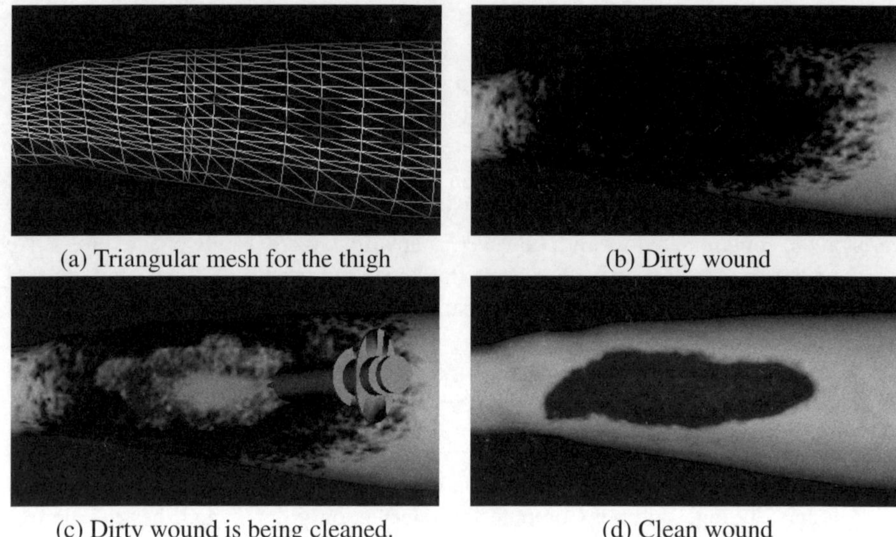

(a) Triangular mesh for the thigh   (b) Dirty wound

(c) Dirty wound is being cleaned.   (d) Clean wound

Figure 1. Wound irrigation visualization

cleaned in Fig. 1(c); it can be seen that the boundary between the dirty area and the cleaned area is smooth, eliminating blocking artifacts exhibited in our previous work; and finally, Fig. 1(d) shows the wound after cleaning, which is ready for further debridement operations such as cutting dead tissue. The results shown in Fig. 1 demonstrate that texture mapping and image processing techniques can provide effective and efficient solutions for irrigation visualization in the surgical wound debridement simulator.

4. Acknowledgement

This project was a collaborative effort between the Virginia Modeling, Analysis and Simulation Center (VMASC) at Old Dominion University and the Eastern Virginia Medical School. Partial funding was provided by the Naval Health Research Center through NAVAIR Orlando TSD under contract N61339-03-C-0157, and the Office of Naval Research under contract N00014-04-1-0697, entitled "The National Center for Collaboration in Medical Modeling and Simulation". The ideas and opinions presented in this paper represent the views of the authors and do not necessarily represent the views of the Department of Defense.

References

[1] J. Seevinck, M. Scerbo, L. Belfore, L. Weireter, J. Crouch, Y. Shen, F. McKenzie, H. Garcia, S. Girtelschmid, E. Baydogan, and E. Schmidt, A Simulation-Based Training System for Surgical Wound Debridement, *Medicine Meets Virtual Reality 14*, Long Beach, CA, 2006.

[2] L. Belfore, J. Crouch, Y. Shen, S. Girtelschmid, and E. Baydogan, A Software Framework for Surgical Simulation Virtual Environment, *Medicine Meets Virtual Reality 14*, Long Beach, CA, 2006.

[3] OpenSceneGraph, http://www.openscenegraph.org

Medicine Meets Virtual Reality 14
J.D. Westwood et al. (Eds.)
IOS Press, 2006

Simulating Bending Behaviour of Thread and Needle

Ofek Shilon [1],

Simbionix Ltd., 6 Hamlacha st., Lod 71520, Israel

Abstract. The traditional approach to modeling bending of a thread consists in adding springs connecting non-neighbouring keypoints. An alternative is introduced, starting by articulating an intrinsic bending energy of an arbitrary joint, and deducing the resultant justification forces. Significant visual appeal is thus gained, with negligible computational costs. We further investigate the bending interaction of a spline with a connected rigid body, and mention several generalization directions.

1. Introduction

Surgical simulation is a relatively young field, and yet is a very rapidly growing one. The benefits of training surgeons by computerized interactive simulation were validated in numerous studies, and the ever-rising computation abilities make this area richer and wider by the day. Simbionix Ltd. is a leading manufacturer of simulators for minimaly-invasive procedures, that have recently launched *Suture-Tutor*^{TM}, an endoscopic suturing simulator.

Out of the various innovations developed for *Suture-Tutor*^{TM}, the one we present here has to do with the behaviour of the suturing thread, modeled as a spline object. Specifically, we present novel results in the simulation of the *justification* behaviour of such a thread.

Our basic approach towards this task is the articulation of a bending energy at a thread point, and the derivation of resulting justification forces. From here, range several discretization schemes that suit a range of needs, from the quick-and-dirty to the thorough and realistic.

2. Spline Justification

Let $\mathbf{x}(s)$ be a C^2 parametrized curve in $\mathbb{R}^3$, with tangent given by $\mathbf{T}(s) = \frac{\dot{\mathbf{x}}(s)}{\|\dot{\mathbf{x}}(s)\|}$. We set the following expression for the total bending energy of the curve :

$$E_{total} = \alpha \int_0^1 \kappa^2(s)ds \tag{1}$$

---

[1] E-mail: ofek@simbionix.com

where $\kappa(s)$ is the curvature at $\mathbf{x}(s)$, and α characterizes the material's rigidness. This expression, beyond being reasonable, has a sound physical basis - cf. [LL], §17. The deduction that follows can easily be made to encompass also non-uniform rigidness $\alpha(s)$. Let us inspect two schemes of discretisizing this expression.

2.1. Successive Tangents Discretization

Assume for a moment that the curve is parametrized by arc-length. Then, by definition $\kappa(s) = \left\|\dot{\mathbf{T}}(s)\right\|$. We approximate this value as follows:

$$\kappa^2(s) = \left\|\dot{\mathbf{T}}(s)\right\|^2 \approx \frac{1}{\Delta s^2}\|\mathbf{T}(s+\Delta s) - \mathbf{T}(s)\|^2 \approx \frac{1}{\Delta s^2}\theta(\mathbf{T}(s+\Delta s), \mathbf{T}(s))^2$$

$$\approx \frac{2}{\Delta s^2}(1 - \cos(\theta(\mathbf{T}(s+\Delta s), \mathbf{T}(s)))) = \frac{2}{\Delta s^2}(1 - \mathbf{T}(s+\Delta s)^T \mathbf{T}(s))$$

where $\theta(\mathbf{T}(s+\Delta s), \mathbf{T}(s))$ is the angle between the vectors. If we discretize the curve into a finite sequence of keypoints, the following energy discretization arises naturally:

$$E_{total} \approx \alpha \sum_{i=0}^{n-1} \frac{2}{\Delta s_i^2}(1 - \mathbf{T}_{i+1}^T \mathbf{T}_i)\Delta s_i$$

where $\mathbf{T}_i = \mathbf{T}(s_i)$. Since the zero-bending energy is arbitrary, we can seperate the expression into bending energies at individual joints:

$$E_i = -\frac{\alpha}{\Delta s_{i-1}}\mathbf{T}_i^T \mathbf{T}_{i-1} \tag{2}$$

Although derived for uniform-speed curves, this result is in fact applicable to a much wider family of (reasonable) curves, and lends itself to different interpretations.

Now, we restrict ourselves further to *linear splines*, i.e. - curves that are given in the form $\mathbf{x}(s) = \sum b_i(s)\mathbf{x}_i$. We'll also make use of a concatenated matrix-vector form: $\mathbf{x}(s) = B(s)\mathbf{x}$, where $B(s) = (b_0(s)I \mid b_1(s)I \mid \cdots \mid b_{n-1}(s)I)$, and $\mathbf{x} = (\mathbf{x}_0^T \mid \mathbf{x}_1^T \mid \cdots \mid \mathbf{x}_{n-1}^T)^T$. Denote $\mathbf{v}(s) = \sum b_i'(s)\mathbf{x}_i = B'(s)\mathbf{x}$ and $\mathbf{a}(s) = \sum b_i''(s)\mathbf{x}_i = B''(s)\mathbf{x}$ and suppose we sample the curve at times s_j, $j = 0, \ldots, m-1$ - times which need not be related to the keypoints $\mathbf{x}_i$, not in location nor in number. For convenience, abbreviate further: $B_j' = B'(s_j)$, $\mathbf{v}_j = \mathbf{v}(s_j)$ and $\mathbf{a}_j = \mathbf{a}(s_j)$. Finally, we can now differentiate directly and gather up terms to obtain the concatenated vector of justification forces at all keypoints $\mathbf{x}_i$:

$$\mathbf{F}^{just} = -\nabla_{\mathbf{x}}(\sum E_j) = \alpha \sum_{i=0}^{m-2} \frac{1}{\|\mathbf{v}_j\|} B_j'^T(I - \mathbf{T}_j \mathbf{T}_j^T)(\frac{\mathbf{T}_{j-1}}{\Delta s_{j-1}} + \frac{\mathbf{T}_{j+1}}{\Delta s_j})$$

Edge effects can be simply accounted for by setting $\mathbf{T}_0 = \mathbf{T}_{n-1} = \mathbf{0}$.

2.2. Local Curvature Discretization

We adhere to the linear spline setup, but now reexamine the approximation of eq. 2 , Dropping the unit-speed assumption. The curvature at a point s is given by -

$$\kappa(s) = \frac{\|\mathbf{v}(s) \times \mathbf{a}(s)\|}{\|\mathbf{v}(s)\|^3}$$

(cf. [Dc]). The seemingly tedious task of calculating $\nabla(\kappa^2)$ was facilitated (as all calculations in this work) by our own Mathematica package *GradPack*, which can be freely downloaded from http://library.wolfram.com/infocenter/MathSource/5901/. The resulting justification force at keypoint i is:

$$\mathbf{F}_i = \alpha \sum_j \left(\frac{6\|\mathbf{v}_j \times \mathbf{a}_j\|^2}{\|\mathbf{v}_j\|^8} b_i'(s_j)\mathbf{v}_j - \frac{2\|\mathbf{v}_j \times \mathbf{a}_j\|}{\|\mathbf{v}_j\|^6}(b_i'(s_j)\mathbf{a}_j - b_i''(s_j)\mathbf{v}_j) \right) \Delta s_j$$

which seems to present a bit smoother behaviour, and is a bit easier to code (since edge keypoints do not require seperate coding), with a bit of performance cost - but still is very much interactive.

3. Conclusion, Implementation and Extensions

This work presented an expression for spline curves' bending energy, along with two novel approaches to its discretization and differentiation. Our implementations of both the schemes depicted utilize implicit integration for robustness, and still achieve highly interactive rates: a 50-knots thread based on Kochanek-Bartels spline, along with a high-res 1600-vertices needle model, achieved ~140 FPS on a 3.2 GHz Pentium-4 machine (including textures and light, not including collision detection/response or interaction with other organs). Several short movies demonstrating our results are available at http://www.simbionix.com/download/Movies/.

Our simulations already utilize several extensions of these results. A first example is the simulation of a needle-thread joint: we formulated a similar bending energy at a curve/rigid body joint, and derived justification forces in a manner similar to that presented above. A second example is the simulation (in a diffirent product) of a hernia mesh: while simulating a rectangular piece of cloth, we mimiced it's tendency to justify by virtually interlacing it with vertical/horizontal justifying splines of the form presented here. Many other subsequent developments will be presented in detail elsewhere.

References

[LL]   Landau L.D., Lifshitz E.M., Theory of Elasticity, Third edition, Butterworth-Heinemann, Oxford 1986.

[LMGC] Lenoir J., Meseure P., Grisoni L., Chaillou C., Surgical Thread simulation, ESAIM Proceedings, November 2002, Vol. 12, p. 102-107.

[Dc]   DoCarmo M., Differential Geometry of Curves and Surfaces. Prentice-Hall, New Jersey 1976.

[LRRV1] Lawton W., Raghavan R., Ranjan S. R., Viswanathan R. , Ribbons and groups: a thin rod theory for catheters and filaments, J. Phys. A: Math. Gen. 32 1709-1735, 1999.

Medicine Meets Virtual Reality 14
J.D. Westwood et al. (Eds.)
IOS Press, 2006

Web-Based Viewer for Systematic Combination of Anatomy and Nomenclature

Jonathan C. SILVERSTEIN (jcs@uchicago.edu), Muhamad AMINE, Fred DECH,
Peter JUREK, Isidore PIRES, Victor TSIRLINE, Colin WALSH
Department of Surgery, The University of Chicago

Abstract. Integrating anatomic nomenclature with geometric anatomic data via a web interface and providing illustration and visualization tools presents numerous challenges. We have developed a library of anatomic models and methods for navigating anatomic nomenclature. Based on the library and tools, we have developed a simple, yet powerful, open web-based tool that uses tree navigation and selection for assembling and downloading self-documenting anatomic scenes in Virtual Reality Modeling Language.

Keywords. Virtual Reality, Nomenclature, Geometric Modeling, Anatomy

1. Problem

With availability of anatomic data in electronic form such as the slice images of the Visible Human Project (VHP) [1] and symbolic naming hierarchies such as in the Systematized Nomenclature of Medicine-Clinical Terms (SNOMED) [2], there arises the need to combine these in a usable fashion for a variety of purposes. For example, combining geometric models with structure names is critical for virtual anatomy teaching [3,4]. Despite many related commercial and academic products, an easily navigable, scalable, free web-based library for assembling virtual reality scenes from standardized nomenclature hierarchies has not appeared. This may be because creating such a resource depends on stepwise integration of many skills:

1. image processing
2. anatomic knowledge
3. medical illustration
4. geometric modeling/processing
5. hierarchy database navigation and management
6. web-application development
7. assigning elemental structures to hierarchy leaves.

We previously reported a system, AutoSCAN, that we used for conducting the first four steps [5]. Here we report completing the last 3 steps and deployment as an entirely open system. A key to feasibility is that structures must be modeled at the elemental level and assigned to hierarchical tree leaves such that they assemble properly up the branches without duplication of geometries.

2. Methods

We chose to focus on accepted open standards with simple semantics in an effort to be both computationally simple and human understandable. Thus, we began with the following widely accepted standard public data: the VHP female anatomic slice images and the SNOMED database. We previously reported our methods for generating a production line of elemental geometric anatomic models [5]. A key feature of those methods is that models are constructed only for leaf nodes such that scenes can be assembled without duplication of geometries (what we call elemental models). We assigned these elemental models to SNOMED concepts, imputed concepts where required (fed back the new concepts to SNOMED) and computed the precise hierarchical tree that would include the elemental models as leaves and their predecessors using a custom-built algorithm. The SNOMED CT database was replicated in MySQL and PHP. As part of the scan browser, two functions were created in PHP: expand and collapse. The expand function would do a breadth first traversal to find a parent's immediate children, add these nodes to a display tree, and then return the tree as XML. Similarly, the collapse function would remove a parent's children from the tree.

In order to selectively display the leaves that had models, a flag (modelexists) was added to the database. In order for a leaf to appear in the scan browser, it must be flagged as well its parents, up to the root node. To accomplish this task, a recursive function was developed that performed a bottom up depth first traversal of the SNOMED tree from these leaves, through their parents, up to the root node. In this way, all paths from the root node leading to these leaves would be visible by the scan browser. Future models can be added and made visible in a similar fashion.

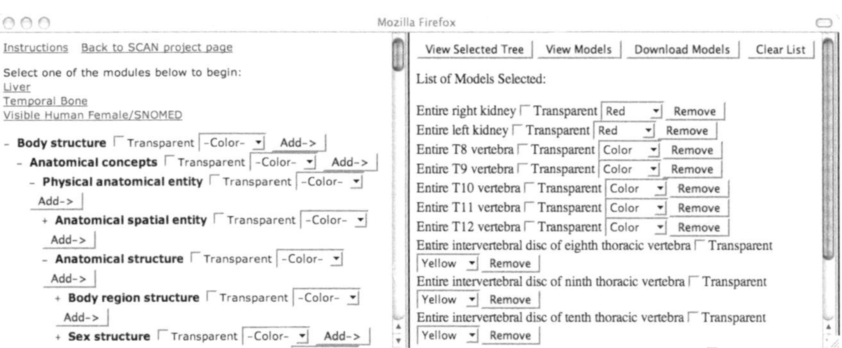

Figure 1. Web VRML authoring system in use – http://cci.uchicago.edu/projects/scan/.

The resulting sub-tree that precisely overlays SNOMED and includes exactly what was required then became the basis for our system. On Linux, Apache, MySQL, PHP, we built a web-application that assembles and displays the navigable tree and options to select concepts or their branches, transparency, and color for passing to the VRML generation sub-system which appears in a separate frame, as shown in the Figure 1 (left frame shows tree navigation and right frame shows individual model editing, tree and model generation). A key feature is that selections of branches cascade down the tree. For example, to collect models of the thoracic spine, instead of selecting each level, the available thoracic spine concept is selected once and cascades to generate the models available (in the examples, Figures 1,2,3, because only the abdomen is included, this adds models T8 through T12 vertebra). Once assembled, these scenes can be freely downloaded for use in a variety of applications (using open formats).

3. Results

The user can generate arbitrary scenes using simple tree navigation of available models, colors, and transparency. Branches can be selected and the color and transparency selections cascade. However, visualization characteristics of individual models can still be subsequently modified. The "View Selected Tree" button allows one to assemble and view the simplest tree that precisely represents the selected models and their predecessors (see Figure 2). The "View Models" button allows one to view the resulting combined scene (see Figure 3). Alternatively, one can download the VRML for use in other applications via the "Download Models" button. Finally, the names of each model are included as standard VRML attributes in each node in the .wrl as the server assembles it. Thus, the name of each model self-documents by clicking on the model in the resulting VRML scene.

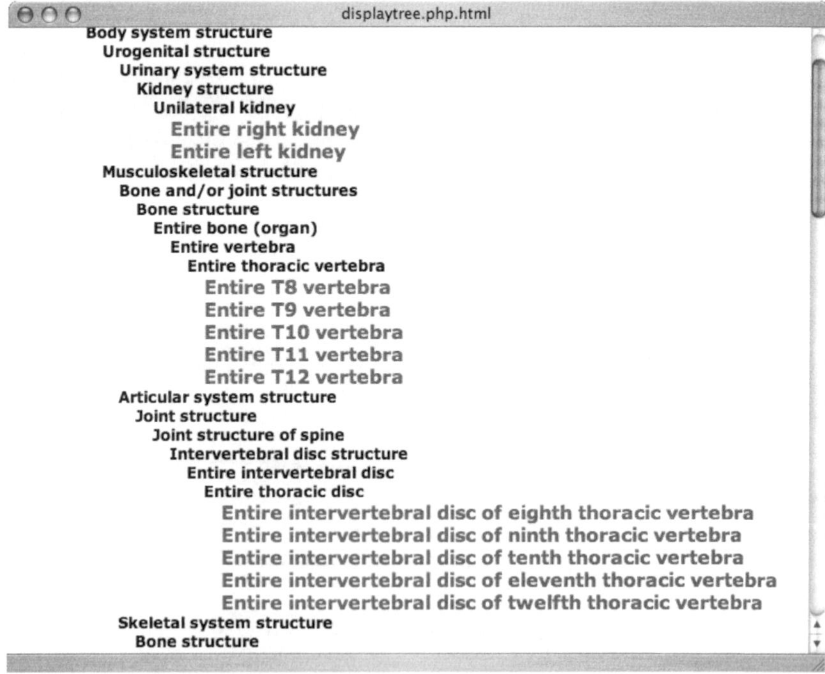

Figure 2. Example tree constructed via the authoring interface (Figure 1) by pressing button "View Selected Tree". This shows the selected hierarchical paths in human readable tabular format in a separate scrolling browser window.

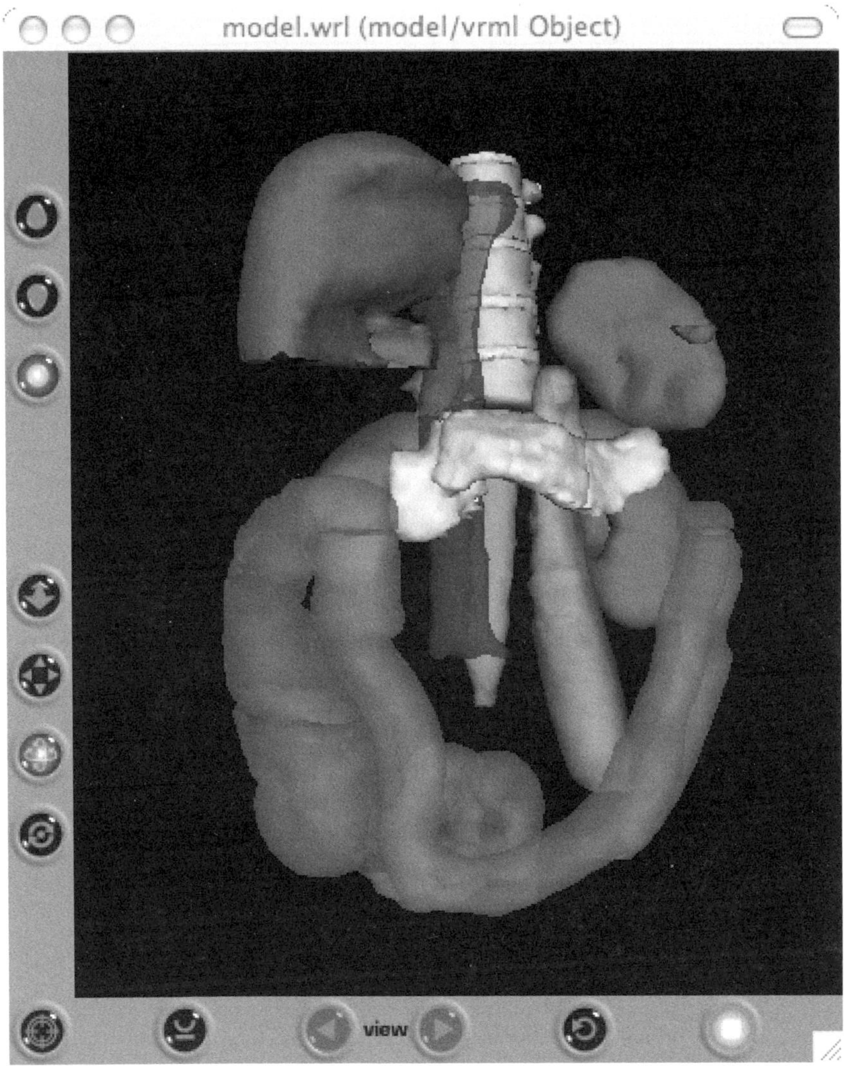

Figure 3. Example VRML scene constructed via the authoring interface (Figure 1) by pressing button "View Models". This shows the .wrl file rendered in a browser with the free cross-platform Cortona plugin (available at http://www.parallelgraphics.com/products/cortona).

To date, we have integrated over 300 elemental anatomic structures into our system and provided it free (and source available) online at http://cci.uchicago.edu/projects/scan/. The system has also been applied to other models using ad hoc hierarchies including previously constructed liver models [4] and temporal bone structures assembled from a histological dataset (also available on-line). Simply by navigating a hierarchy (a familiar process to computer users) and selecting structures, colors, and transparency, Internet users can assemble interactive virtual reality anatomic scenes that self-document structure names. The only system requirements at the desktop are the cross-platform Firefox browser and a VRML plugin if models are viewed online (rather than simply downloaded). Because models are elemental, hierarchy traversal algorithms are not computationally intensive, and VRML can be assembled via concatenation, system performance is high with interactive speed and instantaneous scene generation. If scenes are generated that contain numerous models, the bottleneck appears to be network speed because VRML is a text-based format and thus large files can represent complex geometries. Adding model size feedback to the interface may be desirable.

4. Conclusion/Discussion

The system described serves as a useable navigable library of anatomic structures for assembling virtual anatomic scenes. Such a library, provided in an open access and curated fashion can enable educators, researchers, and even clinicians to rapidly assemble interactive medical illustrations from arbitrary viewpoints for communicating complex anatomic relationships.

Future steps include geometric improvements of the elemental models, expansion of the model library, and expansion of the hierarchy via submissions to SNOMED. Also, we will explore the feasibility of combining this tool with our previously described AutoSCAN modeling system in a web-based portal thereby allowing upload and publishing of user-supplied slice data with modeling, concept assignment, hierarchical navigation, and visualization capabilities.

Acknowledgement

This work was supported by NIH/National Library of Medicine grant R01-LM06756.

References

[1] Ackerman. The Visible Human Project: a resource for education. Acad Med 1999;74(6), 667–670.
[2] http://www.snomed.org/ – College of American Pathologists.
[3] Hoffman H, Vu, D. Virtual Reality: Teaching tool of the 21st Century? Acad Med 1997;72(12):1076–81.
[4] Silverstein et al. Virtual Reality: Immersive Hepatic Surgery Educational Environment. Surgery. 2002;132(2):274–7.
[5] Silverstein et al. Automated Renderer for Visible Human and Volumetric Scan Segmentations. Stud Health Techno Inform 2005: 111:473–6.

Medicine Meets Virtual Reality 14
J.D. Westwood et al. (Eds.)
IOS Press, 2006

Haptic Feedback for the GPU-Based Surgical Simulator

Thomas Sangild SØRENSEN [a,1] and Jesper MOSEGAARD [b]
[a] Centre for Advanced Visualisation and Interaction, [b] Department of Computer Science, University of Aarhus, Denmark

Abstract. The GPU has proven to be a powerful processor to compute spring-mass based surgical simulations. It has not previously been shown however, how to effectively implement haptic interaction with a simulation running entirely on the GPU. This paper describes a method to calculate haptic feedback with limited performance cost. It allows easy balancing of the GPU workload between calculations of simulation, visualisation, and the haptic feedback.

Keywords. Haptic feedback, GPU, surgical simulation, congenital heart disease.

Introduction

Surgical simulators have traditionally been implemented on the CPU and many algorithms have been proposed in order to calculate realistically looking soft-tissue deformations in real-time. An overview of the field is provided in [1]. Haptic feedback is often used to increase the realism of user interactions. This provides an additional challenge as force feedback must be provided at least at 500 Hz to feel smooth. To achieve such an update rate from a simulation running at a much lower frequency, extrapolation schemes have been developed, e.g. [2,3]. Overall,

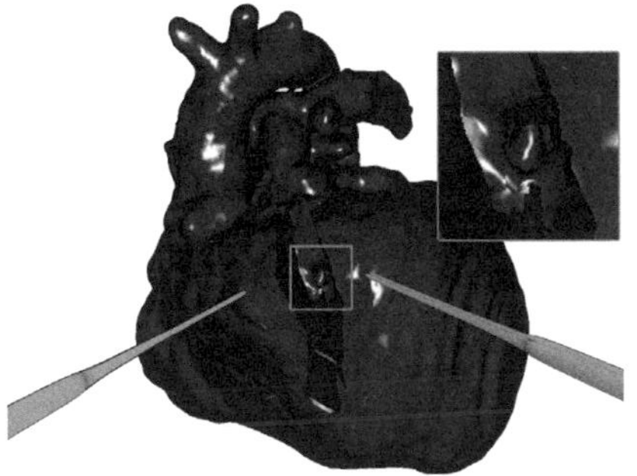

Figure 1. Surgery simulation on a congenitally malformed heart. The simulator runs entirely on the GPU. The surgical instruments provide haptic feedback.

speed has been a major concern as many time-consuming tasks all had to be handled on the CPU. Motivated by this issue, it was shown in [4] that a twenty to thirty fold acceleration of a spring-mass based surgical simulation could be achieved when moving computations from the CPU to the GPU (i.e. the graphics card). This allowed real-time

---

[1] Corresponding author: Thomas Sangild Sørensen, CAVI, University of Aarhus, Aabogade 34, 8200 Aarhus N, Denmark; E-mail: sangild@cavi.dk

surgical simulation on very complex organs, such as the heart, for the first time. Calculating tissue deformations on the GPU does however expose some previously unaddressed problems on how to resolve haptic interaction. Since communication with the haptic devices must be handled on the CPU, synchronization and data transfer between the GPU and the CPU is necessary. Unfortunately this is a relatively slow operation. Hence, we must carefully design the communication scheme to avoid new performance bottlenecks.

In this paper we describe and evaluate an efficient method of haptic interaction with the GPU based surgical simulator [4]. Haptic feedback is provided in response to collisions between instruments and tissue. The overall design criterion is to allow efficient, smooth, two-handed haptic interaction and easy balancing of the workload between simulation, visualisation, and delivery of force feedback.

A driving force behind the described simulator and proposed tools is an effort to develop a surgical simulator dedicated to procedures in congenital heart disease, hence the illustration at the front page (Figure 1).

1. Materials and Methods

1.1. Hardware and Software Platforms

The hardware platform used to evaluate the simulation was a personal computer running Windows XP on an AMD FX-55 CPU, and 2 GB of memory. The graphics bus was PCI Express x 16. The proposed algorithms were tested on three different graphics cards, a Geforce 6800 Ultra, a Quadro FX 4400, and a Geforce 7800 GTX, all from Nvidia. Two Phantom Omnis (Sensable Technologies) were used to achieve haptic interaction by low-level access through the accompanying OpenHaptics Toolkit. All programming was done in C++ using OpenGL and Cg with some manual modifications of the compiled vertex and fragment programs. The cardiac model used throughout this paper were obtained from three-dimensional MRI [5] using the segmentation algorithm described in [6]. The marching cubes algorithm was used for all surface reconstructions. Throughout this paper we will consider a spring mass simulation of 20.270 particles visualised by a surface of 137.490 faces.

1.2. Spring Mass Simulation on the GPU

This section provides a short description of our GPU based simulator, since some terminology from its implementation is necessary to explain the extension with haptic interaction. Further details of the GPU implementation can be found in [4]. First we discretise the volume of the concerned organ, e.g. the heart muscle mass, into a set of particles arranged in a regular three-dimensional grid (Figure 2). Each particle is connected in a fixed pattern to its 18 nearest neighbours. The grid is mapped to a 2D-texture such that each particle is represented by a single

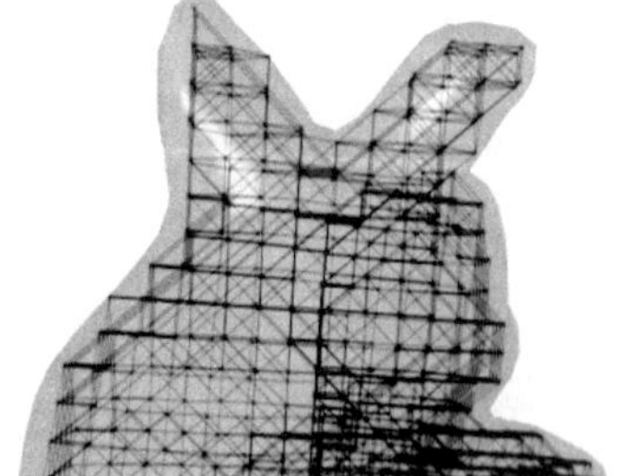

Figure 2. Particles in the spring mass system are connected in a regular, three-dimensional grid (black). Each particle is allowed to move, but constrained by the springs to neighbouring particles.

texel (Figure 3). We name this texture the *position-texture.* Conceptually, parallel computation of the spring mass system is invoked by rendering a single quad covering the entire position-texture. Processing of the white (void) particles is avoided by a depth test. A fragment program computes the forces that influence each particle due to its spring connections and the spring mass differential equation is solved by numerical integration to obtain updated particle positions. We refer to one pass of these calculations as a *simulation-step* in the remaining paper. A surface is

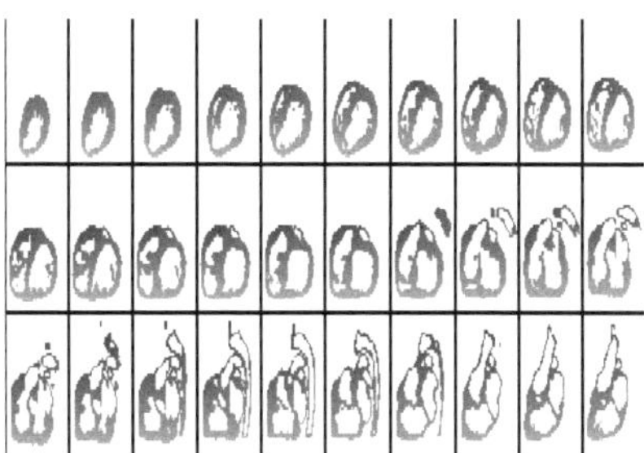

Figure 3. Excerpt of the position-texture. Each particle in the three-dimensional grid (Figure 2) is mapped to a unique texel (non-white). White texels correspond to void simulation particles outside the tissue.

constructed from the boundary nodes in the spring mass system and used for visualisation. During visualisation, a vertex program performs texture lookups in the position-texture to obtain the most recent particle positions. This allows us to use a static display list of the initial surface to also render it deformed. Rendering this surface is subsequently referred to as a *visualisation-step.* In [7] a mapping that decouples the visualised mesh from the physical simulation was presented. This allows for arbitrarily detailed surface meshes to be deformed by an underlying physical simulation (Figure 1 and Figure 2).

1.2.1. Probing and Grabbing

The probing gesture (i.e. touching the tissue with an instrument) was realised entirely on the GPU by extending the fragment program responsible for the simulation-step. Prior to writing the final position to the position-texture, each fragment determines if the corresponding particle has moved inside the bounding ellipsoid of an instrument. In that case the particle is projected to the boundary of the ellipsoid before updating the position-texture.

The grabbing gesture was designed to make use of both the CPU and the GPU. At the beginning of the gesture we read back the position-texture to the CPU *once* to identify particles inside the instrument's bounding volume and store pointers to these. For the duration of the grabbing gesture a dedicated fragment program writes the absolute positions of the grabbed particles into the position-texture based on the current position of the instrument.

1.2.2. Haptic Feedback

Communication with the haptic device is handled by the haptic thread on the CPU. We are consequently required to continuously read back data from the GPU to the CPU in order to provide haptic feedback. We could transfer the entire position texture and let the CPU compute the relevant forces from the current simulation state. It is much cheaper however to compute these forces on the GPU and read back only the result. In the following we describe how to achieve this for the grabbing and probing gestures:

During a grabbing gesture the CPU holds a list of the grabbed particles and corresponding coordinates in the position-texture as described in section 1.2.1. We create an off-screen *force-buffer* at the size of this list and for each particle a dedicated fragment program is run. This fragment program looks up the position of all neighbours to the current particle in the position-texture and calculates the force stored in each spring connection. The individual spring forces are summed to find the overall force vector affecting the particle. This vector is stored in the force-buffer at the position corresponding to the processed particle. Finally the force-buffer is read back to the CPU and passed to the haptic thread. If two hands are active both sets of corresponding forces are returned in a single readback. This is an optimisation as each readback implies a relatively costly synchronisation between the GPU and the CPU.

During a probing gesture the situation is more difficult since the set of particles contributing to the force feedback is no longer constant during the gesture, but changes in each frame depending on the position of the instrument. We can re-use the force-buffer approach however, if we extend it with a fast method to pick the particles that collide with the instrument. Note that instruments can only collide with surface particles. As a fast picking algorithm, we propose to render a *simulation-surface* into an offscreen *picking-buffer*. A simulation-surface is a mesh that connects the boundary particles in the spring mass simulation. It is not necessarily identical to the high-resolution mesh used in the visualisation-step due to the mapping presented in [7]. The

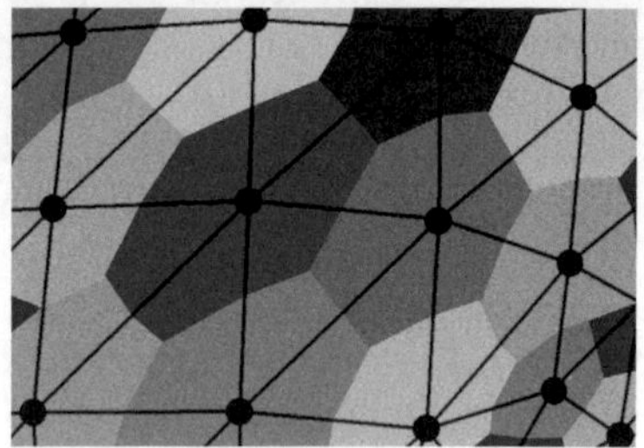

Figure 4. Contents of the picking-buffer. The simulation-surface is projected into the picking-buffer as represented by the black mesh. The surface is "shaded" with a colour representing the texture coordinate in the position-texture (Figure 3) of the corresponding particle in the spring-mass system (Figure 2).

simulation-surface is rendered as seen from the base of the associated instrument. It will be "shaded" with colours that provide texture coordinates to the nearest simulation node in the position-texture. The result is a Voronoi-like diagram as illustrated in Figure 4. During force-buffer calculations we use this diagram to identify which particles in the spring mass system that are potentially touching the instrument. Consider a point on the boundary of the instrument. Transforming this point with the modelview and projection matrices that were used when rendering the picking-buffer results in a *picking-coordinate*. Using this picking-coordinate for a texture lookup in the picking-buffer provides the texture coordinate to the corresponding particle in the position-texture due to the shading of the simulation-surface. To determine if the instrument is actually near the picked node, the third colour-component of the picking-buffer stores the distance from the picked point on the simulation-surface to the instrument.

The discussion above describes how to use the picking-buffer to find the position-texture coordinates of the particles colliding with the probing instrument. It boils down to a single texture lookup for each sampling point on the boundary of the instrument. In the previously described case of grabbing, these position-texture coordinates were given directly as input to the fragment program which updated the force-buffer. When probing, we extend this fragment program to use instead a texture lookup in the picking-buffer to obtain the desired position-texture coordinate. The calculation of probing forces is initialised from the CPU, which keeps a list of sampling points on each instrument's boundary. One by one, the sampling points are projected onto the picking buffer and the resulting picking-coordinates passed to the force computing fragment program. Each resulting force is stored in the corresponding entry in the force-buffer, which is finally read back to the haptic thread on the CPU.

Table 1. GPU rendering times on selected graphics cards.

[1] One simulation-step in a spring mass system of 20.270 nodes (18 neighbours each).
[2] One visualisation-step according to [7] (90.868 vertices / 137.490 faces).
[3] One rendering step of the off-screen picking-buffer (12.031 vertices / 46.928 faces).
[4] One calculation and subsequent readback of force feedback from 50 particles.

	Geforce 6800 Ultra	Quadro FX 4400	Geforce 7800 GTX
Simulation-step [1]	2.5 ms	3.5 ms	0.9 ms
Visualisation-step [2]	19.9 ms	20.8 ms	11.1 ms
Picking-buffer [3,4]	6.3 ms	5.3 ms	2.6 ms
Force-buffer [4]	0.3 ms	0.7 ms	0.2 ms

2. Results

Table 1 summarises the performance measurements obtained from the simulator for each of the tested graphics cards. As expected the newest GPU, the Geforce 7800 GTX, is the fastest for fragment and vertex processing (rows 1-3). It performs significantly better than the other two cards. To calculate and read back the accumulated spring forces the cards perform comparably due to the relatively high synchronisation cost of initiating a data transfer (row 4).

A simulator was developed to support haptic interaction with cardiac models. One example from the running simulator is shown in Figure 1, where an incision was made to reveal the exact location of a ventricular septal defect in a congenitally malformed heart. A movie of the running simulator is available at http://www.daimi.au.dk/~sangild/MMVR06.wmv.

3. Discussion

It is clear from Table 1 that surface visualisation is the single most expensive task in the simulator. In fact, several simulation-steps could be performed for each visualisation-step while maintaining an overall frame rate of at least 30 Hz. Here the term *overall frame rate* covers the accumulated cost of a number of simulation-steps, a visualisation-step, rendering of the picking-buffers, and finally calculation and readback of the force buffers. Each simulation-step should be followed by rendering and readback of the force-buffer to ensure the highest update frequency of the haptic devices. When probing, the additional cost of updating the picking-buffers must also be considered. As seen from the 3rd row in Table 1, updating the picking buffer after each simulation-step significantly reduces the number of simulation-steps possible per overall frame. We briefly mention two strategies for high-frequency haptic rendering that do not necessitate picking-buffer updates after each simulation-step. The first strategy is to read back the force feedback from the GPU at e.g. 30 Hz and use the algorithms presented in [2,3] to extrapolate this data to the desired update frequency on the CPU. Another strategy is to allow the use a slightly outdated picking-buffer but proceed with the update and readback of the force-buffer based on updated instrument positions. We have chosen the latter of these two strategies.

Using the Geforce 7800 GTX as an example, we describe a combination of steps that will lead to an overall frame rate of 30 Hz running the simulator with haptic interaction. An overall frame rate requirement of 30 Hz corresponds to 33 ms available per frame. 11.1 ms are used for surface visualisation. Two picking-buffers (one for each hand) will be updated once in each overall frame, leaving 17 ms for simulation and force readback. During this period we can perform approximately 15 simulation-steps with subsequent rendering and readback of the force-buffers. This corresponds to a simulation-step frequency of 450 Hz.

Comparing the overall system performance to a similar implementation on the CPU, the GPU implementation is much faster. With the work presented in this article we believe to be one step closer to a fully functional cardiac surgery simulator. As a next step we are planning to extend the simulator with support for suturing of patches to close e.g. septal defects.

Acknowledgments

We kindly acknowledge the funding we obtained from the Danish Research Agency (grant #2059-03-0004). Likewise we deeply appreciate the clinical feedback provided by pediatric heart surgeons Ole Kromann Hansen and Vibeke Hjortdal from the Department of Cardiothoracic Surgery at Aarhus University Hospital.

References

[1] A. Liu, F. Tendick, K. Cleary and C. R. Kaufmann. A survey of surgical simulation: applications, technology, and education. Presence: Teleoperators and Virtual Environments. 2003;12(6):599–614.

[2] F. Mazzella, K. Montgomery, J. C. Latombe. The Forcegrid: A Buffer Structure for Haptic Interaction with Virtual Elastic Objects. ICRA 2002:939-46.

[3] G. Picinbono, J-C. Lombardo, H. Delingette, N. Ayache. Improving realism of a surgery simulator: linear anisotropic elasticity, complex interactions and force extrapolation. Journal of Visualisation and Computer Animation, 13(3):147-67.

[4] J. Mosegaard, P. Herborg, T.S. Sørensen. A GPU accelerated spring-mass system for surgical simulation. Medicine Meets Virtual Reality 13, 2005:342-8.

[5] T.S. Sørensen, H. Körperich , G.F. Greil, J. Eichhorn, P. Barth, H. Meyer, E.M. Pedersen, P. Beerbaum. Operator-independent isotropic three-dimensional magnetic resonance imaging for morphology in congenital heart disease: a validation study. Circulation. 2004;110(2):163-9.

[6] T.S. Sørensen, E.M. Pedersen, O.K. Hansen, K. Sørensen. Visualization of morphological details in congenitally malformed hearts: Virtual, three-dimensional reconstruction from magnetic resonance imaging. Cardiology in the Young. 2003;13(5):451-60.

[7] J. Mosegaard, T.S. Sørensen. Real-time Deformation of Detailed Geometry Based on Mappings to a Less Detailed Physical Simulation on the GPU. IPT & EGVE Workshop 2005:105-10.

Medicine Meets Virtual Reality 14
J.D. Westwood et al. (Eds.)
IOS Press, 2006

Avionics-Compatible Video Facial Cognizer for Detection of Pilot Incapacitation

Morris STEFFIN, MD
VRNEUROTECH
Email
msteffin@morrissteffinmd.com

Abstract. High-acceleration loss of consciousness is a serious problem for military pilots. In this laboratory, a video cognizer has been developed that in real time detects facial changes closely coupled to the onset of loss of consciousness. Efficient algorithms are compatible with video digital signal processing hardware and are thus configurable on an autonomous single board that generates alarm triggers to activate autopilot, and is avionics-compatible.

Keywords. Video Cognizer; Behavioral monitoring; Loss of consciousness; High-acceleration; Pilot incapacitation; Triggered autopilot; Video digital signal processing.

Introduction

High-acceleration loss of consciousness (HGLOC) is a particularly severe hazard in the operation of modern military aircraft, particularly in the case of supermaneuverable planes [1]. Immediate and automatic detection prior to complete pilot blackout is essential to trigger autopilot functions. However, the false alarm rate must be kept low to avoid interference with mission-critical pilot responses. It has long been known that characteristic facial changes accurately reflect state of consciousness. Eye blink rate is been well established along with a blank stare [1], and characteristic mouth movements are reliable indicators of HGLOC. More recently, additional monitoring techniques have been tested [2, 3, 4, 5], but these are not deployable in an actual aircraft. The approach developed in this laboratory circumvents this limitation by means of a video facial cognizer operating in real time to detect the characteristic facial changes at the onset of HGLOC and to provide an electrical trigger allowing the appropriate corrective response, such as switching to autopilot. The system is flexible enough to allow pilot interaction for the prevention of inappropriate overrides. The algorithms will run on video digital signal processing (DSP) board technology which functions in a stand-alone, compact, and avionics-compatible configuration.

Methods

The cognizer utilizes techniques previously described [6] to convert multidimensional video data to scalar values that can be processed by standard scalar filters and transforms, thus allowing for much more efficient data processing and statistical analysis [7,8].   The approach to rapid detection of facial expression changes is shown in Figure 1A, **Results** (see real time animation at Steffin [9]).

This detection scheme is based upon resolution of the pattern of mouth movements and eye movements, with particular reference to discriminating physiologically significant cessation of movement. The cognizer operates on two images: eyes and mouth. By employing two stages of digital filtering of the scalar movement signals, the system provides adequate signal-to-noise ratio from the images to detect physiologically relevant cessation of movement, as shown in **Results**.

Results

Detection of signals related to behavioral patterns is facilitated by passing the scalar signals through a digital high-pass filter, as demonstrated in Figure 1B, thus stabilizing the baseline and improving signal-to-noise ratio.

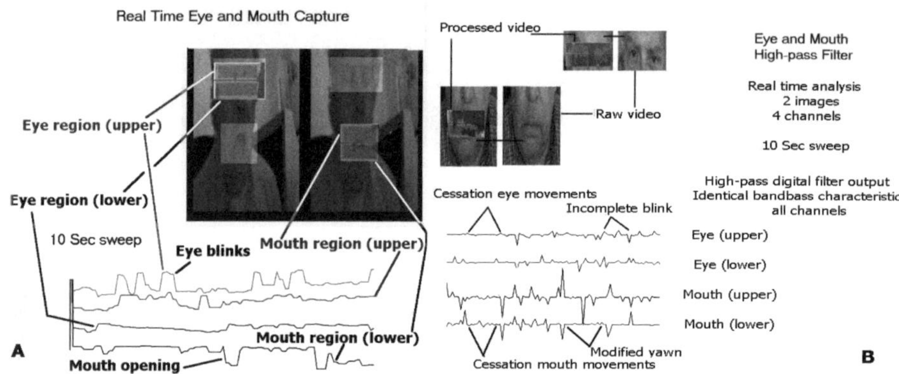

Figure 1. A. Simultaneous capture of eye and mouth configurations, two channels each, from video in a frontal dual image format; full sweep is 10 Sec (See also Steffin [9]). Processed video regions are within rectangular marked areas. **B.** Video capture technique as in **A** with high-pass filtering. Output demonstrates improved baseline drift and signal-to-noise ratio for movement discrimination . Note particularly the quiet baseline post-filtering during the period of movement cessation. Low amplitude movements are thus more reliably measured.

The output of the high-pass filter is further processed with the addition of exponential decay that is activated on cessation of movement and cancelled on return of movement, as shown in Figure 2. Eye and mouth cessation triggers for autopilot are generated when movement signals fall below critical amplitude (see Figure) and are reset for autopilot deactivation when amplitudes increase with resumption of movement. The most reliable trigger is generated from correlation of *combined* eye and mouth behavior, as shown.

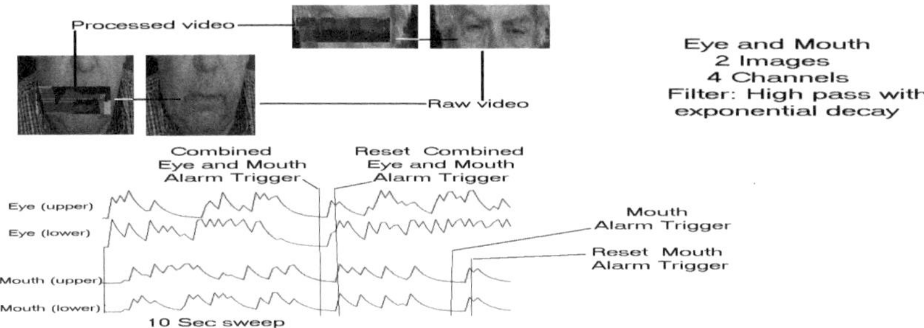

Figure 2. High pass filtering as in Figure 1B with exponential decay added. Separate triggers can be derived from eye and mouth behavior, although the most reliable trigger would depend on correlation between eye and mouth behavior, as shown for the combined eye and mouth trigger case

Discussion

This efficient video cognizer generates triggers for autopilot activation upon cessation of movement indicative of loss of consciousness. The algorithms are DSP compatible in an avionics environment. Deployment of this incapacitation monitor would thus increase the safety of high-performance aircraft operation.

References

[1]   Siuru, W. Supermaneuverability fighter technology of the future. *Aerospace Power Journal.* Spring, 1988. http://www.airpower.maxwell.af.mil/

[2]   Benni, P. NIRS monitoring of pilots subjected to +Gz acceleration and G-induced loss of consciousness. *Tufts EECS Colloquium 2002.* http://www.ece.tufts.edu/colloquia/archives/fall02/10_2.html.

[3]   Chen, H., Wu, Y., and Kuo, M. An electromyographic assessment of the anti-G straining maneuver. *Aviation Space and Environmental Medicine* **75:2** (2004), 162-167.

[4]   Krishnamurthy, A. Current concepts in acceleration physiology. *Indian Society of Aerospace Medicine.* www.isam-india.org

[5]   Modak, S., Tyagi, P. K., Singh, A. K., and Plate, J. Centrifuge training vis-à-vis G-LOC incidents - an update. *Ind. J Aerospace Med* 46:1 (2002), 42-50.

[6]   Steffin, M. Method and apparatus for detection for drowsiness and quantitative control of biological processes. *US Patent Application.* USPTO Application Number US-2004-0234103. Publication date: November 25, 2004.

[7]   Steffin, M. and Wahl K. Occam's approach to video critical behavior detection: a practical real time video in-vehicle alertness monitor. In: Westwood, J. M., Haluck R. S., et al. eds. *Medicine Meets Virtual Reality 12 Proceedings* (Newport, California, January 13-16, 2004). IOS Press, (Amsterdam, The Netherlands) 2004:370-375.

[8]   Steffin, M. VRNEUROTECH Technology: Video drowsy driver detection system. *VRN Science.* www.vrneurotech.com

[9]   Steffin M. Virtual reality biofeedback in chronic pain and psychiatry. In Lorenzo NY, Lutsep H. (eds.). www.emedicine.com: *Neurology* 2004.

Medicine Meets Virtual Reality 14
J.D. Westwood et al. (Eds.)
IOS Press, 2006

TRUS-Fluoroscopy Fusion for Intraoperative Prostate Brachytherapy Dosimetry

Yi SU[a], Brian J. DAVIS[b], Michael G. HERMAN[b], Richard A. ROBB[a,1]
[a]Biomedical Imaging Resource, Mayo Clinic College of Medicine, Rochester, Minnesota, 55905 USA
[b]Division of Radiation Oncology, Mayo Clinic College of Medicine, Rochester, Minnesota, 55905 USA

Abstract. A fluoroscopic to TRUS fusion based approach for intraoperative prostate brachytherapy dosimetry was developed. Seed images were identified from multiple fluoroscopic images and reconstructed to determine the three dimensional distribution of the implanted seeds. Seeds identified from the TRUS images were used as fiducials for the registration between fluoroscopic and TRUS images. Dose analysis was then performed based on the fused images. A phantom study was performed to test this approach and a 3 mm registration error was observed. Radiation isodose contours were generated and superimposed on the TRUS images.

Keywords. prostate brachytherapy, fluoroscopy, dosimetry

1. Introduction

Permanent prostate brachytherapy (PPB) is a common method for treating early stage prostate cancer. Despite the improvement in implantation techniques in recent years, exact replication of the treatment plan in the operating room (OR) remains difficult [1, 2]. Thus, intraoperative dosimetry (ID) is an important improvement for the current practice [3] in order to monitor the quality of the implantation. ID can be achieved by reconstruction of three dimensional (3D) seed coordinates from several angles of fluoroscopic images followed by registration of fluoroscopic and ultrasound images. Several prior studies on the reconstruction of 3D seed locations from multiple fluoroscopic images have been published[4-7]. Several groups have reported the registration of fluoroscopic images to ultrasound images either using specifically designed fiducials [8] or using needle tips as the basis for registration [9]. Based on the observation that a portion of the seeds can be visualized by trans-rectal ultrasound (TRUS) [10], the hypothesis that these seeds can be used as the fiducials for registration is tested. This paper reports a TRUS-fluoroscopy fusion based dose analysis approach for PPB using implanted seeds as fiducials.

---

[1] Corresponding Author: Richard A. Robb, Biomedical Imaging Resource, Mayo Clinic College of Medicine, Rochester, Minnesota, 55905, USA; E-mail: Robb.Richard@mayo.edu.

2. Methods and Materials

A thresholding based technique was implemented to segment the seed images from fluoroscopic images. The raw images were filtered by a predefined filter, which enhance the contrast between seeds and their background. Both the filtered and the original images were interactively thresholded and combined by a logical AND operation to form the segmented images. Manual editing was performed to remove false positives.

Self-connected components in the segmented fluoroscopic images are referred to as clusters. During the segmentation process, before the manual editing step, size analysis was conducted to remove any components outside a user defined size range. A cluster analysis [4] was performed to determine the number of seeds inside each cluster. Each cluster was then divided into individual seeds based on the primary axis of the components [4] to determine the location of each seed image.

A seed reconstruction method reported earlier [4] was used to determine the 3D location of implanted seeds based on the seed image locations. This method can accurately reconstruct 3D seed locations from incomplete sets of two dimensional distributions determined from three fluoroscopic images acquired at different angles.

The fusion of the 3D seed locations with the TRUS images was realized by a registration mechanism using seeds identified from the TRUS as fiducials. A downhill simplex algorithm was used to minimize the sum of the squared distance between nearest neighbors. Dose calculation was then performed based on the revised AAPM protocol [11] using the reconstructed seed locations. Isodose contours were then generated based on the dose calculation.

A graphical user interface (GUI) was implemented which integrated the above mentioned steps. The image data was processed and dose analysis was performed based on the work flow illustrated in Fig. 1. Controls were provided in the GUI for interactive segmentation of the fluoroscopic images and manual editing of the segmented results.

A phantom study was performed to validate the fluoroscopic-TRUS fusion based dose analysis system. TRUS images of a prostate phantom with 64 implanted seeds (Fig. 2) were acquired at 5 mm intervals. Fluoroscopic images of the phantom were taken using a radiation simulator at 30 degree intervals. The fluoroscopic images were segmented and then reconstructed to determine the 3D seed locations. Seeds were manually identified from the TRUS images to be used as fiducials for TRUS-fluoroscopy fusion. Based on the registered seed coordinates in the TRUS images, radiation dose was calculated and isodose contours were displayed by superimposing them on the TRUS images.

3. Results

The seed images identified from the projections at 0, 30 and 60 degrees were 57, 64 and 64 respectively. The reconstruction algorithm was able to determine implanted seed locations with only three false positive seeds (Fig. 3). The mean distance between TRUS seeds and the reconstructed seeds was 3mm at registration. The isodose contours superimposed on the TRUS images are shown in Fig. 4.

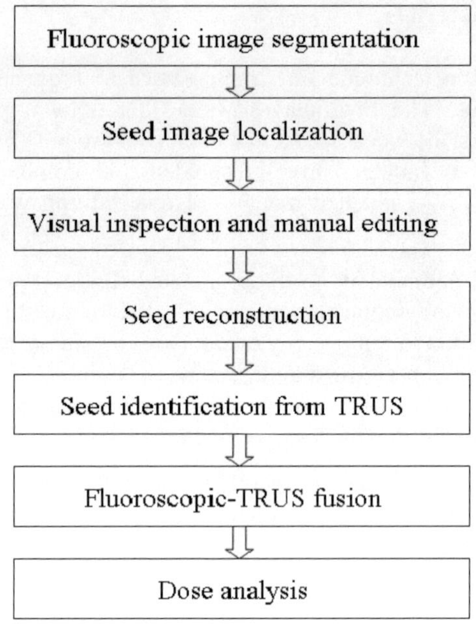

Figure 1. Work flow of the fluoroscopy-TRUS fusion based dose analysis for PPB

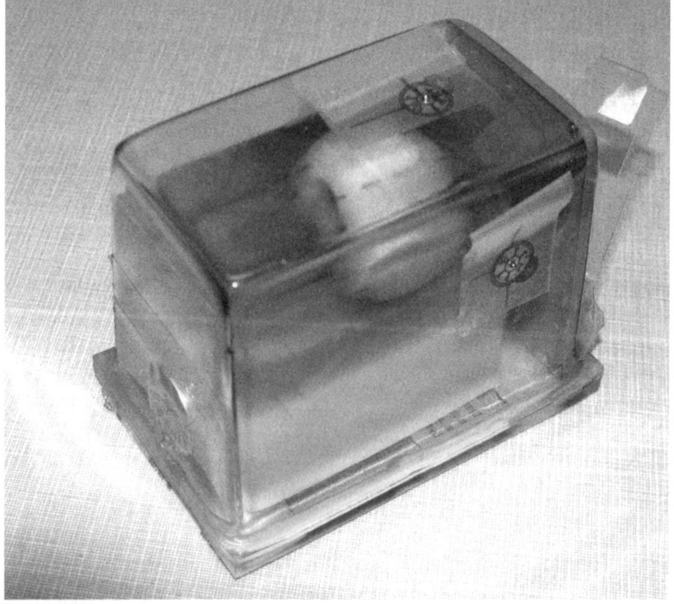

Figure 2. A picture of the prostate phantom used in this study.

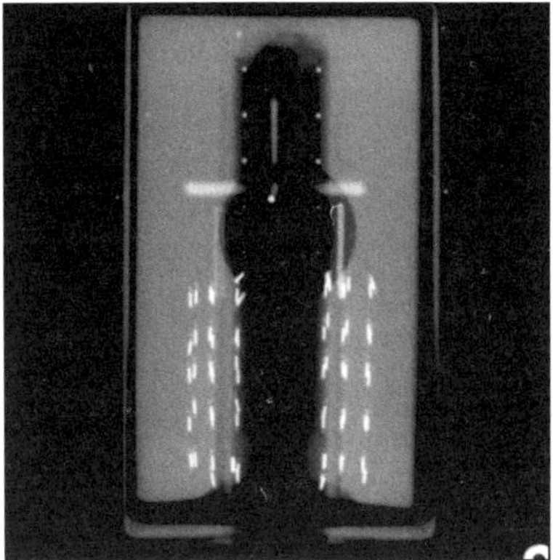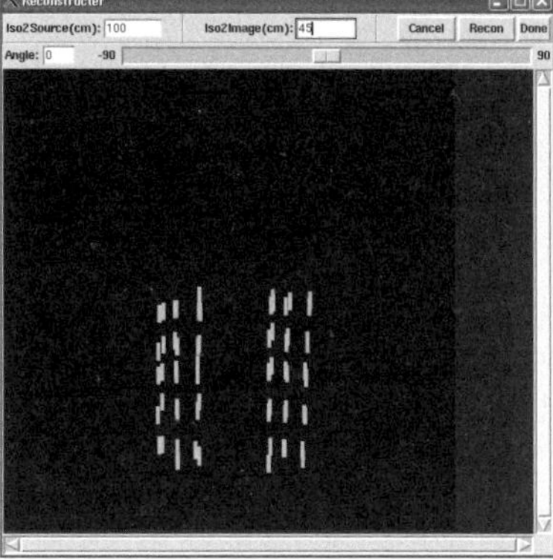

Figure 3. An example of a fluoroscopic image of the phantom (Left) and the reconstructed seed locations (Right).

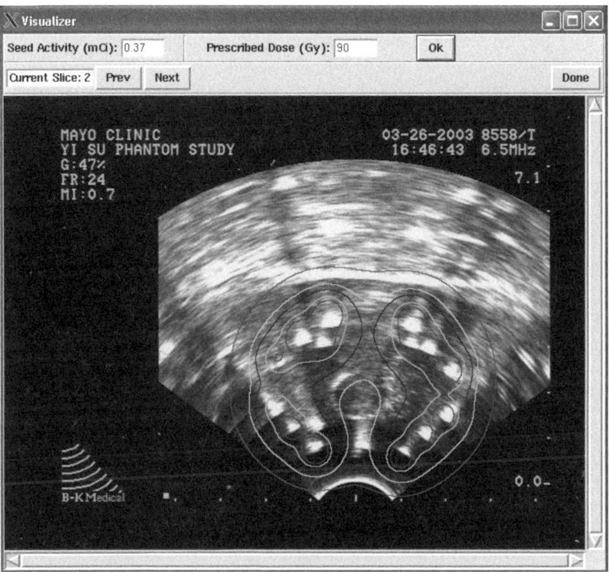

Figure 4. Isodose contours superimposed on the TRUS image at registration.

4. Discussion

Considerable human interaction is needed for the seed image identification process to remove false positives in the segmentation results. False positive seed images identified from the fluoroscopic images will cause false positives in the reconstructed 3D seeds. Although the seed reconstruction algorithm can compensate for the undetected seeds due to overlapped seed images, it does not have the capability of eliminating false positives. Another source of false positives is caused by the action of the seed reconstruction algorithm whereby a single seed image may be reused more than once. A more advanced technique is needed to reduce the likelihood of generating false positives and detect all the implanted seeds. However, it should be noted that unless a significant number of seeds are undetected or a large number of false positives are generated, the resulting dosimetry parameters will not be significantly affected [12].

The relatively high level of registration error can be improved by using more sophisticated registration algorithms that have outlier rejection capabilities, since artifacts in the TRUS images can be mistaken as seeds. Due to the fact that the correspondence of seeds between TRUS images and fluoroscopic images can not be easily established, the number of seeds identified from TRUS should be large enough to represent the seed distribution for meaningful registration. Fortunately, it has been shown that 40% or more seeds are usually identified from TRUS [13].

Ongoing efforts to integrate prostate contouring tools into the system are under way so that clinically meaningful dosimetry parameters such as D90, and V100 can be calculated.

5. Conclusion

A TRUS-fluoroscopic fusion based intraoperative dosimetry method for prostate brachytherapy has been developed. Preliminary phantom studies show promising results. With further validation, this approach will significantly improve the current PPB procedure in the OR.

References

[1]   Beyer, D. C., Shapiro, R. H. and Puente, F., *Real-time optimized intraoperative dosimetry for prostate brachytherapy: a pilot study.* Int. J. Radiat. Oncol. Biol. Phys., 2000. **48**(5): p. 1583-1589.

[2]   Prestidge, B. R., Prete, J. J., Buchholz, T. A., Friedland, J. L., Stock, R. G., Grimm, P. D., and Bice, W. S., *A survey of current clinical practice of permanent prostate brachytherapy in the United States.* Int. J. Radiat. Oncol. Biol. Phys., 1998. **40**(2): p. 461-465.

[3]   Nag, S., Ciezki, J. P., Cormack, R., Doggett, S., DeWyngaert, K., Edmundson, G. K., Stock, R. G., Stone, N. N., Yu, Y., Zelefsky, M. J., and Clinical Research Committe, A. B. S., *Intraoperative planning and evaluation of permanent prostate brachytherapy: report of the American Brachytherapy Society.* Int. J. Radiat. Oncol. Biol. Phys., 2001. **51**(5): p. 1422-1430.

[4]   Su, Y., Davis, B. J., Herman, M. G., and Robb, R. A., *Prostate brachytherapy seed localization by analysis of multiple projections: identifying and addressing the seed overlap problem.* Med. Phys., 2004. **31**(5): p. 1277-1287.

[5]   Todor, D. A., Cohen, G. N., Amols, H. I., and Zaider, M., *Operator-free, film-based 3D seed reconstruction in brachytherapy.* Phys. Med. Biol., 2002. **47**(12): p. 2031-2048.

[6]   Tubic, D., Zaccarin, A., Beaulieu, L., and Pouliot, J., *Automated seed detection and three-dimensional reconstruction. II. Reconstruction of permanent prostate implants using simulated annealing.* Med. Phys., 2001. **28**(11): p. 2272-2279.

[7]   Altschuler, M. D. and Kassaee, A., *Automated matching of corresponding seed images of three simulator radiographs to allow 3D triangulation of implanted seeds.* Phys. Med. Biol., 1997. **42**(2): p. 293-302.

[8]   Todor, D. A., Zaider, M., Cohen, G. N., Worman, M. F., and Zelefsky, M. J., *Intraoperative dynamic dosimetry for prostate implants.* Phys. Med. Biol., 2003. **48**(9): p. 1153-1171.

[9]   Gong, L., Cho, P. S., Han, B. H., Wallner, K. E., Sutlief, S. G., Pathak, S. D., Haynor, D. R., and Kim, Y., *Ultrasonography and fluoroscopic fusion for prostate brachytherapy dosimetry.* Int. J. Radiat. Oncol. Biol. Phys., 2002. **54**(5): p. 1322-1330.

[10]   Han, B. H., Wallner, K., Merrick, G., Butler, W., Sutlief, S., and Sylvester, J., *Prostate brachytherapy seed identification on post-implant TRUS images.* Med. Phys., 2003. **30**(5): p. 898-900.

[11]   Rivard, M. J., Coursey, B. M., DeWerd, L. A., Hanson, W. F., Huq, M. S., Ibbott, G. S., Mitch, M. G., Nath, R., and Williamson, J. F., *Update of AAPM Task Group No. 43 Report: A revised AAPM protocol for brachytherapy dose calculations.* Med. Phys., 2004. **31**(3): p. 633-674.

[12]   Su, Y., Davis, B. J., Herman, M. G., Manduca, A., and Robb, R. A., *Examination of dosimetry accuracy as a function of seed detection rate in permanent prostate brachytherapy.* Med. Phys., 2005. **32**(9): p. 3049-3056.

[13]   Davis, B. J., LaJoie, W. N., McGee, K. P., Geyer, S. M., King, B. F., Wilson, T. M., Mynderse, L. A., Herman, M. G., and Robb, R. A. *Seed identification rates as a function of imaging modality in permanent prostate brachytherapy using CT-MR-TRUS image fusion.* in *American Brachytherapy Society 2002.* 2002.

Medicine Meets Virtual Reality 14
J.D. Westwood et al. (Eds.)
IOS Press, 2006

Augmented Reality with Fibre Optics

Gunther SUDRA+, Georg EGGERS*, Sebastian SCHALCK+, Bjoern GIESLER+,
Ruediger MARMULLA*, Ruediger DILLMANN+

[+] *Institute of Computer Science and Engineering (CSE)*
Universität Karlsruhe (TH), 76128 Karlsruhe, Germany
Email: Sudra@ira.uka.de

[*] *Department of Cranio-Maxillofacial Surgery*
University of Heidelberg, 69120 Heidelberg, Germany
Email: Ruediger.Marmulla@med.uni-heidelberg.de

Abstract. In this paper we present the concept and the first results of the Fibre
Optic Pointer – a miniaturized Augmented Reality system for craniofacial surgery.
The objective is the integration into surgical instruments.

Keywords. Augmented Reality, Craniofacial Surgery, Fibre Optic

1. Introduction

Craniofacial surgery is a highly complex medical discipline with various risks for
surgeon and patient. The objective of our system is to support the surgeon's spatial
cognition by using Augmented Reality (AR) techniques to directly visualize virtual
objects in the surgical site. Thus the surgeon does not need to turn his head from the
patient to the computer monitor and vice versa [1]. However, the inflexible handling of
existing AR systems [2,3,4,5] (e.g. occlusion of video-beamers, calibration of see-
through devices) reduce the benefit for the surgeon. Hence we present the concept of a
small AR technique which acts very close to the patient and therefore does not impede
persons and devices in the operation room. The objective is the integration into surgical
instruments.

2. Methods

The experimental hardware setup has been built up at the Institute of Computer Science
and Engineering, Universität Karlsruhe (TH). The main components of the system are a
light source, a miniature TFT display and a fibre optic bundle (Figure 1).
Miniaturization is realized using the fibres to separate image generation from image
output coupler. The current demonstration device projects small structures (e.g. arrows
for navigation) on a surface.

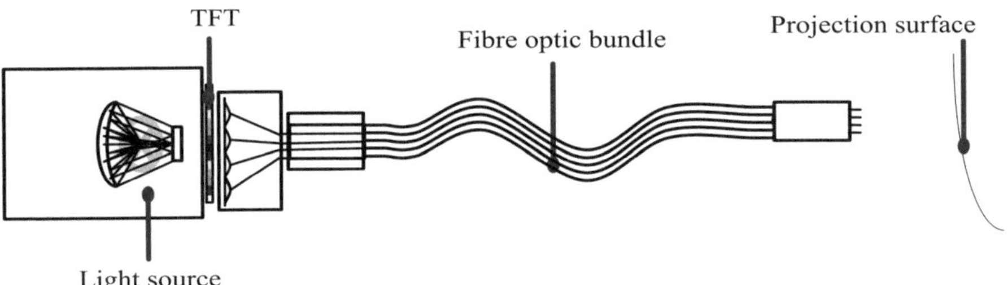

Figure 1. Concept of the system

2.1 Calibration

For correct projection of symbols the system has to be calibrated once using a CCD camera behind a semi-transparent projection screen. The result of the calibration defines a correspondence between a pixel of the miniature TFT display and a "pixel" of the projection. One advantage of this approach is the opportunity to use randomly arranged fibres on both sides of the bundle.

Our attempt splits the TFT display area into small regions and uses a quadtree data structure for representation. In the first stage a single region is illuminated and the resulting luminous fibres in the fibre optic bundle are detected. If more than a single luminous fibre is found, the region will be splitted into four child regions and the algorithm repeats until an area can be assigned to a single fibre. In some cases the detection of these regions fails, e.g. due to effects from other pixels. To correct this, the second stage of the algorithm uses combinations of adjacent regions and attempts to assign these combinations to a fibre. In the third stage all regions belonging to a single fibre are simultaneously illuminated. With this, effects on adjacent regions which are assigned to other fibres, are summed up. They are prevented by readjusting the boundary between this regions.

2.2 Tracking and Registration

Tracking is performed using passive sphere markers and the wide spread optical tracking system NDI Polaris. For registration we use an active pointer and landmarks on the CAD model of the fibre optic pointer.

3. Results

The first evaluation of the demonstration device in laboratory environment included tests to project navigation information (e.g. arrows to visualize the direction to a target structure, Fig.2). The intensity of the projection is sufficient for an augmentation under normal conditions and provides the user with helpful information in a flexible way.

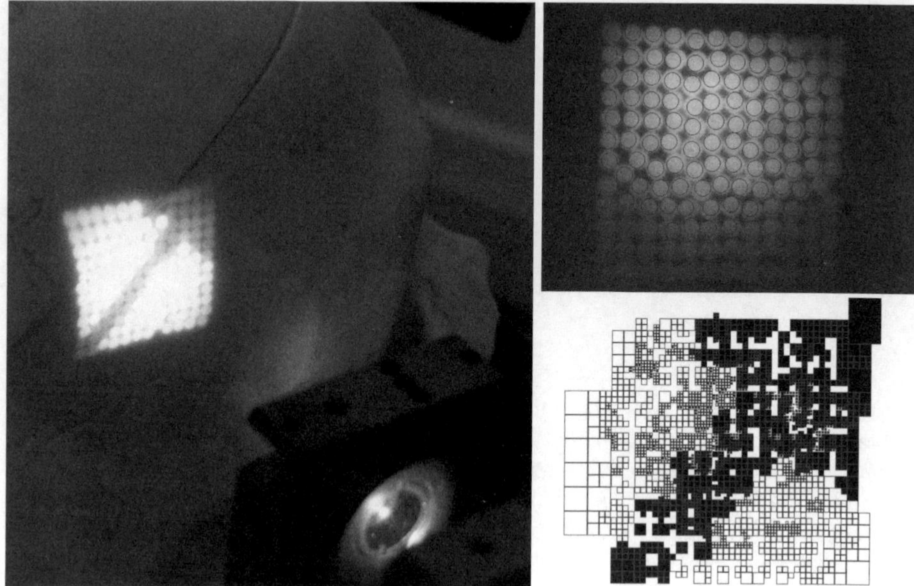

Figure 2. left: Projection of navigation information on a plastic skull, top right: CCD image for calibration, bottom right: Calibration mask of TFT display

4. Conclusion

We presented a novel concept for a small and flexible AR tool for the surgery room. We also report on the results of testing the calibrated and tracked demonstration device in laboratory environment. This can be seen as proof of concept.

However, objective of our work is the integration of the projection device into surgical instruments. Therefore future work will focus on a more sophisticated hardware which allows a further miniaturization. Compared to established AR projection systems the proposed method avoids occlusions and allows projections into areas which are only accessible by a narrow path. The clinical evaluation will be accomplished at the Department of Cranio-Maxillofacial Surgery, Heidelberg.

5. References

[1] G. Goebbels, K. Troche, M. Braun et al: Development of an Augmented Reality System for intra-operative navigation in maxillo-facial surgery. Proceedings AR/VR-Statustagung, Leipzig 2004
[2] N. Glossop, C. Wedlake, J. Moore et al: Laser Projection Augmented Reality System for Computer Assisted Surgery. Proceedings of MICCAI03, Montréal 2003
[3] B. Mansoux, L. Nigay, J. Troccaz et al : The Mini-Screen : An Innovative Device for Computer Assisted Surgery Systems. Studies in Health Technology and Informatics Medicine Meets Virtual Reality, Long Beach 2005
[4] M. Rosenthal, A. State, J. Lee et al.: Augmented reality guidance for needle biopsies: an initial randomized, controlled trial in phantoms, J Med Imag Anal 6(3): 313-320, 2002
[5] F. Sauer, A. Khamene, B. Bascle et al.: An Augmented Reality System for Ultrasound Guided Needle Biopsies, Studies in Health Technology and Informatics, Medicine Meets Virtual Reality, Newport Beach 2002

Medicine Meets Virtual Reality 14
J.D. Westwood et al. (Eds.)
IOS Press, 2006

Bubble Packing Application in Computerized Planning of Cryosurgery

Daigo Tanaka[b], Kenji Shimada[a, b], and Yoed Rabin[a]
[a] *Department of Mechanical Engineering*
[b] *Department of Biomedical Engineering, Carnegie Mellon University,*
5000 Forbes Ave, Pittsburgh, PA, 15217, USA

Abstract. Among many factors, the effectiveness of the cryoprocedure is determined by the quality of the cryoprobes layout. A computerized planning tool for optimizing this layout has the potential of improving the outcome of cryosurgery, reducing post-operative complications, and reducing the cost of the clinical operation. As part of an ongoing effort to develop planning tools for cryosurgery, the current study takes a novel approach, based on bubble-packing method. This study shows that the application of bubble-packing shortens runtime by an order of magnitude. In this study, the bubble-packing method is integrated with bioheat transfer simulations to demonstrate the quality of planning.

1. Introduction

Minimally-invasive cryosurgery is typically performed by means of cryoprobes in the shape of long hypodermic needles. Prostate cryosurgery was the first minimally-invasive cryosurgical procedure to pass from the experimental stage and become a routine surgical treatment. The minimally-invasive approach created a new level of difficulty in cryosurgery planning, in which a pre-defined 3D region of tissue must be injured while leaving the surrounding tissues unaffected.

The difficulties in planning a minimally-invasive cryoprocedure have been widely acknowledged by other researchers, and efforts to develop computerized planning have been reported in the literature [1, 2]. Recently, a prototype of a computerized cryoprobe placement tool was presented by Lung et al. [3]. This tool operates iteratively and relies on a series of bioheat transfer simulations of the cryosurgical procedure. At the end of each simulation, defective regions are identified, which consist of cryoinjured tissue external to the target region and uninjured tissue internal to the same region. Using a force-field analogy, these defective regions repel or attract the cryoprobes, iteratively moving them to better locations prior to the next bioheat transfer simulation. This force-field analogy technique has been proven numerically efficient for 2D problems [3].

The ultimate goal of the current study is to develop a computerized planning tool for cryosurgery that takes as input a 3D target region, reconstructed from ultrasound or MRI images, and suggests the optimal cryoprobe placement within a few minutes, during a surgery. Toward this goal, this report presents a new technique for computerized planning of cryosurgery using the bubble-packing method [5]. The new technique is faster by an order of magnitude than the aforementioned previous techniques. The quality of planning is at a similar level or only slightly inferior to that of the previous techniques.

2. Computational Method for Cryoprobe Layout

When thermal conductivity, blood perfusion rate, and metabolic heat generation rate are virtually uniform throughout the simulated region, the shape of target tissues becomes the most dominant factor in planning the layout of cryoprobes. It is thus reasonable to assume that an evenly spaced layout of cryoprobes would be close to the optimal one. The current method adopts a technique, called the bubble packing method [5], to evenly distribute the cryoprobes.

Bubble packing first generates spherical elements, called bubbles, inside the domain. It then defines proximity-based inter-bubble forces that make two adjacent bubbles attract each other when they are located too far and repel each other when they are located too close. Such force is defined by a piecewise cubic polynomial function:

$$f(l) = \begin{cases} al^3 + bl^2 + cl + d & 0 \le l \le 1.5l_0 \\ 0 & 1.5l_0 < l \end{cases} \tag{1}$$

$$f(l_0) = f(1.5l_0) = 0, \quad f'(0) = 0, \quad f'(l_0) = -k_0, \tag{2}$$

where l is the distance between two bubbles, l_0 is the stable distance, and k_0 is the corresponding linear spring constant at l_0.

Given the inter-bubble forces, the physically-based relaxation finds a bubble configuration, that yields a static force balance. Assuming a point of mass at the center of each bubble, and the effect of viscous damping, the proposed relaxation method finds a force-balanced configuration of bubbles by solving the equation of motion:

$$m_i \frac{d^2 x_i(t)}{dt^2} + c_i \frac{dx_i(t)}{dt} = f_i(t), \qquad i = 1...n \tag{3}$$

where m_i, x_i and c_i denote the mass, position, and damping coefficient of the i–th bubble, respectively. Note that $f_i(t)$ is the sum of inter-bubble forces exerted on bubble i by all its adjacent bubbles. This second-order ordinary differential equation is numerically integrated by the fourth-order Runge-Kutta method.

At the end of planning, bioheat transfer simulations of the cryoprocedure are executed to evaluate the quality of the cryoprobe layout. For simulation purposes, heat transfer is modeled with the classical bioheat transfer equation [6]:

$$C\frac{\partial T}{\partial t} = \nabla(k\nabla T) + \dot{w}_b C_b (T_b - T), \tag{4}$$

where C is the volumetric specific heat of the tissue, T is the temperature, t is the time, k is the thermal conductivity of the tissue, $\dot{w}_b$ is the blood perfusion rate (measured in volumetric blood flow rate per unit volume of tissue), C_b is the volumetric specific heat of the blood, and T_b is the blood temperature entering the thermally-treated area. The classical bioheat equation is solved using a finite difference method [4].

3. Results

The positions of the cryoprobes were determined for the 2D and 3D prostate models segmented from ultrasound images. The -22.5°C isotherm was used to represent the freezing threshold temperature to calculate the defective region. The runtime and the defective region for 2D planning were compared with force-field method [3]. For 3D planning, the runtime and the defective region are measured (Table 1). Figure 1 shows the graphical representation of the cryosurgery with the computed cryoprobe layout. The quality of planning is at a similar level or only slightly inferior to that of the force-field method with 14 and 12 cryoprobe cases in 2D planning. 3D planning is also accomplished around 30 seconds.

Table 1 Evaluation of planning. RT: runtime (min), DR: defective region (defect volume divided by prostate volume, %), BP: bubble-packing method, FF: force-field method

No of CP	RT 2D BP	RT 2D FF	DR 2D BP	DR 2D FF	RT 3D BP	DR 3D BP
10	0.10	306	18.9	8.2	0.48	26.0
12	0.13	349	10.6	7.2	0.55	25.7
14	0.15	144	6.8	5.4	0.62	26.6

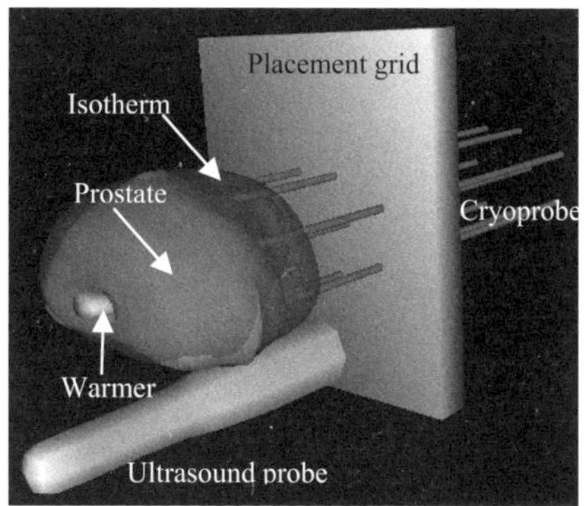

Figure 1 Graphical representation of cryosurgery

4. Conclusions

Compared with a previous planning technique based on the force-field analogy, the bubble packing method shortens the planning runtime by an order of magnitude, while compromising the quality of the layout by only a small percentage.

Acknowledgements

This project is supported by the National Institute of Biomedical Imaging and Bioengineering (NIBIB) – NIH, grant # R01-EB003563-01. We would like to thank Dr. Aaron Fenster from the Robarts Imaging Institute, London, Canada, for providing ultrasound images, and Dr. Ralph Miller at Allegheny General Hospital, Pittsburgh, PA for clinical advice.

References

[1]   Keanini, R.G., and Rubinsky, B., 1992, "Optimization of Multiprobe Cryosurgery," ASME Trans. J. of Heat Transfer, 114, 796-802.
[2]   Baissalov, R., Sandison, G.A., Reynolds, D., Muldrew, K., 2001, "Simultaneous Optimization of Cryoprobe Placement and Thermal Protocol for Cryosurgery," Phys. in Medic. Biol., 46, 1799-1814.
[3]   Lung, D.C., Stahovich, T.F., and Rabin, Y., 2004, "Computerized Planning for Multiprobe Cryosurgery using a Force-field Analogy," Comp. Methods in Biomech. and Biomed. Eng., 7 (2), 101-110.
[4]   Rabin, Y., and Shitzer, A., 1998, "Numerical Solution of the Multidimensional Freezing Problem During Cryosurgery," ASME Trans. J. of Heat Transfer, 120, 32-37.
[5]   Shimada, K., 1993, "Physically-Based Mesh Generation: Automated Triangulation of Surfaces and Volumes via Bubble Packing," Ph.D. thesis, Massachusetts Institute of Technology.
[6]   Pennes, H.H., 1948, "Analysis of tissue and arterial blood temperatures in the resting human forearm," J. App. Phys., 1, 93–122.

Medicine Meets Virtual Reality 14
J.D. Westwood et al. (Eds.)
IOS Press, 2006

Tracking Endoscopic Instruments Without Localizer: Image Analysis-Based Approach[1]

Oliver Tonet [a,2], T.U. Ramesh [b] Giuseppe Megali [a] and Paolo Dario [a]

[a] *CRIM Lab - Scuola Superiore Sant'Anna*
[b] *Indian Institute of Technology, Kharagpur, India*

Abstract. In this paper we present an approach to localize endoscopic instruments with respect to the camera position, purely based on video image processing. No localizers are required. The only requirement is a coloured strip at the distal part of the instrument shaft, to facilitate image segmentation. The method exploits perspective image analysis applied to the cylindrical shape of the instrument shaft, allowing to measure five degrees of freedom of the instrument position and orientation. We describe the method theoretically and experimentally derive calibration curves for tuning the parameters of the algorithm. Results show that the method can be used for applications where accuracy is not critical, e.g. workspace analysis, gesture analysis, augmented-reality guidance, telementoring, etc. If this method is used in combination with a robotic camera holder, full localization with respect to the operating room can be achieved.

Keywords. Localization, Tracking, Shape analysis, Pinhole camera, Laparoscopy

1. Introduction

Localization of objects in space is one of the key prerequisites for providing computer assistance in the operating room. By tracking position and orientation of the surgical instruments and the patient in the surgical workspace, it is possible to measure distances, compute trajectories, analyze gestures, etc. The positioning of localizers in the notably cluttered operating room (OR) is a critical issue. Also, during laparoscopy, the surgeon uses many different instruments; providing all instruments with sensors for localization is troublesome and hampers their movements.

In this paper we describe a novel method for localization of laparoscopic instruments with respect to the camera position, purely based on laparoscope image processing. No localizers are required. The method exploits perspective image analysis applied to the cylindrical shape of the instrument shaft, allowing to measure five degrees of freedom (DOFs) of the instrument position and orientation. The only requirement to be able to track conventional surgical instruments is a colored strip at the distal part of the instrument shaft, to facilitate image segmentation.

---

[1]This work has been supported in part by the FIRB-2001 Project *ApprEndo* (no. RBNE013TYM) and by *EndoCAS*, the Centre of Excellence for Computer-Assisted Surgery (COFINLAB-2001), both funded by MIUR, the Italian Ministry of Education, University and Research.

[2]Correspondence to: Oliver Tonet, CRIM Lab, Scuola Superiore Sant'Anna, v.le Rinaldo Piaggio 34, 56025 Pontedera (PI), Italy. Tel.: +39 050 883405; Fax: +39 050 883402; E-mail: oly@sssup.it.

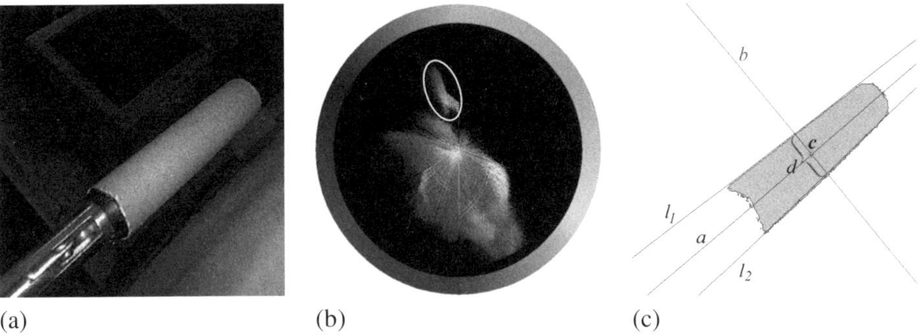

(a)   (b)   (c)

Figure 1. The colour-coded instrument (a); the averaged colour distribution in the H-S plane of 3000 laparoscopic images (b); the segmented image with superimposed geometric features needed for localization (c).

2. Methods

The method operates in two steps: first, image analysis is performed to estract relevant geometrical features from the color-coded region on the endoscope image; subsequently, object coordinates are computed starting from these features.

2.1. Image analysis

To perform geometrical analysis on the instrument shaft, we need to distinguish the endoscopic instrument with respect to the operative scene. For this purpose, we exploit the HSV (hue-saturation-value) segmentation method proposed in [1]. The distal part of the instrument shaft is colour-coded with a strip of azure adhesive tape that occupies a free region in the HSV space of endoscopic images. Figure 1.a shows the colour-coded instrument. Figure 1.b shows a typical color distribution in the H-S plane of laparoscopic images of a surgical procedure. By selecting pixels with the HS values in the highlighted area, the colored strip can be segmented automatically.

With reference to Figure 1.c, we now show how to compute the relevant geometrical features needed for localization, starting from the segmented image. Point c is defined as the centroid (center of mass) of the segmented region S, highlighted in gray in Figure 1.c. Let $\mu(S)$ be the characteristic function of the segmented region S:

$$\mu(\vec{p}) = \begin{cases} 1 & \text{if } \vec{p} \in S \\ 0 & \text{if } \vec{p} \notin S \end{cases}$$

The centroid $\vec{c}$ can be computed as:

$$\vec{c} = \frac{\sum_{\vec{p} \in H} \mu(\vec{p})\vec{p}}{\sum_{\vec{p} \in H} \mu(\vec{p})}.$$

The line direction a, corresponding to the axis of the instrument shaft, is computed as the axis of minimum inertia of the segmented region S. The moment of inertia tensor of S is defined as I_{ij}:

$$I_{ij} = \sum_{\vec{p} \in H} \mu(\vec{p})(p^2 \delta_{ij} - p_i p_j)$$

where $i, j \in x, y$, H is the whole image, δ_{ij} is the Kronecker delta and $p = \|\vec{p}\|$. a is computed as the eigenvector corresponding to the smallest eigenvalue of the moment of I_{ij}. b is the straight line through $\vec{c}$ and perpendicular to a: $b \perp a$, $\vec{c} \in b$.

To find lines l_1 and l_2, Hough transform is used. Applying edge detection to the segmented image, we isolate the contours of the segmented region S, obtaining S', a 1-pixel wide outline of the colour-coded region. Collinear pixels transform to peaks in the Hough plane. In S', the most collinear points are found in the two line segments that belong to lines l_1 and l_2. Therefore, the first two global maxima of the Hough transform of S' correspond to the convergent lines l_1 and l_2 tangent to the instrument shaft (see Figure 3).

2.2. Localization

Neglecting the opening/closing movement of the end-effector, the kinematics of the endoscopic instrument is characterized by 4 DOFs: two rotation angles around the access point, insertion depth, and rotation of the instrument around it's axis. Referring to Figure 2.a, the measurement of X, Y, Z, θ, and φ univocally determines position and orientation of the surgical instrument, except for the roll angle. However, since instruments have cylindrical symmetry, the roll angle can be neglected for several surgical assistance tasks.

2.2.1. Measuring position: X, Y, Z

A simple geometric model for describing an endoscope camera is the pinhole camera model [2], depicted in Figure 2.b: the image $p(x, y)$ of a point $P(X, Y, Z)$ in the 3-D space is defined as the intersection of the image plane I with the ray from P through a centre of projection $C(0, 0, \lambda)$. This projection can be described best by means of perspective geometry involving homogeneous coordinates (for convenience, the axes of the reference frames are defined to be coincident):

$$\begin{cases} x = \frac{x_h}{w_h} \\ y = \frac{y_h}{w_h} \end{cases} , \quad \begin{pmatrix} x_h \\ y_h \\ z_h \\ w_h \end{pmatrix} = \begin{vmatrix} 1 & 0 & 0 & 0 \\ 0 & 1 & 0 & 0 \\ 0 & 0 & 1 & 0 \\ 0 & 0 & -\frac{1}{\lambda} & 1 \end{vmatrix} \begin{pmatrix} kX \\ kY \\ kZ \\ k \end{pmatrix} = \begin{pmatrix} kX \\ kY \\ kZ \\ \frac{-kZ}{\lambda} + k \end{pmatrix} , \tag{1}$$

where λ is the focal length of the camera, w is the 4th homogeneous coordinate, and k is an arbitrary non-zero constant. Real cameras are not geometrically exact, since lenses introduce minor irregularities into images, typically radial distortions. Several camera calibration techniques are available for compensation of these distortions.

For reconstructing the position of a point $P(X, Y, Z)$ in 3-D space, $p(x, y)$ coordinates of its projection on the image plane are not sufficient, since this only allows to reconstruct the optical ray through p and P. If also the Z coordinate is known, P can be determined univocally.

Perspective projection scales down objects with distance along the Z axis. From (1), the distance of the image points $\vec{p_1}(x_1, y_1)$ and $\vec{p_2}(x_2, y_2)$, corresponding to two points

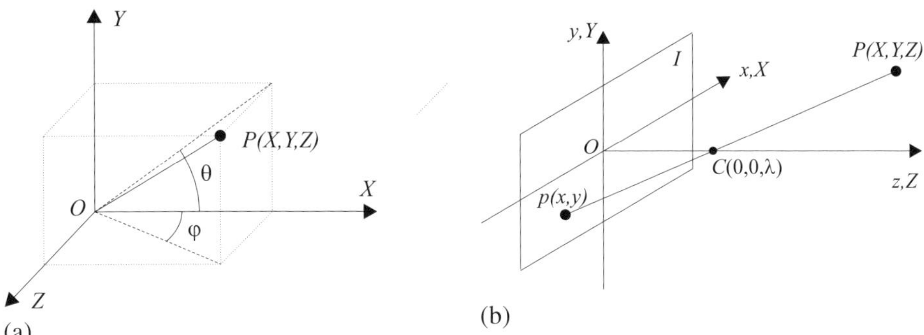

Figure 2. Angles defining local orientation of an object (a); Pinhole camera model (b).

$\vec{P_1}(X_1, Y_1, Z)$ and $\vec{P_2}(X_2, Y_2, Z)$, lying on a plane parallel to the image plane, is reduced by the ratio:

$$\frac{\|\vec{p_1} - \vec{p_2}\|}{\|\vec{P_1} - \vec{P_2}\|} = \frac{1}{1 - Z/\lambda}$$

To determine the Z coordinate of a point we exploit the size reduction of the circular sections of the instrument shaft. Due to the perspective model, the shape of S changes with instrument orientation, making it difficult to estimate a circular section at the borders of the coloured strip. We therefore preferred estimating the diameter of the circular section through $\vec{c}$. The diameter d (in pixels) of the circular section is estimated as the length of the line segment given by the intersection of b with the lines l_1 and l_2. The relation $Z(d)$ is determined experimentally in the results.

$$d = \|(l_1 \cap b) - (l_2 \cap b)\|, \ b \perp a, \ \vec{c} \in b$$

2.2.2. Measuring orientation: θ and φ

θ is the angle formed by line a with the x axis of the endoscopic image.

Perspective projection makes parallel lines converge. The shaft of an instrument, when placed at an angle with respect to the image plane, progressively appears more conical (see Figure 3.a and 3.b). By measuring this convergence, it is possible to compute φ, the rotation of the instrument around the Y axis. Having previously computed l_1 and l_2, we define the convergence angle α, as the angle between two unit vectors lying on these two lines: $\alpha = \cos^{-1}(\hat{l}_1 \cdot \hat{l}_2)$. The angle φ can be computed by measuring α, since the relationship between α and φ can be derived from Eq. (1). In the results section, we will derive this relation experimentally.

3. Experimental setup

For measuring experimentally the relation $\varphi(\alpha, d)$ Storz 0° and 30° laparoscopes were used, connected to a Storz TRICAM 3-chip camera. A Y/C connection to a Matrox RT 3000 frame grabber was used to capture the images at 640×480 pixel. Images were

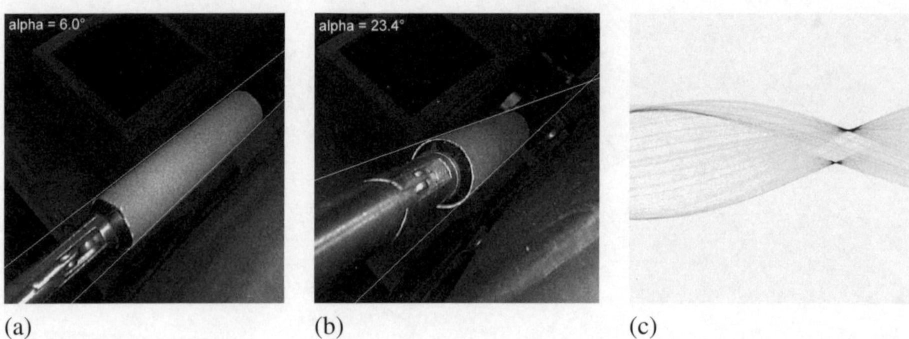

(a)   (b)   (c)

Figure 3. Line convergence due to perspective transform: two images of the instrument, placed at different angles with respect to the image plane (a), (b); the highlighted lines correspond to the first two global maxima of the Hough transform of the images (c).

calibrated using Camera Calibration Toolbox, based on [3]. This equipment is used routinely in the operating room. After analyzing the HSV domain of images from recorded laparoscopic surgeries we selected our colour-code which was well away from the usual HSV domain of these images. Azure adhesive tape (45 mm width) of this chosen colour was attached cylindrically on the shaft of a laparoscopic instrument (10 mm in diameter), near the operative end but separated from the active part. Using a sterile adhesive tape will make the procedure simple, without any specific pre-operative preparation or much disturbance to the actual surgical setup.

8 series of 24 images were acquired at various orientations and distances from the camera using a specially designed setup, to accurately measure the distances (accuracy ± 1 mm) and angles (accuracy $\pm 0.25°$). φ was varied from $0°$ to $72°$ at $3°$ increment in the following setups:

- $0°$ camera, at $Z = \{50, 70, 90, 100\}$ mm and $\theta = 0°$,
- $30°$ camera, at $\theta = \{22°, 45°, 67°, 90°\}$ and $Z = 75$ mm,

where Z is the distance between the camera lens and center of the colour-coded region.

The images obtained, after distortion correction, were binarized by passing through a window filter for the coded colour in the HSV space. Sobel filter was used to detect edges in the segmented images. Radon transform, closely related to Hough transform, was used to detect straight lines in the images.

4. Results

The measurements taken are represented graphically in Figure 4. From relation $\alpha = \alpha(\varphi, \theta)$ (Figure 4.a) we deduce independence of measurements from θ, which is in line with the cylindrical symmetry of the optical system and the pinhole camera model. Also the curves $d = d(\varphi, \theta)$ at fixed Z and varying θ (not shown) exhibit the same behaviour.

Relation $\alpha = \alpha(\varphi, Z)$ (Figure 4.b) shows monotonous behaviour in the full range and is nicely approximated by a 2nd order polynomial. At $Z \geq 70$ mm, the curves are overlapping, allowing to estimate φ from measured α by inverting the plotted function, without need for knowing Z. Laparoscopy is performed by using two instruments for

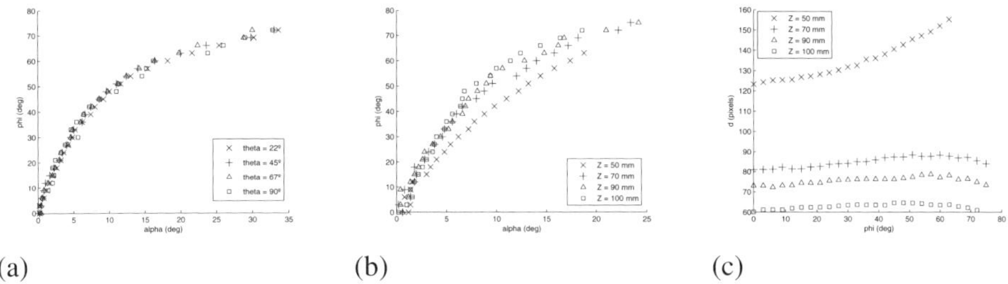

(a)   (b)   (c)

Figure 4. Experimental relations: $\varphi = \varphi(\alpha, \theta)$ (a), $\varphi = \varphi(\alpha, Z)$ (b), $d = d(\varphi, Z)$ (c).

intervention: to be able to view the colour-coded strips of both instruments, with the viewing angle of typical laparoscopic cameras, $Z \gtrsim 100$ mm is required.

Measurement of instrument size $d = d(\varphi, Z)$ (Figure 4.c) is quite independent of φ, except for very close distances. It is therefore possible to estimate the Z coordinate of the instrument, independently from the instrument orientation given by θ and φ.

5. Conclusions

We presented a method for localizing 5 DOFs of an endoscopic instrument, based on shape analysis and requiring only a coloured strip at the distal part of the instrument shaft. Optical localizers achieve higher accuracy. Yet, the proposed method is simple, does not require any specific pre-operative preparation, and does not cause disturbance to the actual surgical setup. Position and orientation are measured in the reference frame of the endoscope camera. The method can be optimal if used in combination with a robotic camera holder, since the robot position is easily measured, thus achieving full localization with respect to the world reference frame, and since no unwanted camera motion will occur. The method can be suitable for applications where accuracy is not critical, such as workspace analysis, surgical navigation assistance tasks like proximity warnings [4], offline analysis of video recordings for performance assessment [5].

References

[1] G. Wei, K. Arbter, and G. Hirzinger, Automatic tracking of laparoscopic instruments by color coding, *Proc. CVRMed-MRCAS'97* (1997), 357–366.

[2] K.S. Fu, R.C. Gonzales, and C.S.G. Lee, *Robotics*, McGraw-Hill, New York, 1987.

[3] J. Heikkilä and O. Silvén, A four-step camera calibration procedure with implicit image correction, *Proc. IEEE Comp Soc Conf CVPR'97* (1997), 1106–1112.

[4] S. D'Attanasio, O. Tonet, G. Megali, M.C. Carrozza, and P. Dario, A semi-automatic hand-held mechatronic endoscope with collision-avoidance capabilities, *Proc. IEEE International Conference on Robotics and Automation - ICRA*, **2** (2000), 1586–1591.

[5] S. Sinigaglia, G. Megali, O. Tonet, and P. Dario, Defining metrics for objective evaluation of surgical performances in laparoscopic training, *Proc. CARS-ISCAS* (2005), 509–514.

Medicine Meets Virtual Reality 14
J.D. Westwood et al. (Eds.)
IOS Press, 2006

Computer–Aided Forensics: Facial Reconstruction

Wesley Turner[a], Peter Tu[a], Timothy Kelliher[a], Rebecca Brown[a]
[a]Imaging Technologies, GE Global Research, Niskayuna NY

Abstract. The 3D reconstruction of facial features from skeletal remains is a key component to the identification of missing persons and victims of violent crime. A comprehensive Computed Tomography (CT) head-scan database is currently being collected which will enable a new approach to forensic facial reconstruction. Using this unique resource, we show how a face space can be tailored to a specific unknown, or questioned skull. A set of database derived estimates of the questioned face is constructed by first computing non-rigid transformations between the known head-scan skulls and the questioned skull followed by application of these transformations to the known head-scan faces. This effectively factors out influences due to skeletal variation. A tailored face space is formed by applying Principal Component Analysis (PCA) to this ensemble of estimates of the questioned face. Thus, the face space is a direct approximation of correlated soft tissue variance indicative of the population. Ours is the first mathematical representation of the face continuum associated with a given skull. Embedded in this space resides the elements needed for recognition.

1. Introduction

The forensic identification of human remains is often aided by the three-dimensional reconstruction of a face model from an unknown or questioned skull. In many cases subtle traces of resemblance to the questioned face can be enough to trigger recognition in someone familiar with the deceased.

The tissue-depth approach uses knowledge acquired from the population regarding the soft tissue thickness at key points on the skull in order to constrain the reconstruction. In the United States, forensic artists commonly employ the tissue-depth approach in manual clay-based reconstruction. The artist consults an average tissue-depth table for a chosen population such as female Caucasoid. Markers with the appropriate depth are affixed to the landmark positions of the skull. Due to the scarcity of the tissue depth locations, the artist is required to use their professional judgment to fill in the gaps between the markers with clay [1].

Tissue-depth tables present limited information such as the mean and standard deviation at several locations on the skull. Concerns have been raised regarding the validity of these measurements [2]. In particular these tables do not contain sufficient information to characterize the major modes of correlated soft tissue variation expressed by the population. This paper introduces a new statistical soft-tissue model in the form of a tailored face space by making extensive use of a database of CT scans of the entire head.

Bone and soft-tissue are well discriminated in a CT volume. As a consequence it is possible to automatically extract surfaces for skulls and soft tissue. The diversity of faces observed in the general population is based on a combination of both skeletal and soft-tissue variation. The main challenges to our data-driven approach are to remove the influences of skeletal variance, to capture and model the main modes of soft-tissue variation and to define methods by which the user can use expert knowledge to mold the soft-tissue model into a specific reconstruction.

It has been shown that an estimate of the questioned face can be generated by first warping a known skull onto the questioned skull and then applying the same transformation to the known face [3]. Instead of performing this procedure on just a single known skull, we propose the application of this procedure to an entire set of suitably selected skulls. Thus skeletal variance is effectively factored out of the transformed database. This application requires fully automatic and robust registration. We have developed algorithms that meet these requirements.

The transformed faces of the database represent an ensemble of estimates of the questioned face and can be used to directly approximate the correlated variance of soft-tissue depth. PCA is used for this purpose with the major eigenvectors forming the basis of a face space tailored to the questioned skull.

The legitimacy of facial reconstruction as a forensic technique has been questioned [4]. Our work presents compelling results that directly address these concerns, opening up the prospect of increased objectivity and effectiveness of this field.

2. Related Work

At first, the tissue-depth approach was adapted directly to the computer by digitizing the skull, digitally adding the same tissue depths to the skull, and computing the interpolation between the markers [5]. Others used markers to constrain a generic head model consisting of muscles and skin in a deformable framework [6].

With the availability of skull and face surfaces from CT volumes, researchers have moved beyond the sparse landmark-based techniques to deformable dense registration algorithms that map the entire surface or volume of a known skull onto the surface of the questioned skull. These new algorithms generate a more subtle and refined warping field. Already methods have been developed which identify landmarks on both the known and the questioned skull [3]. A warping function is defined so as to bring the known landmark point set into correspondence with the questioned landmarks. The same function is applied to the known CT facial surface to warp it to the questioned skull, giving a reconstruction. Other researchers avoid the problem of establishing landmarks by defining a warping function in terms of crest lines, or areas of high curvature, on the skulls [7]. The warping algorithms developed in our work advances on existing techniques by being fully automatic and by using both crest-lines and points in smoothly varying regions of the skull.

It has been shown that PCA can effectively capture the main modes of deformation within a human shape space [8]. More specifically it has been shown the effectiveness of PCA for modeling shape variation of 3D faces [9]. Our face space is unique in that it is tailored to a specific skull as opposed to the facial variation associated with the entire population.

3. Algorithms

The construction of a soft tissue model for a questioned skull is based on the information from a number of known heads in the database. Consequently it is necessary to register each known skull with the questioned skull. Since the variation of the soft tissue is estimated using PCA each transformed face from the database needs to be embedded into a linear space. Finally, *a priori* anthropological knowledge can be used to mold this face space into a specific reconstruction.

3.1. Skull Registration

The CT head-scans are captured with a slice thickness of 2.5 millimeters. For each head-scan an isosurface is extracted representing the known skull and an isosurface is extracted representing the known face. The questioned skull is also represented by an isosurface that is extracted from a CT scan of the questioned skull. The marching cubes algorithm is used to generate all the isosurfaces [10]. An example of the distribution of tissue depth defined by a pair of known skull and face isosurfaces can be seen in figure 1.

Figure 1: The distribution of tissue depth from skin to skull for a caucasoid female. Depths are in millimeters

The goal is to find a deformation which when applied to the known face gives an approximation to the questioned face. The deformation should preserve the soft tissue structure of the known face while removing the variation due to the difference in skeletal structure. An appropriate method for generating the deformation is to select the transformation such that it maps the known skull in to the questioned skull. Thus the deformation is designed to robustly and automatically register a known skull to the questioned skull. Figure 2 outlines the 4-stage skeletal registration algorithm. [11]

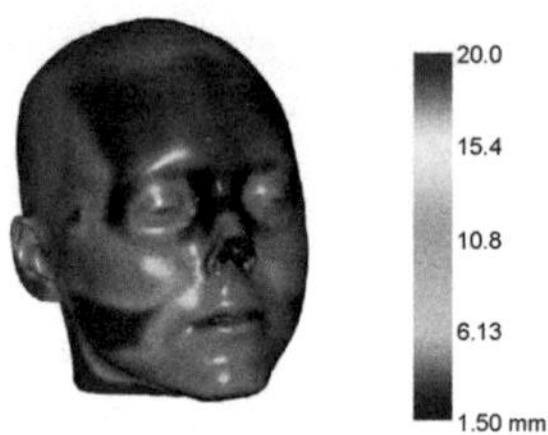

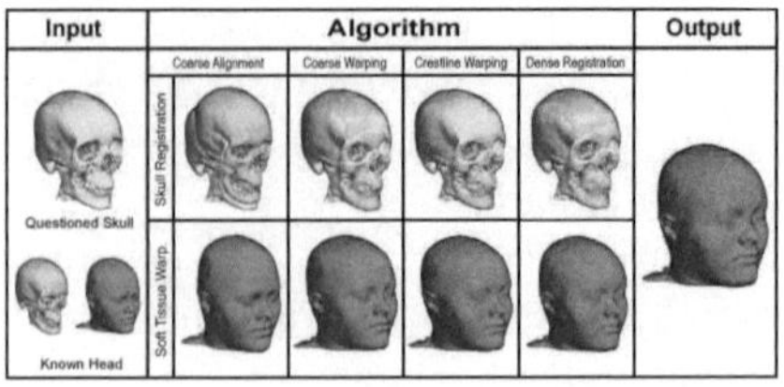

Figure 2: Example flow through the skull registration algorithm

3.2. Generating a Tailored Face Space

An ensemble of estimates of the unknown face is generated by applying the registration algorithm to an appropriate subset of the head-scan database. Each of these estimates needs to be represented as a vector and the ensemble forms a matrix on which PCA can be performed. The resulting face space approximates correlated soft tissue variation of the population without the influences of skeletal variance. We define a vector representation of an estimated face. A cylindrical representation is used to represent a warped isosurface as a vector. Let the origin of a Cartesian coordinate system be placed at the center of the base of the head. The Z axis points toward the top of the head. The X axis points toward the left side of the head and the Y axis points toward the front of the head. A point can be defined by its Cartesian coordinate (x,y,z) or by its cylindrical coordinates.

An important property of the cylindrical representation is that it effectively isolates flesh depth in its own dimension. Using this representation PCA can be carried out on the set of estimates gained from the deformation of each of the known faces from the database to the questioned skull. This results in a face space that is used to understand the most likely face and the ways that the face would vary within the population. Figure 3 shows a slice of the tailored face space for the questioned face shown at the bottom right of the figure.

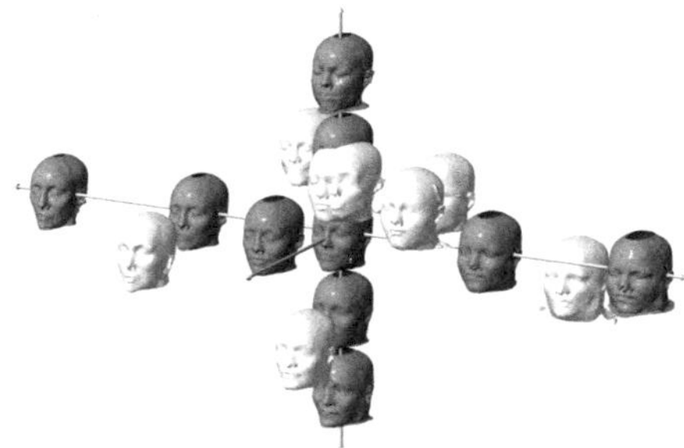

Figure 3 Cross-section of a tailored face space: Each face is positioned based on its face space coordinates, which are defined by the projection of the face onto the first three dominant eigenvectors. The gray faces are various samples from the database after they have been warped onto the questioned skull. The tan faces are generated by adding 0 to 2 standard deviations of a single eigenvector to the mean. As can be seen, the horizontal eigenvector appears to be representative of the potential thickness of the face. The vertical eigenvector captures more subtle features of the cheeks and neck.

To investigate the ability of the face space to approximate the true face, the projection of the true face onto the face space was computed. Since the true face was not used in the construction of the face space, the projected face will not be an exact match of the true face. The face to the left of the average face in figure 3 is the projected face positioned based on its face space coordinates. In this case it is very close to the mean face.

3.3. Face Space Navigation Using Prior Knowledge

Each reconstruction is a weighted sum of the eigenvectors added to the mean. When the weights are all equal to zero, the reconstruction is reduced to the average face. In the absence of any *a priori* knowledge, this is the most likely and hence a reasonable estimate of the questioned face.

There are a number of techniques that have been developed to estimate various spatial properties of the questioned face based on measurements made on the questioned skull. Each one of these heuristics can generate a set of constraining points in space such that the reconstruction should be as close to these points as possible. Each of these points can be represented in the cylindrical coordinate system.

Defining specific methods for deriving anthropological constraints is beyond the scope of this paper. However, in order to show the additional value of credible local information, we have simulated expert knowledge by sampling a small number of points from regions of the true face such as the tip of the nose, the apex of the eyes and the center of the mouth. The results show the effect with and without this information.

4. Results

Six data sets from the database were selected to represent examples of questioned skulls. For each example a tailored face space was generated after exclusion of the head-scan under consideration. The mean face, a constrained reconstruction based on simulated *a priori* knowledge and the projected face was generated for each case. These along with the skull and the true face are shown in figure 4.

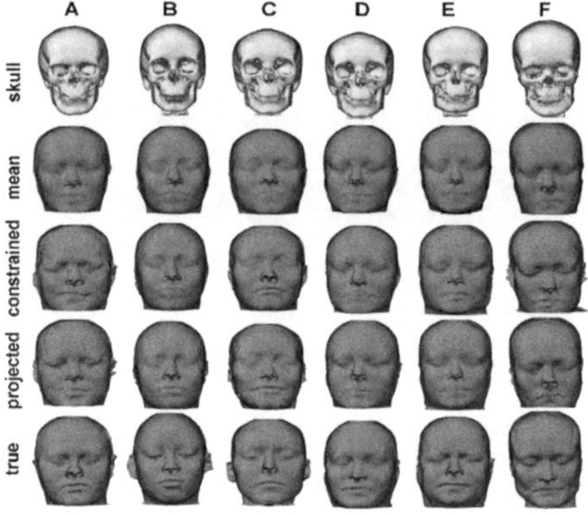

Figure 4 The skull, mean estimation, constrained, projected and true face for six samples from our database.

Selection criteria such as race, age, weight and sex must be defined so that a tailored face space can be generated using appropriate samples from the database. The quality of the samples is more important than the quantity. In the examples shown, approximately ten samples satisfied all the constraints and these were used to generate the face spaces. Much of the gross soft tissue variation was captured. When collection of our CT database is complete, the number of eligible samples for a face space will increase. Deformation modes associated with finer details will be generated.

In previous work assessors unfamiliar with a targeted individual were asked to identify the target from a range of faces after examining a facial reconstruction[4]. Only 1 out of 16 facial reconstructions were identified above chance at statistically significant levels. It was concluded that facial reconstruction appeared to be an unreliable and inaccurate aid to identification. However in the forensic context most successful applications rely on people familiar with the target. Given the striking resemblances in Figure 4 between the true faces and our various reconstructions, including the mean face, we believe that when our system enters in to general usage, success may be achievable even without reliance on familiarity.

5. Discussion

A tailored face space can only provide a basis for possible reconstructions. In order to hone in on a specific reconstruction, *a priori* knowledge is required. While it is beyond the scope of this paper to discuss the validity of these forensic rules of thumb, we believe that the head-scan database will serve as an important resource for this vetting process.

Clearly there are limits to what can be inferred about the appearance of an individual based solely on their skeletal structure. However our purpose is not to generate exact facsimiles, rather as the last voice for the victim we are endeavoring to spark recognition in someone who is familiar with the deceased so that identity can be established.

Since manual methods for face reconstruction are extremely time consuming, forensic artists have been limited to one or two reconstructions. Using our face space methods, large sets of reconstructions that span many possibilities can be automatically generated. This leads to the exciting question of how best to present a continuum of possibilities in an optimal manner. The work presented in this paper will fuel the pursuit of many of these important lines of scientific inquiry.

References

[1] Taylor, K. T. 2001. Forensic Art and Illustration. CRC Press, New York.

[2] Brown, R. E., Kelliher, T. P., Tu, P. H., Turner, W. D., Taister, M. A., and Miller, K. W. P. 2004. A survey of tissue-depth landmarks for facial approximation. Forensic Sci. Comm. 6, 1.

[3] Nelson, L. A., and Michael, S. D. 1998. The application of volume deformation to three-dimensional facial reconstruction: A comparison with previous techniques. Forensic Sci. Int. 94, 167 - 181.

[4] Stephan, C. N., and Henneberg, M. 2001. Building faces from dry skulls: are they recognized above chance rates? J. Forensic Sci. 46, 3, 432 - 440.

[5] Vanezis, P., Blowes, R. W., Linney, A. D., Tan, A. C.,Richards, R., and Neave, R. 1989. Application of 3d computer graphics for facial reconstruction and comparison with sculpting techniques. Forensic Sci. Int. 42, 69 - 84.

[6] Kahler, K., Haber, J., and Seidel, H.-P. 2003. Reanimating the dead: reconstruction of expressive faces from skull data. In ACM Transactions on Graphics. Proceedings of ACM SIGGRAPH 2003; 2003 July 28 - 31; San Diego (CA), ACM SIGGRAPH, New York, 554 - 561.

[7] Quatrehomme, G., Cotin, S., Subsol, G., Delingette, H., Garidel, Y., Gr_evin, G., Fidrich, M., Bailet, P., and Ollier, A. 1997. A fully three-dimensional method for facial reconstruction based on deformable models. J. Forensic Sci. 42, 4, 649 - 652.

[8] Allen, B., Curless, B., and Popovi_c, Z. 2003. The space of human body shapes: reconstruction and parameterization from range scans. In ACM SIGGRAPH 2003.

[9] Blanz, V., and Vetter, T. 1999. A morphable model for the synthesis of 3d faces. In Computer Graphics Proceeding, Annual Conference Series, ACM SIGGRAPH, New York, 187 - 194.

[10] Lorensen, W. E., and Cline, H. E. 1987. Marching cubes: A high resolution 3d surface construction algorithm. In Computer Graphics, ACM, vol. 21, 163 { 169.

[11] Turner, W.D., Brown, R.E.B., Kelliher, T., Tu, P.H., Taister, M.A., Miller,K.W.P. 2005. A novel method of automated skull registration for forensic facial approximation Forensic Sci. Int. 154/2-3, 149-158.

Medicine Meets Virtual Reality 14
J.D. Westwood et al. (Eds.)
IOS Press, 2006

Registration and Segmentation for the High Resolution Visible Human Male Images

Sreeram Vaidyanath[a] and Bharti Temkin[a, b]
[a]*Department of Computer Science, Texas Tech University*
[b]*Department of Surgery, Texas Tech University*
Bharti.Temkin@ttu.edu

Abstract. The Visible Human project by National Library of Medicine (NLM) resulted in two sets of cryosection images of a human male (VHM): low (LR) and high (HR) resolution. By leveraging the already registered and segmented LR images, we have successfully achieved the same for the entire HR image set. 3D models of human anatomical structures generated using this HR image set, presented in this paper, provide qualitative demonstration of the high accuracy of the HR registration and segmentation.

Keywords. Image Registration, Segmentation, Visible Human, Anatomical model

Introduction

High quality 3D models of human anatomical structures are useful in many applications such as anatomical training, medical simulation etc. It is possible to build these models using the existing cryosection images of the visible human available from NLM [1]. However, creating the 3D digital anatomical models – virtual body structures (VBS) - requires the images to be registered with respect to each other and the structures of interest to be segmented within all the slices containing the structures. An important benefit of segmentation is that the structures of interest can be highlighted and labeled. Many applications have been created using the LR VHM images of 1760 x 1024 pixels[4, 5]. For harnessing the better anatomical details of the HR images, having a resolution of 4096 x 2700 pixels, we have registered the entire HR VHM [2, 3] and segmented many major structures of interest. This paper qualitatively demonstrates the accuracy of the HR registration and segmentation by building 3D models of human anatomy.

1. Three-dimensional models of human anatomical structures using HR images

For validating the accuracy of the HR registration and segmentation, 3D models of human anatomy have been generated with our v-vbs system [4]. Structures created from the head region are shown in Fig. 1 and structures created from the torso are shown in Fig. 2. Models of these structures include the brain and the face as well as heart and kidneys. Structures from the leg region are presented in Figs. 3 and 4, which present models of cross section of leg and knee respectively.

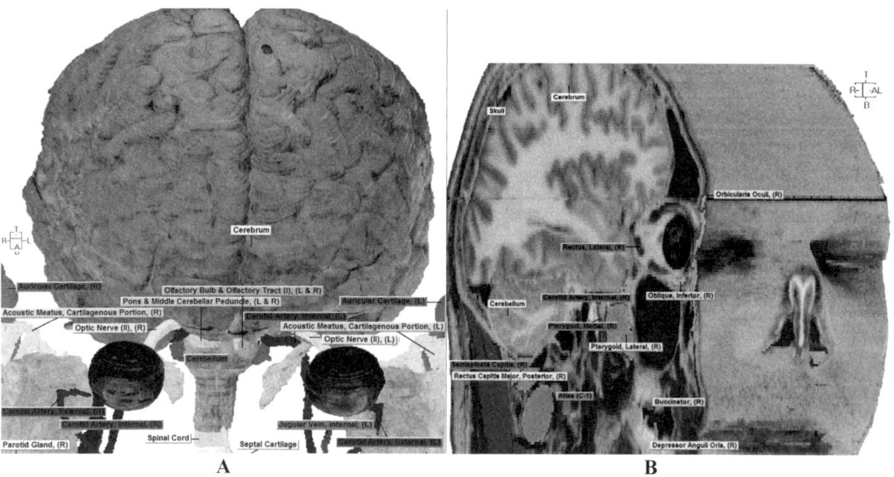

Figure 1. 3D models from the head region; A) Brain and B) Face

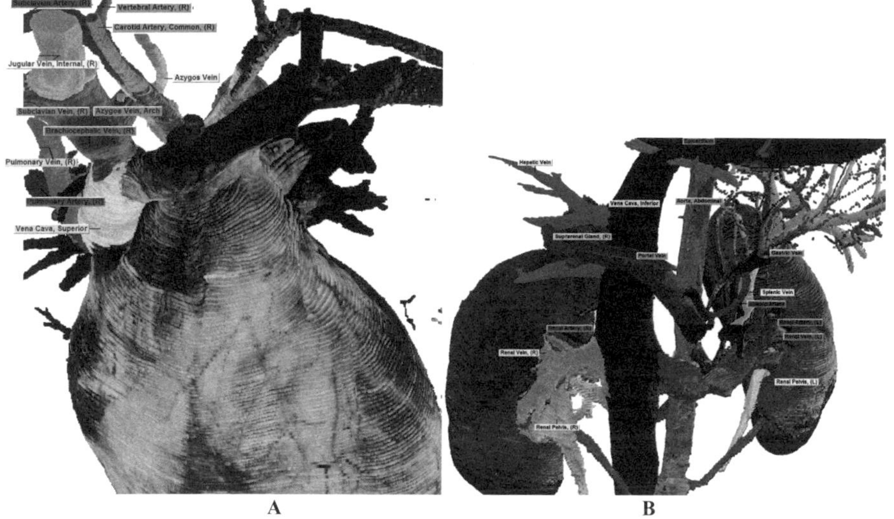

Figure 2. 3D models of the torso region; A) Heart and B) Kidneys

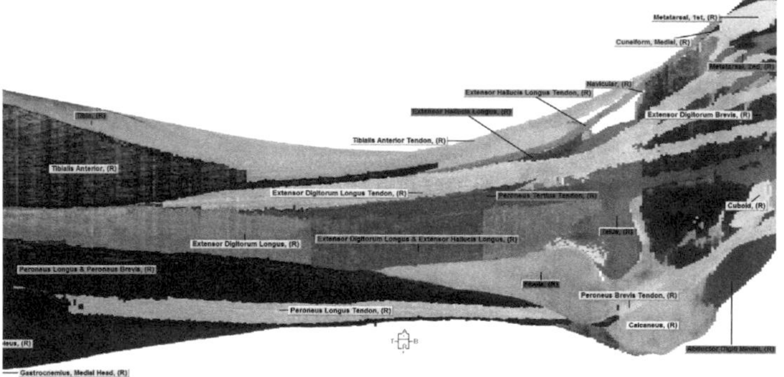

Figure 3. 3D models of section of leg showing tibia and fibula with muscles

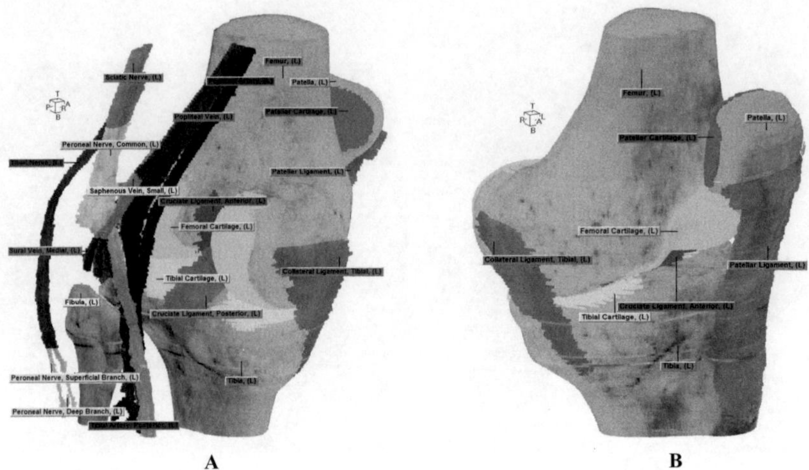

Figure 4. 3D models of the knee showing skeletal, articulation, circulation, and nervous systems with different views

2. Conclusions/Discussions

The 3D models of anatomical structures from various regions of the human body provide a visual verification of the high level of accuracy with which the HR images have been registered and segmented. Small structures seen in HR images, but not visible in the LR images, are not yet segmented and this problems remains to be resolved [6]. Our registration and segmentation process has worked well for above 97% of the 1821 VHM images. Manual refinement of edges of individual structures was required only for images with distortions, assumed to be a result of slicing issues.

Acknowledgement

We fully acknowledge the contributions of Mr. Eric Acosta, whose assistance was instrumental in completing this paper in a timely manner.

References

[1]   http://www.nlm.nih.gov/research/visible/visible_human.html
[2]   Temkin B., Vaidyanath S. and Acosta E., "A high accuracy, landmark-based, sub-pixel level image registration", *Computer Assisted Radiology and Surgery*, pp 254—259, June 2005
[3]   Vaidyanath S. and Temkin B., "High accuracy registration of images with different resolutions," *To be published*
[4]   Temkin B., Acosta E., et al. "An Interactive Three-dimensional Virtual Body Structures System for Anatomical Training over the Internet." *Accepted for publication in Journal of Clinical Anatomy*
[5]   Temkin B., Acosta E., et al., "Web-based Three-dimensional Virtual Body Structures," *JAMIA 9* (5): pp 425—436, 2002.
[6]   Malvankar A. and Temkin B., "Segmenting the Visible Human images", *To be published*

Medicine Meets Virtual Reality 14
J.D. Westwood et al. (Eds.)
IOS Press, 2006

Flatland Sound Services Design Supports Virtual Medical Training Simulations

Victor M. VERGARA[1], PANAIOTIS[1,2], Tim EYRING[1], John GREENFIELD[1],
Kenneth L. SUMMERS[3], and Thomas Preston CAUDELL[1]
*[1]Dept. of ECE, [2]Dept. of Music, [3]Center for High Performance Computing,
University of New Mexico*

Abstract. This paper describes the evolution of the design of Flatland Sound
Service (FSS), a sound system for virtual reality required to support Project
TOUCH (Telehealth Outreach for Unified Community Health), a multi-year
collaboration between the Schools of Medicine at the state Universities of Hawaii
and of New Mexico. Two virtual sonic environments specific case scenarios, a
neurological trauma (Toma) and a virtual kidney nephron (Nephron), were
developed using integrated services provided by FSS. Flatland is an open source
visualization and virtual reality application development tool created at the
University of New Mexico.

Keywords. Auditory Icons, Earcons, Sonification, Virtual Sonic Environments,
Sound Rendering, Semitone, Octave, Avatar.

Introduction

The importance of sound in virtual reality systems increases as interactive applications
evolve into holistic interchanges of information between users and software tools. In
every day life, sound constitutes an important source of information about the world
that surrounds us. Sound must perform a similar task in virtual reality by providing
meaningful information [1]. This concept of adding meaning to sound and combining it
with graphical systems is an active research topic [2] that requires adequate tools.
Flatland Sound Service (FSS) was created to provide these tools. Flatland is an open
source visualization and virtual reality application development tool created at the
University of New Mexico [3].

Advanced sonification techniques require the integration of sound services that
surpass simple sound playback. The creation of informative virtual sonic environments
requires an integrated, unified sound system capable of managing the variety of devices,
software and libraries available today, without significantly affecting graphical
performance.

FSS includes the standard synthesis and sound rendering capabilities commonly
found in other virtual sonic environment systems ([4] and [5]). These capabilities
support many standard sonification techniques ([1] and [6]) including earcons, auditory
icons, audification, sound-parameter mapping, and localization. In addition, the FSS
modular design provides extensibility to support atypical sonification techniques that
include algorithmically generated music and other specialized systems.

The remainder of this paper is organized as follows: section II describes the tools and methods used to implement FSS; section III presents the two examples of project TOUCH that utilize Flatland and FSS; section IV is the conclusion.

1. Tools and Methods

The Flatland Sound Services is of a modular design that supports diverse sound and music related software and hardware tools and devices. It is composed of three main components: the Sound Management Application (SMA), Resident Sound Servers (RSS), and a Resident Open Sound Control Server (ROSCS). (See Figure 1.)

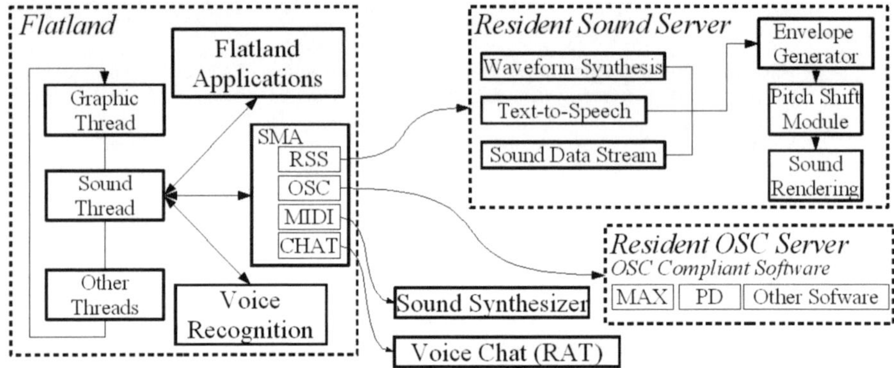

Figure 1. Basic block diagram of Flatland Sound Service system.

The SMA is an interface link between Flatland and available sound servers. It receives input from Flatland Sound Library calls and communicates to the sound servers using network protocols. This enables a Flatland project to arbitrarily use resident servers on the host computer, or servers on networked computers.

In Flatland, every virtual object has an associated sound function that is called during sound-control thread execution. The sound function communicates with SMA using the Flatland Sound Library, a high-level set of instructions designed to coordinate sound and graphics. Virtual objects may or may not have an associated visual representation, and could simply be relevant virtual environment or process data. The SMA determines what sound servers are available to handle the FSL call (or launches a resident server such as RSS), translates the input to an appropriate output protocol, and sends it to the server (attached MIDI software or hardware device, RSS, or ROSCS).

The Resident Sound Server (RSS) is an independent application module designed to handle most VR sound-related functions: sound file playback, additive synthesis, pitch shifting, and sound localization among others. Because the SMA communicates to the RSS using TCP/IP, the RSS application can run on a remote computer, reducing the Flatland host CPU load.

All other sound calls are translated either to MIDI or OSC for communication to respectively compliant software and hardware devices. While MIDI is an industry standard, the OSC protocol [7] is a more flexible and extensible command language protocol designed to communicate with high-level sound and music software such as PD ([8] and [9]), Max/MSP [10] and other software that supports it. UDP is typically used as the network protocol that transmits OSC data.

1.1. Resident Sound Server Functions

Functionality of the RSS depends on which base development library is used: either Open Audio Library (OpenAL [10]) or Simple Direct media Layer (SDL, [12] and [13]). OpenAL is an audio API optimized for virtual reality and is recommended for most applications. SDL provides low-level access to audio devices and is more suitable for some specialized and experimental purposes. The RSS has three stages of production: sound generation, sound modification, and sound rendering.

1.1.1. Sound Generation

Sound generation includes sound file playback, additive synthesis, wave table synthesis, text to speech synthesis, and external signal streaming.

Sound playback loads sound data from files into a buffer to be manipulated and played. It can be used for audio icons, earcons, sound effects, ambient sounds, and recorded music. Of the possible sound sources, this is currently the most common form of sound generation in Flatland because it is the least CPU intensive form of producing a wide range of sounds, and it conforms to the basic Flatland paradigm that a defined sound, or set of sounds, is associated with each graphic object.

Sound synthesis is useful for audification, parameter mapping, and musification. Flatland RSS supports additive synthesis. Additive synthesis [14] builds complex waveforms by producing the sine-tone components that define the wave. Each sine wave is specified by frequency and amplitude. Additive synthesis is quite flexible if controlled properly. However, for complex waveforms, this is a CPU intensive form of synthesis.

Wave table synthesis and audio streaming is in development. While streaming provides the capability to use external sound sources (e.g. microphones and network audio), wave table synthesis is an efficient way to use more realistic instrument sounds to play music. These sound generating capabilities will open Flatland to more versatile interaction with users, and provide a larger palette of sounds for music synthesis within Flatland.

Flite [15], which converts text strings into synthesized voice sound-data, is Flatland's main text-to-speech engine. It was chosen for its simplicity, speed, and portability.

1.1.2. Sound Modifiers

Once a sound is generated it is then routed through the Sound Modification stage. There are currently two modifiers in RSS: a pitch shifter and an envelope generator.

Pitch shifting is primarily used in the context of generating music. However, it can also provide variety to otherwise repetitive sounds by making pitch changes each time they are played. Any sound source can be shifted up or down as much as one octave in pitch (0.5 to 2.0 times the frequency of the source, which is equal to -12 to 12 semitones). Resolution of the shift can be defined as an integer in the range 48 to 72, where 60 is considered to be "no shift" and each number increments the pitch by one equal-tempered semitone. For finer resolutions, a floating-point number is used instead to specify the pitch shift as a frequency ratio between 0.5 and 2.0.

The envelope generator takes care of fast time-varying intensity changes of sounds. This modifier is also typically used for music synthesis. Musical instruments are not only identified by their spectral content, but by their loudness change over time. Many percussive sounds and plucked strings have a sharp attack with quick decay and release. Sustained strings generally have a slow attack, slight decay, indefinite sustain, and slow release.

1.1.3. Sound Rendering

The final stage of the RSS renders sound in a 3D virtual space. It is here that a sound is given spatial characteristics providing an enhanced realism. Aside from 3D positioning, sounds are modified using a Doppler effect to simulate movement and echo and reverberation to suggest surfaces and room characteristics.

Some sounds do not require spatial localization, for example background music. Such sounds are positioned relative to the user's head instead of localized in the virtual space.

1.2. External Devices

Flatland's RSS provides developers with substantial sound-related tools for virtual environments. However, there are situations that call for more sophisticated hardware and software tools and devices that have been optimized for particular sound and music applications. For this reason, Flatland's SMA supports direct MIDI communication to internal music software or external sound synthesis modules. SMA can open a MIDI channel through the operating system to communicate to the default MIDI device. It can also be set up to control MIDI software synthesizers like those commonly used by web browsers.

In addition to MIDI, network communication with applications such as Max/MSP, PD, and other sound and music creation software is achieved by providing OSC command protocol via UDP sockets. These applications offer graphic, object-oriented algorithmic programming environments and support the OSC protocol, which has a much more flexible communication structure than MIDI.

1.3. Voice Chat

Multi-user collaborative applications [16] require not only graphical representations of distant users (Avatars) but also their voices. Voice chatting in Flatland is provided using the Robust Audio Tool (RAT [17]), an open-source audio conferencing application. Flatland's sound server launches RAT at initialization, which works independently and as long as Flatland is running.

1.4. Speech Recognition

Text-to-speech is complemented by speech recognition. Flatland utilizes Sphinx-2 [18] for speech recognition. Sphinx-2 offers continuous speech decoding, and separates words by analyzing pauses in speech. It does not need to be "trained" for each user, but recognition requires that a limited, predefined list of words be used for a particular context.

2. Implementation and Results

Virtual sonic environments were developed for two medical applications: a simulation of evolving epidural hematoma (TOMA project) and the modeling of a renal nephron (Nephron project) [19].

2.1. TOMA

The first development stage of the TOMA case included audio icons. Relevant sounds associated with medical tools enhanced user interaction with the virtual patient. These sounds included patient breath and heartbeat, application of neck brace and bandages, and patient sounds associated with breathing difficulties and seizure, among others.

Verbal communication is necessary in multi-user systems. The second development stage was intended to improve the TOMA collaborative mode [16]. The chat module with RAT was added to FSS, allowing users to speak to each other in a remote-sight collaborative setup in which participants of the same virtual environment were actually in different parts of the world.

2.2. Nephron

The Nephron project features algorithmically generated music. FSS sends the user's position and chemical gradient data to a networked computer running a program in Max/MSP called SoundCycler ([20] and [21]). Max/MSP uses the incoming data to influence algorithmic creation of musical textures, which provide users with orientation cues and indications of chemical balances in the nephron.

3. Conclusion and Future Work

Flatland's current sound system provides developers with tools for creating a wide range of interactive sound and music content while minimizing their need to write new code. Some of these tools are in early stages of development while others will improve with future hardware and algorithm optimization.

The synthesis module will be improved with more sophisticated synthesis methods. Chatting will be added into SSA to place distant users' voices at avatar mouths. The most ambitious improvement is to build a module to create algorithmically generated music within Flatland. This module will provide non-musicians with tools to sonify information using music.

Acknowledgements

This publication was made possible by Prime Contract No. V549P-4828-02 from the Pacific Telehealth and Technology Hui. Its contents are solely the responsibility of the authors and do not necessarily represent the official views of the Pacific Telehealth and Technology Hui or the US Department of Defense.

References

[1]   T. Hermann and H. Ritter. *Sound and Meaning in Auditory Data Display.* Proceeding of the IEEE, Vol. 92, No.4, April 2004.

[2]   Panaiotis, V. M. Vergara, T. P. Caudell, et al., "Algorithmically Generated Music Enhances VR Nephron Simulation." MMVR 14 Proceedings, IOC Press, The Netherlands, 2006.

[3]   Caudell, T.P, Summers*, K.L., Holten*, J., Hakamata*, T. Mowafi*, M., Jacobs, J., Lozanoff, B.K., Lozanoff, S., Wilks, D., Keep, M.F., S., Saiki, S, Alverson, A., "Virtual Patient Simulator for Distributed Collaborative Medical Education", The Anatomical Record (Part B: New Anat.) V. 270B, pp. 23-29 (Jan., 2003)

[4]   A. de Campo, C. Frauenberger and R. Höldrich. *Designing a Generalized Sonification Environment.* Proceedings of ICAD 04-Tenth Meeting of the International Conference on Auditory Display, Sydney, Australia, July 6-9, 2004.

[5]   J. Cardoso, J. Carvalho, Luís Texteira and Álvaro Barbosa. *SoundServer: Data sonification on-demand for Computacional Instantes* Proceedings of ICAD 04-Tenth Meeting of the International Conference on Auditory Display, Sydney, Australia, July 6-9, 2004

[6]   T. Hermann and A. Hunt. Guest editors' introduction: *An introduction to Interactive Sonification.* IEEE MultiMedio Vol. 12. Apr-June 2005, 20-24.

[7]   W. Matt. *Open Sound Control Specification.* March 26, 2002. http://www.cnmat.berkeley.edu/OpenSoundControl/OSC-spec.html

[8]   M. Puckette. *"Pure Data."* Proceedings, International Computer Music Conference. San Francisco: International Computer Music Association, pp. 269-272. 1996.

[9]   M. Puckette. *PD Documentation.* http://www-crca.ucsd.edu/~msp/Pd_documentation/index.htm

[10] Miller Puckette, David Zicarelli, et al., Max/MSP. IRCAM and Cycling74.

[11] *OpenAl Specification and Reference,* Loki software. http://www.openal.org/openal_webstf/specs/oalspecs-specs.pdf

[12] Sam Latinga, Stephanie Peter and Ryran Gordon. *SDL_mixer 1.2.* http://jcatki.no-ip.org/SDL_mixer/

[13] Sam Latinga. *Simple Direct media Layer Introduction.* http://www.libsdl.org/intro.php

[14] M. Russ. *Sound Synthesis and Sampling.* Focal Press. 1996.

[15] A. W. Black and K. A. Lenzo. Flite: a small fast run-time synthesis engine. In Proceedings of the 4th ISCA Workshop on Speech Synthesis, page 204, Scotland, August-September 2001. Available Online: http://www.ssw4.org/system,papers/flite.pdf.

[16] M. Y. Mowafi, K.L. Summers, J. Holten, J.A. Greenfield, A. Sherstyuk, D. Nickles, E. Aalseth, W. Takamiya, S. Saiki, D. Alverson, and T. P. Caudell. *Distributed Interactive Virtual Environments for Collaborative Medical Education and Training: Design and Characterization.* JIAMSE 2004.

[17] V. Hardman, Kouvelas I., M.A. Sasse and A. Watson, *A packet loss Robust-Audio tool for use over the Mbone.* Research Note RN/96/8. Dept. of Computer Science, University College London, England, 1996.

[18] Xuedong Huang, Fileno Alleva, Mei-Yuh Hwang, and Ronald Rosenfeld. *An overview of the sphinx-II speech recognition system.* In ARPA Human Language Technology Workshop, pages 81--86. Morgan Kaufmann, March 1993. published as Human Language Technology.

[19] D. C. Alverson, S.M. Saiki Jr, T. P. Caudell, K. Summers, T. Goldsmith, D. S. Wax, M. Bowyer, A. Liu, D. Wilks, *Distributed Immersive Virtual Reality Simulation Development for Medical Education.* JIAMSE 2005, Vol. 15. pag. 19.

[20] Panaiotis, V. M. Vergara, T. P. Caudell, et al., "Algorithmically Generated Music Enhances VR Nephron Simulation." MMVR 14 Proceedings, IOC Press, The Netherlands, 2006.

[21] Panaiotis, S. Smith, V. E. Vergara, S. Xia, T. P. Caudell, "Algorithmically Generated Music Enhances VR Decision Support Tool," Science and Technology for Chem-Bio Information Systems (S&T CBIS) Conference, Oct. 2005.

Medicine Meets Virtual Reality 14
J.D. Westwood et al. (Eds.)
IOS Press, 2006

565

Simulating Tele-Manipulator Controlled Tool-Tissue Interactions Using a Nonlinear FEM Deformable Model

D A WANG[1], A FARACI, F BELLO and A DARZI
Department of Biosurgery and Surgical Technology, Imperial College London

Abstract. Enhanced visualization of an operating scene presented by a robotically assisted tele-manipulator system such as the *da Vinci*™ can be provided through the use of augmented reality facilities. Generating overlays from 3D models and the intra-operative video allows the surgeon to acquire greater information about the surgical scene. Tool-tissue interactions must be tracked to ensure the overlays are updated regularly and accurately. The work presented here describes how these interactions may be modelled by integrating a nonlinear finite element model with the 3D reconstruction and using the tool kinematic data as input to the deformation.

Keywords. Augmented reality, deformation, simulation, tracking

1. Background

Robotic minimally invasive surgery provides the surgeon with great manoeuvrability within a limited working volume. Although the reduced traumas to patient tissue and speedy recovery times have shown to be advantageous, such procedures present the surgeon with a restricted field of view. Augmented reality is a technique that can be used to enhance this narrow view by superimposing additional information onto the surgeon's view.

This work concentrates on providing augmented reality for the *da Vinci* tele-manipulator system. The operating scene is displayed to the surgeon via an endoscopic camera and visual enhancement is presented by overlaying 3D reconstructions of the organs within the operating scene. Previous work in this area focused on cardiac surgery [1] and cholecystectomy operations [2].

An important aspect of accurate augmented reality is the tracking of the objects within the scene. An operating scene is highly dynamic, constantly changing due to interactions with the surgical instruments. Taking into account these changes ensures that the data displayed is accurate and useful.

2. Methods

In order to simulate tool-tissue interactions between an organ and the *da Vinci* instrument, this work integrates a 3D reconstruction from pre-operative CT/MRI scans with a nonlinear finite element model (FEM) using the multi-resolution approach in [3].

---

[1] Corresponding Author: D A Wang, Dept. of Biosurgery and Surgical Technology, 10th Floor QEQM Building, St Mary's Hospital, Praed St, London W2 1NY, UK; E-mail: dorothy.a.wang@imperial.ac.uk

The model is then deformed using data corresponding to the movements of the *da Vinci* instrument.

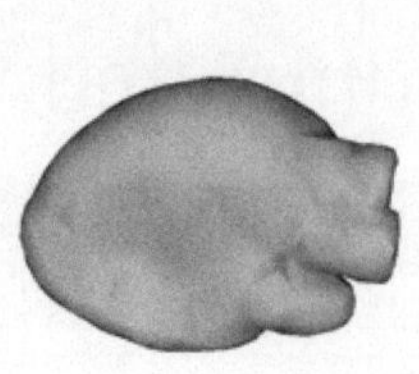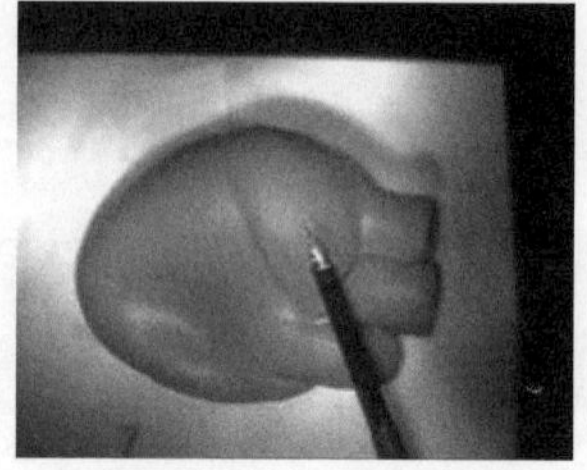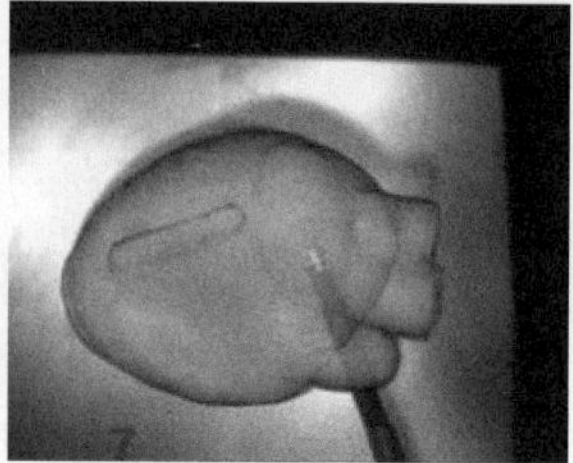

Figure 1. Illustrations of the 3D reconstruction model, the first video frame in the sequence and the overlay of the 3D model registered with the video frame.

Preliminary experiments have been carried out on a phantom heart model manufactured by Limbs & Things [4]. A video sequence of the heart being probed using a *da Vinci* instrument was captured. The 3D reconstructed model of the heart phantom was manually registered to the first frame of the video sequence using a rigid transformation (Figure 1).

A camera calibration and a video-based instrument-camera calibration technique were implemented for the *da Vinci* system as presented in [5]. The instrument-camera calibration determined the transformation between the *da Vinci* coordinate system and the camera coordinate system that was defined during the camera calibration.

The position of the tool tip during the interaction was determined by applying forward kinematics to the collected instrument data. These coordinates were computed with respect to the *da Vinci* coordinate frame. To establish how these positions relate to the virtual 3D heart model, they were converted into camera coordinates using the previously computed *da Vinci* to camera transformation. Any changes in camera pose were taken into account and applied accordingly.

The positions of the instrument with respect to the camera coordinate frame were used to calculate the force of the interaction between the tool and the tissue. The 3D heart surface model was used to build a tetrahedral mesh through an automatic tetrahedral mesh generator [6] to be integrated with a nonlinear FEM to produce a volumetric soft tissue deformation. Inputting the force into the tetrahedral model enabled the reconstruction to be updated and deformed at each time interval. The input force has been generated by constraining the coordinates of the tip of the tool to the point of contact on the surface of the heart model. Corresponding video frames from the simulation and the original sequence were then used to create overlays.

3. Results

Initial results indicate that tool-tissue interactions may be modelled using this offline methodology. Figure 2 illustrates a video frame from the true deformation sequence and the corresponding frame from the simulated deformation sequence. The overlay generated from superimposing the simulated frame onto the video frame is also presented.

The simulation of the interaction was suitable for the overall deformation, although it was found to have reduced accuracy when the deformation involved movement deep within the 3D model. Improving this accuracy depends on identifying the relevant parameters of the FEM model such as elasticity and the Poisson ratio for compressibility. In this work these variables were adjusted empirically.

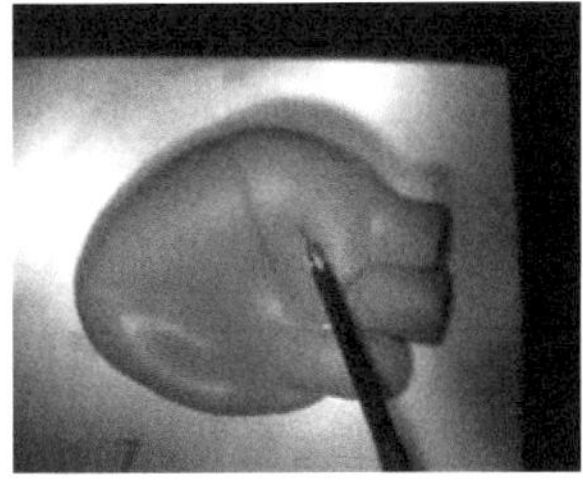 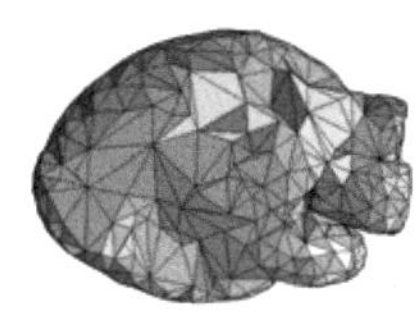 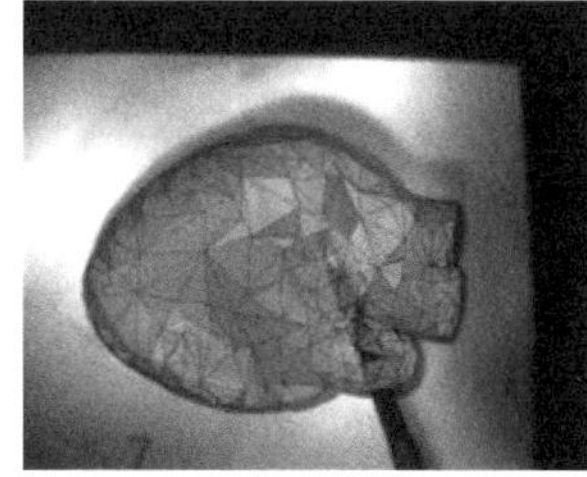

Figure 2. Video frame of the interaction between the *da Vinci* tool and the phantom heart, the rendering of the deformed model and the overlay of the corresponding simulated deformation onto the frame.

4. Discussion

The proposed model-based methodology holds the potential to combine a biomechanical model with information about tool-tissue interaction to dynamically update the augmented reality overlays. Adequate parameter values for this biomechanical model are vital in order to minimize latency and improve the performance of the deformation. The creation of a better quality tetrahedral mesh may allow for more robust deformations during tool-tissue interactions that consist of applying an increasingly large force on a single point along a defined direction. Further work will continue in this area, including real-time simulation of the interactions and overlay generation.

References

[1] Devernay F, Mourgues F, Coste-Maniere E. Towards Endoscopic Augmented Reality for Robotically Assisted Minimally Invasive Cardiac Surgery. Proc. MIAR 2001, pp16-20.
[2] Hattori A, Suzuki N, Hashizume M et al. A Robotic Surgery System (da Vinci) with Image Guided Function – System Architecture and Cholecystectomy Application. MMVR 2003.
[3] A. Faraci, F. Bello, and A. Darzi. Soft Tissue Deformation using a Nonlinear Hierarchical Finite Element Model with Real-Time Online Refinement. Proc. of MMVR 13, pages 137–144, 2005.
[4] Limbs & Things. http://www.limbsandthings.com/
[5] Wang DA, Bello F, Darzi A. Augmented Reality Provision in Robotically Assisted Minimally Invasive Surgery. Proc. CARS 2004.
[6] http://www.distene.com

Medicine Meets Virtual Reality 14
J.D. Westwood et al. (Eds.)
IOS Press, 2006

Physically Accurate Mesh Simulation in a Laparoscopic Hernia Surgery Simulator

Xiuzhong Wang, Yunhe Shen and Venkat Devarajan [1]
Electrical Engineering, University of Texas at Arlington

Abstract. In this paper we use the 2D angular spring based mass-spring-damper (AMSD) model to simulate the plastic mesh in a laparoscopic hernia surgery simulator. We propose a physically based method to systematically derive the optimal parameters of the 2D AMSD model. While the traditional 2D MSD model lacks resistance against bending, the 2D AMSD model with optimized parameters can provide correct bending resistance as well as stretching resistance. The simulated mesh is demonstrated to be much more realistic.

Keywords. Mass-spring-damper Model, Parameter Optimization, Angular Spring, Physical Accuracy, Surgery Simulation

1. Introduction

In a laparoscopic hernia surgery, the surgeon makes small incisions and inserts a miniature video camera and surgical instruments through tubes. He operates while watching a television monitor. He first locates and pulls the hernial sac back into the abdominal cavity, exposing the defect in the abdominal wall. Then he covers this weakened portion with a plastic mesh. Finally, he staples the mesh onto the abdominal wall, taking advantage of the natural pressure of the abdomen to secure the repair and promote healing.

The advantage of laparoscopy from the patients's point of view is that only the smallest incisions are required. However, this approach is more difficult for surgeons to perform successfully than the traditional open surgery. Because the surgeon works 'remotely' with these instruments and is guided only by what he sees on a monitor, he has less control than otherwise. Thus, laparoscopy requires extensive and specialized training. A virtual reality based surgery simulator is a potential answer for this need.

In the laparoscopic hernia surgery simulator, the simulation of the plastic mesh is very crucial. During a real surgery procedure, the mesh is rolled into a cylinder by hand, then inserted into the abdominal area where it unrolls itself. The plastic mesh can be modeled by a 2D mass-spring-damper (MSD) model. However, the traditional 2D MSD model provides too weak a resistance against bending [5] and it flattens out very slowly. In our previous work [5], we applied preload on the springs to provide correct bending resistance. The mesh is much more responsive but undesired boundary effects arise because of the preload. In this paper, we use the 2D angular spring based MSD (AMSD)

---

[1]Correspondence to: Venkat Devarajan, Electrical Engineering, University of Texas at Arlington, Arlington TX, 76010. Tel.: +1 817 272 3485; Fax: +1 817 272 2253; E-mail: venkat@uta.edu.

model [1][2][3] and optimize its parameters by viewing the mesh as an isotropic plate to achieve physically accurate simulation. Note that our parameter optimization method is different from those in [2][3] where the relationship between the parameters and mesh geometry of the model and the material properties of the real object was not addressed, and it is also different from that in [6] where the relationship was not explicitly obtained.

2. Parameter Optimization for the 2D AMSD Model

The 2D AMSD model of the plastic mesh is constructed on equilateral triangle meshes (Fig. 1(a)) by assigning masses to the vertices, structural springs to the edges of the triangles and angular springs between opposite vertices of each pair of triangles sharing an edge. Note that the angular spring, which is used to produce bending resistance, is different from the flexion spring in the traditional MSD model. The angular spring is a more abstract spring. It provides force perpendicular to the corresponding triangle at its two vertices to resist the change of the dihedral angle between adjacent triangles. Since the internal force must be balanced, we assume that the angular spring also produces force on the two vertices of the common edge so that the resultant force and torque the angular spring exerts on the two triangles are zero. In Fig. 1(b), the angular spring between vertices B and H produces forces $\mathbf{F}_B$, $\mathbf{F}_H$, $\mathbf{F}_G$ and $\mathbf{F}_J$ at the four vertices. $\mathbf{F}_B$ and $\mathbf{F}_H$ are determined according to the dihedral angle change α and the geometry of the mesh. Since the meshes are symmetric, we have $\mathbf{F}_G = \mathbf{F}_J = -(\mathbf{F}_B + \mathbf{F}_H)/2$.

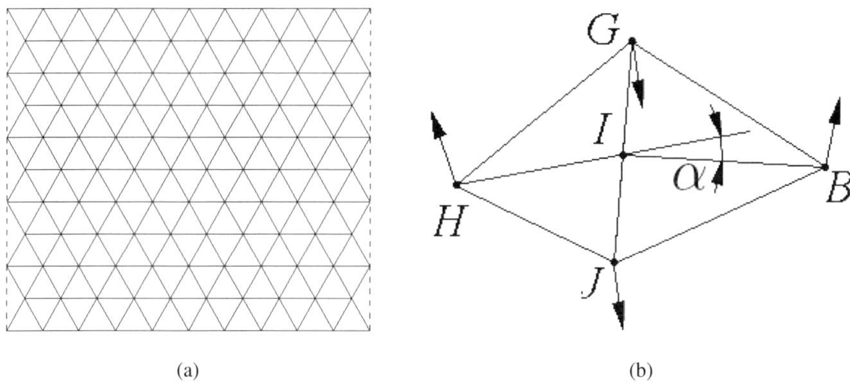

(a)　　　　　　　　　　　　　(b)

Figure 1. (a) Equilateral triangle meshes; (b) the forces that the angular spring produces on adjacent triangles.

2.1. Modeling Stretching Stiffness

Let the length of the side of the equilateral triangle mesh be U. By matching axisymmetric stretching of a continuum circular plate of isotropic material, we can obtain the Hooke's constant of the structural spring [5].

$$k = \frac{\sqrt{3}Eh}{3(1 - \nu)} \tag{1}$$

where E is the Young's modulus of the plate material, ν is the Poisson constant and h is the depth of the plate.

2.2. Modeling Bending Stiffness

Similar to our previous work [5], we match axisymmetric bending of a circular plate for accurate modeling of bending stiffness. According to the elasticity theory of plates [4], when an isotropic circular plate is bent by moments uniformly distributed along its edge, it deforms into a parabolic surface, which can be approximated by a spherical cap [5].

For the AMSD model to be physically accurate, it should also approximately bend into a spherical cap under axisymmetric bending. Let the bending curvature of the plate and the model be ρ. Figure 2(a) shows a structural spring between vertices B and J and the corresponding great circle. Since the neutral plane of the plate has no strain under axisymmetric bending, arc $\overset{\frown}{BJ}$ should not change its length, i.e. $\overset{\frown}{BJ} = U$. Then $\gamma = U\rho$ and the displacement of the structural spring is

$$u = \frac{2}{\rho} \sin \frac{U\rho}{2} - U \tag{2}$$

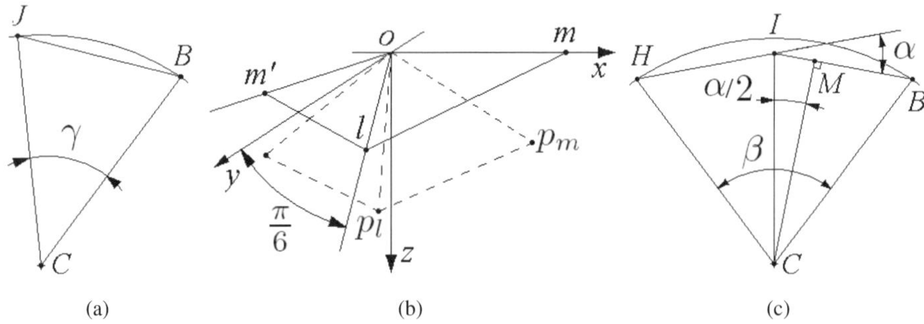

Figure 2. (a) The great circle passing through a structural spring; (b) the displacements of the vertices of adjacent triangles; (c) the great circle passing through two opposite vertices of adjacent triangles.

We restrict to use linear springs. Thus, the elastic energy of the structural spring is

$$W_s(\rho) = \frac{\sqrt{3}Eh}{6(1-\nu)}\left(\frac{2}{\rho} \sin \frac{U\rho}{2} - U\right)^2 \tag{3}$$

where the subscript s indicates the structural spring.

According to [4,5], the bending energy of the plate corresponding to one triangle of the AMSD model is

$$E_T(\rho) = (1+\nu)DA\rho^2 = \frac{\sqrt{3}(1+\nu)DU^2}{4}\rho^2 \tag{4}$$

where the subscript T denotes the triangle mesh, $D = Eh^3/(12(1-\nu^2))$ is the flexural stiffness of the plate and $A = \sqrt{3}U^2/4$ is the area of the triangle.

Since each triangle has three structural springs and angular springs and each of these springs are shared between two triangles, the bending energy of the AMSD model corresponding to one triangle is $W_T(\rho) = 3(W_a(\rho) + W_s(\rho))/2$, where $W_a(\rho)$ is the energy function of the angular spring with respect to the axisymmetric bending curvature.

The model and the plate should have the same bending stiffness. Therefore, $W_T(\rho) = E_T(\rho)$, from which we can obtain

$$W_a(\rho) = \frac{\sqrt{3}(1+\nu)DU^2}{6}\rho^2 - \frac{\sqrt{3}Eh}{6(1-\nu)}\left(\frac{2}{\rho}\sin\frac{U\rho}{2} - U\right)^2 \tag{5}$$

Next, we are going to derive the force function $F_a(\rho)$ of the angular spring. Let the x-y-z Cartesian coordinate system be aligned with the equilateral triangle meshes so that one vertex of a triangle coincides with the origin of the coordinate system, another vertex (m) of the triangle falls on the x-axis and the third (vertex l) falls in the first quadrant of the x-y plane (Fig. 2(b)). When the AMSD model is axisymmetrically bent into a spherical cap tangent to the x-y plane, vertex m moves to p_m and its coordinates are

$$(x(\rho), y(\rho), z(\rho)) = \left(\frac{1}{\rho}\sin U\rho, 0, \frac{1}{\rho}(1 - \cos U\rho)\right) \tag{6}$$

Then, the tangent direction of the trajectory of vertex m is $\mathbf{t} = (U\rho\cos U\rho - \sin U\rho, 0, U\rho\sin U\rho + \cos U\rho - 1)$.

Similarly, the coordinates of vertex l are $\left(\frac{1}{2\rho}\sin U\rho, \frac{\sqrt{3}}{2\rho}\sin U\rho, \frac{1}{\rho}(1 - \cos U\rho)\right)$. Therefore, the normal of the triangle is $\mathbf{n} = (\sqrt{3}\sin U\rho(1 - \cos U\rho), \sin U\rho(1 - \cos U\rho), -\sqrt{3}\sin^2 U\rho)$, which is also the direction (or opposite direction) of the resistant force from the angular spring.

The angle between vector $\mathbf{n}$ and $\mathbf{t}$ should be a function of curvature ρ. We denote it by $\theta(\rho)$. We have $\cos\theta(\rho) = \mathbf{t} \cdot \mathbf{n}/(\|\mathbf{t}\|\|\mathbf{n}\|)$. Then the energy of the angular spring, which is the summation of the work of its four associated forces, is

$$W_a(\rho) = \int_0^\rho F_a(\kappa)\sqrt{\left(x'(\kappa)\right)^2 + \left(z'(\kappa)\right)^2}\cos\theta(\kappa)d\kappa \tag{7}$$

Thus

$$F_a(\rho) = \frac{W_a'(\rho)}{\sqrt{\left(x'(\rho)\right)^2 + \left(z'(\rho)\right)^2}\cos\theta(\rho)} \tag{8}$$

Further, we are going to derive the force function of the angular spring in terms of the dihedral angle change α. Figure 2(c) shows the great circle passing through the two opposite vertices B and H (also see Fig. 1(b)). $\angle BIH$ is the dihedral angle because the meshes are equilateral triangles, and its complementary angle is the change of the dihedral angle relative to the rest state of the model. Since there is no strain on the neutral plane of the plate, the length of the arc on the great circle between two opposite vertices of two adjacent triangles of the model should not change either. Therefore, the angle it faces to the center of the sphere is $\beta = \sqrt{3}U\rho$. Let CM be perpendicular to BI. Then M should be the center of the corresponding triangle mesh. Thus, $BM = 2IM$. Therefore, we obtain $\beta = \alpha + 2\arctan(2\tan(\alpha/2))$. Further, we obtain

$$\rho = \frac{\sqrt{3}}{3U}\alpha + \frac{2\sqrt{3}}{3U}\arctan(2\tan\frac{\alpha}{2}) \tag{9}$$

From (8) and (9), when α is small, by Taylor's expansion, we can obtain

$$F_a(\rho(\alpha)) = \frac{Eh^3}{6(1-\nu)U}\alpha + O(\alpha^3) \approx \frac{Eh^3}{6(1-\nu)U}\alpha \approx \frac{Eh^3}{6(1-\nu)U}\sin\alpha \qquad (10)$$

3. Validation

First, we simulate a $32\,\mathrm{cm}\times24\,\mathrm{cm}$ plate with depth $0.1\,\mathrm{cm}$ ($E = 1.0 \times 10^7\,\mathrm{N/cm^2}$, $\nu = 0.3$) clamped horizontally at one short end and loaded by a force $F = 1\,\mathrm{N}$ at one corner on the other end. We test both the AMSD model and the MSD model with preload [5] and compare the deformations with that obtained by ANSYS (an FEM software package). The deformations are shown in Fig. 3(a), in which the top surface is the deformation obtained by FEM, the middle surface is the deformation of the AMSD model and the bottom surface is the deformation of the MSD model with preload. The root mean square errors of the AMSD model and the MSD model with preload are $0.080\,\mathrm{cm}$ and $0.082\,\mathrm{cm}$ respectively. Thus, the two models can achieve approximately the same accuracy.

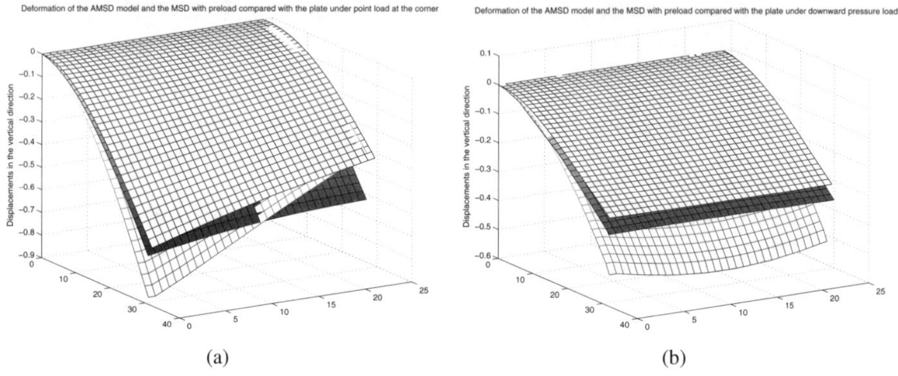

(a)   (b)

Figure 3. (a) Comparison of the results from the AMSD model (middle gray), the MSD model with preload (bottom plain) and the FEM (top plain) under point load; (b) comparison of the results from the AMSD model (middle gray), the MSD model with preload (bottom plain) and the FEM (top plain) under pressure load.

Second, we simulate the clamped plate under pressure $P = 0.002\,\mathrm{N/cm^2}$ (downward). The deformations are shown in Fig. 3(b), in which the top surface is the deformation obtained by FEM, the middle surface is the deformation of the AMSD model and the bottom surface is the deformation of the MSD model with preload. For the AMSD model and the MSD model with preload, the root mean square errors are $0.04\,\mathrm{cm}$ and $0.09\,\mathrm{cm}$ respectively. Again, we can see that the AMSD model with optimized parameters is very accurate, which validates our parameter optimization scheme.

4. Simulation

We start with a spirally rolled 2D AMSD model for the plastic mesh in a laparoscopic inguinal hernia scenario as shown in Fig. 4(a). When the simulation starts, the AMSD model begins to unroll itself quickly (Fig. 4(b) and Fig. 4(c)). Then the mesh is manipulated by two instruments to cover the defective area (Fig. 4(d)). Finally, the mesh is stapled at a proper position. The AMSD model with the optimized parameters allows very realistic mesh behavior.

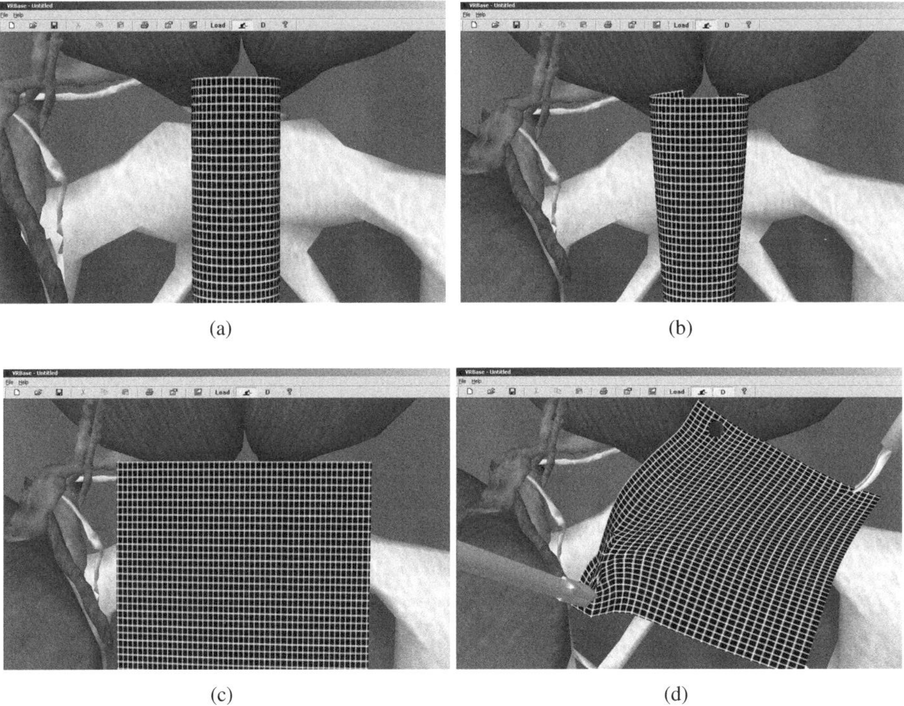

(a)

(b)

(c)

(d)

Figure 4. Initially rolled mesh (a), partially unrolled mesh (b), completely unrolled mesh (c) and mesh manipulating and stapling (d) in a laparoscopic inguinal hernia surgery scenario.

5. Conclusion

In this paper, we have been able to derive optimal parameters for structural springs and angular springs of the 2D AMSD model by matching a continuum plate under axisymmetric stretching and bending. The 2D AMSD model with optimized parameters is shown to be able to simulate the real plate with very high physical accuracy, which results in much more realistic simulation of the mesh placement procedure in the laparoscopic inguinal hernia surgery simulator.

References

[1] D. Baraff and A. Witkin, Large Steps in Cloth Simulation, *Proc. SIGGRAPH'98*, pp. 43–54.

[2] R. Bridson and S. Marino and R. Fedkiw, Simulation of Clothing with Folds and Wrinkles, *Proc. 2003 ACM SIGGRAPH/Eurographics Symposium on Computer animation*, pp. 28–36.

[3] E. Grinspun and A. N. Hirani and M. Desbrun and P. Schröder, Discrete Shells, *SCA '03: Proc. 2003 ACM SIGGRAPH/Eurographics Symposium on Computer animation*, pp. 62–67.

[4] V. Panc, *Theory of Elastic Plates*, Noordhoff International Publishing Leyden, 1975.

[5] X. Wang and V. Devarajan, 1D and 2D Structured Mass-spring Model with Preload, *The Visual Computer*, vol. 21 (2005), no. 7, pp. 429–448.

[6] A. Maciel and R. Boulic and D. Thalmann, Deformable Tissue Parameterized by Properties of Real Biological Tissue, *Proc. International Symposium on Surgery Simulation and Soft Tissue Modeling*, pp. 74–87, 2003.

Medicine Meets Virtual Reality 14
J.D. Westwood et al. (Eds.)
IOS Press, 2006

3D Surface Accuracy of CAD Generated Skull Defect Contour

RJ WINDER [a,1], W MCKNIGHT [a], I MCRITCHIE [a], D MONTGOMERY [b], J WULF [c]
[a] University of Ulster, United Kingdom
[b] Queen's University, [c] University of Lübeck

Abstract. The creation of a satisfactory cosmetic outcome in the repair of cranial defects relies on manual skill. However, computer aided design is gaining acceptance in the creation of custom cranial implants. The purpose of this work is to demonstrate the accuracy of a CAD generated skull defect contours using 3D difference maps. 3D multi-slice CT scanning was carried out on a life size plastic skull. Surface models were generated of the original skull and of temporofrontal and parietal defects. Surface contours were interpolated towards the centre of the defect from the edges where it was blended. The CAD contour deviation ranged from 0.0 mm to 2.0 mm with 80% of the total defect area less than 0.66 mm as measured by difference maps. CAD techniques can be used to produce contours for the repair of cranial defects with minimum deviation from the original skull contour. This enables accurate design and production of cranial implants.

Keywords. CAD, cranioplasty, 3D surface accuracy, virtual surgery, NURBS

Purpose

The creation of a satisfactory cosmetic outcome in the repair of large cranial defects mainly relies on manual skill. Computer aided design (CAD) and computer assisted manufacture (CAM) are gaining acceptance in the creation of custom made cranial implants (1-2). Previously, mirror imaging has been used to create a contour for a defect from the contra-lateral side of the head. However, this may be limited for patients with an asymmetrical skull or where the defect crosses the skull mid-line. Computer assisted design of a skull defect repair has been successfully implemented in a number of centres (3). The accuracy of CAD implants is generally measured in simple linear terms using distance as the main indicator of fit (4). However, no data exists as to the accuracy of a 3D CAD generated contour for the repair of large skull defects. We have previously demonstrated the efficacy of CAD/CAM in virtual neurosurgical planning (5) and have subsequently developed a methodology whereby the 3D surface contour of the implant may be accurately assessed. The purpose of this work is to demonstrate how accurate CAD generated skull repair can be achieved for two commonly occurring defects.

---

[1] Corresponding author: Dr John Winder, Room 15J13, School of Health Sciences, University of Ulster, Shore Road, Newtownabbey, Co. Antrim, BT37 0QB, UK; E-mail rj:.winder@ulster.ac.uk.

1. Methods

3D volumetric multi-slice CT scanning was carried out using a Siemens 16 slice Volume Zoom CT scanner on a life size plastic skull. CT imaging parameters were as follows; slice thickness = 0.75 mm, pixel size = 0.457 mm, 176 mA and 0.5 second rotation time. Two common skull defects, a large temporofrontal and a parietal, which crossed the skull mid-line, were created in the original surface rendered CT data using 3D image editing. Figure 1 shows the simulated defects in which the bone has been deleted in the skull to simulate typical defects. Surface models (STL format) of the original skull and the two defects were generated using Mimics software (www.materialise.com, Leuven, Belgium). A CT number threshold was applied to segment the plastic skull. Reverse engineering using CAD software (CopyCAD, V6.004, Delcam, UK) was applied to generate an accurate contour of the defect from which a custom made titanium or acrylic implant may be generated. The CAD contour was generated using non-uniform rational B-splines (NURBS). To generate a suitable NURBS surface, contour profiles of the undamaged skull were produced and interpolated across the defect using the bone surface around the edge as a starting point. The NURBS surface was interpolated towards the centre of the defect from all directions where it was blended with the surface from the opposite edge. The resulting NURBS surface was compared to the original skull surface to determine how well the CAD generated surface preformed. A colour coded difference map was generated where the distance of one surface from the other was computed and presented as a colour coded map.

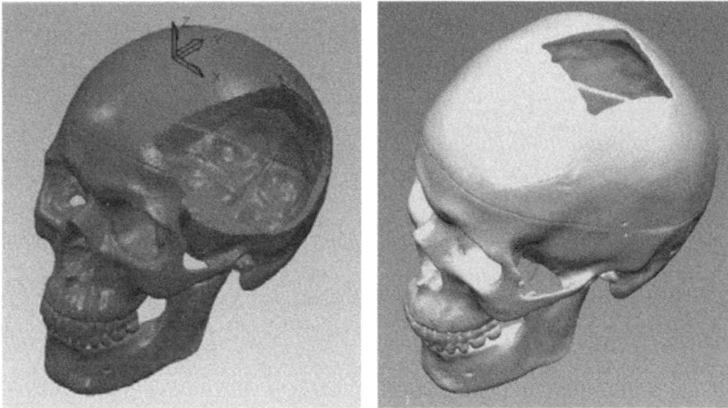

Figure 1 showing computer generated temporofrontal and parietal defects

2. Results & Discussion

Figure 2 shows the CAD generated contour for the large temporofrontal defect. Also, shown in figure 2 is the difference map for the CAD contour compared to the original skull surface. The dark areas represented deviation of the repair contour of between 1 and 2 mm, whilst the lighter areas represent deviations of less than 1 mm. Note that there is no deviation at the edge of the repair as the NURBS surface uses the original skull to engineer the repair, therefore the two are coincident in this region. The CAD contour deviation, for the temporofrontal defect, ranged from 0.0 mm at the edge of the defect to a maximum of 2.0 mm near the centre. 80% of the total contour area deviated less than 0.66 mm from the desired surface. Similar results were obtained for the parietal defect.

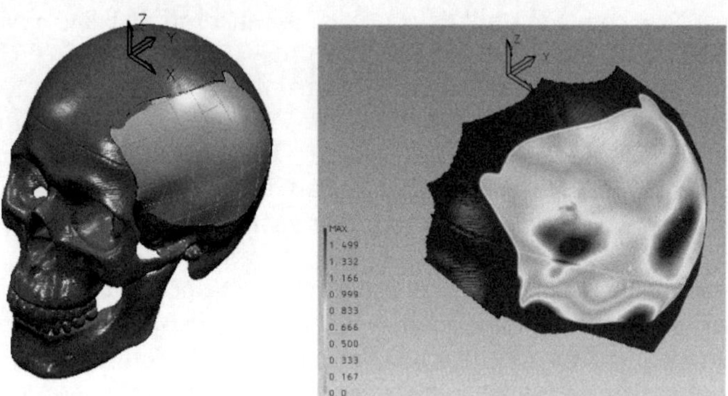

Figure 2 showing a CAD generated repair and 3D contour difference map.

CAD of skull contours provides a successful way of creating a good cosmetic outcome for the repair of skull defects. The contour is blended from the patient's own skull and conforms well to complex surfaces. This is apparent around the supra-orbital ridge and the zygomatic arch where deviations of 0.2 – 0.4 mm were observed. Implants designed using this technology will have an excellent fit. This may have the effect of reducing time in theatre as implants will not require physical manipulation and may be fitted more rapidly. The maximum deviation observed was not greater than 2.0 mm and this may be further reduced with some manual intervention by the operator.

3. Conclusion

CAD techniques can be used to produce accurate 3D contours for the repair of cranial defects with minimum deviation from the original skull contour. This enables accurate design and production of custom made cranial implants.

References

[1]   Hoffmann B, Sepehrnia A.   Taylored implants for alloplastic cranioplasty-clinical and surgical considerations. *Acta Neurochir* 93 (2005), 127-9.
[2]   Dean D, Min K-J, Bond A. Computer aided design of large-format prefabricated cranial plates. Journal of Craniofacial Surgery, 14 (2003), 819-832.
[3]   Hieu LC, Bohez E, Vander Sloten J, Oris P, Phien HN, Vatcharaporn E, Binh PH. Design and manufacture of cranioplasty implants by 3-axis CNC milling. *Technol Health Care* 10 (2002), 413-23.
[4]   Joffe J, Nicoll S, Richards R, Linney, A, Harris M. Validation of computer assisted manufacture of titanium plates for cranioplasty. *Int J Oral Maxillofac Surg* 28 (1999), 309-13.
[5]   Winder J, McRitchie I, McKnight W, Cooke S. Virtual surgical planning and CAD/CAM in the treatment of cranial defects. *Stud Health Technol Inform.* 111 (2005), 599-601.

Medicine Meets Virtual Reality 14
J.D. Westwood et al. (Eds.)
IOS Press, 2006

"Virtual Unwrapping"
of a Mummified Hand

RJ WINDER [a1], W GLOVER [b], T GOLZ [c], J WULF [c], S MCCLURE [a], H CAIRNS [d],
M ELLIOTT [d]
*[a] University of Ulster, [b] Ulster Museum, [c] University of Lübeck,
[d] Musgrave Park Hospital*

Abstract. The purpose of this work is to demonstrate the feasibility of medical
virtual reality technologies in the investigation of a mummified hand. The Ulster
Museum obtained the mummy hand, which originated from Thebes, without any
identifying information. The mummified hand was investigated using
conventional X-ray and 3D multi-slice Computed Tomography (CT). Imaging
revealed a range of fractures of the wrist, metacarpals and phalanges whilst 3D CT
demonstrated internal structures using volume rendering. The absence of any
features of bone healing at the fracture sites would imply that they occurred just
prior to death or in the mummified state possibly during excavation. Conventional
X-ray imaging indicated that the hand, although small, was likely to have
originated from an adult. Medical imaging and virtual reality display will enable
us to produce a rapid prototyped model using fused deposition technology.
Therefore, further paleopathological research can be performed on the replica
without the need to handle the original specimen.

Keywords. Virtual, mummified hand, 3D CT, anthropology, FDM

1. Purpose

The purpose of this work is to demonstrate the feasibility of medical virtual reality
technologies in the investigation of a mummified hand. Medical imaging and VR
display has been used in the past to reveal internal mummified structures in a range of
objects (1). This work was to attempt to determine additional information regarding
the identification of a mummified hand without disturbing the wrapping of linen
bandages and removing any of its soft tissues.

2. Background

The Ulster Museum obtained the wrapped left hand of an Egyptian mummy, which
originated from Thebes, Egypt, without any identifying information. It was donated to
the Museum by a member of the Macoun family who were well known in Northern
Ireland and had been in linen manufacturing since the 1880s. It was part of a donation
of some 50 objects in total. It is no surprise to find an object from Egypt turning up in

[1] Corresponding author: Dr John Winder, Room 15J13, School of Health Sciences, University of Ulster,
Shore Road, Newtownabbey, Co. Antrim, BT37 0QB, UK; E-mail rj.winder@ulster.ac.uk.

the hands of a linen trader in Belfast as the mummified objects were often wrapped in the finest linen material.

The preparation of bodies for mummification was very thorough and involved the following steps,

- The body was cleaned and dried out by packing the cavity with Natron (this is a preservative material based on sodium carbonate)
- The skin was painted several times with perfumed oils to keep it supple
- The abdomen and chest were filled out with pieces of resin-soaked cloth or sawdust to create a life-like appearance
- The eyes were often replaced with small rolls of linen
- The nails were stained with henna which gave them a reddish colour
- Often a ring was placed on the little finger of the left hand.

The hand was wrapped in bandages as shown in Figure 1. An examination of the wrappings of the hand and a consideration of its provenance allows us to make the following observations. The hand has the fingers and thumb wrapped separately and the bandages are in alternate bands of faded red and white. It is known from the 21st Dynasty onwards, circa 1085 BC, that the body before it was wrapped in bandages was painted with ochre mixed with gum arabic; yellow for women and red for men. However, this colouring was not extended to the outer bandages and there is no evidence to suggest a correlation between the sex of a mummy and the manner in which its hands were wrapped. In Ptolemaic and Roman times mummification became very elaborate.

There were a number of unanswered questions about the hand. What age was the person from whom it came? What social standing were they? What was the approximate date of mummification? Was the hand removed before or after death?

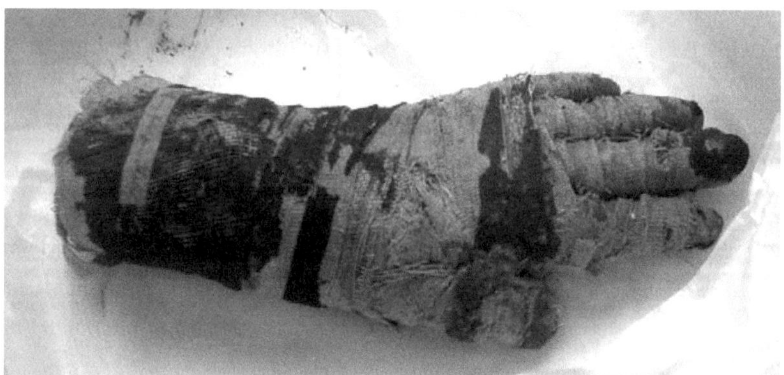

Figure 1. Showing the mummified hand wrapped in linen

3. Methods

The mummified hand was investigated using conventional X-ray imaging and 3D multi-slice Computed Tomography (CT) using a Siemens Somatom Sensation 16. The 3D CT was acquired with a slice thickness of 0.75 mm and a pixel size of 0.27 mm. Firstly, the conventional X-rays were compared to reference hand X-ray images (2) to determine the age of the body from which the hand originated. Secondly, CT number measurements were made on individual tissues to determine their origin. These figures were compared with CT numbers of tissues identified by Ruhli et al, 2004 (1). Thirdly, commercial 3D visualisation software was used to segment and render both soft and hard tissue structures. Finally, a rapid prototyped (RP) fused deposition model was built using the FDM 3000 system from Stratasys®. This system uses a soluble support structure which allowed safe removal of the support structures without damaging the model.

4. Results and Discussion

Often bandages of different colours were arranged in quite complex geometrical patterns and often the bodies had the fingers wrapped separately. For these reasons it is likely that the mummified hand dates to the Ptolemaic (332-30 BC), or Roman period and that it was the hand of a wealthy person since this degree of mummification was only afforded to rich members of ancient Egyptian society.

The specimen, which was a left hand, included a few centimetres of the distal radius and ulna together with the carpus and all five digits. There was excellent preservation of mineralisation. The physeal plates were fused and the overall development was that of a skeletally mature individual (2). The conventional X-ray revealed a range of fractures of the wrist, metacarpals and phalanges. 3D CT also demonstrated the fractures using volume rendering and also demonstrated more fractures than were apparent on the original conventional x-ray. Comminuted fractures were present through the distal radius and ulna. Further fractures in the first three metacarpals and the proximal phalanx of the middle finger were also demonstrated. The absence of any features of bone healing at the fracture sites would imply that they occurred either just prior to death or in the mummified state possibly during excavation. There is no radiographic evidence of inflammatory or degenerative arthritis or of a focal destructive bone lesion. This may indicate that the person was young or was not a manual worker. The conclusion drawn about the fractures within the hand is that they occurred after death. It is possible that a full mummy was broken up after its initial discovery. The value of the individual parts would have been greater than the mummy as a whole artefact.

Figure 2 shows a coronal reformat indicating the preservation of internal hard tissue structures, although soft tissues like fat, muscle and tendons were less well preserved. Table 1 shows CT number measurements for internal tissues and other substances present. There is a significant amount of air within the hand as indicated by

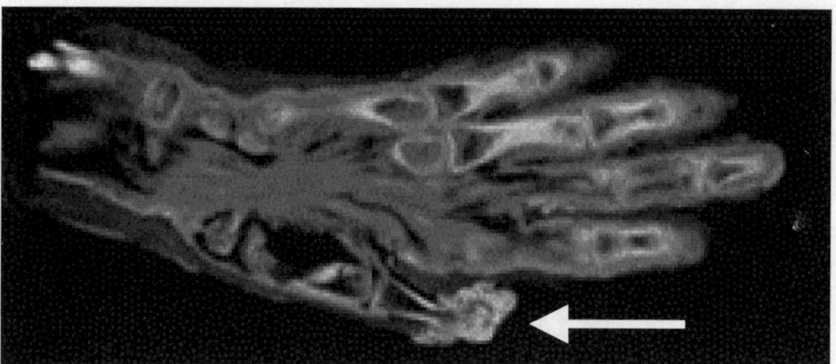

Figure 2. Showing a coronal multi-planar reformat

the black areas within both the bone and soft tissue. The presence of air has biased the CT number ranges quoted in table 1. It is interesting to note that the CT number reduced, on average, from the phalanges to the carpal bones. It can be seen from the photograph in figure 1 that the thumb looks relatively short. On internal inspection it was revealed that the top of the thumb was missing. It had been replaced by another material that had a higher density than most of the cortical bone present in the fingers. It was also quite uniform in appearance. Careful investigation of the material, by measuring its CT number revealed, it had a range of +1000 to +1300. This is equivalent to the dense cortical bone present. The CT number range was similar to a ceramic toe prosthesis found in another specimen and also to plaster (3). It was not possible to accurately identify the material without removing the linen covering, but we believe a prosthesis was made to correct the broken thumb.

Figure 3 shows a "virtual unwrapping" of the hand by removing both the linen wrapping and soft tissue. The method of unwrapping included identification of a CT number threshold which was applied to the CT data volume. Application of the threshold removed most of the linen and soft tissue. However, further manual editing was performed by setting specific pixels to a value of air (-1024). This was carried out on a slice-by-slice basis to delete fragments of data that were not successfully deleted by thresholding. The surface rendering in figure 3 shows the individual fingers clearly, the gross fracture at the wrist and the prosthesis on the thumb.

Table 1. CT number ranges for tissues/substances within the hand

Tissue / substance	CT number range
Linen covering	-820 to −720
External soft tissue	-800 to −530
Internal soft tissue	-120 to +300
Bone	0 to +1200
Thumb prosthesis	+1000 to +1300

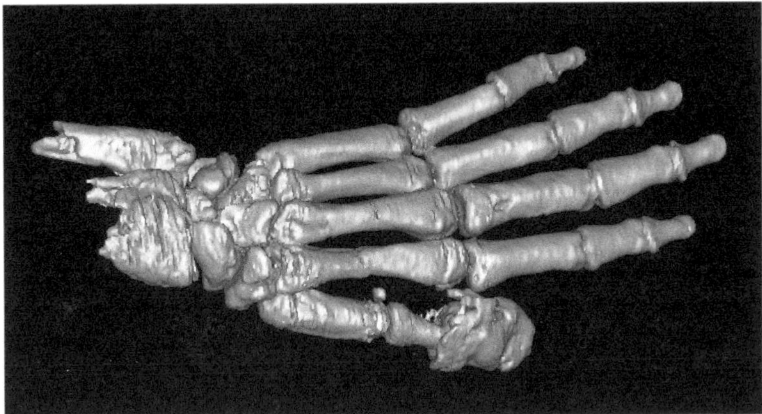

Figure 3. Showing "unwrapped" surface rendering of the bones

Finally, the 3D surface rendered data was surface modelled and the data saved as an "STL" file. This data format was useful as it enabled the original CT slices to be imported to CAD software for the production of a rapid prototyped fused deposition model (FDM). Figure 4 shows the FDM model which took 24 hours to build at a cost of 750 Euro. The metacarpal fractures and thumb repair are clearly visible. In addition, the solid model can provide a haptic experience of the mummy hand. Our findings support the investigation of other authors [4,5] whereby VR in combination with RP technologies provide useful tools to improve research on paleopathological and paleoanatomical specimens by reducing the chance of irreversibly destroying them.

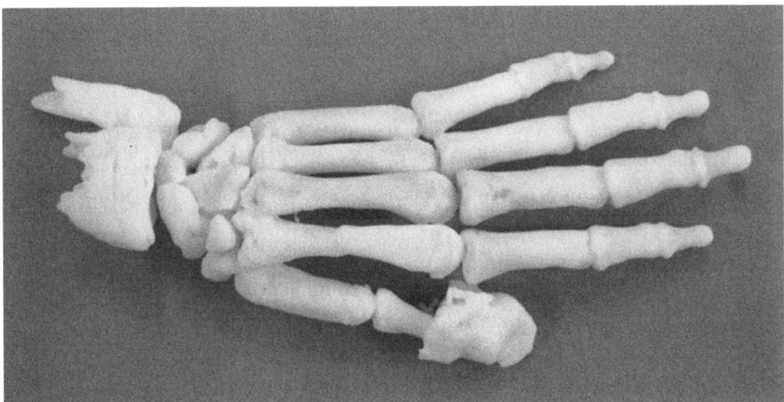

Figure 4. Showing fused deposition model of the mummy hand bones

5. Conclusion

Medical imaging and VR display has been used to investigate a mummified hand. Conventional X-ray imaging indicated that the hand, although small, was likely to have originated from an adult. This procedure has enabled us to produce a rapid prototyped model using fused deposition technology. Final conclusions lead us to speculate that the hand was removed from a mummy from the Ptolemaic or Roman period and was probably from a high social standing. The hand was likely removed from a complete mummy after excavation.

References

[1]   Ruhli FJ, Chhem RK, Boni T. Diagnostic paleradiology of mummified tissue: interpretation and pitfalls. *Journal of the American College of Radiology* 55 (2004), 218-227.
[2]   *Radiographic Atlas of Skeletal Development of the Hand and Wrist.* 2nd Edition. William Walter Greulich, S Idell Pyle, Stanford University Press 1959.
[3]   Sigmund G, Minas M. The Trier mummy: radiological and histological findings. *European Radiology* 12 (2002), 1854-1862.
[4]   Recheis W, Weber GW, Schafer K, Prossinger H, Knapp R, Seidler H, zur Nedden D. New methods and techniques in anthropology. *Coll Antropol* 23 (1999), 495-509.
[5]   Hjalgrim H, Lynnerup N, Liversage M, Rosenklint A. Stereolithography: potential applications in anthropological studies. *Am J Phys Anthropol* 97 (1995), 329-33.

Medicine Meets Virtual Reality 14
J.D. Westwood et al. (Eds.)
IOS Press, 2006

583

A Haptics Based Simulator for Laparoscopic Pyeloplasty

Haisheng Wu [a,1], Craig Hourie [a], Roy Eagleson [a] and Rajni Patel [a]

[a] *Canadian Surgical Technologies & Advanced Robotics (CSTAR),*
339 Windermere Rd., London, Ontario, Canada, N6A 5A5; and
Department of Electrical and Computer Engineering,
University of Western Ontario, London, ON., Canada, N6H 5B9

Abstract. We present a methodology for modeling the surgical procedures involved in robotics-assisted Pyeloplasty, which is a minimally invasive surgical procedure for correcting a kidney ureteropelvic junction obstruction. The simulator facilitates surgical training of laparoscopic pyeloplasty by providing both visual and haptic feedback to the trainee.

Keywords. Haptics, visualization, pyeloplasty, minimally invasive surgery simulator

1. Introduction

Unlike conventional open pyeloplasty, robotics-assisted minimally invasive surgery (MIS) requires only a few small incisions. Through these incisions, a surgeon uses a set of remotely operated tools, including an endoscopic camera, clamps, sutures, and an ultrasonic scalpel to mobilize the renal pelvis and proximal ureter, and then remove the obstruction. While laparoscopic surgery has the advantage of reduced hospital stay, decreased postoperative pain, and faster healing for patients, it also has the limitation that performing laparoscopic procedures requires extensive training and experience on the part of surgeons [1].

The goal of the research described in this paper is to provide tools that surgeons can use to acquire such training for the specific case of pyeloplasty. In our knowledge, no comprehensive simulators exist for pyeloplasty and other similar procedures.

2. Related work

For the purpose of real-time soft tissue simulation incorporating realistic physical models several methods have been developed [2]. Recently, Basdogan et al. [3] have developed a haptics based simulator that involves inserting a catheter into the cystic duct using a pair of laparoscopic forceps. France et al. [4] have developed an intestine simulator based on a mass-spring model. Zhong et al. [5] have developed a pre-computed finite element

---

[1]Correspondence to: Haisheng Wu. Tel.: +1 519 685 8500 ext. 36492; Fax: +1 519 663 8401; E-mail: hwu25@uwo.ca.

method (FEM) for modeling soft tissue deformation. However, the forces generated with the last two approaches were only rendered visually without haptic feedback.

3. Methods and implementation

The experimental pyeloplasty simulator is composed of three components: The Haptic device interface, a 3D deformable visual model of the kidney and ureter, and a hyperelastic force model of the ureter.

3.1. Haptic device

Haptic input and output, including force and position information, are provided using the Pantograph, a 5 degrees of freedom (DOF) haptic device manufactured by Quanser (see Figure 1a). The haptic device can provide 5DOF input and output comprised by translation in x, y, z directions and orientation with pitch and roll.

3.2. Deformable tissue/organ model

In this paper, a 3D Graphic deformable tissue/organ model, including the renal pelvis, proximal ureter, aorta, and vena cava, are represented by smooth meshes wrapped with texture surfaces for visualization. All the meshes are generated by using a uniform 3D cubic B-spline interpolation algorithm. Given $(n + 1) \times (m + 1)$ control points, $P_{0,0}$ to $P_{n,m}$, the parametric B-spline point, $P(u, v)$ can be computed as follows:

$$P(u, v) = \sum_{i=\lfloor nu-2 \rfloor}^{\lceil nu+2 \rceil} \sum_{j=\lfloor mv-2 \rfloor}^{\lceil mv+2 \rceil} P_{ij} B(nu - i) B(mv - j) \tag{1}$$

where B is the cubic blending function. Note that the lower and upper limits of this loop prevent the calculation of B values that are definitely 0 since 3rd order cubic B-Splines only take into account at most 4 control points. However, Equation 1 only approximates the control points, where the splines do not pass through all the control points.

To interpolate the $(n + 1) \times (m + 1)$ control points, we can replace them with $(n + 3) \times (m+3)$ phantom control points (consider clamped end condition), as $P_{i,j} = MA_{i,j}$, where M is a coefficient matrix. The linear equations are solved using the Gaussian elimination approach so that the spline that approximate $A_{i,j}$ interpolates $P_{i,j}$.

3.3. Force model

When surgical tools interact with the simulated renal pelvis and proximal ureter, the tissue deformation can be very large due to hyperelasticity. The nonlinear biomechanical parameters of soft tissue are critical in this simulation. Recently, Farshad et al. [6] have reported the elastic properties of a fresh pig kidney. Based on the their results (see Figure 1b), a nonlinear force model is extracted by using cubic splines model as $\sigma = a\varepsilon^3 - b\varepsilon^2 + c\varepsilon + d$, where σ is stress, ε is strain, and a, b, c, d are coefficients. The surface area of laparoscopic clamp is about $15mm^2$, so the reflection force is usually less than 4.5N.

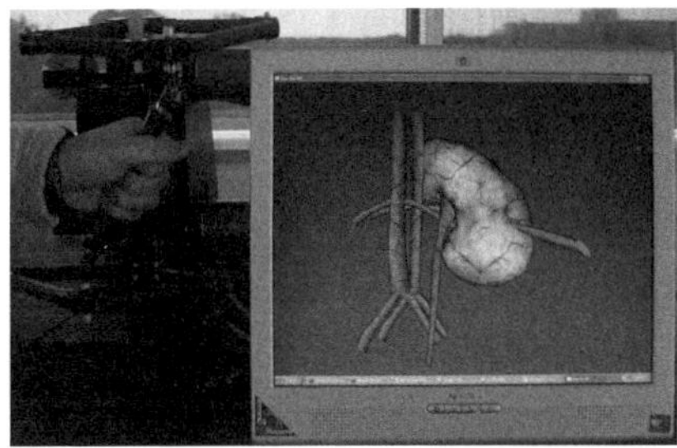

(a) Deformable graphic model and haptic device.

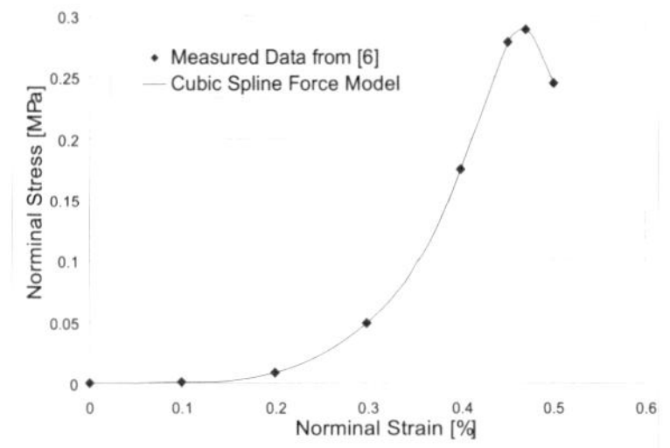

(b) Stress/strain curve caused by uni-axial compression on a pig kidney and the corresponding force model.

Figure 1. Deformable graphical model, haptic device and force model

The pyeloplasty simulator is implemented using C++ and the Reachin API on a PC platform with an Intel P4 2.8GHz CPU. The Reachin API offers a graphics rendering loop updated at 50Hz and a haptics rendering loop updated at $1K$Hz, as well as an interface with the Pantograph haptic device.

4. Concluding remarks

The simulator discussed in this paper allows surgeons to manipulate the ureter and kidney, including pulling and touching. This simulator can be used to expedite surgical training. Future work will focus on interactions with tissue while mobilizing the ureter.

Acknowledgements

This research was supported by the Ontario Research and Development Challenge Fund under grant 00-May-0709, and by an infrastructure grant from the Canada Foundation for Innovation awarded to the London Health Sciences Centre (CSTAR).

References

[1] S. Dad and E. Crawford. *Urologic Laparoscopy*. W.B. Saunders Co., Philadelphia, 1994.
[2] A. Liu, F. Tendick, K. Cleary, and C. Kaufmann. A survery of surgical simulation: Applications, Technology, and Education. *MIT Press* (12)(6), 2003.
[3] C. Basdogan, C. Ho, and M. Srinivasan: Virtual environment in medical training: Graphical and haptic simulation of laparoscopic common bile duct exploration. *IEEE/ASME Transactions on Mechatronics* (6) (3): 269-285, 2001.
[4] L. France, J. Lenoir, P. Meseure, and C. Chaillou. Simulation of a minimally invasive surgery of intestines. In *Virtual Reality International Conference* (VRIC-Laval Virtual), June, 2002.
[5] H. Zhong, M. Wakchowiak, and T. Peters. Enhanced pre-computed finite element models for surgical simulation. *Stud. Health Technol. Inform.*(111):622-628, 2005.
[6] M. Farshad, M. Barbezat, P. Flueler, F. Schmidlin, P. Graber and P. Niederer. Material characterization of the pig kidney in relation with the biomechanical analysis of renal trauma. *Journal of Biomechanics* (32), 417-425, 1999.

Medicine Meets Virtual Reality 14
J.D. Westwood et al. (Eds.)
IOS Press, 2006

Effects of Assembling Virtual Fixtures on Learning a Navigation Task

Bin Zheng [1,2], Alex Kuang [1], Frank Henigman[1], Shahram Payandeh [1], Alan Lomax[1],
Lee Swanström[2], Christine L. MacKenzie[1]

[1]Schoosl of Kinesiology and Engineering Science, Simon Fraser University, CANADA
[2] Minimally Invasive Surgery, Legacy Health System, Portland, Oregon, USA

Abstract: An approach to enhance navigation task performance is to integrate sensory guidance (virtual fixtures) into a virtual training system. To evaluate the effects of adding virtual fixtures to skill acquisition, 32 subjects were required to use a PHANToM   input device, to transport a virtual object through a computer generated 3-D graphic maze. Subjects practiced navigation under 4 conditions: the maze was augmented with either a graphic fixture (G), attractive force field (F), both graphic and force field (GF), or no (N) virtual fixture. Fifteen practice trials were given before subjects were transferred to a situation with no virtual fixtures. Results showed that the implementation of the force field assisted task performance during practice; however, it failed to show positive transfer effects. In contrast, adding a graphic fixture to the virtual maze helped subjects to define the optimal pathway throughout navigation, which facilitated skill acquisition.

Keywords: motor learning, virtual fixture, navigation, human-computer interaction, specificity hypothesis

1. Introduction:

Navigation is a common procedure during angiograph, catheterization, endoscopic, and teleoperation. Navigation training using a computer-based simulation, sensory guidance can be implemented with the goal to enhance task performance. Sensory guidance tools, are also called virtual fixtures, can be rendered with either graphics (visual) and/or force (haptic) features. Integration of virtual fixtures with simulation has been documented to improve task performances in navigation by increasing movement speed and accuracy [1-3]. In this study, we are interested in investigating the role of virtual fixtures in skill acquisition. The research question was when subjects are trained in an environment with augmented virtual fixtures, will the skill be transferred to a similar environment without virtual fixtures?

2. Methods:

2.1. Virtual Fixtures and 3-D maze

This study was conducted in the Enhanced Virtual Hand Lab at Simon Fraser University (Figure 1A), with stereoscopic, head coupled graphics 3-D display, or with 2-D display of the maze. In this context, virtual fixtures are computer-generated with haptic, or graphical features or both to provide sensory guidance along a preferred path. We defined a Virtual Fixture Library (Figure 1B) and a set of Virtual Fixture Assembly Languages (Figure 1C), which allowed the virtual fixtures to have different properties and behaviors. The Virtual Fixture Library consisted a set of primitive shapes, including Cone, Sphere, and Cylinder (Figure 1B). With these items, a tunnel was assembled with abilities to display attractive force fields and/or light green color. The tunnel was then built into a 3-D virtual maze (Figure 1D). The maze was constructed using SGI Open Inventor scene graph with two levels, four rooms, and enclosed by transparent glass ceilings and a red floor. The scene graph was then translated into Ghost scene graph to compute the force rendering.

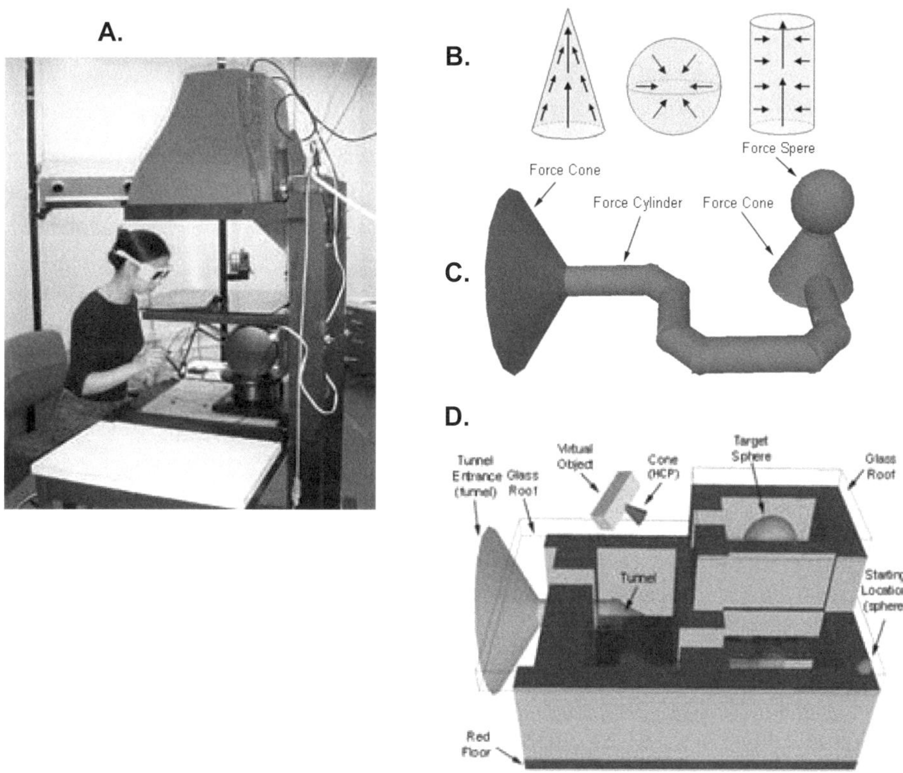

Figure 1. A) Experiment layout. B) Virtual fixture library. C) Assembled virtual tunnel. D) 3-D maze with augmented virtual tunnel.

Since the main focus for this project was to examine the navigation performance of a virtual object through the maze, object-to-object collision detection and force feedback were the major issues for our implementation. We chose an approximation algorithm – voxel sampling [4] – that applies a finite set of points on object's surface and computed the force vector based on collision forces between the object and the components that make up the maze. This force vector was rendered as a point force outputting to the PHANToM stylus. This allowed fast approximation of collision detection and still achieved the haptic rendering rate of 1000Hz.

2.2. Tasks

The task was to grasp a virtual object from its start position outside the maze using a PHANToM, bring the object to the entrance of the maze, navigate it through the rooms inside the maze, and transport the virtual object to the second floor of the maze.

Thirty-two university students (ages 19 to 30 yrs) were recruited and randomly assigned to one of four practice groups, the no graphic and force virtual fixture group (N group), graphic only (G group), force only (F), the graphics and force (GF) group. They performed task for 15 trials then were transferred to a neither graphic nor force virtual fixture condition for 5 more trials. Participants provided Informed Consent, and the protocol was approved by the Simon Fraser University Office of Research Ethics.

2.3. Measures

A navigation trial was divided into 12 phases, corresponding to the transport of the virtual object through different sections of the maze. Movement time and number of collisions were computed for each phase. A summed movement time and number of collisions were computed for each trial.

Collision detection was computed by using voxel sampling [4]. In this experiment, 16 points were equally distributed to the virtual object's surface. When any point touched the maze it would be recorded as a collision. Data were sampled at 100 Hz, while haptic rendering was at 1000 Hz. We sampled one data frame in each 10 haptic frames. In each sampling phrase, we treated the data with all continuous 1's in the data file as one collision, regardless of the duration of each collision.

For example, if a file for collision was recorded as below, 5 collisions were reported.

"111111111111111110000011000000000000000000101011100"

Note that we only considered the collision within a sampling phase. If one collision spanned two sampling phases, we consider it as one collision for each phase and sum it as two collisions in total for that trial.

2.4. Data analyses

In order to examine the learning effect, we blocked the 15 practice trials into 3 phases, i.e., the initial phase (trials 1-5), the middle phase (trials 6-10), and the late phase (trials 11-15). We included a transfer phase for trials 16 - 20, with no virtual fixtures added to the maze.

A 4 virtual fixture group (N, G, F, GF) x 4 learning phase (initial, middle, late, transfer) x 2 dimension (2-D vs. 3-D) mixed factorial ANOVA with repeated measure on the last two factors was used for each of temporal and collision measures. Means and standard errors are reported for significant effects, with a priori alpha level of 0.05.

3. Results

Statistical analyses disclosed effects for learning phase and dimensions on several temporal and collision measures. Basically, as practice increased, the movement times and the number of collisions reduced. Also, tasks were performed quicker and less collisions in 3-D than 2-D display environments.

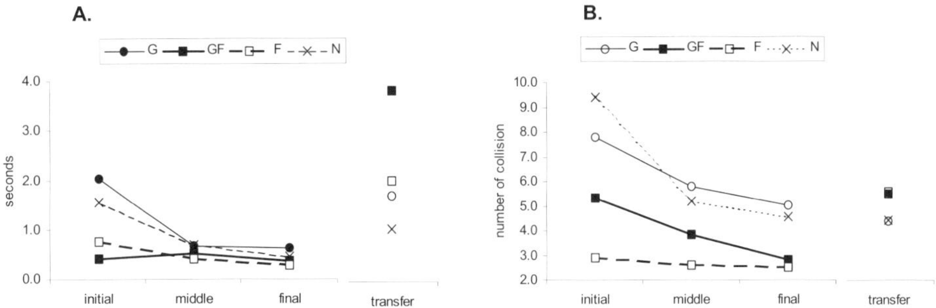

Figure 2. The movement time and number of collisions reduced as practice went on. Interaction between learning phase and virtual guidance was revealed on time12 (A) and number of collision at segment 5 (B).

Interactions between learning phase and virtual fixture group were also revealed for movement times and number of collisions (Figure 2A, 2B). Figure 2A illustrated the phase and guidance interaction found from time 12, where the virtual object was transported out of the maze. With attractive force fields (F and GF groups), subjects transported objects faster during the practice. However, such superior performance could not be carried to the transfer trials, where the force field was not available. In contrast, when practicing in N and G conditions, subjects built skills through practice and carried some of this skill to the transfer trials. Figure 2B illustrated that subjects in F and GF groups transported the object with less collisions during segment 5 of practice. However, when subjects performed in the transfer trials where the force field was not available, the number of collisions increased dramatically compared to the N and G group. In contrast, when practicing in condition with no virtual guidance (N group) and graphic guidance (G group), subjects were able to reduce the number of collisions through practice. Subjects kept a lower rate of collision during the transfer trials. Similar results were found for total time and collisions.

4. Discussion

The primary goal of this study was to investigate the role of virtual fixtures on skill acquisition. Specifically, we examined the effects of implementation of virtual fixtures (either haptic or graphic) on learning a navigation task. We hypothesized that adding virtual fixtures would facilitate task performance and the skills would be transferred to a no-virtual-fixture environment. However, the results from this study demonstrated that adding a force field indeed facilitated the task performance during practice but did not have positive effects on skill acquisition.

Although the result contradicted our expectation, it supports the prediction of the *specificity hypothesis* for motor learning. The specificity hypothesis addresses the skill specific to feedback conditions during which the skill was learned [5]. If a designed task requires subjects to navigate throughout a maze without virtual fixtures, adding extra sensory feedback during the practice phase would not help build specific motor skills.

In this study, subjects trained in the F and GF conditions showed no positive transfer effects to the condition with no virtual fixtures. In contrast, practicing in the N group, subjects positively transferred parts of their skill to the transfer trials because the sensory feedback they experienced was identical. Therefore, an optimal training environment should match the sensory feedback for the designed environment. Skills built in such a training environment would have higher transfer rate to the designed work environment.

Our second comment focuses on the outcome of G group where the virtual fixture was rendered with graphic features. Implementation of graphical guidance (a green tunnel, in this study) did not facilitate task performance (Figure 2A, 2B). This maybe due to the design of graphic guidance itself: the cross-sectional area of the graphic guidance was smaller than the gates and rooms of the maze. Transporting the object into a graphic tunnel in G group was actually more challenging than moving the object throughout the maze itself.

Surprisingly, after being trained with a graphic fixture in the G group, subjects did better in transfer trials than those subjects in F and GF group. It seemed that increasing the task difficulty on practice (i.e., adding visual constraints in this case) might help build specific motor skills. Obviously, the above statement does not agree with the specificity hypothesis; however, earlier research found similar results, indicating skills built in a tough practice environment could be transferred to an amiable environment [6, 7].

Recently, a study on motor learning was conducted by Burdet et al (2001). The task was to move a mechanical lever between the start and end position as quickly and accurately as possible. In one training condition, a divergent force field was applied during the movement. If the lever moved out of an ideal but invisible neutral line, the divergent force field would further deviate the movement trajectory. Being trained in such an unpleasant environment, subjects built better skills compare to subjects trained in a normal environment. Subjects were forced to define the optimal pathway throughout the practice.

In conclusion, adding virtual fixtures has contrasting effects on skill acquisition. Increasing task constraints during the practice such as introducing restricted graphic guidance may not be good for task performance initially, but does help subjects to define the optimal pathway throughout navigation, which subsequently helps with skill acquisition. These results have important implications for the design of an optimal virtual training environment.

ACKNOWLEDGEMENTS: This research was supported by the Natural Sciences and Engineering Research Council (NSERC) Strategic Project, Canada to C.L. MacKenzie and Michael Smith Foundation for Health Research of British Columbia through Post-graduate Scholarship to B. Zheng. The authors would like to thank Virginia Hankins for kind assistance on preparing the drafts of this paper.

References:

[1]. M.P. Fried, V.M. Moharir, J. Shin, M.Taylor-Becker, P. Morrison. Comparison of endoscopic sinus surgery with and without image guidance. Am J Rhinol **16**, 2002. 193-7.

[2]. S. Park, R. Howe, and D. Torchiana, Virtual fixtures for robotic cardiac surgery. Proc of 4th MICCAI. Utrecht, The Netherlands, 2001.

[3]. D. Yi and V. Hayward. Augmenting computer graphic with haptics for the visualization of vessel networks. 10th conf on computer graphic and application. Beijing, China, 2002.

[4]. W. McNeely, K. Puterbaugh, and J. Troy, Six degree-of-freedom haptic rendering using voxel sampling. Proc. of ACM SIGGRAPH, 1999, 401-408.

[5]. L.Proteau, R.G. Marteniuk, and L. Levesque, A sensorimotor basis for motor learning: evidence indicating specificity of practice. The Quarterly Journal of Experimental Psychology. A, Human Experimental Psychology **44**, 1992, 557-75.

[6]. E. Burdet, R. Osu, D.W. Franklin, T.E. Milner, and M. Kawato, The central nervous system stabilizes unstable dynamics by learning optimal impedance. Nature **414**, 2001, 446-9.

[7]. H.T.A.Whiting, G.J.P. Savelsbergh, and J.R. Pijpers, Specificity of motor learning does not deny flexibility. Applied Psychology **44,** 1995, 315-322.

Medicine Meets Virtual Reality 14
J.D. Westwood et al. (Eds.)
IOS Press, 2006

Zero-Dose Fluoroscopy-Based Close Reduction and Osteosynthesis of Diaphyseal Fracture of Femurs

Guoyan Zheng[a,1], Xiao Dong[a], Frank Langlotz[a], and Paul Alfred Gruetzner[b]
[a]MEM Research Center, University of Bern, Switzerland
[b]BG Trauma Center for Orthopedic Surgery, University of Heidelberg, Germany

Abstract. This paper presents a novel technique to create a computerized fluoroscopy with zero-dose image updates for computer-assisted fluoroscopy-based close reduction and osteosynthesis of diaphyseal fracture of femurs. With the novel technique, repositioning of bone fragments during close fracture reduction will lead to image updates in each acquired imaging plane, which is equivalent to using several fluoroscopes simultaneously from different directions but without any X-ray radiation. Its application facilitates the whole fracture reduction and osteosynthesis procedure when combining with the existing leg length and antetorsion restoration methods and may result in great reduction of the X-ray radiation to the patient and to the surgical team. In this paper, we present the approach for achieving such a technique and the experimental results with plastic bones.

Introduction

One of the difficulties with minimally invasive technique in fractural treatment is caused by the absence of direct visual contact to the implant and the accuracy of the achieved reduction. As a consequence, the fluoroscope is used more intensively during modern surgical techniques. For that reason, both patient and surgical staffs are exposed to high radiation doses [1]. The integration of conventional fluoroscopes into computer-assisted navigation systems has been established as one means to partially reduce the radiation.

Although a number of authors reported excellent experience with currently existing systems for virtual fluoroscopy [2][3], two disadvantages of these devices can be identifier during routine clinical use. The purely, two-dimensional (2D) representations of surgical tools represent the tracked object in a rather abstract way. Moreover, changes in the bony anatomy due to fracture reduction or osteotomy can only be analyzed by the re-acquisition of C-arm images causing additional radiation to patient and surgical staffs and requiring re-positioning of the fluoroscope at the patient during the surgery.

---

[1] Corresponding Author: Dr. Guoyan Zheng, MEM Research Center, University of Bern, Stauffacherstrasse 78, CH-3014 Bern, Switzerland; Email: Guoyan.Zheng@MEMcenter.unibe.ch

1. Methods and Tools

To avoid the re-acquisition of images after bony manipulation, the simultaneous dynamization of conventional fluoroscopic images in different projection planes was developed. Dynamization here denotes that the repositioning of X-ray projection of each fragment in each image plane during close fracture reduction and osteosynthesis. It is carried out in two steps. The first step is to prepare data for image repositioning right after image acquisition. And the second step is to reposition the X-ray projection of each fragment according to bony manipulation.

1.1. Data Preparation

The tasks of this step are automated identification, pose and size estimation, projection contour extraction, and interpolation weights computation of each diaphyseal bone fragments of femur. An automatic fragment identification algorithm has been proposed to estimated its pose and size through 3D morphable object fitting using a parametric cylinder model [4]. The projection of each identified cylinder onto into imaging plane, a quadrilateral, is then fed to a region information based active contour model to extract the fragment projection contour. And for each point on the contour, four interpolation weights relative to the four vertexes of the cylinder projection were calculated as follows, which completed the data preparation for dynamization.

Let's denote the four vertices of the quadrilateral as $P_0 = (x_0, y_0)$, $P_1 = (x_1, y_1)$, $P_2 = (x_2, y_2)$, $P_3 = (x_3, y_3)$, any point $P = (x, y)$ inside this quadrilateral can be interpolated by these four vertices with following equations:

$$P = \sum_{i=0}^{3} W_i * P_i \quad \text{and} \quad \begin{cases} W_0 = (1-r)*(1-s) \\ W_1 = r*(1-s) \\ W_2 = r*s \\ W_3 = (1-r)*s \end{cases} \tag{1}$$

where W_i is the interpolation coefficients for P_i.

To further calculate the parametric coefficients (r, s), a Newton-type downhill iterative optimization algorithm is used by reformulating the problem as:

$$\begin{cases} f(r,s) = x - \sum_{i=0}^{3} W_i * x_i = 0 \\ g(r,s) = y - \sum_{i=0}^{3} W_i * y_i = 0 \end{cases} \tag{2}$$

1.2. Image Dynamization

Spatial changes in repositioning of the associated bone objects (as determined by the navigation system) resulted in the positional change of each cylinder as well as the four vertexes of its projection onto each image plane. Based on the new position of its projection and the interpolation weights calculated in the first step, the virtual projection of the fragment could be determined and was used to warp the segmented sub-image of the fragment projection over the static background.

2. Results

For experimental evaluation, we applied our method to registered C-arm images of plastic femur with simulated fractures as shown in Figure 1.

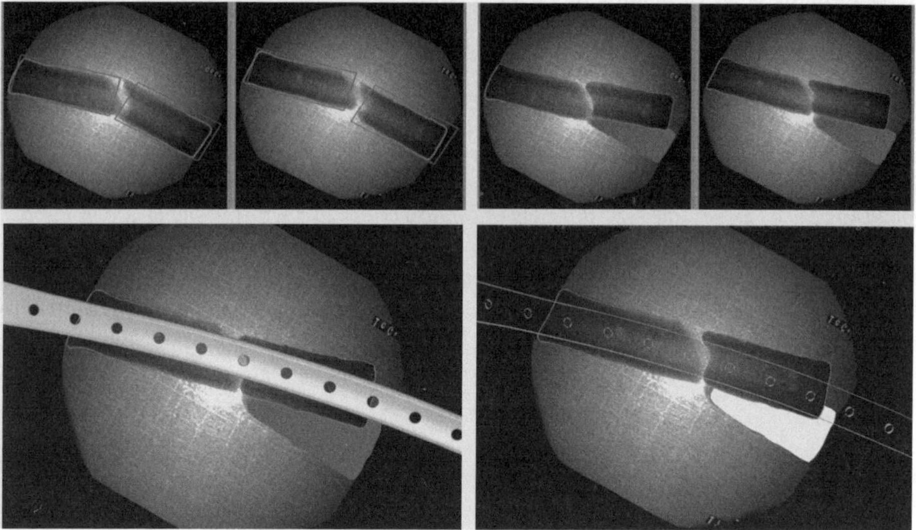

Figure 1. Fragment identification and projection contour extraction (top left); image dynamization for close fracture reduction (top right); photorealistic rendering of osteosynthesis plate (bottom left) and non-photorealistic rendering of osteosynthesis plate (bottom right)

3. Conclusions

The persisting problem in minimally invasive fracture reduction is related to the precise and atraumatical reduction of the main fragments. The repetitive checking of reduction during surgery and interference between reduction and the fixation of implants are the most demanding and time consuming steps. The proposed technique provides a means to achieve zero-dose fluoroscopy-based close reduction and osteosynthesis.

References

[1] Y.R. Yampersaud, K.T. Foley, A.C. Shen, et al. Radiation exposure to the spine surgeon during fluoroscopically assisted pedicle screw insertion. *Spine* 2000, 2637 - 2645
[2] R. Hofstette, M. Slomczykowski, C. Krettek, et al. Computer-assisted fluoroscopy-based reduction of femoral fractures and antetorsion correction. *Comp Aid Surg* 2000, 311 – 325
[3] L.Joskowicz, C. Milgrom, A. Simkin, et al. FRACAS: a system for computer-aided image-guided long bone fracture surgery. *Comp Aid Surg* 1998, 277 – 288
[4] G. Zheng, X. Dong, X. Zhang, L.-P. Nolte. Automated detection and segmentation of diaphyseal bone fragments from registered C-arm images for long bone fracture reduction. Proceedings of the 2005 IEEE Engineering in Medicine and Biology, September, 2005

Medicine Meets Virtual Reality 14
J.D. Westwood et al. (Eds.)
IOS Press, 2006

Author Index